WITHDRAWN FROM STOCK

Chesley's Hypertensive Disorders

— *in* Pregnancy —

Second Edition

Edited by

Marshall D. Lindheimer, MD
Professor of Medicine, Obstetrics and Gynecology,
and Clinical Pharmacology
Department of Obstetrics and Gynecology and Medicine, and
the Committee on Clinical Pharmacology
The University of Chicago
Chicago, Illinois

James M. Roberts, MD
Professor and Vice Chairman (Research)
Department of Obstetrics, Gynecology, and Reproductive Sciences
University of Pittsburgh
Elsie Hilliard Hillman Chair of Women's and Infants' Health
Research
Director, Magee-Womens Research Institute
Pittsburgh, Pennsylvania

F. Gary Cunningham, MD
Professor and Chairman
Department of Obstetrics and Gynecology
University of Texas Southwestern Medical Center
Dallas, Texas

With 20 contributors

Appleton & Lange
Stamford, Connecticut

Copyright © 1999 by Appleton & Lange
A Pearson Education Company
Copyright © 1978 by Appleton-Century-Crofts as *Hypertensive Disorders in Pregnancy* by Leon C. Chesley.

www.appletonlange.com

99 00 01 02 03 / 10 9 8 7 6 5 4 3 2 1

Prentice Hall International (UK) Limited, *London*
Prentice Hall of Australia Pty. Limited, *Sydney*
Prentice Hall Canada, Inc., *Toronto*
Prentice Hall Hispanoamericana, S.A., *Mexico*
Prentice Hall of India Private Limited, *New Delhi*
Prentice Hall of Japan, Inc., *Tokyo*
Simon & Schuster Asia Pte. Ltd., *Singapore*
Editora Prentice Hall do Brasil Ltda., *Rio de Janeiro*
Prentice Hall, *Upper Saddle River, New Jersey*

Library of Congress Cataloging–in–Publication Data

Chesley's hypertensive disorders in pregnancy / edited by Marshall D.
  Lindheimer, F. Gary Cunningham, James M. Roberts. -- 2nd ed.
      p.   cm.
    Rev. ed. of: Hypertensive disorders in pregnancy / Leon C.
  Chesley. c1978.
    Includes bibliographical references and index.
    ISBN 0–8385–3970–X (case : alk. paper)
    1. Hypertension in pregnancy.   I. Lindheimer, Marshall D., 1932–   .
      II. Cunningham, F. Gary.   III. Roberts, James M., 1941–   .
  IV. Chesley, Leon C., 1908– Hypertensive disorders in pregnancy.
  V. Title: Hypertensive disorders in pregnancy.
    [DNLM: 1. Pregnancy Complications, Cardiovascular.
  2. Hypertension--in pregnancy.   3. Eclampsia.   WQ 244 C5245 1998]
  RG580.H9C48   1998
  618.3--dc21
  DNLM/DLC   98-49703
  for Library of Congress   CIP

ISBN 0-8385-3970-X

90000

9 780838 539705

Production Editor: Elizabeth Ryan
Designer: Mary Skudlarek

PRINTED IN THE UNITED STATES OF AMERICA

Contents

Contributors

Phyllis August, MD
Professor of Medicine
Chief, Hypertension Division
Department of Medicine
Cornell University Medical Center
Attending Physician
Division of Hypertension
Department of Medicine
New York Presbyterian Hospital
New York, New York
*Chapter 19, "Chronic Hypertension and
Pregnancy"*

**Philip N. Baker, BMedSci, BM, BS, DM,
MRCOG**
Department of Obstetrics and
  Gynaecology
University of Nottingham
City Hospital
Nottingham, United Kingdom
*Chapter 10, "Platelet and Coagulation
Abnormalities"*

Kirk P. Conrad, MD
Associate Professor
Division of Maternal-Fetal Medicine
Department of Obstetrics, Gynecology,
  and Reproductive Sciences
Department of Cell Biology and
  Physiology
University of Pittsburgh
Magee-Womens Research Institute
Pittsburgh, Pennsylvania
*Chapter 8, "Renal and Cardiovascular
Alterations"*

F. Gary Cunningham, MD
Professor and Chairman
Department of Obstetrics and
  Gynecology
University of Texas Southwestern
  Medical Center
Dallas, Texas
Section Editor

Jacques A. Dürr, MD
Associate Professor of Medicine
Division of Nephrology
Department of Medicine
University of South Florida College of
  Medicine
Tampa, Florida
Chief of Nephrology
Department of Medicine
Bay Pines Veterans Administration
  Medical Center
Bay Pines, Florida
*Chapter 4, "Control of Volume and Body
Tonicity"*

Susan J. Fisher, PhD
Professor
Departments of Stomatology, Anatomy,
  Pharmaceutical Chemistry and
  Obstetrics, Gynecology and
  Reproductive Sciences
University of California at San Francisco
San Francisco, California
*Chapter 11, "Defects in Placentation and
Placental Perfusion"*

Steven A. Friedman, MD
Associate Professor of Obstetrics and
 Gynecology
Department of Obstetrics and Gynceology
Oregon Health Sciences University
Staff Perinatologist
Division of Perinatology
Department of Obstetrics and Gynecology
Kaiser Permanente Northwest Region
Portland, Oregon
*Chapter 6, "Prediction and Differential
 Diagnosis"*

Lillian W. Gaber, MD
Associate Professor
Department of Pathology
University of Tennessee
Memphis, Tennessee
*Chapter 7, "Pathology of the Kidney, Liver,
 and Brain"*

Eileen D.M. Gallery, MD, FRCP
Clinical Professor
Division of Medicine, Obstetrics, and
 Gynaecology
Department of Renal Medicine
Sydney University at Royal North Shore
 Hospital
St. Leonards, New South Wales, Australia
*Chapter 9, "Alterations in Volume
 Homeostasis"*

John C. Hauth, MD
Professor and Director
Center for Research in Women's Health
Vice Chairman for Research
Division of Maternal-Fetal Medicine
Department of Obstetrics and
 Gynecology
University of Alabama at Birmingham
Birmingham, Alabama
Chapter 5, "Preeclampsia–Eclampsia"

Carl A. Hubel, PhD
Research Assistant Professor
Department of Obstetrics, Gynecology,
 and Reproductive Services
University of Pittsburgh
Magee-Womens Research Institute
Pittsburgh, Pennsylvania
*Chapter 14, "Lipid Metabolism and
 Oxidative Stress"*

Kenneth J. Leveno, MD
Director of Maternal-Fetal Medicine
Gilette Professor of Obstetrics
Department of Obstetrics and
 Gynecology
University of Texas Southwestern
 Medical Center
Chief of Obstetrics
Department of Obstetrics and
 Gynecology
Parkland Memorial Hospital
Dallas, Texas
Chapter 17, "Management of Preeclampsia"

Marshall D. Lindheimer, MD
Professor of Medicine, Obstetrics and
 Gynecology, and Clinical Pharmacology
Department of Obstetrics and
 Gynecology and Medicine, and the
 Committee on Clinical Pharmacology
The University of Chicago
Chicago, Illinois
Section Editor

Margaret K. McLaughlin, PhD
Associate Professor
Department of Obstetrics, Gynecology,
 and Reproductive Sciences
University of Pittsburgh
Associate Director
Magee-Womens Research Institute
Pittsburgh, Pennsylvania
Chapter 3, "Hemodynamic Changes"

Roberta B. Ness, MD, MPH
Assistant Professor
Women's Health Program
Departments of Epidemiology,
 Medicine, and Obstetrics and
 Gynecology
University of Pittsburgh
Magee-Womens Research Institute
Pittsburgh, Pennsylvania
Chapter 2, "Epidemiology of Hypertension"

James M. Roberts, MD
Professor and Vice Chairman (Research)
Department of Obstetrics, Gynecology,
 and Reproductive Sciences
University of Pittsburgh

Elsie Hilliard Hillman Chair of Women's
and Infants' Health Research
Director, Magee-Womens Institute
Pittsburgh, Pennsylvania
Section Editor

Baha M. Sibai, MD
Professor and Chief
Division of Maternal-Fetal Medicine
Department of Obstetrics and
Gynecology
University of Tennessee, Memphis
Memphis, Tennessee
Chapter 16, "Prevention of Preeclampsia"

Robert N. Taylor, MD, PhD
Associate Professor
Reproductive Endocrinology Center
Department of Obstetrics, Gynecology,
and Reproductive Sciences
University of California at San Francisco
San Francisco, California
Chapter 12, "Endothelial Cell Dysfunction"

Jason G. Umans, MD, PhD
Associate Professor of Medicine and
Clinical Pharmacology
Division of Biological Sciences
Department of Medicine and Committee
on Clinical Pharmacology
University of Chicago
Chicago, Illinois
Chapter 18, "Antihypertensive Treatment"

Rocco C. Venuto, MD
Professor
Co-Director, Nephrology Division
Department of Medicine
State University of New York at Buffalo
School of Medicine and Biomedical
Science
Director, Nephrology Unit
Department of Medicine
Erie County Medical Center
Buffalo, New York
Chapter 15, "Animal Models"

Kenneth Ward, MD
Associate Professor
Division of Reproductive Genetics
Department of Obstetrics and Gynecology
University of Utah
Director
Division of Reproductive Genetics
Department of Obstetrics and Gynecology
University of Utah Hospital
Salt Lake City, Utah
Chapter 13, "Genetic Factors"

Frederick P. Zuspan, MD
Professor and Chairman Emeritus
Department of Obstetrics and Gynecology
Ohio State University
Columbus, Ohio
Co-Editor in Chief
American Journal of Obstetrics
and Gynecology
"Foreword"

Foreword

I am privileged to have personally known the authors of two landmark texts on hypertension in pregnancy. The first was William Diekmann, MD, from the University of Chicago, whose text was first published in 1941, and revised in 1952. The second was Leon Chesley, PhD, an admirer of Diekmann, whose book *Hypertensive Disorders in Pregnancy* appeared in 1978. These two texts, published approximately a quarter century apart, were single authored by unique and scholarly giants of their generation. Their compendiums were the result of careers devoted to studying a disease that afflicts 10% of all pregnancies and is a leading cause of maternal mortality, especially in underdeveloped parts of the world.

Now, two decades later, we have a third landmark text, the second edition of *Chesley's Hypertensive Disorders in Pregnancy.* Though no longer single authored (a virtual impossibility given the current pace of science), this edition is unique for several reasons. First, each of the three editors are particularly known for their expertise as well as for signal contributions to the field of hypertension in pregnancy. Gary Cunningham, Chair of Obstetrics and Gynecology at the University of Texas Southwestern Medical Center and senior editor of *Williams' Obstetrics,* is the ultimate clinician who has published extensively on the clinical spectrum of pre-eclampsia, and in his most recent studies has focused on the correct management of eclampsia. Marshall Lindheimer is unique in that he is a physician-scientist whose discipline is internal medicine and nephrology but has devoted his research career to the study of renal physiology, volume homeostasis, and the control of blood pressure in pregnancy, and his clinical skills to the management of medical disorders during gestation. James Roberts, an obstetrician, trained at, and for many years part of the faculty of, the renowned Cardiovascular Institute at the University of California, San Francisco, currently heads the Magee-Womens Research Institute in Pittsburgh. The prolific scientific contributions of this research institute have made it the leader in the field of hypertension in pregnancy for over a decade, and I am sure this leadership will continue for some time to come. Also, it is fair to say that Dr. Roberts and his colleagues are responsible for the current focus on the role of the endothelium in the pathophysiology of preeclampsia. In my opinion, it would be difficult to find a more articulate and scholarly group of editors, and I am sure that Leon Chesley is pleased to know that his book is in good hands and will continue to be so.

Another feature, perhaps unique, is the way the second edition was designed. The editors divided the text into three "pies," then recruited gifted authors, all well-known scholars in the area, to contribute, one editor writing each chapter in collaboration with them, so as to achieve continuity and avoid (as much as possible) redundancy. I suspect, however, from the years when I chaired the Obstetrics and Gynecology Department at the University of Chicago, that my ex-faculty member Marshall D. Lindheimer just could not keep his fingers out of the entire pie!

The book has 19 chapters divided into six sections of variable length, each also supervised by an editor. They are:

1. Orientation
2. Cardiovascular Adaptation to Normal Pregnancy
3. Clinical Spectrum of Preeclampsia
4. Pathology and Pathophysiology of Preeclampsia
5. The Etiology of Preeclampsia
6. Prevention and Management of Preeclampsia

Though the text focuses on preeclampsia, the potentially malicious pregnancy-specific disorder, there are also chapters devoted to chronic hypertension as well as to antihypertensive medications. One fortunate decision of the editors was to reprint in its entirety the classic chapter entitled "History" from Leon Chesley's 1978 text (within Chapter 1). This will be a treat to newer generations of investigators who may not be able to find the out-of-print first edition. This chapter has also been updated by the three editors as well as by Leon, and represents a true passing of the baton by the old master.

It is particularly timely to honor our dear friend Leon Chesley, the guru behind today's scientific and clinical approach to the hypertensive disorders complicating pregnancy. The editors and most of the authors know Leon, have heard him lecture, and consider him their role model. However, I am the only one among them to have had a protracted personal day-to-day relationship with "Ches," when from 1960 to 1966, he periodically visited the Medical College of Georgia, several times each year, usually for a period of four weeks, to perform collaborative clinical studies on our hypertensive patients. My faculty and I profited greatly from these visits, learning from Ches his impeccable approach to investigation and to medical writing. These are among the reasons I feel so honored to pen this Foreword to my dear friend Leon Chesley and to my contemporary editor-contributor colleagues and friends whose names adorn this text.

I predict that this book will have a special place in history, akin to that of the first edition, as well as to the Diekmann text. It will be extremely useful to all interested in hypertensive disorders in pregnancy, including obstetrician-gynecologists, internists (especially those who specialize in hypertension and nephrology), practitioners of family medicine, and clinical and basic science investigators. The text is not only expertly written and timely, but it underscores a vast amount of progress regarding hypertension in pregnancy during the past two decades.

Frederick P. Zuspan, MD

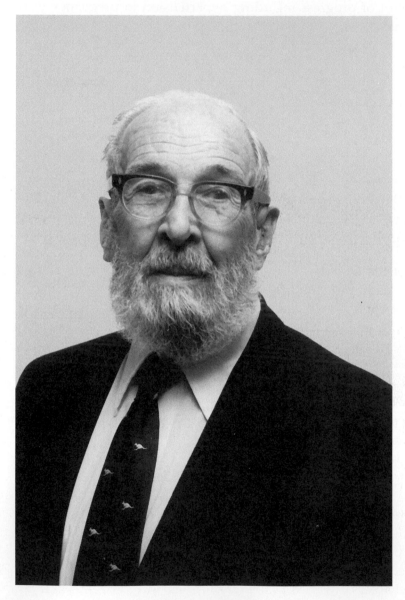

Leon C. Chesley, PhD

Preface

In 1996, Gary Cunningham, senior author of *Williams' Obstetrics*, approached me with the idea of organizing a second edition of *Chesley's Hypertensive Disorders in Pregnancy*. This first edition, though published in 1978, was still a major reference text for investigators in the field, often kept locked in drawers for safe-keeping, as this out-of-print classic was difficult to locate. Next we contacted Dr. James Roberts, Director of the Magee-Womens' Research Institute, whose investigative team is among the leading contributors to the literature on preeclampsia this decade. Of interest, their conference room dedicated by Leon Chesley, and bearing his name, contains his framed photograph positioned to keep a watchful eye on the quality of their deliberations. With three enthusiastic editors on board the second edition was born.

The 1999 edition is a multiauthored text, reflecting the enormous progress in the field since 1978 (and the editors' recognition that there are few Leon Chesleys among us today as well!). To stay in the spirit of the initial edition, your editors developed the following strategy. Each chapter would be first-authored by an acknowledged expert in the topic assigned, and would also be co-authored by one of the editors. This was meant to insure the timeliness of the material, increase cohesiveness, minimize redundancy, and above all, to achieve the goals set for the text. We believe that the strategy worked, though it may have been taxing to the co-author editor, especially when the topic deviated several degrees from his own area of expertise.

This edition is aimed both at investigators and practicing physicians. Thus, one will find chapters designed primarily as scholarly assessments of a given research area, and others with didactic advice for the care of pregnant women with hypertension. Of interest is the considerable variability in focus from chapter to chapter, some authors reviewing the literature, primarily as those cited have presented it, others combining this with commentary, at times almost philosophical (in Chapter 4, an editors' comment was inserted to tell the reader why!). Some authors tried to mimic the encyclopedic approach (with all encompassing tables) in Chesley's first edition, others preferred a more concise approach, (but with extensive bibliography). Your editors decided to leave these approaches intact, the co-editor comparing the chapter's goal and the initial Chesley text in the introductory comments. Finally, Chesley's Chapter 2 in the first edition, "History," is reprinted in its entirety as part of our own first chapter. This historical review is a must read, and we doubt if it will be equaled for quite some time.

We consider Leon Chesley the father of modern research in the hypertensive disorders of pregnancy (some might say of modern research in obstetrics as well). He is now over 90 years of age, having weathered two strokes with mind and sense of humor intact. We visited him several times during the genesis of this edition, receiving his blessing on each occasion. We are proud to honor him with this edition.

Marshall D. Lindheimer, MD

I

Orientation

1

Introduction, History, Controversies, and Definitions

Marshall D. Lindheimer, James M. Roberts,
F. Gary Cunningham, and Leon Chesley

Leon Chesley's *Hypertensive Disorders in Pregnancy* was first published in 1978.[1] Then, as now, hypertension complicating pregnancy was a major cause of fetal and maternal morbidity and death, particularly in less developed parts of the world. Most of this morbidity has been associated with preeclampsia, a disorder in which high blood pressure is but one aspect of a systemic disease. The first edition was single authored, written entirely by Dr. Chesley, a PhD in physiology, who originally found employment during the Great Depression as a chemist at the Margaret Hague Maternity Hospital, in Newark, New Jersey. Curious as to why certain tests were being performed on convulsing pregnant women, Dr. Chesley went to the wards, and the research that followed resulted in signal contributions about preeclampsia–eclampsia published from the late 1930s through the early 1980s. His many works included major observations in such diverse areas as epidemiology, remote prognosis, vascular and renal pathophysiology, and treatment, all focusing on hypertension in pregnancy. A compendium of his achievements is but one aspect of the initial edition of this text, which for two decades has been a major resource for clinicians and investigators who have endeavored to learn more about high blood pressure in pregnant women.

In 1978 a text devoted to the hypertensive disorders in pregnancy could be single authored, due in part to the energy, intellect, and other attributes of Leon Chesley, but also because at that time research in this important area of reproductive medicine was still sporadic and unfocused, and progress regrettably slow. Leon almost singly energized the field, and the three editors of this text are among many of those for whom he served as a role model, nurturing us in early and mid-career. The result has been logarithmic progress in such areas as prevention, pathogenesis, and management, and thus this second edition, to be useful, must be multiauthored. We hope that this text will do scholarly justice to Dr. Chesley's 1978 *tour de force* and its effects on the field for these past 20 years.

The remainder of this introductory chapter will focus on historical perspectives, a guide to controversial issues, and definitions. The format will be as follows: Dr. Chesley's original chapter entitled "History" is reprinted in its entirety. Unable to improve on it, we have added a short update where his classic text ends. The chapter ends with a reprint of Dr. Chesley's banquet address before a workshop held in 1976[2] entitled, "False Steps in the Study of Preeclampsia." This meeting led to the formation of the International Society for the Study of Hypertension in Pregnancy, and Dr. Chesley's message about how to study preeclampsia remains valid today.

HISTORY (FROM ORIGINAL TEXT)[1] (FIG. 1–1)

Several German authors, such as von Siebold (1839, 1845), Knapp (1901), Kossmann (1901), Fasbender (1906), Fisher (1924), and Bernhart (1939) have written on the history of eclampsia, but all too often they did not document their sources and made errors that live on in second-, third-, and nth-hand reviews.[3-8]

Bernhart (1939) wrote that eclampsia was mentioned in the ancient Egyptian, Chinese, Indian, and Greek medical literature.[8] One of the oldest sources that he cited, without specific reference, was the Kahun (Petrie) papyrus dating from about

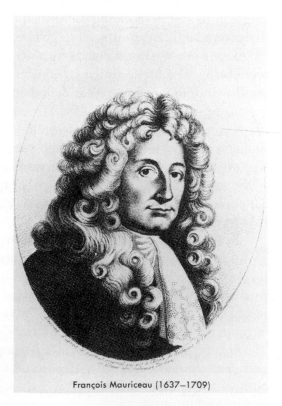

François Mauriceau (1637–1709)

Figure 1–1. This portrait of Francois Mauriceau inaugurated the "History" chapter in the first edition of this text.

2200 BC. His source is likely to have been Menascha (1927).[9] Griffith (1893) had translated Prescription No. 33, on the third page of the papyrus, as: "To prevent (the uterus) of a woman from itching (?) auit pound—upon her jaws the day of birth. It cures itching of the womb excellent truly millions of times."[10] Menascha cited the paper of Griffith but rendered the translation (in German) as: "To prevent a woman from biting her tongue auit pound—upon her jaws the day of birth. It is a cure of biting excellent truly millions of times."[9] He suggested that the untranslated word "auit" means "small wooden stick." In a later book on the Kahun papyrus, Griffith (1898) changed his translation to: "To prevent a woman from biting (her tongue?) beans, pound—upon her jaws the day of birth." Curiously, Menascha did not cite Griffith's later translation and he included the word "auit" from the first version. Possibly the ancient scribe had eclampsia in mind, but that interpretation is tenuous at best.[11]

Bernhart (1939) also wrote, again without references, that both the Indian Atharva-Veda and the Sushruta, of old but unknown dates, mention eclampsia. He said that the Atharva-Veda described an amulet to be worn in late pregnancy for warding off convulsions during childbirth.[8] There are several references to pregnancy in the Atharva-Veda (translated by Whitney, 1905).[12] One is a description of a protective amulet to be put on in the 8th month of gestation (Bk. VIII, 6, pp. 493–498), but there is not the remotest indication of any specific disorder such as convulsions. The ceremonial verses are clearly directed toward protecting the woman's genital organs against demons and rapists, who are characterized by such epithets as "after-snuffling," "fore-feeling," and "much licking" (to name the milder ones).

There are two possible references to eclampsia in the Sushruta (English translation edited by Bhishagratna, 1911).[13] In Volume II, Chapter 8, page 58: "A child, moving in the womb of a dead mother, who had just expired (from convulsions etc.)—" should be delivered by cesarean section. The parenthetic "from convulsions etc." was supplied by the editor and comparison with the Latin translation (Hessler, 1864)[13] indicates that it probably was not in the original text. In Chapter 1, page 11 of Volume II: "An attack of Apatànkah due to excessive hemorrhage, or following closely upon an abortion or miscarriage at pregnancy (difficult labor) or which is incidental to an external blow or injury (traumatic) should be regarded as incurable." Again the parenthetic words are editorial explanations and the "Apatànkah (convulsions) might well be those associated with severe hemorrhage. By comparison with the Latin translation, the English version seems to have been embellished, for the Latin version specifies only abortion and hemorrhage. An editorial note (pp. 58–60, Vol. II) asserts that the ancient Indians delivered living eclamptic women by cesarean section, but the editor provided no documentation whatever.

Bernhart's (1939) reference to the old Chinese literature was to Wang Dui Me, whose work was translated into German by Lo (1930).[14] The work, originally published in 1832 AD, was thought to be free of any influence of Western medicine but even it if were, there is no indication that it recorded only ancient observations. In several respects it seems to have been contemporary; the author described what Lo translated as "Eklampsie" and wrote: "I use recipe No. 232. . . ."

Several of the German authors cite Hippocrates as commenting on the susceptibility of pregnant women to convulsions and on their prognosis. None of the quotations appears in *The Genuine Works of Hippocrates* as translated by Adams (1849), or in any of the half-dozen other translations that I have seen. Some of the quotations can be found in other Greek sources.[15] Earlier translators, for instance, had attributed the *Coacae Praenotiones* to Hippocrates, but most scholars agree that it was written before Hippocrates's time. One such quotation, appearing in several German papers is: "In pregnancy, drowsiness and headache accompanied by heaviness and convulsions, is generally bad." It comes from the *Coacae Praenotiones* (Coan Prognosis), XXXI, No. 507. The Greeks of that time recognized preeclampsia, for in the Coan Prognosis, XXXI, No. 523, we find: "In pregnancy, the onset of drowsy headaches with heaviness is bad; such cases are perhaps liable to some sort of fits at the same time" (translated by Chadwick and Mann, 1950).[16] Hippocrates (4th century BC), in his Aphorisms (Sec. VI, No. 30), wrote: "It proves fatal to a woman in a state of pregnancy, if she be seized with any of the acute diseases." Galen, in the 2nd century AD commented that epilepsy, apoplexy, convulsions, and tetanus are especially lethal (Vol. 17, pt. II, p. 820, Kühn [ed]: 1829).[17] It may be significant that Galen specified convulsive disorders and perhaps he had in mind what we now call eclampsia, which was not to be differentiated from epilepsy for another 1600 years.

Celsus, in the first century AD, mentioned often fatal convulsions in association with the extraction of dead fetuses (Bk. VII, Chap. 29, translated by Lee, 1831).[18] In the same connection, Aetios, in the 6th century AD, wrote: "Those who are seriously ill are oppressed by a stuporous condition . . . ," "Some are subject to convulsions . . . ," and "The pulse is strong and swollen" (Chaps. 22, 23, translated by Ricci, 1950).[19]

There is a possible reference to eclampsia in Rösslin's (1513) *Der Swangern Frawen und Hebammen Rosengarten,* a book that was the standard text of midwifery in Europe and England for almost two centuries.[20] In discussing the maternal prognosis in difficult labor with fetal death, Rösslin listed among the ominous signs unconsciousness and convulsions (Bk. I, Chap. 9, p. 67). The book was largely based upon the older classics, and the relevant section is reminiscent of Celsus, Aetios, and, especially, Paul of Aegina (translated by Adams, 1844).[21] The book was translated into English from a Latin version of what probably was the second edition and appeared in 1540 as *The Byrth of Mankinde.* Raynalde revised and amplified the second edition of 1545, and the text was little altered thereafter. Ballantyne's (1907) quotation of the relevant paragraph in Book II, Chapter 9, from the edition of 1560 is virtually identical with that published 53 years later (Raynalde, 1613), except for the variable and carefree spelling of the times.[22,23]

Gaebelkhouern (variously, Gabelchoverus, Gabelkover, 1596) distinguished four sorts of epilepsy in relation to the seats of their causes, which he placed in the head, the stomach, the uterus, and chilled extremities.[24] He further specified that only the pregnant uterus causes convulsions, particularly if it carries a malformed fetus. The mothers feel a biting and gnawing in the uterus and diaphragm that leads them to think that something is gnawing on their hearts (epigastric pain? The description of that symptom is usually credited to Chaussier, 1824, 228 years later).[25]

Although eclampsia is dramatic, it is not astonishing that there are so few references to it in the older writings, which covered the whole field of medicine. Eclampsia had not been differentiated from epilepsy, and obstetrics was largely in the hands of midwives. Even some relatively modern textbooks of obstetrics have barely noticed eclampsia, and those of Burton (1751) and Exton (1751) made no mention whatever of convulsions.[26,27] In the first edition of Mauriceau's (1668) book, the only comment on convulsions relates to those associated with severe hemorrhage, of which his sister died.[28] The literature of eclampsia, for practical purposes, began in France because it was there that male physicians first took up the practice of obstetrics on a significant scale. Viardel, Portal, Peu, and de la Motte each published notable books in the late 17th and early 18th centuries.

In later editions of his book, Mauriceau devoted more and more attention to what we now call eclampsia. Hugh Chamberlen published purported translations of Mauriceau's later editions, but they seem to have been impostures and really were reissues of the translation of the first edition (1673).[29] Such fraud befits a family that kept so important an invention as the forceps secret through three generations for personal profit, and befits the man who sold the secret. In the edition of 1694, and possibly earlier, Mauriceau set forth several aphorisms dealing with the subject. Among them were (No. 228): The mortal danger to mother and fetus is greater when the mother does not recover consciousness between convulsions.[30] (No. 229): Primigravidas are at far greater risk of convulsions than are multiparas. (No. 230): Convulsions during pregnancy are more dangerous than those beginning after delivery. (No. 231): Convulsions are more dangerous if the fetus is dead than if it is alive. He attributed the convulsions to an excess of heated blood rising from the uterus and stimulating the nervous system and thought that irritation of the cervix would aggravate the situation. He also believed that if the fetus were dead, malignant vapors arising from its decomposition might cause convulsions. His assigning convulsions to such specific causes carries the implication that he had distinguished eclampsia from epilepsy.

Kossmann (1901) wrote that in 1760, before he had bought (gekauft hatte) his title "de Sauvages," Bossier first introduced the word *eclampsia*.[5] He said that de Sauvages was a typical Frenchman in that he took it badly whenever his title was omitted, that he had mistaken the meaning of the Greek word from which he derived eclampsia, that none of the supporting references that he cited was correct, and that we owe the word to de Sauvages's slovenly scholarship.

Kossmann was in error. De Sauvages published under that name at least as early as 1739, and there is no indication in the *Biographisches Lexikon* (Hirsch, 1887) that he had not been born as de Sauvages.[31] He did acquire the title "de Lacroix" later. De Sauvages (1739) differentiated eclampsia from epilepsy in his *Pathologia Methodica,* the three editions of which were forerunners of his *Nosologia* that Kossmann cited. He indicated that epilepsy is chronic and that the fits recur over long periods of time; all convulsions of acute causation, de Sauvages called *eclampsia,* spelled with one *c* in the first and second editions and with two in later publications.[32,33] He attributed the source of the words to Hippocrates, in the sense of *Epilepsia puerilis,* which Kossmann considered to be erroneous. In later editions, he cited de Gorris's *Definitionem Medicarum,* Hippocrates, and the *Coan Prognosis,* in none of which the word occurs, according to Kossmann.

Part of the discrepancy is explained by the questionable authorship of many writings that have been attributed to Hippocrates.[15,16,34] Most scholars do not accept the sixth book of *Epidemics* as being his, but in Section I, No. 5, the word does appear and has been translated as "epilepsy," both before and after de Sauvages's time. Galen (Vol. 17, pt. I, p. 824, Kühn [ed]: 1829) translated εχλαμψιες as "fulgores" (lightning, shining, brilliance) but after four half-pages of discussion as to its significance, concluded that here it means epilepsy.[17] Nearly a century after de Sauvages, Grimm (1837) translated the word as "Fallsucht" (epilepsy).[34] The word does not appear in the edition of de Gorris's definitions (1578) that I have seen, but it may be in others.[35] Perhaps de Sauvages cited the wrong dictionary, for he is vindicated by another one. Castelli (1682), in his *Lexicon Medicum,* defined *eclampsis* as brightness, lightning, effulgence, or shining forth, as in a flashing glance ("splendorum, fulgorum, effulgescentium et emicationem, qualis ex oculis aliquando prodeunt").[36] He cited several writings attributed to Hippocrates in which the word was used metaphorically to mean the shining vital flame in puberty and the vigorous years of life ("emicatione flamme vitalis in pubertate et aetatis vigora"). Under *Effulgescentia* he wrote "vide eclampsis." In an earlier edition (1651), *eclampsis* did not appear, but *effulgescentia* had several definitions, the first of which is a disorder characteristic of boys, the most familiar being epilepsy ("quas Graeci εχλαμψιας vocant Hipp. praesertim significant morbum puerorum proprium, aut certè perquam familiarissimum, id est, Epilepsium").[37] Castelli, who followed Galen's discussion just mentioned, wrote that to some the word denoted the temperamental change to warmth, or the effulgent vital flame of youth and early manhood. Others considered the interpretation to be the bodily development and perfection during early adulthood.

Blancard (variously Blancardo, Blankaard, 1683) in his *Lexicon Medicum,* defined *eclampsis* as "effulgio" and wrote that some authors had called the circulation eclampsis because they thought that a flashing principle in the heart ("luminoso principe in corde") impelled the blood.[38] The word disappeared from his later editions.

In the third edition (1759) of *Pathologia Methodica,* de Sauvages listed several species of eclampsia in relation to such acute causes as severe hemorrhage, various sources of pain, vermicular infestations, and other such factors as had been noted by Hippocrates.[33] One species was *Eclampsia parturientium* and de Sauvages indicated that Mauriceau had described the disease.

Vogel (1764), Cullen (1771), and Sagar (1776), in their classifications of diseases, adopted de Sauvages's *Ecclampsia parturientium*, but dropped one of the two *c*'s.[39-41] Interestingly, the taxonomists defined both *Convulsio gravidarum* and *Eclampsia parturientium* (or *parturientes*) as different genera and without cross-reference between the two.

Gutsch (1776), a student of J. C. Gehler in Leipsig, may have been the first German obstetrician to take up the word, and for a generation the German use of it seems to have been confined to that center.[42] Kossmann (1901) wrote that the word reappeared in France in 1844, but Ryan (1831) said that it was generally used there in his time.[5,43] That is confirmed by the listing of publications in the *Index-Catalogue of the Library of the Surgeon General's Office* (1890), where the word *eclampsia* appears in the titles of 31 books or monographs from six European countries before 1845; there were many from France.

Ryan (1831) recognized the specificity of what he called dystocia convulsiva: He gave as synonyms "labor with convulsions," "convulsio apoplectica," "apoplexia hysterica," "apoplexia lactusa," "apoplexia sympathetica," and "eclampsia."[43] When consciousness returned between fits, Ryan called them epileptiform; when coma or stertor supervened, he called them apoplectic or eclamptic convulsions. He wrote that the convulsions may occur during the last 3 months of pregnancy, in labor, or after delivery and that the prognosis is unfavorable "as a third of those afflicted are destroyed." Postpartum eclampsia is less dangerous, he said.

Bossier de Sauvages's (1739) use of the word *eclampsia* as a generic term for convulsions having an acute cause persisted for more than 200 years.[32] *Stedman's Medical Dictionary* (1957) defined eclampsia as "convulsions of an epileptoid character" and listed several varieties. Puerperal eclampsia was defined as "convulsions of uremic or other origin, occurring in the latter part of pregnancy or during labor;" there was no mention of the puerperium. The 20th edition, in 1961, discarded all but the obstetric definition; "Coma and convulsions that may develop during or immediately after pregnancy, related to proteinuria, edema, and hypertension." Puerperal eclampsia was described as following delivery, which is technically correct, but a misleading guide to interpretation of much of the literature of the 19th century.

SIGNS

Edema

Fasbender (1906) wrote that Demanet (1797) was the first to relate convulsions with edema.[6,44] An anonymous author (1855) included Demanet's entire paper in a review that is more accessible than the original.[45] All six of Demanet's eclamptic patients were edematous, and he suggested that anasarca be added to the three recognized causes of convulsions, i.e., depletion, repletion, and labor pains. Most eclamptic women have such marked edema that it could not have escaped notice before 1797 and, in fact, several writers had commented on it before then. Mauriceau (1694) remarked on the severe edema of one of his patients (Observation No. 90), but he usually did not describe the women other than to specify age and parity.[30] De la Motte (1726) considered edema to be benign unless associated with convulsions.[46] Smellie (1756) presented his cases as exemplifying methods of delivery and said nothing about the appearance of the patients.[47] Van Swieten (1745), in his commentary on Boerhaave's Aphorism No. 1302, specified edema as one of the indications for phlebotomy in women threatened with convulsions.[48]

Proteinuria

Rayer (1840) found protein in the urines of three pregnant edematous women.[49] From his descriptions, it seems probable that the first one had preeclampsia and the other two had Bright's disease.

Lever (1843) is generally credited with the discovery of proteinuria in eclampsia.[50] He was stimulated to look for it by the clinical resemblance between eclampsia and Bright's disease, and he found it in nine of ten convulsive women. The description of the postmortem findings in the one woman who did not have proteinuria is suggestive of meningitis and perhaps her convulsions were not of eclamptic origin. Because of the rapid abatement of the proteinuria after delivery, Lever concluded that eclampsia is different from Bright's disease, although others of his era were not so astute. Lever attributed the proteinuria to renal congestion caused by compression of the renal veins by the bulky uterus. He speculated that such compression might be absent in the "upwards of 50" normal women in labor whose urines he found to be normal, unless "symptoms have presented themselves, which are readily recognized as precursors of puerperal fits."

Simpson (1843) should share credit with Lever, for in the same year he wrote: "(I) had publically taught for the last two sessions, viz., that patients attacked with puerperal convulsions had almost invariably albuminous urine, and some accompanying, or rather, preceding dropsical complications."[51] Unfortunately, one of his fatal cases of eclampsia did have chronic nephritis and he found granular kidneys at autopsy, which led him to believe that eclampsia was a manifestation of nephritis.

Hypertension

Old-time clinicians surmised the presence of eclamptic hypertension from the hard, bounding pulse, but confirmation was long delayed for want of methods for measuring the blood pressure. Sphygmographic tracings were interpreted as showing arterial hypertension, but no absolute values could be specified. Mahomed (1874) reported that such tracings indicated the presence of hypertension in nearly all pregnant women, and he concluded that "Puerperal convulsions and albuminuria were accounted for by the predisposing condition of high tension in the arterial system existing during pregnancy."[52,53] The sphygmographic features pointing to hypertension were: (1) the increased external pressure required to obtain optimal tracings, (2) a well-marked percussion wave separated from the tidal wave, (3) a small dicrotic wave, and (4) a prolonged tidal wave. We now know that the hemodynamic changes of normal pregnancy do not include hypertension, but the increased cardiac output changes the character of the pulse. The ancient Chinese recognized the altered pulse perhaps as long as 4500 years ago; in the *Yellow Emperor's Classic of Internal Medicine* we find: "When the motion of her pulse is great she is with child" (translation by Veith, 1949).[54]

Ballantyne (1885), from sphygmograms made in two eclamptic and one severely preeclamptic women, concluded that arterial blood pressure is considerably increased.[55] One of the patients died 10 hours after delivery, and the tracings suggested that "after the completion of labor there is a great tendency to complete collapse (of the arterial pressure) and that unless checked will go on till death closes the scene." His description of terminal hypotension is descriptive of many cases of fatal eclampsia, although he generalized too broadly. Galabin (1886) wrote: "From sphygmographic tracings taken during the eclamptic state, I have found that the pulse is . . . one of abnormally high tension, like that in Bright's disease."[56] In discussing the management of eclampsia, he wrote: "The first treatment should be to give an active purgative. This lowers arterial pressure. . . ."

Despite the efforts of earlier investigators, indirect methods for the measurement of arterial blood pressure did not become available until 1875. The instruments of Marey, Potain, von Basch, and others led to overestimates of the blood pressure but did give relative values. Thus, Lebedeff and Porochjakow (1884), using von Basch's sphygmomanometer, found that the blood pressure is higher during labor than in the early puerperium.[57] Vinay (1894), using Potain's device, observed that the blood pressure was increased in pregnant women with proteinuria (180–200 mm Hg as compared with the normal of up to about 160, by his method).[58] The discovery of eclamptic hypertension is widely credited to Vaquez and Nobécourt (1897), who remarked that they had confirmed Vinay's observations published in his textbook 3 years earlier.[59] Vinay (1894), however, said nothing about the blood pressure in eclampsia and regarded his hypertensive albuminuric patients as having Bright's disease.[58] Wiessner (1899) reported that the blood pressure fluctuates widely during eclampsia.[60]

Cook and Briggs (1903) used an improved model of Riva Rocci's sphygomomanometer that has not been greatly changed to this day.[61] They observed that normal pregnancy has little effect on the blood pressure until the onset of labor, when it increases with uterine contractions. Women with proteinuria were found to have hypertension, and the authors wrote that the detection of increased blood pressure in a pregnant woman should "excite the apprehension of eclampsia." They observed that proteinuria was usually associated with hypertension and thought that the blood pressure was the better guide to prognosis.

The differentiation of preeclampsia–eclampsia from renal disease and essential hypertension was long delayed, and although we now recognize that they are separate entities, the correct diagnosis is often difficult. Although Lever (1843) looked for proteinuria in eclamptic women because of their clinical resemblance to patients with glomerulonephritis, he concluded that the diseases are different because eclamptic proteinuria cleared rapidly after delivery.[50] Others of that era, however, cited his discovery of proteinuria as evidence for the identity of the diseases. Frerichs (1851), in his textbook, wrote that eclampsia represents uremic convulsions and the concept persisted for half a century.[62] Autopsies of women dying of eclampsia often uncovered no renal abnormalities detectable by methods then available, but that objection was countered by Spiegelberg (1878),[63] for example. He wrote, in italics, *True eclampsia depends upon uremic poisoning in consequence of deficient renal excretion.* He attributed the deficiency to chronic nephritis aggravated by pregnancy or to disease of the renal arteries secondary to vasospasm. He suggested, as had others before him, that the renal vasospasm arose reflexively from stimulation of the uterine nerves, a hypothesis revived in modern times by Sophian (1953).[64] The *Zeitgeist* was reflected in the 1881 issue of the *Index-Catalogue of the Library of the Surgeon General's Office.* Under "Bright's disease" it specified "see, also, —Puerperal *convulsions.*"

Toward the end of the 19th century the development of cellular pathology and of improved histologic methods led to the detection of a characteristic hepatic lesion and the recognition of eclampsia as an entity, distinct from Bright's disease (Jürgens, 1886; Schmorl, 1893).[65,66] The differentiation of the nonfatal, nonconvulsive hypertensive disorders remained confused for many years. The terms "nephritic toxemia," "Schwangerschaftsniere," and "Nephropathie" persisted through the 1930s and the term "low reserve kidney" was introduced as late as 1926.

The recognition of primary or essential hypertension is relatively recent, but its relevance to pregnancy was not appreciated for many years after it had been accepted as an entity. Allbutt (1896) observed that middle-aged and older men and especially women often develop hypertension and that the increase in blood pressure is not accompanied by any other evidence of renal disease.[67] He referred to the condition as "senile plethora" or "hyperpiesis;" later it was termed "essential hypertension" by Frank (1911) or "hypertensive cardiovascular disease" by Janeway (1913).[68,69] The appellation "senile" had a lingering effect, and obstetricians thought that women of childbearing age were not old enough to have developed essential hypertension.

Herrick and coworkers (1926–1936) recognized essential hypertension as an important and frequent component of the hypertensive disorders in pregnancy.[70-72] They showed that what the obstetricians called chronic nephritis in and following pregnancy was more often essential hypertension. Herrick (1932) wrote: "Viewed largely, then, the toxemias of pregnancy are probably not toxemias.[70] Rather they are evidences of underlying tendencies to disease." He thought that about a quarter of the cases have renal disease, either frank or brought to light by pregnancy. The rest, he thought, have frank or latent essential hypertension. In some papers, he seemed not to have decided whether eclampsia and severe preeclampsia caused vascular disease or were manifestations of it that were revealed and peculiarly colored by pregnancy. In one of his last papers on the subject (Herrick and Tillman, 1936), he wrote: "When these are fully delineated it is our opinion that we shall find nephritis concerned in but a small fraction of the toxemias; that the larger number, including the eclampsias, the preeclampsias, and the variously designated milder types of late toxemia . . . will be found to have unit characteristics based upon cardiovascular disease with hypertension."[72]

Fishberg (1939), in the fourth edition of his book *Hypertension and Nephritis*, denied the specificity of preeclampsia–eclampsia, which he regarded as manifestations of essential hypertension.[73] Although he retreated from that view in the following edition (1954), he continued to regard eclampsia as "a typical variety of hypertensive encephalopathy."[74]

Dieckmann (1952) in his book *The Toxemias of Pregnancy*, said that about half of the women with hypertensive disorders in pregnancy have either nephritis or essential hypertension, but that primary renal disease accounted for not more than 2%.[75] That opinion, in which he both followed and led, gained wide acceptance. Herrick's estimate of the prevalence of chronic renal disease, however, seems to have been closer to the truth. Several studies of renal biopsies have indicated that 10 to 12% of women in whom preeclampsia is diagnosed clinically have the lesions of primary renal disease, usually chronic glomerulonephritis.

HYPOTHESES AND RATIONAL MANAGEMENT

Zuspan and Ward (1964) wrote that in the treatment of the eclamptic patient, "she has been blistered, bled, purged, packed, lavaged, irrigated, punctured, starved, sedated, anesthetized, paralyzed, tranquilized, rendered hypotensive, drowned, been given diuretics, had mammectomy, been dehydrated, forcibly delivered, and neglected."[76] Many procedures could be added to the list. Aside from the great variety of medications, surgical approaches have included ureteral catheterization, implantation of the ureters in the colon, renal decapsulation, drainage of spinal fluid, cisternal puncture, trepanation, ventral suspension of the uterus, postpartum curettage, oophorectomy, and so on. I do not rehearse the list in any spirit of levity, for it is important to remember that each of the treatments was rational in the light of some hypothesis as to the cause or nature of eclampsia. That is more than we can say for our present management, which is purely empiric, perhaps too often symptomatic, and in some respects based upon imitative magic.

Eclampsia was not differentiated from epilepsy until 1739, and the distinction was not generally accepted for another century. Merriman (1820) discussed dystocia convulsiva and wrote: "The cases alone deserving the appellation of puerperal convulsions, which have fallen under my observation, have borne a very exact resemblance to the epilepsy."[77] Ryan, in his *Manual of Midwifery* (1831), recognized eclampsia as an entity, but 25 years later his countryman Churchill, in his *Theory and Practice of Midwifery* (1856), classified gestational convulsions as hysteric, epileptic, and apoplectic.[43,78] By the time the differentiation from epilepsy was generally accepted, eclampsia had been confused with uremic Bright's disease, and the proliferation of hypotheses as to its cause was delayed until late in the 19th century.

Hippocrates, in his Aphorisms, Section VI, No. 39, wrote: "Convulsions take place either from repletion or depletion" (translated by Adams, 1849).[15] Hippocrates referred to convulsions generally, as did Galen who iterated his view (Vol. 18, pt. I, p. 61, Kühn [ed]: 1829).[17] Accordingly, obstetricians divided on the question of which factor accounted for convulsions in childbirth. Mauriceau (1694) recommended bloodletting, except in the convulsions associated with severe hemorrhage.[30] According to Gutsch (1776), who did not give a reference, van Swieten wrote that depletion was the cause and attributed the convulsions to collapse of the cerebral blood vessels.[42] Gutsch was completely wrong, but virtually every history of eclampsia has perpetuated his error. Van Swieten (1745), in commenting on Boerhaave's Aphorism No. 1322, was in agreement with the concept that the sudden reduction in intraabdominal pressure at delivery might lead to a pooling of blood diverted from the brain and thus account for weakness and syncope.[48] Van Swieten went on to say that if the uterus did not contract, "then lying-in women run with blood, and, by the sudden inanition of the (cerebral) vessels, die in convulsions; pretty nearly in the same manner that the strongest animals, when their arteries are cut open by the butcher, their blood being entirely exhausted, are seized with violent convulsions before they die" (English translation of 1776).[48] Clearly, van Swieten was not referring to eclamptic convulsions. In his comments on Aphorisms Nos. 1010, 1295, and 1302, van Swieten indicated unequivocally that cerebral congestion is the cause of what we now call eclamptic convulsions. He attributed the cerebral repletion to compression of the abdominal organs by the large uterus, to blockage of the aorta by the uterus, and to the violent expulsive efforts at delivery, all of which diverted blood to the brain. Accordingly, he wrote: "no one can doubt but the letting of blood must prove of the greatest service, especially if these symptoms (including edema) happen near the time of delivery; for then by the violent efforts of labour, the blood may be forcibly thrown into the vessels of the encephalon, and all its functions thereby suppressed; or even a fatal apoplexy may ensue from a rupture of the vessels; convulsions too may often follow" (comment on Aphorism No. 1302).

In addition to the factors specified by van Swieten as leading to repletion, other writers had suggested reflex effects arising from stimulation of the uterine nerves and suppression of the menses during pregnancy. The opposite hypothesis, that the convulsions were caused by depletion or cerebral anemia, had its proponents and still lingers on in terms of cerebral vasospasm and edema.

Old-time physicians and barber-surgeons resorted to bloodletting in the treatment of many disorders and they noted the extraordinary tolerance of pregnant women for hemorrhage. By the end of the 18th century the "plethora of pregnancy" was a widely accepted concept that seems to have tipped the scales in favor of repletion and cerebral congestion as the cause of gestational convulsions. Phlebotomy and purgation, which were the sheet anchors in the management of eclampsia one and two centuries ago, probably were of late origin. Section V of Hippocrates's Aphorisms specified contraindications to those measures. No. 29: "Women in state of pregnancy may be purged, if there be any urgent necessity, from the fourth to seventh month, but less so in the latter case. In the first and last periods it must be avoided." No. 31: "If a woman with child be bled, she will have an abortion, and this will be the more likely to happen, the larger the foetus" (translated by Adams, 1849). Galen agreed (Vol. 17, pt. II, pp. 652, 821, Kühn [ed]: 1829).[17]

Although Celsus, in the first century AD, disputed the adverse effect of bleeding, the doctrine persisted (Bk. II, Chap. 10, translated by Lee, 1831).[18] In the 6th century, Aetios reiterated the deleterious effect of phleobotomy; he cited Hippocrates when he recommended bleeding as a means of inducing abortion (Chap. 18, translated by Ricci, 1950).[19] Avicenna, in the 11th century, advised against both bleeding and purgation during pregnancy (translated by Krueger, 1963).[79] Maimonides, in the 12th century, seems to have contradicted himself.[80] His 12th Treatise, Aphorism 5 is: "The conditions and complications that mitigate [sic] against bloodletting, although signs of filling may be apparent, are as follows: Convulsive disorders. . . ." But Aphorism 22 says: "Venesection is an utmost necessity at the very onset: (in) patients suffering from . . . convulsions . . ." (translated by Rosner and Muntner, 1970).

The prime object of phlebotomy was to decrease cerebral congestion and to that end, some physicians preferred bleeding from the temporal artery or jugular vein. Leeches and cups were applied to the scalp, neck, and even face to draw blood away from the brain. Blisters and sinapisms were placed in various areas for the same purpose, and the scalp was shaved for the closer application of cold packs. Sometimes the physician recognized that repeated phlebotomies had so weakened the woman that another would be hazardous, so that rather than subject her to another general hemorrhage, he placed leeches or cups on the head for the local diversion of blood from the brain. Ryan (1831), who attributed eclampsia to cerebral congestion, wrote: "In these kingdoms, copious depletion with camphor mixture, ether, etc, are chiefly employed," along with repeated bleedings.[43] Ether, which was popular in France, was given in mixtures by mouth or subcutaneously.

Those who believed that the convulsions were caused by irritation of the uterus also used sinapisms, blistering, and the like as counterirritants, and they bled patients from veins in the feet, which they believed to be a revulsive measure.

Later, when a circulating toxin was postulated as the cause of eclampsia, phlebotomy was retained as a rational treatment because it directly removed the noxious substance. To the same end, all of the emunctories were stimulated and the use of diuretic, purgative, emetic, and sudorific drugs became popular. High colonic irrigation and gastric lavage were used for the same purpose. Tincture or extract of jaborandi was used to induce intense sweating and when its most active alkaloid was identified as pilocarpine, that drug came into use. It was tried for a time in Edinburgh, but abandoned when it was found to have doubled the maternal mortality from 30 or 35% to 67%; the women drowned in their own secretions (Hirst, 1909).[81] A parallel situation exists today in the common use of potent diuretic drugs, which probably do no real good and are dangerous, though not so dramatically as in the case of pilocarpine.

The concept of eclampsia as a toxemia is more than a century old. The earliest reference that I have found is by William Tyler Smith (1849), who wrote: "It deserves to be borne in mind, that the depuratory functions ought, in order to preserve health, to be increased during gestation, as the *debris* of the foetal, as well as the maternal system, have to be eliminated by the organs of the mother.[82] Besides these forms of toxaemia, the state of the blood which obtains during fevers, or during the excitement of the first secretion of milk, may excite the convulsive disorder." He used the word *toxaemia* so casually as to suggest that it might have been a current concept. Murphy (1862), in his *Lectures on the Principles and Practice of Midwifery*, wrote 13 years later: "Predisposing causes of convulsions are hyperaemia, anaemia, and toxaemia" and *"The direct proximate cause* of convulsions is impure blood" (his italics).[83] Mahomed (1874), explaining the hypertension that he thought to be present in all pregnant women, wrote: "The blood of the mother is overcharged with effete material, for she has to discharge the excrementitious matters of the fetus by her own excretory organs; her blood is therefore in a measure poisoned . . ." and "Thus puerperal eclampsia and albuminuria were accounted for. . . ."[52,53] The later controversy as to whether Fehling (1899) or van der Hoeven (1896) had priority in suggesting fetal waste products as the cause of eclampsia was obviously an exercise in futility.[84,85] Actually, Mauriceau (1694) had attributed convulsions in many cases to decompositional products of the dead fetus.[30]

In the symposium on eclampsia, held in Giessen in 1901, the almost unanimous opinion was that the disease is caused by a toxin, but there was no agreement as to its source. The uremic hypothesis had not yet succumbed, and some writers held out renal insufficiency, either intrinsic or secondary to uterine compression of the renal veins or ureters, as the cause. As previously mentioned, a variant explanation was renal vascular spasm arising as a reflex from nervous stimulation in the uterus. Other hypotheses included fetal catabolic products, bacterial toxins, autointoxication by noxious substances absorbed from the gut, toxins from the placenta released directly or by lytic antibodies against it. Several French investigators, of whom Delore (1884) was probably the first, suggested bacterial infection.[86] Gerdes (1892) attributed eclampsia to a bacillus that was later identified as *Proteus vulgaris* and Favre (1891) alleged the same role for *Micrococcus eclampsiae*.[87,88] That hypothesis was quickly overthrown, but the idea that bacterial toxins released in focal infections had a role was advocated for another half century. Proponents of autointoxication as the cause of eclampsia pointed to the predominance of the hepatic lesion in the periportal areas of the hepatic lobules, which receive most of the blood draining the gut.

Rosenstein (1864), adopting Traube's explanation of uremic convulsions, suggested that the proteinuria depleted the plasma proteins and that the combination of watery blood and hypertension led to cerebral edema, convulsions, and coma.[89] Munk (1864) tested Traube's hypothesis by ligating the ureters and jugular veins of dogs and injecting water through the carotid artery, thereby evoking convulsions and coma that he regarded as uremia.[90] A modern clinical counterpart is the water intoxication produced in an occasional patient by the injudicious and prolonged infusion of oxytocin in large volumes of dextrose solution.

An enormous amount of work was expended in trying to identify the toxin. Frerichs (1851), who equated eclampsia with uremic convulsions, postulated an enzyme that converted urea to ammonium carbonate.[62] Some thought that a precursor of urea, carbamic acid, was the toxin. Other substances "identified" as the toxin included creatine, creatinine, xanthine, acetone, lactic acid, urobilin, leucomaines akin to ptomaines, globulins, and water.

Then, as now, new hypotheses were introduced with supporting observations or experiments that either could not be confirmed or were interpreted differently by other investigators. Many examples could be cited. The French school developed the concept that pregnant women excreted less than normal amounts of endogenous toxins, which therefore accumulated in the bloodstream. In support of their hypothesis, they reported that the urine of eclamptic women was less toxic and the serum more toxic than the same fluids from normal pregnant and nonpregnant subjects. Volhard (1897) and Schumacher (1901) reviewed their work critically, repeated their experiments, and demolished their conclusions.[91,92] Dixon and Taylor (1907) reported pressor activity in alcoholic extracts of placenta, but Rosenheim (1909) showed that bacterial contamination accounted for the effect.[93,94] More recently, the many reports of antidiuretic activity in blood, urine, and cerebrospinal fluid of women with preeclampsia–eclampsia have been called into question for the same reason (Krieger, Butler, and Kilvington, 1951).[95] The earlier reports of the lethal effect of placental extracts, press juices, and autolysates given intravenously or their production of proteinuria when injected into the abdominal cavity were largely explained by Lichtenstein (1908).[96] He found (1) that extracts of other organs are equally toxic, (2) that the particulate matter in the preparations blocked the pulmonary capillaries, (3) that the lethal effect and intravascular coagulation could be duplicated by the injection of inorganic particles suspended in saline solution, (4) that the proteinuria could be duplicated by the injection of other foreign proteins, and (5) that filtered extracts were innocuous. Schneider (1947) identified the "toxin" in placental extracts free of particles as thromboplastin, which causes intravascular coagulation.[97]

PROPHYLAXIS

Mauriceau (1694) recommended two or three phlebotomies during the course of pregnancy as prophylaxis against eclampsia, but he disparaged a colleague who had bled one woman 48 times and another 90 times.[30]

Dietary taboos originated in the superstitions of antiquity and have persisted, with modifications, to the present day. Meat, especially red meat, has had a bad name and has been forbidden or restricted in the dietary treatment of many disorders, including preeclampsia–eclampsia. Thus Miquel (1824), in discussing prophylaxis against convulsions in pregnancy, recommended a farinaceous vegetable diet in the form of a slop or, preferably, one of milk products together with avoidance of spices.[98] De Wees (1828) attributed to overeating the one case of eclampsia that he mentioned in his *Treatise on the Diseases of Females*. Prenatal care was unusual in the first half of the 19th century, but some physicians did see private patients before labor.[99] Johns (1843) wrote that every physician should see his obstetric patients at intervals during the latter months of pregnancy. He described edema of the hands and face, headache, giddiness, ringing in the ears, loss of vision, pain in the stomach, and a flushed face as denoting an increased risk of convulsions.[100] He wrote that the risk was converted to certainty if (1) the women were pregnant for the first time or had had convulsions in a previous pregnancy; (2) if the head of the child presented, or (3) if the women were of full and plethoric habit. (In passing, it was widely believed at that time that convulsions occurred only in association with vertex presentations.) To prevent convulsions, Johns advocated a diet of fruits, vegetables, and milk, as well as laxatives or purgatives, diuretics, moderate exercise and plenty of fresh air, phlebotomy, and, if the signs and symptoms were marked, emetics. Meigs (1848) boasted that although he had seen a good many cases of eclampsia, he was very sure that he had prevented a far greater number.[101]

Sinclair and Johnston (1858) wrote that admittances of women to the Dublin Lying-in Hospital, in all cases except dire emergencies, were by arrangement made before the end of pregnancy. Each woman was given a ticket to be signed by a priest or by a respectable citizen, which she then took to the Dispensary for the countersignature of a physician.[102] The physician checked on her signs and symptoms, and if she had edema, headaches, dizziness, or proteinuria, she was either admitted to the hospital or seen regularly in the Dispensary. She was purged freely and repeatedly, kept in bed, and allowed nothing but the mildest and lightest nutriment. The authors stated: "Very often have convulsions been most certainly warded off altogether." When convulsions had not been prevented, they thought that the severity of the disease had been decreased by their treatment.

After Lever's (1843) discovery of proteinuria in eclamptic and preeclamptic women, more and more physicians recommended periodic urinalyses in the latter months of pregnancy.[50] When proteinuria was found, they prescribed dietary restrictions along with laxative and diuretic agents and, often, phlebotomy. The diet usually was limited to fruits, vegetables, and milk and was low in protein. Low protein diets were advocated for an ever-increasing number of reasons. They were thought to be more easily digestible and to minimize gastric irritation; nervous stimuli from the uterus and gastrointestinal tract were long thought to cause cerebral repletion (or depletion) and thus to trigger convulsions. Another objective was to lessen the "plethora of pregnancy." When eclampsia came to be regarded as uremic Bright's disease, the diets seemed rational because they reduced the load of nitrogenous catabolites and supposed toxins to be excreted by the kidney. Still later, the Dublin school, especially, argued that incompletely digested fragments of the protein molecule were absorbed from the intestine and had a toxic effect. The bodily defenses against the so-called split proteins were normally adequate but during pregnancy the fetus and placenta represented an additional source of such noxious substances. When the combined invasions overwhelmed the defenses, toxemia and eclampsia resulted. Another hypothesis was that the amino acids from the digested proteins were decarboxylated but not deaminated, with the production of toxic amines.

One of the circumstantial evidences for the efficacy of low protein diets was the observation that eclampsia was predominantly a disease of middle- and upper-class women. That widely held opinion may have been influenced by the fact that many physicians who published had private practices, but Fitzgibbon (1922), who saw all classes in Dublin's Rotunda, wrote: "Toxaemia is unquestionably a disease of the well-to-do classes of society."[103] Ruiz-Contreras (1922), of Barcelona, reported that the incidences of proteinuria and eclampsia were far greater in his private patients than in the charity patients he managed in the clinic.[104] When the nutrition improved and the dietary intake of protein increased among the masses, the incidences of proteinuria and eclampsia rose.

During World War I the incidence of eclampsia decreased significantly in Germany and rose again after the Armistice. Germans are reputed to eat heavily, and the nutritionists reasoned that in good times they eat too much. During the war years they might have eaten less protein and benefited by a relative immunity to eclampsia. An editorial (1917) in the *Journal of the American Medical Association* stated: "The conclusion seems inevitable that restrictions of fat and meat tend to ward off eclampsia."[105] That interpretation had an effect that persists to the present day. As late as 1945, Stander, in the ninth edition of *Williams' Obstetrics*, advocated the dietary restriction of protein in the treatment of hypertensive disorders in pregnancy.[106] Many obstetricians prescribed such diets for all of their patients as prophylaxis against preeclampsia. The current practice of nearly all American obstetricians in limiting weight gain during pregnancy to 15 or 20 lbs stems from the same source.

CLASSIFICATION OF THE HYPERTENSIVE DISORDERS IN PREGNANCY

Classifications are of relatively recent origin. Women with prodromal signs of gestational or puerperal convulsions were designated as having threatening or imminent eclampsia, but a specific name of the condition was long delayed. During much of the latter half of the 19th century, eclampsia was thought to be uremic Bright's disease and women with proteinuria and edema were thought to have nephritis, although a few authors simply called it "albuminuria," a term that persisted for many years in England.

Leyden (1881) described "the kidney of pregnancy" (Schwangerschaftsniere) and, in 1886, pointed out that the renal changes in eclampsia are similar (Chap. 4).[107,108] He reviewed the meager literature, citing several authors who had suggested that prolonged duration of the kidney of pregnancy sometimes leads to chronic nephritis and wrote that he had seen several such cases. Probably the most vigorous proponent of that view was Schroeder (1878), who thought that what we call preeclampsia was acute nephritis.[109] He wrote that prompt termination of pregnancy would prevent the progression to chronic nephritis, whereas delay would favor it. Needless to say, the kidneys of survivors were not examined during pregnancy and the differential diagnosis was highly uncertain.

As a result of Leyden's work, nonconvulsive hypertensive disorders in pregnancy were called "kidney of pregnancy" or "nephropathy," and later, "nephritic toxemia." Some of those terms still persist. In the United States, just after 1900, the most common designation was "the toxemia of pregnancy." Webster (1903), in his *Textbook of Obstetrics*, referred to the "pre-eclamptic state" and Bar (1908) introduced the word "éclampsisme" as meaning eclampsia without convulsions or threatening eclampsia.[110,111]

Once the concept of circulating toxins gained acceptance at the turn of the century, many disorders of obscure origin came to be classified as toxemias of pregnancy. Included were such diverse conditions as hyperemesis, acute yellow atrophy of the liver, ptyalism, gingivitis, pruritus, herpes, severe dermatitides, neuritis, psychosis, chorea, anemia, abruptio placentae, and all forms of hypertension. We see a comparable situation today, when so many physicians attribute almost any disorder of unknown origin, or even malaise, to "a virus."

The unitarians thought that a single toxin might be responsible for the array of effects and suggested that hyperemesis protected a woman from eclampsia because she vomited out much of the noxious substance. Williams (1912), in the third edition of his *Obstetrics*, wrote that the unitarians were impeding progress and that investigators should look for toxins specific for each disorder.[112] His classification of the "toxemias of pregnancy" was: *pernicious vomiting, acute yellow atrophy of the liver, nephritic toxemia, preeclamptic toxemia, eclampsia, presumable toxemia* (under which he included most of the diverse array just cited).

The many classifications proposed before 1940 were essentially variations on Williams' theme, although there was a progressive disappearance of the presumable toxemias. Some writers differentiated hepatic eclampsia from renal eclampsia.

In 1940, the American Committee on Maternal Welfare (Bell et al, 1940)[113] proposed the following classification:

Group A. Diseases not peculiar to pregnancy
      I. Hypertensive disease (hypertensive cardiovascular disease)—benign, mild, severe, or malignant
      II. Renal diseases
        a. Chronic vascular nephritis (nephrosclerosis)
        b. Glomerulonephritis, acute or chronic
        c. Nephrosis, acute or chronic
        d. Other forms of renal disease

Group B. Disease dependent on or peculiar to pregnancy
        I. Preeclampsia, mild or severe
      II. Eclampsia
          a. Convulsive
          b. Nonconvulsive (coma with findings at necropsy typical of eclampsia)

Group C. Vomiting of pregnancy

Group D. Unclassified toxemia, in which the above categories cannot be separated for want of information.

Acute yellow atrophy was dropped, but vomiting was retained "because of precedent." Mild hypertensive disease was defined by the absence of marked vascular changes and blood pressures below 160/100; no lower limit of blood pressure was specified. Mild preeclampsia was defined by the appearance after the 24th week of blood pressures of 140 to 160 systolic and 90 to 100 diastolic, proteinuria of less than 6 g/L, and slight or no edema.

In 1952, another subcommittee of the American Committee on Maternal Welfare (Eastman et al, 1952) revised the classification.[114] They dropped vomiting as unrelated to the hypertensive disorders and deleted renal diseases in the mistaken belief that they are easily differentiable from essential hypertension and preeclampsia. Two new categories were added: preeclampsia or eclampsia superimposed upon chronic hypertension, and recurrent toxemias. Clumsy diction inadvertently permitted the diagnosis of preeclampsia on the basis of any one of the three cardinal signs, even persistent edema or rapid weight gain alone.

Obstetricians in Aberdeen, and in some other areas, follow Nelson's (1955) definition of preeclampsia.[115] Edema is ignored and the diagnosis is made if the diastolic pressure rises to 90 mm Hg or more after the 25th week and is found on at least 2 days. In the absence of proteinuria, the disorder is called mild; if proteinuria appears, it is called severe preeclampsia. The mildly preeclamptic group, thus classified, must include many women with latent hypertension brought to light by pregnancy, as well as chronic hypertensive women whose blood pressures have abated during midgestation. The severe group would include many cases that would be called mild in other classifications.

Various schemes of classification have been published within the past few years in *Gynaecologia*. They have been compared by Rippmann (1969) who has compiled a list of more than 60 names in English and more than 40 in German that have been applied to the hypertensive disorders in pregnancy.[116]

EDITORS' UPDATE

The reprinted chapter was actually composed prior to 1975, and at approximately the same time, inspired by and with Leon's blessing and support, Drs. Marshall Lindheimer and Fred Zuspan were organizing an International Workshop through

nstitutes of Health (USA) focusing on the Hypertensive Disorders of
e meeting held September 25–27, 1975, was convened to solve the fol-
problem: "Hypertension, especially preeclampsia, is a major complication
of pregnancy causing significant morbidity and mortality in both fetus and mother.
Nevertheless, research on the hypertensive complications of pregnancy has been
sporadic, and scientists studying this and related fields have rarely communi-
cated."[117] The workshop's aim was stated as an attempt to "stimulate investigative
efforts in the field and to establish avenues of communication between clinical and
laboratory scientists in various disciplines."

The meeting achieved its immediate goals, and its long-term influence was
even more startling. Approximately 60 invited participants from diverse research
fields and clinical disciplines, including many academic "stars," shared their views
and data, argued profusely at times, and parted energized with new perspectives. A
text of the symposium published in 1976 is still liberally cited.[117] Of importance, the
enthusiasm generated by the workshop culminated in the establishment of a new
group, the International Society for the Study of Hypertension in Pregnancy. Its inaugural congress was held in Dublin, Ireland, in 1978, with subsequent meetings
every 2 years thereafter. More important, the long-term goals of Leon Chesley, implicit in this text's initial edition as well as those of the 1976 workshop organizers,
appear to have been realized, namely, those focusing attention on a critical but neglected area of maternal and fetal health. Thus, as stated in introductory paragraphs
of this chapter, the 1980s and 1990s have been characterized by an explosion of research accomplishments which increase exponentially as we approach the millen-
nium. Both physicians and investigators now recognize a continually increasing
panoply of pathophysiological changes associated with preeclampsia, and recognize
that this disease is more than just hypertension, it is a systemic disorder.[118,119] The
chapters which follow include among other topics, attention to and new findings in
placental studies, the roles of autocoids and a host of circulating substances, as well
as the vascular endothelium. New, also is a rapidly expanding interest in the contribution of the maternal constitution, both genetic and environmental, to the genesis
of preeclampsia. These latter studies are guided to a large degree by Leon Chesley's
landmark of the outcome of preeclampsia which included women whose clinical
courses were followed for over 40 years after an eclamptic convulsion.[120] All of the
accomplishments alluded to above will be amply cited in the chapters that follow.

This optimistic introduction, however, must be tempered a bit, as there are still
many unsolved problems and controversies, and the cause(s) of hypertension complicating gestation, especially preeclampsia and eclampsia is (are) yet to be definitively established. We will discuss but two of the controversies here, measurement
of blood pressure during gestation, and continuation of our inability to agree on
classification schemas.

Measurement of Blood Pressure

Until the 1990s, literature regarding measurement of blood pressure in pregnancy
was quite confusing. Controversies included the preferable posture for testing the

subject (such as lateral recumbency or quiet sitting), and most important which Korotkoff sound, either K_4 (muffling of sound) or K_5 (disappearance of audible beats), was a better measurement of diastolic pressure in pregnant women.[121] The debate over posture related to observations that blood pressure rises in some women destined to develop preeclampsia when they change from a lateral to a supine posture (once called the "roll over" test),[122] which led many to observe that the lowest blood pressures were obtained when pregnant women were positioned on their sides. It is now believed that lower values with the woman in lateral recumbency merely reflect the difference in hydrostatic pressure when the cuff is positioned substantially above the left ventricle.[123] In this respect, the "roll over" phenomenon as a predictor of preeclampsia seems to have been discredited, but there are still occasional claims that the difference in blood pressure when measurements in lateral and supine recumbency are compared are more than just a postural phenomenon.[124]

The controversy of K_4 vs. K_5 stems from a belief that the hyperdynamic circulation of pregnant women frequently leads to large differences between these sounds, with the latter often approaching zero. As recently as the early 1990s, groups such as the World Health Organization and the British Hypertension Society defined diastolic blood pressure in pregnant women as K_4, and others, including the National High Blood Pressure Education Program (NHBPEP) recommended K_5.[125-127] Even more confusing was the omission in many publications of which sound was actually used. The newly formed International Society for the Study of Hypertension in Pregnancy became the forum for this debate and of course new research ensued. We now know that large differences between the two sounds are very infrequent, that K_5 more closely approximates true (intraarterial) diastolic levels, that K_4 is often unreliable, and that even where the latter sound has been designated to define diastolic levels, the majority of health providers continue to measure K_5, the putative descriptor of diastolic blood pressure in nonpregnant populations worldwide.[128-130] Thus, current recommendations appear more unanimous; that is, blood pressure should be measured in pregnant women in a manner similar to that in nonpregnant populations: the patient should be seated and rest for about 5 minutes, and the cuff over the arm should be at the level of the heart.

In 1969 Rippman stated that a major detriment to our understanding of hypertension in pregnancy was the multiple conflicting terminologies, a fact underscored in Chesley's original chapter.[1,116] The situation is not much better today. For example, perusing the literature, one encounters terms such as toxemia, pregnancy-induced hypertension or pregnancy-associated hypertension, preeclampsia, and preeclamptic toxemia. This plethora of terminology leads to confusion, especially when the same term, e.g., pregnancy induced hypertension (PIH) is defined differently by various authors. Furthermore, questions regarding the definition of increased blood pressure elevation, including whether to consider absolute blood pressures or incremental changes and the necessity of including proteinuria to differentiate the pregnancy-specific disorder or to include systemic changes other than those of renal function for this differentiation are all still controversial.[127,131-135]

Of note, the primary goal of each of these classification schemas is similar, that is, they are attempts to differentiate a pregnancy-specific disorder associated with increased fetal and maternal risk from other more "benign" preexisting or gestational forms of hypertension. Why then are there so many classifications, some quite discrepant? First, it appears that the signs and symptoms selected to identify preeclampsia were often chosen for convenience rather than relevance to the pathophysiology or outcome. Second, the values used to discriminate normal from abnormal were often selected arbitrarily, and remain to be validated. These include cut-off levels for systolic ($\geq$ 140 mm Hg) and diastolic ($\geq$ 90 mm Hg) blood pressure, and the qualitative and quantitative definitions for abnormal proteinuria. Another, and perhaps the most important confounder is that the purpose for which the classification is used will determine whether sensitivity or specificity is the most important criterion of the classification scheme. *Thus, for clinical care sensitivity is paramount while for research specificity is and should be the primary concern.*

Concerning absolute levels vs. incremental increments in blood pressure: a pathophysiologic approach supports incremental rises because the predominant pathological change is a pregnancy-specific profound vasoconstriction. But an equally compelling argument against incremental blood pressure is that it is too nonspecific, and will lead to substantial overlabeling of normal gravidas as gestational hypertensives. The problem of specificity and sensitivity becomes even more complicated when proteinuria is omitted as a diagnostic requirement in the classification of preeclampsia. For instance, one current classification in many texts and in the National Institutes of Health Working Group report uses hypertension and *proteinuria* or *edema* in their definition; the Australasian Hypertension Society defines de novo hypertension alone in late pregnancy as *mild* preeclampsia; and a recent position paper in the *Journal of Hypertension* recommends that a number of other signs or symptoms alone, e.g., renal insufficiency, as well as neurologic, hematologic, or hepatic system signs or laboratory abnormalities, be combined with hypertension for the diagnosis.[127,133,135]

For clinical care alone we believe that it is appropriate to overdiagnose preeclampsia. This is because gestational hypertension alone can be an early sign or forme fruste of true preeclamptic syndrome, and clinical overdiagnosis ensures proper surveillance. For research, however, classification schema must be stricter. Leon Chesley continually underscored how our understanding of preeclampsia has been both compromised and impeded by the use of the broad clinical criteria described above for research purposes.[136] He continually advocated rigorous diagnostic criteria which included de novo hypertension, proteinuria, and hyperuricemia in nulliparous women who have a normal medical history or preferably with all of the abnormalities returning to normal postpartum.[137] We agree with this definition, adding for further accuracy the definition of hypertension as 140/90 mm Hg, and that of proteinuria as $\geq$ 300 mg/24 hours, or a qualitative value of 2+ on two occassions 4 hours apart.

Finally, we cite the recommendations of the NHBPEP Working Group, in which all three editors of this text participated, as a framework for the taxonomy of the hypertensive disorders of pregnancy as they should be approached *clinically*, recalling, that it, as others, is arbitrary with obvious limitations.[127] We further note, that as this chapter is being finalized, the National Institutes of Health, in conjunction with the NHBPEP, is planning to revisit these suggestions, it is hoped using the rapidly growing databases from recently finished and ongoing multicenter trials which include longitudinal determinations of blood pressures, protein excretion, and a variety of "markers." (The new report is scheduled for late 1999.)

National High Blood Pressure Education Program's Working Group Classification (1990 Report)

The Working Group's clinical classification schema has but four categories: (1) *chronic hypertension (of any cause)*, (2) *preeclampsia–eclampsia*, (3) *preeclampsia superimposed upon chronic hypertension*, and (4) *transient hypertension*.

Chronic Hypertension

Defined as hypertension ($\geq 140/90$ mm Hg) present and observable prior to conception or diagnosed before the 20th week of gestation. In addition high blood pressure presenting in late pregnancy which persists beyond the 42nd day postpartum is also classified as chronic hypertension.

Preeclampsia–Eclampsia

The diagnosis of preeclampsia is determined by de novo increases in blood pressure accompanied by proteinuria, edema, or both. Here *hypertension* is diagnosed by an increase of ≥ 30 mm Hg systolic, or 15 mm Hg diastolic from levels measured prior to the 20th week of gestation, as well as the appearance of a value of $\geq 140/90$ mm Hg (especially when early or prepregnancy values are unknown). The abnormal values must be recorded during two measurements performed 6 hours apart. *Edema* is diagnosed as clinically evident swelling, but fluid retention may also manifest as a rapid increase of weight without evident swelling, e.g., "pitting edema." *Proteinuria* is defined as a qualitative measurement of $1+$ (30 mg/dL), or ≥ 300 mg in a 24-hour collection.

Preeclampsia occurs as a spectrum but is arbitrarily divided into *mild* and *severe* forms. This terminology is useful for descriptive purposes but does not indicate "different diseases" nor should it indicate arbitrary cut-off points for therapy. Severe preeclampsia is diagnosed when the following criteria (or ominous signs and symptoms) are present:

- blood pressure ≥ 160 mm Hg systolic or ≥ 110 mm Hg diastolic, recorded on two or more occasions 6 hours apart, with the patient resting in bed
- proteinuria of ≥ 5 g/24 hours or 3 or $4+$ qualitatively
- oliguria (≤ 500 mL/24 h)
- cerebral or visual disturbances
- epigastric pain
- pulmonary edema or cyanosis

Eclampsia

Eclampsia is the occurrence of seizures in a preeclamptic patient that cannot be attributed to other causes. These issues are discussed further in Chapter 5.

Preeclampsia Superimposed upon Chronic Hypertension

There is ample evidence that preeclampsia may occur in women already hypertensive and that the prognosis for mother and fetus is much worse than with either condition alone. The Working Group recommended that the diagnosis be made on the basis of increases of blood pressure (increments of or exceeding 30 mm Hg systolic and 15 mm Hg diastolic, or 20 mm Hg mean arterial pressure) together with the appearance of abnormal proteinuria or generalized edema.

Transient Hypertension

This describes the development of de novo elevated blood pressure during late pregnancy or in the first 24 hours postpartum without other signs of preeclampsia or preexisting hypertension.

DENOUEMENT

This update would be incomplete without a commentary by Leon Chesley made two decades ago at the banquet of the 1975 Workshop on Hypertension in Pregnancy[2] and reprinted below. Bear it in mind as you read the ensuing chapters.

False Steps in the Study of Preeclampsia

A century ago, an American humorist, Josh Billings, made a good generalization that applies to our views of preeclampsia–eclampsia when he said: "The trouble with people isn't that they don't know, but that so much of what they know ain't so." In talking about false starts in the study of eclampsia, I am acutely aware that much of what we believe today will be added to the list.

An observation by Mauriceau,[30] made in the 17th century, has stood the test of time: preeclampsia–eclampsia is predominantly a disease of primigravidas. It does occur in multiparas, but when it does, there is usually some predisposing factor such as multiple gestation, diabetes, or preexisting primary or secondary hypertension. Hinselmann's analysis of 6498 cases from the literature showed that 74% of cases occurred in primigravidas, although they contributed only a quarter to a third of all pregnancies.[138] He calculated that primigravidas are six times as likely to develop eclampsia as are multiparas.

McCartney has made an outstanding contribution in his electron microscopic studies of renal biopsies.[139] He carefully selected 152 multiparas with known chronic hypertension, all of whom fulfilled the criteria of the American Committee on Maternal Welfare for the diagnosis of superimposed preeclampsia. Renal biopsies of only five of the women showed the pure "preeclamptic lesion" of glomerular capillary endotheliosis, while in another 16 the lesion was superimposed upon renal arteriolar sclerosis. If the definitive diagnosis were based upon anatomic findings, the clinical diagnosis would be erroneous in 86% of the cases.

Admittedly, it has not been proven that every woman with preeclampsia has the typical lesion, and the uncertainties of clinical diagnosis are such that a one-to-one ratio is not likely to be established. Nearly half of the multiparas had lesions of renal disease, usually nephrosclerosis, and it seems that preeclampsia was grossly overdiagnosed clinically.

There are diagnostic difficulties in primigravidas as well. McCartney selected 62 women who were apparently normal in midpregnancy and who developed hypertension, proteinuria, and edema in the third trimester. The clinical diagnosis was preeclampsia. Only 71%, however, had the renal lesion of preeclampsia. That finding might mean merely that the lesion is not always present in preeclampsia, except that 26% had lesions of chronic renal disease and 13 of these 16 women had chronic glomerulonephritis that had been silent during much of pregnancy. Three had no renal lesion at all, and they may have had latent essential hypertension revealed by pregnancy.

The finding of lesions of chronic renal disease in women who were apparently normal in midpregnancy is consistent with certain older clinical observations. Theobald found the prevalence of proteinuria to be lower in midpregnancy than in nonpregnant women of the same ages as the pregnant subjects.[140] In a later paper, he suggested that both proteinuria and hypertension present before conception often disappear during midpregnancy and reappear in the third trimester.[141] Thus, apparently normal women may have a seemingly acute onset of hypertension and proteinuria in the third trimester, and the erroneous diagnosis of preeclampsia is likely to be made. Reid and Teel, in studying women with known hypertension, observed that a significant proportion of them had normal blood pressures during the 2nd trimester; characteristically, the pressure rose again early in the third trimester.[142]

Neither Theobald nor Reid and Teel specified the frequency of such changes, and when I first read their papers I naively dismissed their observations as curiosities of no statistical significance in the differential diagnosis of the hypertensive disorders in pregnancy. In 1946, however, John Annitto and I analyzed 301 pregnancies of women with known hypertension and found that in 39% the blood pressures were significantly decreased until the third trimester.[143] Many had normal pressures during midpregnancy. One extreme case was that of a woman whom we saw during five pregnancies and many times between pregnancies. She was always severely hypertensive while not pregnant, and always normotensive during pregnancy. Near term, she might have a pressure such as 140/84 in one pregnancy and 130/90 in another. In short, we had her in the hospital at bedrest and under sedation for 8 days at about 18 months after her 4th pregnancy. Her lowest diastolic pressure was 150 mm Hg, and it ranged up to 180, with systolic pressures always greater than 250 mm Hg. Nearly a year later, she registered in the antepartum clinic in the 4th month of pregnancy; her blood pressure was 110/60, and she remained normotensive throughout pregnancy, as she had in her earlier gestations. She deviated from the usual pattern in not becoming hypertensive early in the 3rd trimester.

In brief, hypertension of apparently acute onset seldom justifies the diagnosis of preeclampsia in a multipara, who is much more likely to have frank essential hypertension or renal disease that abated during midpregnancy, or latent essential hypertension that is brought to light and sometimes peculiarly altered by gestation. I have developed this theme at some length because now that eclampsia has become rare, most studies of the disease are made in women bearing the diagnosis of preeclampsia. Any study of preeclampsia that includes multiparas will lead to erroneous conclusions, and I have done more than my share to confuse the field. The Pennsylvania Dutch have a saying that describes my situation: "Too soon Oldt, too late Schmart."

The relation between preeclampsia–eclampsia and later chronic hypertension has been a source of contention and confusion for many years. In 1940, our group at the Margaret Hague Maternity Hospital reexamined most of the women who had had hypertensive disorders in their pregnancies during 1935 and 1936.[144] The prevalence of hypertension among the 319 thought to have had preeclampsia was about 36%, and there seemed to be an almost linear relation between the duration of the supposed preeclampsia and the frequency of hypertension at follow-up. A similar relation had been described by Harris,[145] Gibberd,[146] Peckham,[147] and others, and we erroneously accepted their conclusion that prolonged preeclampsia had caused chronic hypertension.

When Annitto and I completed our study of pregnancies in women with documented essential hypertension, I looked again at the data in the follow-up study of 1940. Multiparas constituted about half of the patients who had satisfied the criteria for the diagnosis of preeclampsia as laid down by the American Committee on Maternal Welfare. Many of them had had hypertension in earlier pregnancies, and they undoubtedly had latent or frank hypertensive disease, rather than preeclampsia.

The woman with chronic hypertension whose blood pressure falls to normal levels in midpregnancy and rises again early in the 3rd trimester is the patient who is likely to be carried for several weeks with supposed preeclampsia. Termination of the pregnancy when the pressure rises would jeopardize the fetus, and so the physician temporizes. The clinical picture does not worsen as weeks go by, because all the patient has is hypertension. When she is found to have hypertension at follow-up, she has it because she had it before pregnancy and *not* because she was carried for several weeks with preeclampsia.

We dropped our follow-up studies of women with nonconvulsive hypertensive disorders and retracted our conclusion that prolonged preeclampsia causes chronic hypertension. In an effort to ascertain the relation, if any, between acute gestational hypertension and chronic hypertension, we have reexamined at intervals of 6 or 7 years nearly all of the 270 women who survived eclampsia at the Margaret Hague Maternity Hospital from 1931 through 1951. Only one of these patients has had no follow-up, and in 1974 we traced all but three. The diagnosis of eclampsia is not always correct, but it is far more reliable than that of preeclampsia. Moreover, 75% of the patients were primigravidas, and the multiparas have been analyzed separately. The greatly different prognoses for primiparous and multiparous eclamptic women are instructive.

In brief, the prevalence of chronic hypertension among women who had eclampsia as primiparas is not different from that in unselected women of the same ages. Eclampsia, then, is not a sign of latent hypertension, as some internists had believed, and eclampsia, whatever the duration of the acute hypertensive phase, does not cause chronic hypertension. That conclusion has been drawn by Theobald,[148] Browne,[149] Adams and MacGillivray,[150] and others in the British Isles and by Dieckmann,[75] Tillman,[151] Bryans,[152] and others in the United States. Tillman's study is notable, for he accumulated a large group of women whose blood pressures were known before, during, and after pregnancies. He found that whether the pregnancies were normotensive or hypertensive they had no effect on blood pressure at follow-up.

Women who had eclampsia as multiparas have had a remarkably different prognosis. Nearly three times the expected number have died, and 80% of the remote deaths have resulted from the lethal consequences of hypertensive disease. The prevalence of chronic hypertension among the survivors is increased over that found in several series of unselected women matched for age. The high prevalence of hypertensive disease among women having eclampsia as multiparas is explained by their having had hypertension before pregnancy, which predisposed them to eclampsia.

Clearly, women who have eclampsia as multiparas are different from those who have eclampsia as primiparas, and the two groups must be analyzed separately. The inclusion of multiparas in studies of preeclampsia or eclampsia leads to erroneous conclusions, and, as a result, I now regard many of my own earlier publications as virtually worthless.

I should mention one paper that has received wide attention. Epstein,[153] an internist then at Yale, reexamined 48 women at about 15 years after hypertensive pregnancies thought to be preeclamptic. He found a higher prevalence of hypertension among them than in control women selected because their pregnancies had been normotensive, and he concluded that prolonged preeclampsia causes hypertension. One of his tables shows that 24 of the 48 women were multiparas at the time the pregnancies were studied. It seems probable that few of the women really had preeclampsia, and history has repeated itself. Moreover, the selection as controls of women who had escaped gestational hypertension constituted a strong bias, for it excluded many who would develop hypertension as they grew older. Many future hypertensive women manifest the diathesis by gestational hypertension, and such women have apparent but not "true" preeclampsia.

Many of the hypotheses about the cause of eclampsia cannot stand in light of the predominant occurrence of the disease in nulliparas. When I came into the field 40 years ago, the standard management of preeclampsia was restriction of dietary protein, and many obstetricians put all of their patients on low protein diets as prophylaxis against preeclampsia. It was a time-honored custom, reinforced by the 200-year-old obstetric belief that eclampsia is a disease of upper-class women and by the observation that the incidence of eclampsia decreased in some parts of Germany during World War I. Germans are reputed to eat heavily and, according to the nutritionists, too much. During the war they might have eaten less, and the nutritionists seized on protein as the source of the eclamptic toxin because protein had long been anathema. An editorial in the *Journal of the American Medical Association* said "The conclusion seems inevitable that restriction of fat and meat tends to ward off eclampsia."[105] Ruiz-Contreras wrote that the incidence of proteinuria and eclampsia was far higher among his private patients than in the women whose pregnancies he managed in the charity wards.[104] He observed a rise in the incidence of proteinuria and eclampsia in ward patients when their nutrition improved, as the intake of dietary protein increased among the masses.

The restriction of protein seemed rational a century ago, when eclampsia was thought to be a form of uremia. When that hypothesis was disproved, others took its place. One proposed incomplete digestion of proteins with the production of toxic "split products." That led to the Dublin or Rotunda method of management, in which gastric lavage, high colonic irrigation, and purgation were aimed at washing out all toxins within reach. In addition, an initial phlebotomy removed some of the circulating toxin; a second bleeding 2 hours later was aimed at getting toxins that had been mobilized into the bloodstream in the interim. Another hypothesis was that the amino acids resulting from the digestion of protein were decarboxylated but not deaminated, thus resulting in toxic amines.

The decreased incidence of eclampsia in some parts of Germany during the war was explained in various ways. Some thought that increased physical activity in pregnant working women was the answer. Others postulated toxins or antigens in semen as the cause of eclampsia; with the men away at the front, the women supposedly were not realizing their wonted (and perhaps wanted) chronic exposure to poisoning. The hypothesis relating eclampsia to dietary protein prevailed, with effects that persist to the present day.

Germany suffered no serious shortage of food during the war; however, the incidence of eclampsia began to decline toward the end of the first year of the war. The severe shortages occurred during the first year following the armistice, while the Allies continued the blockade, and the incidence of eclampsia then rose. The converse of the German experience occurred during the siege of Madrid, about 30 years later. The incidence of eclampsia rose strikingly, only to subside in the following year.

Lehmann[154] obtained the statistics for all of Baden, from the Landsamt in Karlsruhe, and found that the proportionate representation of primiparous deliveries had decreased in proportion to the reduction in incidence of eclampsia during the war. Some months after the armistice, the proportion of primiparous deliveries rose dramatically, with a parallel increase in the incidence of eclampsia. During the war, many of the men remaining home were fathers of large families, and their wives continued to have pregnancies as multiparas. After the young men came home there were, in due course, parallel surges in primiparous deliveries and eclampsia. Hinselmann,[138] however, did note a decrease in the incidence of eclampsia in primigravidas, but Lehmann's study explains most of the fluctuation.

Díaz del Castillo found that in Madrid there had been a surge in primiparous deliveries in proportion to the high incidence of eclampsia.[155] During the siege, the boys had been cooped up with the nubile nulliparas, and in due time there was a wave of primiparous deliveries.

Fifty years ago eclampsia was common in New York City, and it had a seasonal incidence, with the peak in March and April. The followers of Hippocrates attributed it to the variable, unsettled weather and the nutritionists to the lack of fresh vegetables and fruit. In Denmark in the 1920s, there were two seasonal peaks, 6 months apart. Many young women worked as domestic servants under contracts that expired the same day throughout the nation. Lehmann wrote that at the expiration of the contracts, many of the women quit and married.[154] The peak incidence of primiparous deliveries and of eclampsia occurred together, 9 to 10 months later. To return to New York, March and April fall at just the right interval after June weddings.

It has been known for more than two centuries that the incidence of eclampsia is higher in city women than in their country cousins. The moralistic nutritionists have explained the phenomenon by saying that the effete city woman lounges around her apartment drinking cocktails, smoking cigarettes, and eating snacks of junk food, for which she pays the penalty of an increased susceptibility to eclampsia. The country wife, supposedly, is out in the fresh air and sunshine, does physical labor such as shoveling hay, and eats a wholesome diet. Again, Lehmann found that the incidence of eclampsia follows the incidence of primiparous deliveries.[154] In those days, the average family size in the cities was smaller than in the countryside, where the farmers begat their future farm hands. The proportion of primigravidous deliveries accounted for nearly all of the difference, and admittance of country women to hospitals in the city accounted for the rest.

The nutritionists are now taking a different approach and attributing eclampsia to a dietary deficiency of protein, or of this or that vitamin or one or another of various minerals. As one example, Siddall[156] pointed out that the highest incidence of eclampsia in the nation was in the southeastern block of states, the region in which almost all cases of pellagra occurred. He concluded that deficiency of thiamin is the cause of eclampsia. H. L. Mencken once assessed the cultural level of each of the then 48 states, using criteria such as the prevalence of literacy, high school and college education, libraries, musical organizations, etc. The states came out in nearly the same order by each criterion, and the final evaluation put Massachusetts, Connecticut, and New York at the top, with Mississippi, Arkansas, and Alabama at the bottom. Characteristically, Mencken put another column into the table showing the prevalence of membership in churches. There was a good inverse correlation—the higher the membership in churches, the lower the cultural level. About 25 years ago, some joker put in a third column showing eclamptic deaths, and from the correlation concluded that the cause of eclampsia must be church membership. This conclusion seems as valid as the one drawn by the nutritionists.

The difficulty with the nutritional hypothesis as to the cause of eclampsia is that the disease is predominantly one of the first viable pregnancy. Impoverished and malnourished women are the very ones who have pregnancies in rapid succession. The fetal drain thus imposed upon whatever poor reserves they begin with must deplete them progressively. If malnutrition were the cause of eclampsia, its frequency should rise with parity. It does not.

I have alluded to the high incidence of eclamptic deaths in the southeastern states, which brings up the question of the reliability of statistics and their interpretation. We know nothing of the incidence of preeclampsia anywhere but in our own hospitals, and even there, that knowledge depends upon who makes the diagnoses. In studying the familial factor in eclampsia, I have seen the delivery charts of daughters, daughters-in-law, and granddaughters of eclamptic women in well over 100 different hospitals. Considering only first pregnancies, where the risk of preeclampsia is high, no blood pressure was recorded in 23 charts, and there was but a single recording in 27, 7 of which were from 140/90 to 178/110. Twenty-four percent of the charts showed no urinalysis, and 31% carried no notation about the presence or absence of edema. In nine charts, there was no recording of blood pressure, no urinalysis, and nothing about edema. In such hospitals, the incidence of diagnosed preeclampsia must be low. Moreover, many charts bearing the diagnosis of normal pregnancy showed clear evidence of mild or severe preeclampsia and even, in one case, of eclampsia—with nine convulsions, gross proteinuria, anasarca, and acute hypertension in the range of 150–174/100–120 mm Hg; this patient was on the "danger list" for 24 hours. Is that a normal pregnancy?

Even if hospital statistics were accurate, they would not reflect the incidence of preeclampsia in a given community. In many regions, including the southeastern states, many women have no prenatal care and are delivered at home unless some serious complication occurs. I used to visit Frederick Zuspan when he was at the Medical College of Georgia, and I once saw seven eclamptic patients on the wards; not one was from Augusta. They had been brought in from as much as 200 miles away because of convulsions.

The other source of geographic statistics is deaths from eclampsia. These statistics are not any better. What they reflect chiefly is the quality, availability, and utilization of prenatal care, for when preeclampsia is detected early, a progression to severe preeclampsia to eclampsia to death usually can be prevented.

In 1831, Ryan wrote that women particularly susceptible to eclampsia are "those who are in labor for the first time and who are illicitly in this condition."[43] The nutritionists have suggested a poor diet in unmarried pregnant women as the explanation for their predisposition to eclampsia. The psychosomaticists have suggested mental stress. Lehmann confirmed the difference in Danish women, but when he analyzed by parity he found identical incidences in married and unmarried primigravidas.[154] The incidence in multiparas was much lower but the same in married and unmarried women. Except among slum-dwelling relief clients, most illegitimate pregnancies in the past have occurred in young nulliparas. The current wave of sexual liberation may change that, although access to abortion is an ameliorative factor.

As previously mentioned, obstetricians believed for two centuries that eclampsia was a disease of upper-class women. In 1768, Denman wrote that frail, delicate, educated, and highly intelligent city women who cultivated music were at particu-lar risk.[157] Perhaps the belief arose because obstetricians who served upper-class women wrote papers, whereas midwives, who served the lower classes, seldom published. It was not until about 1925 that Kosmak[158] suggested that eclampsia might be equally common in the impoverished and the wealthy, and today the widespread belief is that it is far more common in the poor than in private patients. Reverting for a moment to the undiagnosed case of eclampsia, it was the patient's private physician who wrote on the diagnosis sheet, "Normal pregnancy, normal labor, normal delivery, normal puerperium."

In Aberdeen, Scotland, the medical school has access to data for nearly every delivery in the city, and it appears from Nelson's analysis that there is little differ-ence in the incidence of preeclampsia among the five social classes.[115] A slight in-crease was noted in social class 3, and further analysis has shown an increase in class 3-C, which includes such women as the wives of streetcar conductors.

Another popular belief is that black American women are more susceptible to preeclampsia–eclampsia than are white women, and the belief has been linked to social class as well as to race. Mengert[159] reviewed his wide experience in three dif-ferent major centers and concluded that there is no racial difference; I agree. In the data from the Margaret Hague Maternity Hospital, which I mentioned above, 8% of the eclamptic women were black, and 8% of all deliveries were of black women. At the King's County Hospital, where black women account for 78% of obstetric pa-tients, the incidence of preeclampsia is identical in black women and in white women. The prevalence of chronic hypertension among black women is nearly three times that of white patients, which accords with several epidemiologic stud-ies in nonpregnant populations. Erroneous differential diagnosis has been respon-sible for the idea that black women are more susceptible to preeclampsia.

Old-time obstetricians believed that certain bodily builds predispose to eclampsia, but they could never agree as to what the characteristics were. Denman said frail, delicate women, but others thought that it was strong, plethoric sub-jects.[157] Systematic studies were long delayed, and, when they were made in the late 1920s, they unfortunately were conducted with patients thought to have preeclampsia and included large proportions of multiparas. Another flurry of pa-pers appeared in the early 1960s, and they are not better. The conclusion was that short, squat, obese women are more susceptible than long, lean, lank ones. For the past 40 years I have been seeing formerly eclamptic women in follow-up studies, and there are few obese women among them. In several indices of bodily build, the data for these women fall on normal distribution curves for unselected women. The bodily build alleged to predispose to eclampsia is that often associated with essen-tial hypertension, and the inclusion of multiparas in studies of preeclampsia again seems to have led to an erroneous conclusion.

I have alluded to the German experience during World War I. The nutrition-ists' misinterpretation of the role of dietary protein is now behind us, but for half a century virtually all American obstetricians have tried to limit the weight gained in pregnancy to 20, 15, or even 12 lbs as prophylaxis against preeclampsia. That practice stems from the same source as the restriction of dietary protein. In 1923, Carl Henry Davis was the first to advocate the measure.[160] He wrote that the gain should be limited to 20 lbs and that overweight women should gain less or should even lose weight. "The marked decrease of eclampsia in Central Europe during the period of war rationing led us to realize that eclamptics usually are women who have gained weight excessively during pregnancy."

In the same year, Calvin R. Hannah estimated the "reproductive weight" as 12 lbs which he derived by adding together the average weights of fetus, placenta, and amniotic fluid.[161] He wrote: "Patients whose weight is above standard and who continue to gain over the reproductive weight of 12 lbs, manifest preeclamptic symptoms."[161]

A flood of papers appeared describing the gain in weight during normal and hypertensive pregnancies, usually with no separation of primigravidas from multiparas. Each author ascertained the average gain in his normal subjects, which was 24 lbs when all of the data were pooled. In a statistical maneuver that defies comprehension, each author then set his average as the upper limit of normal, thereby denying the normality of half of his own normal patients. From the pooled data of many papers, it appears that two-thirds of normal women had gained between 13 and 35 lbs, with one-sixth having gained more than 35 lbs, despite frequent attempts to limit the gain.

Most authors found the combined incidence and prevalence of hypertensive disorders to increase somewhat with greater gains in weight. When one evaluates the published data, however, it becomes evident that 90% of women who gained more than 30 lbs did not develop any sort of hypertension. Conversely, 90% of women with what was called preeclampsia had gained less than 30 lbs, and 60% had gained less than 22 pounds. In relation to preeclampsia, the total gain during pregnancy probably means nothing, unless a large component of the gain is fluid, which is detected better by high rates of gain in the latter half of gestation.

The original rationale for the limitation of weight gained in pregnancy was fallacious, and there is no good evidence that it prevents preeclampsia. It may even be harmful. Several recent studies have shown that the average birth weights of the infants are lower when maternal gain is restricted. The Netherlands, the Scandinavian countries, and some other countries have lower rates of perinatal mortality than does the United States, and birth weights tend to be higher in the countries with superior salvage of infants. Some extremists suggest that our general practice of limiting maternal gain has increased the rate of prematurity and the birth of smaller weaklings at all stages of pregnancy.

For many years, obstetricians have been frightened by the appearance of edema in their patients, especially if it involves the hands and face, for they regard it as an early sign of preeclampsia. British studies have shown, however, that such edema usually is physiologic and occurs in a high percentage of pregnancies. Moreover, in the absence of proteinuric preeclampsia, infants born to women with edema of the hands or face weigh more at birth than do infants born to nonedematous women. It is not that the infants share the edema, for they do not lose weight excessively in the crib.

Tentatively, it appears that there may be two sorts of gestational edema—one is physiologic and good; the other may be the edema of preeclampsia. I do not know how to differentiate between them. The prevalence of edema is higher in preeclampsia than in normal pregnancy, and the edema is often more severe in preeclampsia.

Edema of the hands and face has long been accepted as an early sign of preeclampsia, but that may have been another of our false steps. The belief stems from retrospective studies of the charts of women with preeclampsia–eclampsia. One goes back in the record looking for premonitory signs, and in perhaps half the cases one finds that the patient's wedding ring was tight at, say, the 30th week of gestation. Aha! Edema of the fingers pointed to oncoming preeclampsia. But how many such studies have included reviews of the records of patients with normal pregnancies? None that I know of. The edema at 30 weeks' gestation may have been physiologic and have had nothing to do with preeclampsia. Certainly Robertson,[162] in his prospective study of gestational edema, could find no relation between generalized edema and later preeclampsia.

Double-blind studies have shown that prevention or dissipation of gestational edema with saluretic agents has no effect upon the incidence of clinical preeclampsia. The control or prevention of a sign does not strike at the basic disorder and, in this case, we may not even be dealing with a sign. I consider the use of diuretics as another of our false steps and can enumerate eight contraindications to their use in pregnant women, especially in preeclampsia.

The use of diuretics brings pilocarpine to mind. A century ago, the induction of sweating was an integral part of the management of eclampsia. Tincture of jaborandi was widely used for this purpose, and when pilocarpine was identified as the active principle, the purified drug was used. The rather poor results were rationalized in this manner: the intense sweating had distilled off water, leaving the eclamptic toxin behind in higher concentration. The drug was given a controlled trial in Edinburgh and abandoned when the usual case mortality doubled from 30 or 35% to 67%.

Since the space allotted to me is limited, I shall close with a few remarks about the management of eclampsia. Zuspan and Ward, in discussing it, wrote, "The eclamptic patient has certainly tested the ingenuity of physicians throughout the centuries as she has been blistered, bled, purged, packed, lavaged, irrigated, punctured, starved, sedated, anesthetized, paralyzed, tranquilized, rendered hypotensive, drowned, been given diuretics, had mammectomy, been dehydrated, been forcibly delivered, and neglected."[76] The list could be extended considerably. Surgical procedures have included ventral suspension of the uterus, drainage of spinal fluid, cisternal puncture, trepanation, ureteral catheterization, implantation of the ureters in the colon, renal decapsulation, oophorectomy, and postpartum curettage. The medical treatments have been legion.

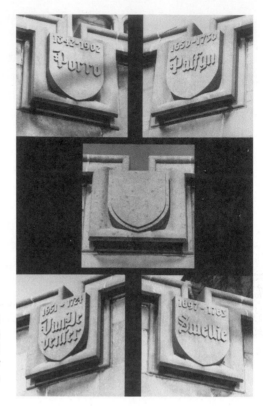

Figure 1–2. Placards honoring famous physicians who made major contributions to the field of obstetrics and gynecology adorn Chicago Lying-in hospital. The empty plaque is reserved for the individual who discovers the cause and/or cure of preeclampsia (perhaps a contributor to this text!).

We should remember that each of the treatments was rational in the light of some hypothesis as to the cause or nature of eclampsia. That is more than we can say for present day management, which is empiric, too often symptomatic, and in some respects, based upon imitative magic (Fig. 1–2).

REFERENCES

1. Chesley LC: *Hypertensive Disorders in Pregnancy.* New York: Appleton-Century-Crofts, 1978:628.
2. Chesley LC: False steps in the study of preeclampsia: In: Lindheimer MD, Katz AI, Zuspan FP, eds. *Hypertension in Pregnancy.* New York: John Wiley and Sons; 1976:1–10.
3. von Siebold ECJ: Versuch einer Geschichte der Geburtshülfe. Berlin: Enslin; 1839, 1845, vols I, II.
4. Knapp L: Bieträge zur Geschichte der Eklampsie. *Mtschr Geburtsh Gynaekol* 1901;14:65–109.
5. Kossmann R: Zur Geschichte des Wortes "Eclampsie." *Mtschr Geburtsch Gynaekol* 1901; 14:288–290.
6. Fasbender H: *Geschichte der Geburtschülfe.* Jena:Fischer;1906;777–804.
7. Fischer I: Geschichte der Gynäkologie. In: Halban J, Sietz L, eds. *Biologie und Pathologie des Weibes.* Berlin: Urban and Schwarzenberg; 1924, vol I.
8. Bernhart F: Geschichte, Wesen und Behandlung der Eklampsie. *Wien Klin Wchschr* 1930;52:1009–1003, 1036–1043.
9. Menascha I: Die Geburtshilfe bei den alten Ägyptern. *Arch Gynaekol* 1927;131:425–461.

10. Griffith FL: The Petrie Papyri. In: Kahun, Gurob, eds. *Hieratic Papyri*. London: Quaritch;1898, vol I, 11.
11. Atharva-Veda Saṁhitā: Whitney WD, trans, Cambridge:Harvard University; 1905, Vols 7, 8, Harvard Oriental Series, Bk VIII, Sec 6, Vol 8. 493–498.
12. Griffith FL: A medical papyrus from Egypt. *Br Med J* 1893;1:1172–1174.
13. Suśrutas: Áyurvédas. *Id est Medicinae Systema a Venerabili d'Hanvantare Demonstratum a Susruta Discipulo Compositum*, Bk II, Sec VIII. Translated and annotated by F Hessler, Erlange Enke; 1853:188.
14. Wang Dui Me: *Schou Schen Hsiau*, Lo JH, trans (into German). Abhandlung Med Facultät Sun Yatsen Universität; 1930:2:19–126.
15. Hippocrates: *The Genuine Works of Hippocrates*, Adams F, trans. London: The Sydenham Society; 1849, vol 2: 715, 743, 758, 766.
16. Hippocrates: *The Medical Works of Hippocrates*, Chadwick J, Mann WN, trans. Oxford: Blackwell Scientific Publications; 1950.
17. Galeni C: *Opera Omnia*. In: Kühn DCG, ed. Leipzig: Car Cnoblochii; 1829, vol 17B, pt II: 652, 821.
18. Celsus AC: *On Medicine*, Lee A, trans. London: Cox; 1831:99, 347.
19. Aetios of Amida: *The Gynecology and Obstetrics of the VIth century AD*, Ricci JV, trans. from the Latin edition of Cornarius, 1542. Philadelphia: Blakeston; 1950:27, 31, 32.
20. Rösslin E: *Der Swangern Frawen und hebammê Rossegarte*. (Facsimile, Eucharius Rösslin's "Rosengarten" gendruckt im Jahre 1513. Beigleit-Text von Gustav Klein.) Munich: Kuhn; 1910:67.
21. Paulus Aegineta: *The Seven Books*, Adams F, trans. London: Sydenham Society; 1844, vol I: 4, 5; vol II:387.
22. Ballantyne JW: The Byrth of Mankind. *J Obstet Gynaecol Br Emp* 1906;10:297–325, 1907; 12:175–194, 255–274.
23. Raynalde T: *The byrth of mankinde, Otherwise Named the Woman's Booke*. London: Adams; 1613.
24. Gabelchoverus: *Artzneybuch, darninnen vast für alle de menschlichen Leibs, anlingen und Gebrechen, ausserlesene und bewehrte Artzneyen usw*. Tübingen: Gruppenbach; 1596.
25. Chaussier F: *Considérations sur les convulsions qui attaquent les femmes encientes*, ed 2. Paris: Compére Juene; 1824.
26. Barton J: *An Essay Towards a Complete New System of Midwifery, Theoretical and Practical*. London: Hodges; 1751.
27. Exton B: *A New and General System of Midwifery*, ed 3. London: Owen (no date given, first edition published, 1751).
28. Mauriceau F: *Des Maladies des Femmes Grosses et Accouchées avec la Bonne et Veritable Méthode, etc*. Paris: Cercle du Livre Précieux; 1668.
29. Mauriceau F: *The Accomplisht Midwife, Treating of the Diseases of Women with Child, and in Childbed, etc*, Chamberlen H, trans. London: Darby; 1673.
30. Mauriceau F: *Traité des Maladies des Femmes Grosses, et celles Qui Sont Accouchées, Einseignant la Bonne et Veritable Méthode pour Bien Aider, etc*. Paris: d'Houry, bk II, chap 28;1694.
31. Hirsch A: *Biographische Lexikon der Hervorragender Aerzte*. Wien and Leipzig, Urban und Schwartzenberg; 1887.
32. de Sauvages F: *Pathologia methodica, seu de Cognoscendis morbis*. Monspelii: Martel; 1739:120.
33. de Sauvages FBS: *Pathologia methodica, seu de Cognoscendis morbis*, ed 3. Leyden: Fratum de Tournes; 1759:286.
34. Hippocrates: *Hippokrates Werke aus dem Grieschischen überselz und mit Erläuterungen*, trans into German by JFC Grimm. Glogau: Prausnitz; 1838.
35. de Gorris J: *Definitionem Medicarum, Libre XXIIII, Literis Graecis Distincti*. Francoforti: Wecheli; 1578.
36. Castelli B: *Castellus Renovatus: Hoc Est, Lexicon Medicum, Quondam à Barth*. Norimbergae: JD Tauberi; 1682:484.
37. Castelli B: *Lexicon Medicum Graeco-Latinum*. Roterodami: Leers; 1651.
38. Blancardo S: *Lexicon Medicum Graeco-Latinum, in Quo Termini Totius Artis Medicae, Secundum*

Neotermicorum Placita Definiunter Vel Circumscribunter Graeca Item Vocabula ex Originibus Suis Deducunter Antehac. Jena: Literis Müllerianis; 1683.

39. Vogel RA: *Definiones Generum Morbum.* Göttingham A:Vandenhöks: Wittwe; 1964.

40. Cullen G: *Synopsis Nosologiae Methodicae. In Usum Studiosorum. Part IV, Genera Morborum.* Edinburgh: Kincaid and Creech; 1771.

41. Sagar JBM: *Systema Morborum Symptomaticum.* Vienensis: Kraus; 1776:437.

42. Gutsch JG: *De Eclampsia Parturientium, Morbo Gravi Quidem Neque Adeo Funesta, Sectio Prior Pathologica,* Inaugural dissertation. Leipzig, 1776.

43. Ryan M: *Manual of Midwifery, or Compendium of Gynaecology and Paidonosology, etc,* ed 3. London: Renshaw and Rush; 1831.

44. Demanet G: Observations sur une cause particulière de convulsions, qui arrivent aux femmes durant la grossesse ou pendant l'accouchement. *Actes Soc Méd Chir Pharmacol Bruxelles an VI* 1797; 1 (pt 2):21–28. Cited by Anonymous: *Arch Gén Méd* 1855;6 (5th series): 464–472.

45. Anonymous: Revue critique. Note pour servir à l'histoire de l'anasarque des femmes encientes et de l'éclampsie puerpérale. *Arch Gén Méd* 1855;6 (5th series): 464–472.

46. de la Motte GM: *Traité Complet des Accouchemens Naturela, non Naturels, et contre Nature. Expliqués dans un Grand Nombre d'Observations et de Réflexions sur l'Arc d'Accoucher.* Paris: Gosse; 1726;307–318.

47. Smellie W: *Theory and Practice of Midwifery,* ed 3. London: Wilson and Durham; 1756:176, 257.

48. van Swieten GLB: *Commentaria in Hermanni. Boerhaave Aphorismos de Cognescendis et Curandis Morbis,* ed 2. Lugduni: Batavorum, Verbeck; 1745. (Translated from the Latin, Edinburgh: Elliot; 1776.)

49. Rayer P: *Traité des Maladies des Reins et des Altérations de la sécrétion urinaire, étudiées en elles-mêmes et dans leurs rapports avec les maladies des uretères, de la vessie, de la prostate, etc.* Paris: Bailière; 1839–1841, vol II: 399–407.

50. Lever JCW: Cases of puerperal convulsions, with remarks. *Guy's Hosp Reports* 1843: (2nd series) 495–517.

51. Simpson JY: Contributions to the pathology and treatment of diseases of the uterus. *London Edinburgh Monthly J Med Sci* 1843;3:1009–1027.

52. Mahomed FA: The etiology of Bright's disease and the prealbuminuric stage. *Med Chir Trans London* 1874;39:197–228.

53. Mohamed FA: The etiology of Bright's disease and the prealbuminuric stage. *Br Med J* 1874;1:585–586.

54. *Yellow Emperior's Classic of Internal Medicine,* Veith I, trans. Baltimore: Williams & Wilkins; 1949:141, 147, 172.

55. Ballantyne JW: Sphygmographic tracings in puerperal eclampsia. *Edinburgh Med J* 1885; 30:1007–1020.

56. Galabin AL: *A Manual of Midwifery.* Philadelphia: Blakiston; 1886:276–280.

57. Lebedeff A, Porochjakow: Basch's sphygmomanometer und der Blutdruck während der Geburt und des Wochenbettes im Zusammenhange mit Puls, Temperatur und Respiration. *Centralbl Gynaekol* 1884;8:1–6.

58. Vinay C: *Traité de Maladies de la Grossesse et des Suites de Couches.* Paris: Baillière; 1894:386.

59. Vaquez, Nobécourt: De la pression artérielle dans l'éclampsie puerperale. *Bull Mem Soc Méd Hôp* Paris 1897;14:117–119.

60. Wiesnner: Über Blutdruckmessungen während der Menstruation and Schwangerschaft. *Centralbl Gynaekol* 1899;23:1335.

61. Cook HW, Briggs JB: Clinical observations on blood pressure. *Johns Hopkins Hosp Rep* 1903;11:451–534.

62. Frerichs FT: *Die Bright'sche Nierenkrankheit und deren Behandlung.* Braunschweig; Friedrich Vieweg und Sohn; 1851:211–220.

63. Spiegelberg O: The pathology and treatment of puerperal eclampsia. *Trans Am Gynecol Soc* 1878;2:161–174.

64. Sophian J: *Toxaemias of Pregnancy.* London, Butterworth; 1953.

65. Jürgens: Berliner medicinische Gesellschaft, Sitzung vom 7 Juli 1886, Discussion. *Berl Klin Wchschr* 1886;23:519–520.

66. Schmorl G: *Pathologisch-anatomische Untersuchungen über Puerperal-Eklampsie.* Leipzig: FCW Vogel; 1893.

67. Allbutt C: Senile plethora or high arterial pressure in elderly persons. Trans Hunterian Soc. London: Headly Brothers; 1896:38–57.

68. Frank E: Bestehen Beziehungen zwischen Chromaffinem System und der chronischer Hypertonie des Menschen? *Deutsch Arch Klin Med* 1911;103:397–412.

69. Janeway TC: A clinical study of hypertensive cardiovascular disease. *Arch Intern Med* 1913;81:749–756.

70. Herrick WW: The toxemias of pregnancy and their end results from the viewpoint of internal medicine. *Illinois Med J* 1932;62:210–220.

71. Herrick WW, Tillman AJB: Toxemia of pregnancy (its relation to cardiovascular and renal disease; clincal and necropsy findings with a long follow-up). *Arch Int Med* 1935;55:643–664.

72. Herrick WW, Tillman AJB: The mild toxemias of late pregnancy: Their relation to cardiovascular and renal disease. *Am J Obstet Gynecol* 1936;31:832–844.

73. Fishberg AM: *Hypertension and Nephritis*, ed 4. Philadelphia: Lea & Febiger; 1939:746.

74. Fishberg AM: *Hypertension and Nephritis*, ed 5. Philadelphia: Lea & Febiger; 1954.

75. Dieckmann WJ: *The Toxemias of Pregnancy*, ed 2. St. Louis: Mosby; 1952.

76. Zuspan FP, Ward MC: Treatment of eclampsia. *South Med J* 1964;57:954–959.

77. Merriman S: *A Synopsis of the Various Kinds of Difficult Parturition: With Practical Remarks on the Management of Labours*, ed 3. London: Callow; 1820:132–133.

78. Churchill F: *On the Theory and Practice of Midwifery: A New American, from the Last Improved (2d) Dublin Edition*. Philadelphia: Blanchard and Lea; 1856:445–446.

79. Avicenna: *Poem on Medicine*, Krueger HC, trans. Springfield, IL: Thomas; 1963:60

80. Maimonides M: *The Medical Aphorisms of Moses Maimonides*, Rosner F, Muntner S, trans. New York: Yeshiva University Press; 1970, vol I: 234–239.

81. Hirst BC: *A Textbook of Obstetrics*. Philadelphia: Saunders; 1909:637.

82. Smith WT: *Parturition and the Principles and Practice of Obstetrics*. Philadelphia: Lea and Blanchard; 1849:281–345.

83. Murphy EW: *Lectures on the Principles and Practice of Midwifery*. London: Walton and Maberly; 1862:497.

84. Fehling: Die Pathogenese und Behandlung der Eklampsie in Lichte der heutigen Anschauung. *Münch Med Wchschr* 1899;46:714–715.

85. van der Hoeven PCT: *Die ätiologie der eklampsie*, inaugural dissertation. Leiden; 1896.

86. Delore: L'eclampsie reconnâitrait une origine bactérienne. *Lyon Méd* 1884;47:186–187.

87. Gerdes E: Zur ätiologie der Puerperaleklampsie. *Centralbl Gynaekol* 1892;16:379–384.

88. Favre A: Über Puerpenaleklampsie. *Virchows Arch [Pathol Anat]* 1891;124:177–216.

89. Rosenstein S: Über Eclampsie. *Mtschr Geburtsk Frauenk* 1864;23:413–426.

90. Munk P: Über Urämie. *Berl Klin Wchschr* 1864;1:111–113.

91. Volhard F: Experimentelle und kritische Studien zur Pathogenase der Eklampsie. *Mtschr Geburtsh Gynaekol* 1897;5:411–437.

92. Schumacher H: Experimentelle Beiträge zur Eklampsiefrage. *Beitr Geburtsch Gynaekol* 1901; 5:257–309.

93. Dixon WE, Taylor FE: Physiological action of the placenta. *Lancet* 1907;2:1158–1159.

94. Rosenheim O: The pressor principles of placental extracts. *J Physiol* 1909;38:337–342.

95. Krieger VI, Butler HM, Kilvington TB: Antidiuretic substance in the urine during pregnancy and its frequent association with bacterial growth. *J Obstet Gynaecol Br Emp* 1951;58:5–17.

96. Lichtenstein F: Kritische und experimentelle Studien zur Toxicologie der Placenta, zugleich ein Beitrag gegen die placentare Theorie der Eklampsieätiologie. *Arch Gynaekol* 1908; 86:434–504.

97. Schneider CL: The active principle of placental toxin: Thromboplastin; its inactivator in blood: Antithromboplastin. *Am J Physiol* 1947;149:123–129.

98. Miquel A: *Traité des Convulsions chez les Femmes Encientes en Travail et en Couche*. Paris: Gazette de Santé; 1824.

99. De Wees WP: *A Treatise on the Diseases of Females*, ed 2. Philadelphia: Carey, Lea, and Carey; 1828:156–157.

100. Johns R: Observations on puerperal convulsions. *Dublin J Med Sci* 1843;24:101–115.

101. Meigs CD: *Females and Their Diseases*. Philadelphia: Lea and Blanchard; 1849:632.

102. Sinclair EB, Johnson G: *Practical Midwifery: Comprizing an Account of 13,748 Deliveries Which*

Occurred in the Dublin Lying-in Hospital During a Period of Seven Years Commencing November, 1847. London: Churchill; 1858.

103. Fitzgibbon G: The relationship of eclampsia to the other toxaemias of pregnancy. *J Obstet Gynaecol Br Emp* 1922;29:402–415.

104. Ruiz-Contreras JM: Bemerkugen über den Einfluss der Lebensmittal auf die Einstetehung der Eklampsie und Albuminerre. *Zentralbl Gynaekol* 1992;46:764.

105. Editorial. Eclampsia rare on war diet in Germany. *JAMA* 1917;68:732.

106. Stander HJ: *Textbook of Obstetrics.* New York: Appleton; 1945:599. (N.B., Actually *Williams' Obstetrics,* ed 9.)

107. Leyden E: Klinische Untersuchungen über Morbus Brightii. *Z Klin Med* 1881;2:133–191.

108. Leyden E: Über Hydrops and Aalbuminurie der Schwangeren. *Z Klin Med* 1886;11:26–49.

109. Schroeder: Discussion. Gesellschaft für Geburtschülfe und Gynaekologie in Berlin, Sitzung von 14 Mai, 1878. *Berliner Klin Wchschr* 1878;15:559.

110. Webster JC: *A Text-Book of Obstetrics.* Philadelphia: Saunders; 1903:375–376.

111. Bar T: Éclampsisme, éclampsie sans attaques. *J Sages-Femmes* 1908;36:153.

112. Williams JW: *Obstetrics,* ed 3. New York: Appleton; 1912.

113. Bell ET, Deckmann W, Eastman NJ et al: Classification of the toxemias of pregnancy. *The Mother* 1940 (April);1:13–17.

114. Eastman NJ, Bell ET, Dieckmann WJ, et al: *Definition and Classification of Toxemias Brought Up-to-Date.* Chicago: American Committee on Maternal Welfare; 1952.

115. Nelson TR: A clinical study of pre-eclampsia. Pts I and II. *J Obstet Gynaecol Br Emp* 1955;62:48–66.

116. Rippmann ET: Prä-eklampsie oder Schwangerschaftsspätgestose? *Gynaecologia* 1969;167:478–490.

117. Lindheimer M, Katz AI, Zuspan FP (Eds): *Hypertension in Pregnancy.* New York: John Wiley & Sons; 1976:443.

118. Roberts JM, Redman CWG: Pre-eclampsia: More than pregnancy induced hypertension. *Lancet* 1993;341:1447–1451.

119. Ness RB, Roberts JM: Heterogenous causes constituting the single syndrome of preeclampsia: A hypothesis and its implication. *Am J Obstet Gynecol* 1996;175:1365–1370.

120. Chesley LC, Annito JE, Cosgrove RA: The remote prognosis of eclamptic women: Sixth periodic report. *Am J Obstet Gynecol* 1976;124:446–459.

121. Johenning AR, Barron WM: Indirect pressure measurement in pregnancy: Korotkoff phase 4 versus phase 5. *Am J Obstet Gynecol* 1992;167:577–580.

122. Gant NF, Chang S, Worley RJ, et al: A clinical test useful for predicting the development of acute hypertension in pregnancy. *Am J Obstet Gynecol* 1974;120:1–7.

123. Van Dongen PWJ, Eskes TKAB, Martin CB, Wan t'Hoff MA: Postural blood pressure differences in pregnancy: A prospective study of blood pressure differences between supine and left lateral position as measured by ultrasound. *Am J Obstet Gynecol* 1980;138:1–5.

124. Hallak M, Bottoms SF, Knudson K, et al: Determining blood pressure in pregnancy: Positional hydrostatic effects. *J Reprod Med* 1997;42:333–336.

125. Petrie JC, Obrien ET, Littler WA, deSwiet M: Recommendations on blood pressure measurement. British Hypertension Society. *Br J Med* 1986;293:611–615.

126. World Health Organization Study Group: The hypertensive disorders of pregnancy. Geneva: World Health Organization; *WHO Tech Bull* 1987;758.

127. National High Blood Pressure Education Program Working Group: Report on high blood pressure in pregnancy. *Am J Obstet Gynecol* 1990;163:1689–1712.

128. Blank SG, Helseth G, Pickering TC, et al: How should diastolic pressure be defined during pregnancy? *Hypertension* 1994;24:234–240.

129. Shennan A, Gupta M, Halligan A, et al: Lack of reproducibility of Korotkoff phase 4 as measured by mercury sphygmomanometry. *Lancet* 1996;347:139–142.

130. deSwiet M, Shennan A: Blood pressure measurement in pregnancy. *Br J Obstet Gynecol* 1996;102:862–863.

131. Redman CWG, Jeffries M: Revised definition of pre-eclampsia. *Lancet* 1988;i:892–898.

132. Davey DA, MacGillivray I: The classification and definition of the hypertensive disorders of pregnancy. *Am J Obstet Gynecol* 1989;158:892–898.
133. Australasian Society for the Study of Hypertension in Pregnancy: Consensus statement management of hypertension in pregnancy: Executive summary. *Med J Australia* 1993; 158:700–702.
134. ACOG Committee on Technical Bulletins: Hypertension in pregnancy. *ACOG Tech Bull* 1996;219:1–8.
135. Brown MA, Buddle ML: What's in a name? Problems with the classification of hypertension in pregnancy. *J Hypertens* 1997;15:1049–1054.
136. Chesley LC: Mild preeclampsia: Potentially lethal for women and for the advancement of knowledge. *Clin Exper Hypertens-Hypertens in Pregnancy* 1989;B8:3–12.
137. Chesley LC: Diagnosis of preeclampsia. *Obstet Gynecol* 1985;65:423–425.
138. Hinselmann H: *Die Elklamsie*. Bonn: Cohen; 1924.
139. McCartney CP: Pathological anatomy of acute hypertension of pregnancy. *Circulation* 1964;30(suppl 2):37–42.
140. Theobald GW: The incidence of albumin and sugar in the urine of normal women. *Lancet* 1931;2:1380–1383.
141. Theobald GW: Further observations on the relation of pregnancy to hypertension and chronic nephritis. *J Obstet Gynaecol Br Emp* 1936;43:1037–1052.
142. Reid DE, Teel HM: Nonconvulsive pregnancy toxemias; their relationship to chronic vascular and renal disease. *Am J Obstet Gynecol* 1939;37:886–896.
143. Chesley LC, Annitto JE: Pregnancy in the patient with hypertensive disease. *Am J Obstet Gynecol* 1947;53:372–381.
144. Chesley LC, Somers WH, Gorenberg HR, McGeary JA: An analysis of some factors associated with posttoxemic hypertension. *Am J Obstet Gynecol* 1941;41:751–764.
145. Harris JW: The after-effects of the late toxemias of pregnancy. *Bull Johns Hopkins Hosp* 1924;35:103–107.
146. Gibberd GF: Albuminuria complicating pregnancy. *Lancet* 1931;2:520–525.
147. Peckham CH, Stout ML: A study of the late effects of the toxemias of pregnancy (excluding vomiting and eclampsia). *Bull Johns Hopkins Hosp* 1931;49:225–245.
148. Theobald GW: The relationship of albuminuria of pregnancy to chronic nephritis. *Lancet* 1933;1:626–630.
149. Browne FJ, Sheumack DR: Chronic hypertension following pre-eclamptic toxaemia: The influence of familial hypertension on its causation. *J Obstet Gynaecol Br Emp* 1956;63:677–679.
150. Adams EM, MacGillivray I: Long-term effect of pre-eclampsia on blood pressure. *Lancet* 1961;2:1373–1375.
151. Tillman AJB: Long-range incidence and clinical relationship of toxemias of pregnancy to hypertensive vascular disease. *Circulation* 1964;30(suppl 2):76–79.
152. Bryans CI Jr: The remote prognosis in toxemia of pregnancy. *Clin Obstet Gynecol* 1966;9:973–990.
153. Epstein FH: Late vascular effects of toxemia of pregnancy. *N Engl J Med* 1964;271:391–395.
154. Lehmann K: *Eklampsien i Danmark i Aarene 1918–1927*. Copenhagen: Busck; 1933.
155. Díaz del Castillo FO: Influencia de la alimentacion sobre la eclampsia (la eclampsia en Madrid durant la guerra). *Rev Clin Esp* 1942;6:166–170.
156. Siddall AC: Vitamin B_1 deficiency as an etiologic factor in pregnancy toxemias. *Am J Obstet Gynecol* 1940;39:818–821.
157. Denman T: *Essays on the Puerperal Fever, and on Puerperal Convulsions*. London: Walter; 1768.
158. Kosmak GW: *The Toxemias of Pregnancy*. New York: Appleton; 1924.
159. Mengert WF: Racial contrasts in obstetrics and gynecology. *J Natl Med Assoc* 1966;58:413–415.
160. Davis CH: Weight in pregnancy; its value as a routine test. *Am J Obstet Gynecol* 1923;6:575–583.
161. Hannah CR: Weight during pregnancy. *Texas State J Med* 1923;19:224–226.
162. Robertson EG: The natural history of oedema during pregnancy. *J Obstet Gynaecol Br Commonw* 1971;78:520–529.

2

Epidemiology of Hypertension

Roberta B. Ness and James M. Roberts

Hypertensive disorders that occur de novo in pregnancy include preeclampsia and transient hypertension. These syndromes, while both marked by elevations in blood pressure that return to normal after delivery, are distinguished clinically by the presence (preeclampsia) or absence (transient hypertension) of proteinuria. Eclampsia is a more life-threatening syndrome, thought to arise from the progression of preeclampsia, that includes preeclampsia plus seizures. Other chapters in this book discuss the clinical and pathologic differences between these two clinical syndromes. Here, we will review the epidemiologic data that characterize the frequency of occurrence, risk factors and predictors for, and the natural history of hypertensive disorders in pregnancy. It is the purpose of this chapter to review these epidemiologic data, critically assess the methods used in conducting previous studies, and indicate areas which are as yet unclear. A particular focus of the chapter will be to discuss the evidence that preeclampsia and transient hypertension in pregnancy are distinct in terms of clinical markers and natural history. We will also review evidence suggesting that preeclampsia, in itself, is a syndrome comprised of at least two etiologies.[1] This is in line with Chesley's cautious admonition in his chapter devoted to epidemiology in this text's first edition, where he noted "The diagnosis of mild preeclampsia is often erroneous in primigravidas and often so in multiparas; yet multiparas have been included in many of the investigations." One etiology may be the result of reduced placental perfusion and is the component of preeclampsia unique to pregnancy. The other may be related to preexisting maternal pathology, in particular, a maternal predisposition to cardiovascular risk, which may not be clinically obvious immediately before or after pregnancy. We have proposed in the past that both of these causes converge to predispose to preeclampsia by the common mechanism of endothelial dysfunction and that the combination of maternal and placental factors is particularly damaging. As such, we will discuss the natural heterogeneity among the risk factors and clinical predictors as well as among the outcomes for mother and infant within the spectrum of preeclampsia.

FREQUENCY OF OCCURRENCE

There is relatively little information on the frequency with which transient hypertension and preeclampsia occur during pregnancy. There are several reasons for this. First, different definitions are used when classifying the hypertensive disorders in pregnancy. One, proposed by the United States National High Blood Pressure Education Program[2] defines preeclampsia as a rise in systolic blood pressure or a blood pressure of ≥ 140/90 mm Hg on two separate occasions at least 6 hours apart plus ≥ 0.3 g/24 hours or 1+ dipstick proteinuria on two occasions at least 6 hours apart. Another, proposed by the International Society for the Study of Hypertension in Pregnancy,[3] defines preeclampsia as an elevated systolic or diastolic blood pressure and the same degree of proteinuria as required for the US definition on at least two consecutive occasions at least 4 hours apart. Furthermore, other, less well-accepted definitions have been used by some authors. Thus, the frequency of hypertensive disorders has been variously estimated based on different definitions. Second, temporal and geographic variation may impact the estimated incidence rates (see below). Third, hypertension in pregnancy is not a reportable condition in the United States and there have been few attempts to estimate the frequency of its occurrence in unselected populations. Finally, most, but not all, studies of hypertension in pregnancy exclude women with preexisting hypertension. Furthermore, women with chronic hypertension are easily misclassified as having one of these reversible conditions during pregnancy.

Nevertheless, two national surveys, one in the United States[4] and one in Great Britain,[5] estimated the incidence of hypertensive disorders in pregnancy. The incidence of eclampsia was estimated in a national survey in Great Britain by Douglas and Redman.[5] All obstetricians and all hospitals with an obstetrics unit were asked to participate in an active surveillance program in 1992. Each presumptive case was reviewed by a single obstetrician and was defined as eclamptic if she had seizures in the setting of hypertension, proteinuria, and either thrombocytopenia or an increased plasma aspartate transaminase concentration. The incidence of eclampsia was estimated to be 0.49 per 1000 pregnancies. Most seizures occurred despite prenatal care (70%) and even after admission to the hospital (77%).

Saftlas et al.[4] estimated the US incidence of preeclampsia and eclampsia from 1979 through 1986 using a nationally representative sample of hospital discharge records. Women with discharge diagnoses of preeclampsia or eclampsia were included in their analysis. Women with preeclampsia superimposed on preexisting hypertension were excluded. The authors estimated that preeclampsia was a complication in 26.1 of every 1000 (2.6%) pregnancies. Eclampsia was diagnosed in only 0.56 per 1000 pregnancies.

The incidence of eclampsia has declined during the 20th century. Chesley showed a marked reduction at Margaret Hague Maternity Hospital from 1931 to 1951 (Table 2–1). Data from the United Kingdom show an almost 20-fold decline in frequency since 1922, almost all of which occurred during the time prior to the 1970s when prenatal care became universally available.[6] Similar data from New

TABLE 2–1. INCIDENCE OF ECLAMPSIA IN CLINIC PATIENTS AT THE MARGARET HAGUE MATERNITY HOSPITAL

	1931–1934	1935–1939	1940–1945	1946–1951	Totals
Registrations	12,604	17,407	12,022	12,208	54,241
Cases of eclampsia	51	41	11	4	107
% incidence	0.40	0.23	0.09	0.03	0.20

Zealand show an incidence rate of 3.2/1000 in 1928 to 1933 and 0.8/1000 in 1956 to 1958.[7] Whereas, the rate of mild preeclampsia was relatively stable during the 8 years of the Saftlas study,[4] the rate of severe preeclampsia increased from 2.9 to 5.2 cases per 1000. This trend was seen in both black and white women.

Because of the decline in eclampsia, much of the recent epidemiologic research has focused on preeclampsia. In a somewhat more selected population in the United States, the incidence of preeclampsia was estimated among control women enrolled in the Maternal Fetal Medicine Network trial of low-dose aspirin to prevent preeclampsia.[8] Included in the study were primiparous women presenting to a series of academic medical centers for prenatal care. Women with a history of chronic hypertension, diabetes mellitus, renal disease, and other medical illnesses as well as women with a baseline blood pressure above 135/85 mm Hg were excluded. Among the 1500 women in the placebo group who were followed throughout pregnancy, 94 (6.3%) developed preeclampsia as defined by hypertension (systolic blood pressure of $\geq$ 140 mm Hg or a diastolic blood pressure of $\geq$ 90 mm Hg) plus proteinuria (either $\geq$ 300 mg/24 h or 2+ or more by dipstick on two or more occasions 4 hours apart). The Maternal Fetal Medicine Network trial also estimated that 5.9% of control women developed transient hypertension in pregnancy (hypertension as defined above without proteinuria). Other randomized clinical trials in the US and Europe have demonstrated similar incidence rates for preeclampsia and transient hypertension.[9-11]

DISCUSSION OF DIFFERENTIAL FREQUENCY ESTIMATES

Hospital-based incidence estimates for preeclampsia systematically differ from national estimates. There are probably five main reasons for this discrepancy. First, many studies, such as that by Saftlas et al., rely on discharge diagnoses. Ales and Charlson[12] performed a validation study of medical records at the New York Hospital and found that 25% of ICD9 codes incorrectly diagnosed preeclampsia and that 53% of true cases were missed by ICD9 coding. Similarly, Eskenazi et al.[13] found that 44% of women who received a discharge diagnosis of severe preeclampsia or eclampsia did not meet a rigorous set of criteria including a change in mean arterial pressure (MAP) of $\geq$ 20 mm Hg from baseline or, if there was no baseline blood pressure reading before 20 weeks' gestation, a MAP $\geq$ 105 mm Hg, two urinary protein dipstick measurements of 1+ or one measurement of 2+, or $\geq$ 300 mg of protein on a 24-hour urine collection. Second, the Maternal Fetal Medicine Network study included only primiparous women, a group known to be at fivefold or greater elevated risk of developing preeclampsia as compared to multiparous women.[14] Third, women electing to enroll in a randomized clinical trial to prevent preeclampsia may also be a group with characteristics that would suggest a tendency to developing hypertension in pregnancy. However, the strict definition of preeclampsia used in the Maternal Fetal Medicine Network trial should have resulted in a decreased incidence estimate. Fourth, women seeking prenatal care at academic medical centers are a selected group who are probably at higher risk of developing pregnancy complications than would be reflected in a national sample. Fifth, data from the British Commonwealth, which uses the Nelson criteria, considers de novo hypertension without proteinuria as mild preeclampsia, and in these studies the diagnosis is most contaminated with gestational hypertensives.

RISK FACTORS AND CLINICAL PREDICTORS

Risk factors consistently shown to be associated with an increased rate of preeclampsia include elevated early pregnancy blood pressure, prepregnancy adiposity, age, family history, preexisting medical conditions such as hypertension or diabetes, obstetric characteristics such as multiple gestation and hydrops fetalis, and primiparity (Table 2–2). The first five of these factors can be understood in relation to a maternal predisposition to cardiovascular disease. The last factors, obstetric characteristics and primiparity, may represent the placental or uniquely pregnancy-related component of preeclampsia. For each of these factors, we will relate the data suggesting its association with preeclampsia. We will also evaluate each factor's ability to accurately predict the development of preeclampsia. In gen-

TABLE 2–2. RISK FACTORS FOR PREECLAMPSIA AND A SUBJECTIVE RATING OF THE WEIGHT OF SUPPORTING EVIDENCE

Risk Factor (References)	Rating of Evidence
Older age[4,15,16]	++
High blood pressure in 2nd/early 3rd trimester[13,17,18,19-24]	++
Prepregnancy hypertension[21,26,30]	+++
Prepregnancy diabetes[25,31,27a,32]	+++
Caloric excess[33-35]	+
Elevated body mass index[13,36-39]	+++
Weight gain during pregnancy[40-44]	+
Family history[45-49]	+++
Primiparity[13,14]	+++
New paternity[51-55,60,61]	++
Lack of previous abortion[13,18,56,57]	++
Barrier contraception[58,59]	++
Excessive placental size[16,64-66]	+++
Lack of smoking[67-72]	+++
Specific dietary factors[73]	+

eral, although each of these factors clearly increases the risk of developing preeclampsia, none is sufficiently sensitive nor specific to warrant its use in defining a high-risk subset of patients.

Age

Several studies have found that hypertensive disorders in pregnancy, including preeclampsia specifically, are more common in women whose pregnancy occurs at an older maternal age (Fig. 2–1). Saftlas et al. reported this observation in their nationally representative cross-sectional study of the US population (see above).[4] As well, it was the general impression of Hansen in a review of studies published before the early 1980s.[15] The risk for a woman over age 35 is about three- to fourfold higher than for a younger woman. Zhang et al. suggested that this effect may occur independent of misdiagnosed chronic hypertension, which is more common in older women, and may reflect collagen replacement of the normal muscle in the walls of myometrial arteries and atrophic changes in the vascular microstructure.[16] The increased percentage of collagen and the undervascularization may then restrict luminal expansion and blood flow to the placenta.

Blood Pressure

Higher blood pressure prior to 20 to 27 weeks' gestation was associated with clinically evident preeclampsia in later pregnancy in healthy, primiparous women in most[17,18] but not all[13] studies. Longitudinal data prior to, during, and after preg-

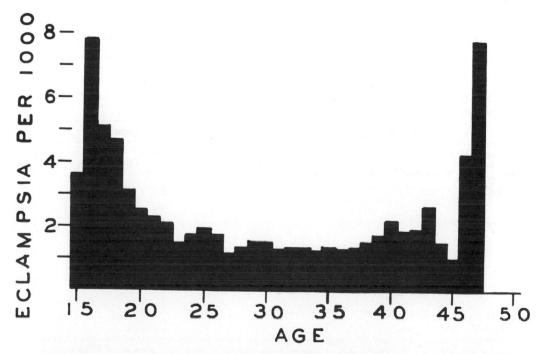

Figure 2–1. Age-specific incidences of eclampsia. (*Source: Lehmann K:* Eklampsien i Danmark i aarene 1918–1927. *Copenhagen: Busck; 1933.*)

nancy in women destined to develop primiparous preeclampsia show that even among nonchronic hypertensives, preeclamptics have a blood pressure that is somewhat higher in the first trimester than normals.[19-22] However, increased early pregnancy blood pressure has not sensitively predicted preeclampsia,[17] perhaps because this indicator is predictive only in women with the maternal genesis of preeclampsia, or perhaps because the normal physiologic decline in blood pressure during the second trimester of pregnancy may mask some women with chronic, undiagnosed hypertension. The largest studies examining the ability of early blood pressure measurements to predict preeclampsia were conducted by Page and Christianson,[23] and by Friedman and Neff[24] (Table 2–3). These studies prospectively evaluated second trimester mean arterial pressure (MAP) in over 14,000 pregnant nulliparous women and in over 22,000 pregnant parous women. Although MAP was related to the development of transient hypertension and preeclampsia in combination (these entities were not separated), a MAP $\geq$ 90 mm Hg was associated with positive predictive values too low to recommend this measure as a useful test: 8.6% and 6.4%, respectively. Similarly, in a smaller, but more methodologically rigorous study of 700 nulliparous women by Villar and Sibai, a MAP of $\geq$ 90 mm Hg had a positive predictive value of 23%.[22]

Preexisting Medical Conditions

Women with preexisting medical conditions such as diabetes[25] and hypertension[26] appear to be at substantially increased risk of developing preeclampsia during pregnancy. Rey and Couturier showed that chronic hypertensive women were about ten times more likely to develop preeclampsia than were normotensive controls after adjustment for obstetric and medical complications.[27] A prospective study by the Maternal–Fetal Network noted superimposed preeclampsia in 25% of

TABLE 2–3. RATE RATIOS FOR FETAL DEATH BY DIASTOLIC PRESSURE AND PROTEINURIA COMBINATIONS

Proteinuria	Diastolic Blood Pressure (mm Hg)						
	<65	65–74	75–84	85–94	95–104	105+	Total
None	2.5[a]	1.5	1.0[b]	1.4	3.1[a]	3.3[a]	1.0[c]
Trace	2.2	1.3	1.2	1.5	2.8[a]	4.5[a]	1.1
1+	1.0	0.9	1.0	3.8[a]	4.3[a]	10.1[a]	1.4
2+	0.0	5.3[a]	3.1[a]	0.0	9.0[a]	11.1[a]	2.7[a]
3+	0.0	6.7[a]	0.0	3.6	18.6[a]	20.2[a]	5.1[a]
4+	0.0	0.0	0.0	0.0	23.1[a]	17.9[a]	6.6[a]
Total	2.0	1.3	1.0[d]	1.5	3.7	6.1	

[a] Statistically significant, $p < 0.01$
[b] Referent rate 0.62%
[c] Referent rate 0.86%
[d] Referent rate 0.68%

Reprinted from Friedman EA, Neff RK: Pregnancy outcome as related to hypertension, edema, and proteinuria. In: Lindheimer MD, Katz AL, Zuspan FP, eds. *Hypertension in Pregnancy*. New York: John Wiley & Sons; copyright © 1976:13–22. Reprinted by permission of John Wiley & Sons, Inc.

chronic hypertensives (35% if the hypertension had been present more than four years before conception).[27a] Also, women with chronic hypertension made up a high proportion of those women who developed severe preeclampsia that was of early onset or was recurrent in one study.[28] Of particular interest is the existence of a dose-response relationship between the severity of preexisting hypertension and the risk of developing preeclampsia. The women with preexisting hypertension who were at greatest risk for developing superimposed preeclampsia were those with disease present for four years or more, evidence of more severe underlying blood pressure elevations as demonstrated by either left ventricular hypertrophy, a serum creatinine greater than 1.0 mg%, or a diastolic BP greater than 100 mm Hg at less than 20 weeks' gestation.[21,27a,29,30]

A history of diabetes mellitus has also been shown to increase the risk for preeclampsia.[31] A prospective study of 334 pregnant diabetic women and control pregnant nondiabetics found the incidence of preeclampsia was higher among diabetics (10%) than controls (4%).[32] Again, there was a relationship between risk during pregnancy and the severity of the underlying condition. The rate of preeclampsia among diabetics increased with the severity and duration of diabetes, from 9% among diet-controlled gestational diabetics to 30% among women with White classes D, F, and R.

Body Size

Data among women living through severe food shortages suggested a reduction in the incidence of preeclampsia.[33] The most convincing study examined births before, during, and after the Dutch famine, a time of severe rations restrictions imposed as a result of a blockade during World War II. During the Dutch famine, the incidence of preeclampsia was lower than that during the preceding and succeeding time periods.[34] However, other ecologic studies of caloric restriction have provided more mixed results,[35] and Chesley has suggested that the Dutch famine data are clouded by a decline of primiparous births during the war (see Chap. 1).

Several more studies confirmed the long-suspected association between baseline body size and preeclampsia with relative risk estimates ranging from 2.3 to 5.5, depending on the definition of overweight used.[13,36,37] Wolfe et al. described the relationship between maternal weight (or body mass index) among 6270 consecutively delivered gravid women. Among women whose body mass index (BMI) was in the 90th percentile or greater, the relative risk of preeclampsia was 2.3.[37] Eskenazi et al., in a carefully designed study of 139 preeclamptic cases and 132 controls, found that a BMI of 25.8 carried a 2.7-fold increased risk for preeclampsia after controlling for other factors.[13] In addition, a recent analysis of data from the Maternal Fetal Medicine Network shows higher rates of preeclampsia with increasing levels of overweight; in that study, overweight was only associated with preeclampsia and not with gestational hypertension.[38] Adiposity may also contribute to the relationships among other maternal predispositions such as hypertension, diabetes, race, and preeclampsia.

However, baseline weight has rarely been rigorously tested as a potential early predictor of preeclampsia.[39] In a model containing BMI measured prior to 20 weeks' gestation as a continuous variable combined with MAP and various readily available biochemical and hematologic markers (mean corpuscular volume, platelet count, antithrombin III, haptoglobin, iron, ferritin, progesterone, uric acid, urine calcium, and microalbumin), the sensitivity, positive, and negative predictive values were 57.1, 26.9, and 93.7, respectively. Test characteristics for BMI alone cannot be estimated from the data.

Body fat distribution appears to have never been examined as a risk factor for or predictor of preeclampsia, despite the known association of increased visceral fat with lipids, hypertension, and clinical coronary heart disease, independent of total body adiposity.

As distinguished from baseline weight or adiposity, weight gain during pregnancy does not appear to consistently predict the occurrence of preeclampsia. At least four studies[40-43] examined the statement made by Hamlin in 1952 that "[should] a young primipara with a low initial blood pressure increase her weight by greater than 8 lbs (between 20–30 weeks) she will proceed almost inexorably towards eclampsia."[44] Nelson retrospectively examined prenatal information among 1457 primigravida women. About two-thirds of the normotensive women and three-fourths of the women who developed preeclampsia gained more than 8 lbs between the 20th and 30th weeks of pregnancy.[40] Similarly, Thomson and Billewicz found that weight gain was not associated with preeclampsia in a second large retrospective study.[41] In two other studies, the weight gain associated with preeclampsia was attributed to edema formation as part of the clinical disease complex.[42,43] Clearly, then, it is important to discriminate between weight after the onset of preeclampsia and prepregnancy weight.

Family History (See also Chap. 13)

Family history also appears to play an important role in the risk for preeclampsia. The incidence of preeclampsia was four times higher in sisters of women who had preeclampsia in their first pregnancy than in sisters of women who did not.[45] Among women who had been eclamptic, Chesley and Cooper[46] found that the rate of preeclampsia was higher in sisters (37%), in daughters (26%), and in granddaughters (16%) than it was in daughters-in-law (6%). These data are supported by Hardy-Weinberg modeling[47] and by HLA typing for given populations.[48,49] However, a specific model of inheritance has not been established. Part of the problem with establishing a specific mode of inheritance is that women with hypertension in pregnancy may have a reduction in the probability of carrying a fetus to term and thus, may not be identified as having the condition. In particular, placental hypoxemia may result in spontaneous abortion.[16] Such a relationship may restrict the appearance of cases and obscure any genetic pattern.

First Birth and Other Placental Factors

Primiparity is one of the strongest risk factors for the development of preeclampsia (Fig. 2–2). MacGillivray noted in 1958 in a well-characterized population in Scotland

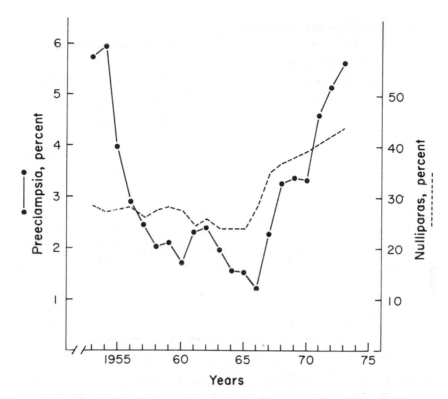

Figure 2–2. Yearly incidence of preeclampsia in the Kings County Hospital, 1953–1974, In relation to proportionate representation of nullipara coming to delivery. (*From Chesley LC:* Hypertensive Disorders in Pregnancy. *New York: Appleton-Century-Crofts; 1978.*)

that preeclampsia occurred in 5.6% of primiparas and in only 0.3% of secundigravidas.[14] Other authors confirmed the observation that primiparas were anywhere from five to ten times more likely to experience preeclampsia than multiparas.[13] Unadjusted data on the relationship between age and preeclampsia have frequently shown younger women to be at an increased risk. However, nulliparity may be the underlying factor driving this apparent association as younger women are more likely to be nulliparous.

The relationship between primiparity and preeclampsia suggests something about the uniqueness of a first placentation vs. a later baby's placental implantation. Redman suggested that in later pregnancies there is the development of protective immunologic mechanisms against paternal antigens.[50] Other epidemiologic data support this suggestion. For example, studies have shown that the relative protection afforded by further pregnancies was reduced or eliminated with new paternity,[51-55] that previous induced abortion was protective,[13,18,56,57] that women using barrier methods of contraception were at increased risk,[58,59] and that risk was reduced with increased duration of sexual activity antedating pregnancy.[55] All of these risk factors would reduce maternal recognition of paternal antigens prior to pregnancy and all of the protective factors would enhance maternal recognition of paternal antigens.

One compelling case study that supports the notion of a lack of sperm-immune recognition in the genesis of preeclampsia describes a patient who had seven pregnancies wherein the fourth and sixth were preeclamptic. These pregnancies represented her first pregnancies by a second and third husband.[60] Furthermore, two case-control studies showed a higher rate of changed paternity among preeclamptics than among controls.[51,61] All of these studies support an immunologic basis for hypertension in pregnancy.

Further support comes from a small number of studies that have examined pregnancies resulting from sperm and oocytes biologically unrelated to the host. In a cohort study by Need et al. involving over 500 pregnancies, insemination with sperm from other than the husband resulted in an increased risk of preeclampsia for both nulliparous and multiparous women.[62] Similarly, pregnancies resulting from donated oocytes were more likely to be complicated by preeclampsia.[63] However, none of these studies adjusted for the potential confounding effects of older maternal age and more frequent multiple births.

Although this epidemiologic evidence, taken as a whole, is highly suggestive, the studies comprising it are not without methodologic limitations. Many of them are quite small, retrospective, and enrolled a highly selected population of women seeking medical care at academic medical centers. Particularly for retrospective studies, referral patterns among preeclamptic women clearly differ from those among women with noncomplicated pregnancies (generally used as controls). In particular, preeclamptic women are more likely to be transported from community institutions and may be more likely to have insurance. Whether these factors might bias findings related to contraception and paternity is unclear. However, it is relevant to point out that in the carefully conducted case-control study by Klonoff-Cohen et al.,[59] patients were more likely to be married, high school educated, and working during pregnancy. When analyzed separately, married women were actually protected from developing preeclampsia by barrier contraception (adjusted odds ratio 0.39, confidence interval 0.26–0.59), whereas single women were at substantially increased risk (adjusted odds ratio 26.08, confidence interval 8.50–79.84).

Obstetric Factors

Even if implantation is normal, relative placental perfusion may be reduced because of excessive placental size. Obstetric complications associated with increased placental size such as twin pregnancies,[64] hydatidiform moles,[65] and hydrops fetalis[66] all markedly increase the risk for developing preeclampsia. Zhang et al. pooled the results from six studies that compared both twin and singleton gestations and found that pregnant women with twin pregnancies were three times more likely to develop hypertension in pregnancy than women with singletons.[16] However, these conditions are sufficiently unusual to account for only a small proportion of all cases of preeclampsia.

Other Risk Factors

Smoking has consistently been found to protect against preeclampsia. Klonoff-Cohen et al.[67] showed that comparing 110 women rigorously defined as being preeclamptic to 115 healthy nulliparous controls, the odds ratio for smoking was 0.71 (confidence interval 0.33–1.50). Although this was not a significant finding, a number of other authors, using case groups consisting of a mixture of women with preeclampsia and transient hypertension in pregnancy, have observed similar effects.[68-72] As well, a dose-response relationship between number of cigarettes smoked per day and the reduction in preeclampsia was shown in a case-control study by Marcoux et al.[70] In this same study, women who smoked, but quit before pregnancy were slightly less likely to develop preeclampsia. Therefore, there does appear to be a modest reduction in hypertensive disorders in pregnancy among smokers. The pathophysiology of this protective effect is not clear.

A number of dietary factors have also been linked to preeclampsia. These include calcium, magnesium and zinc, vitamin E, and n-3 fatty acid supplements, as well as salt restriction.[73] However, randomized clinical trials have not consistently born out the role of any of those studied in preventing preeclampsia. These issues are discussed in more detail in Chapter 16.

Women living at high altitudes appear to have an increased risk of hypertension in pregnancy.[74,75] In one study performed in Colorado, a dose-response relationship between altitude and the frequency of hypertensive disease was demonstrated and the implication was that preeclampsia also increased with increasing elevation.[76] At the same time, women living at higher altitudes had a lower blood volume and lower arterial oxygen saturation, suggesting that this observed effect may be mediated by relative hypoxemia.

Clinical Predictors for Preeclampsia (See also Chap. 6)

Beyond these prepregnancy risk factors, there have been a number of studies evaluating the predictive value for preeclampsia of several readily available clinical maneuvers or of biochemical tests performed during pregnancy. Many of these tests may reflect the pathophysiologic perturbations that link the maternal and placental contributions to preeclampsia.

Roll Over and Other Provocative Tests

A provocative test comparing the diastolic blood pressure while the patient lies on her left side to the diastolic blood pressure after turning onto her back was extensively evaluated as a predictor of preeclampsia.[77-82] Positive predictive values were inconsistent, ranging from 13%[77] to 93%[78] in a series of prospective studies of moderate size. This is likely explained by the fact that the major determinant of difference in brachial blood pressure between the values obtained in the upper arm with the woman on her side and when she is supine is the breadth of the chest. Blood pressure is falsely lowered as the arm is raised above the level of the heart. Also of concern is that the test is performed between 28 and 32 weeks of pregnancy, which may be too late to prevent the consequences of preeclampsia. A number of related provocative tests were proposed on the basis that preeclampsia represents a break in the normal protection afforded by pregnancy to pressor stimuli. In particular, the pressor effects of infusion of epinephrine, norepinephrine, and angiotensin II were assessed, and the effects of isometric exercise and cold were examined.[17] However, infusion tests are generally not sufficiently accurate, and are too complicated, expensive, and time-consuming to be considered as an adequate screen for preeclampsia.

Markers of Endothelial Injury

Many biologic markers have been evaluated as clinical predictors for preeclampsia including ones related to platelets and platelet function, based on the biologically plausible hypothesis that preeclampsia is mediated by a disturbed platelet–endothelium interaction. Included in this group are the concentration and volume of blood constituents and the levels of platelet or endothelial-derived factors. Several studies examined platelet counts and although these were lower in many women with preeclampsia, thrombocytopenia was not found to distinguish between women developing preeclampsia and women with normal pregnancies.[83-86] Several studies suggest that platelet volumes may be a more sensitive measure than platelet numbers of cell turnover secondary to activation within the maternal vasculature in preeclampsia. Platelet volume correlated with the severity of hypertensive disorders in pregnancy.[84,87] In women who developed hypertension and proteinuria, two studies suggest that platelet volume may be predictive. Ahmed et al. evaluated 428 patients from whom four or more platelet measurements were available.[88] The rate of preeclampsia was 17.3%. Sensitivity was 93% and specificity was 97% for a platelet volume $\geq$ 8 fL measured between 24 and 38 weeks. Hutt et al. longitudinally followed 17 women at high risk for preeclampsia, all of whom developed increased platelet volumes of $\geq$ 8 fL at 2 to 5 weeks prior to the onset of signs of disease.[89] Thus, although further work is needed to confirm these initial studies which were performed among nonconsecutive pregnancies in high-risk women, platelet volume may be a good indicator for the later development of preeclampsia.

Platelet function is also abnormal in preeclamptic patients on the whole. For example, a handful of studies have shown that platelet angiotensin II receptors[17] and the sensitivity of platelet intracellular calcium levels to arginine vasopressin[90] are both increased in preeclampsia well before the onset of signs. Changes in the ratio between factor VIII-related antigen and factor VIII activity have been noted in preeclamptic patients, but these related factors appear to predict fetal growth retardation more than they do preeclampsia.[91–94] Also antithrombin III or thrombin–antithrombin III (TAT) complexes were evaluated in preeclamptic and normal pregnancies,[95-97] however, there is substantial overlap in these studies between normal and abnormal groups and because no studies are prospective, it is unclear which comes first, the coagulation factors or the disease.

Fibronectin, a glycoprotein involved in coagulation and platelet function and found in the endothelium, has been the focus of several studies. Fibronectin levels are markedly elevated in preeclamptic patients.[98-101] Ballegeer et al.[102] found that increased levels of fibronectin at 25 to 36 weeks' gestation predicted women developing hypertension with great accuracy (sensitivity 96%, specificity 94%), but did not separately analyze preeclampsia. Taylor et al. proposed that since the majority of fibronectin in the circulation is of hepatic origin, a specific marker of endothelial fibronectin might make for a better laboratory marker. They used an antibody directed against an epitope of fibronectin which is produced by endothelial (and other) cells,[103] but not the liver. Cellular fibronectin (cFN) was found to be strikingly increased in women with preeclampsia 10 to 13 weeks prior to evident disease.[104] Unfortunately, as a single test, this did not distinguish groups destined to develop disease from those destined to have normal pregnancies. However, cFN has never been evaluated in the context of other potential predictors.

NATURAL HISTORY

Maternal Morbidity Immediately Related to Preeclampsia

Transient hypertension in pregnancy, unaccompanied by proteinuria, is not associated with maternal or perinatal morbidity nor mortality.[105]

In contrast, preeclampsia can be a major contributor to maternal morbidity and mortality as an immediate consequence of the progression to eclampsia. Douglas and Redman[5] estimated that among eclamptic women in the United Kingdom in 1992, 1.8% died and 35% had at least one major complication. The most common major complications encountered included a requirement for assisted ventilation (23%), renal failure (6%), disseminated intravascular coagulation (9%), hemolysis, elevated liver enzymes, and low platelets (HELLP syndrome) (7%), and pulmonary edema (5%). The findings from investigators in the United States[106,107] confirmed the very low mortality rates among eclamptic women. Despite the very real morbidity that still accompanies eclampsia, modern day maternal outcomes for this condition are far better than those of the past. In the early 1900s, before the advent of magnesium sulfate therapy, mortality was estimated to be between 10 and 15%.[108] In several case series reported in the late 1800s, 20 to 30% of eclamptic women died from this condition. Roberts[108] points out that these sobering statistics from the past were primarily the result of overaggressive medical management, rather than the result of marked advances in pathophysiologic understanding.

Later Maternal Outcomes

A handful of relatively small studies have shown that women with transient hypertension in pregnancy are at elevated risk for later hypertension. Adams and MacGillivray[109] measured blood pressure in women aged 20 to 35 after their first pregnancies. The authors reported hypertension (diastolic blood pressure ≥ 190 mm Hg) in 60% of women who experienced transient hypertension in their first pregnancies (N = 96) compared to 40% of women with preeclampsia (N = 53), 21% of women who did not have hypertension during pregnancy, and 35% of women who were never pregnant. Follow-up blood pressures were highest among the women with a subsequent hypertensive pregnancy. Similarly, Lindberg et al.[110] reported that the prevalence of hypertension 5 years following their first pregnancy was 51% among 49 women with hypertension in pregnancy compared to 21% among women with preeclampsia and 4% among women with no hypertension during pregnancy. Finally, Jonsdottir et al.[111] showed that women with a history of hypertension in pregnancy had an increased risk of subsequent coronary heart disease.

Cohort studies have repeatedly shown that women with preeclampsia or eclampsia are at risk for developing hypertension and diabetes mellitus later in life. However, this risk is higher among women with recurrent hypertension in pregnancy. Chesley et al. followed from 1931 to 1951 until 1973 to 1974 all but three of 270 women after a baseline episode of eclampsia.[112] They did not find increased rates of hypertension later in life among the overall group of primiparous patients when compared with controls from the general population. However, substantially higher rates of diastolic hypertension at follow-up occurred among women who had eclampsia as multiparas and who had eclampsia as primiparas followed by hypertension in later pregnancies. Most multiparous eclamptics had previous episodes of preeclampsia and thus experienced recurrent disease. In retrospect, about half of the multiparous women had unrecognized chronic hypertension prior to the index pregnancy. Also, the later development of diabetes was two- to fourfold more common among both primiparous and multiparous eclamptics than would have been expected in the general population. Furthermore, Chesley et al.[112] showed that women with eclampsia as multiparas had a mortality rate that was two to five times higher than that of the general population, the result of an excess in cardiovascular deaths (Fig. 2–3).

Other studies confirmed the finding that preeclamptic women who had experienced hypertension in later pregnancies were more likely to develop hypertension later in life than were women who had not experienced recurrent disease.[109,113,114] Sibai et al. followed 406 severe preeclamptics or eclamptics and 409 controls, all primiparous at the index pregnancy, for 7 to 8 years on average.[29] Controls were matched to cases for race (86% were black), age, gestational age at presentation, obstetric complications, and month of delivery. The preeclamptic–eclamptic group had higher rates of preeclampsia in their second pregnancies than did controls (47% vs. 8%). Rates of hypertension later in life were substantially higher in the preeclamptic–eclamptic group, particularly among the women who had a preeclamptic second pregnancy (25% developed hypertension) than among women who had repeated non-preeclamptic pregnancies (2% developed hypertension). Later hypertension was also higher in the group of women who developed preeclampsia at or before 31 weeks' gestation than in women who developed their disease at a more advanced gestational age. As with the Chesley study, rates of diabetes were higher among preeclamptics/eclamptics than controls (6% vs. 4%). Carleton et al. further showed that mean systolic blood pressure was demonstrably higher only a few years after an index preeclamptic pregnancy as compared to a nonhypertensive pregnancy.[115]

Subsequent studies by Sibai et al.[28,116] confirmed these findings and extended them to women who had early disease defined as onset < 28 weeks. This subset of

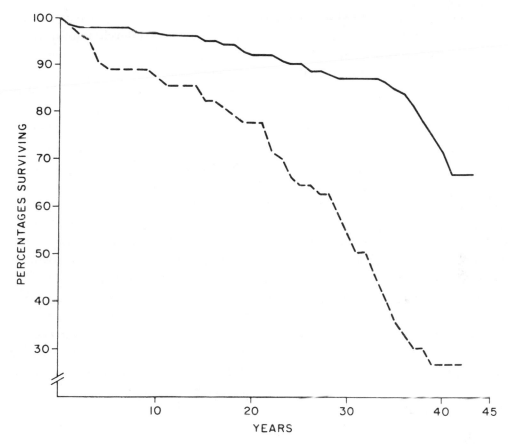

Figure 2–3. Survival following eclampsia. Solid line represents women who had eclampsia in the first pregnancy; broken line represents those who had eclampsia as multiparas. Note the poorer survival in the latter group, their deaths being primarily cardiovascular in origin. (*Reprinted, with permission, from Chesley LC, Annitto JE, Cosgrove RA: The remote prognosis of eclamptic women: Sixth periodic report.* Am J Obstet Gynecol *1976;124:446–459.*)

patients was especially at risk for recurrent preeclampsia (55% in previously normotensive women) in subsequent pregnancies and hypertension in later life.

These data indicate that the development of long-range maternal cardiovascular morbidity after preeclampsia is quite variable. This heterogeneity in maternal outcome is predicted by having preeclampsia as a multipara or as a recurrent event, and by experiencing preeclampsia in the second trimester. In turn, women with underlying disease prior to the index pregnancy were more likely to experience preeclampsia as a multipara, recurrent preeclampsia, and early onset preeclampsia. Conversely, if a woman has been pregnant without preeclampsia her incidence of hypertension is lower than the general population.[117,118]

Perinatal Outcomes

Seventy percent of infants born to preeclamptic women are of normal birth weight for their gestational age.[119,120] Also, data indicate that conditions associated with large infants, such as obesity[13,17,35] and gestational diabetes,[121] increase the risk for preeclampsia. Nevertheless, early onset of preeclampsia heralds not only poor later maternal health but also poor perinatal outcomes in the index pregnancy.[27,28,30,116,122-126] The perinatal mortality rate is higher for infants of preeclamptic women.[127] These demises are the result of intrauterine death from placental insufficiency and abruptio placentae, or the result of prematurity from emergency delivery needed to control the disease.[128] Beyond this, early onset of preeclampsia in the index pregnancy is related to perinatal morbidity in subsequent pregnancies. Lopez-Llera and Horta examined 110 women in whom the onset of eclampsia was divided into gestational ages of < 35 weeks, ≥ 35 to 38 weeks, and ≥ 38 weeks.[122] With earlier onset in the index pregnancy, recurrent preeclampsia and small-for-gestational age infants (SGA) in subsequent pregnancies were more common (42%, 15%, and 10% of infants were SGA in the three groups). Similarly, Sibai et al. showed that earlier onset disease in the first pregnancy was associated with more frequent perinatal death in subsequent pregnancies.[116]

The interaction of underlying maternal disease and preeclampsia results in particularly high perinatal morbidity and mortality. Hypertension detected prior to 20 weeks' gestation without superimposed preeclampsia has been shown to increase the rate of perinatal mortality in most, but not all studies,[30,126] whereas chronic hypertension with superimposed preeclampsia has been associated with high perinatal morbidity and mortality rates in all reports. Page and Christianson prospectively studied 10,074 white and 2,880 black women divided into four groups: with and without chronic hypertension and with and without superimposed preeclampsia.[105] In comparison to women with normal blood pressures without proteinuria, perinatal death rates were two- to threefold higher among chronic hypertensives and six- to tenfold higher among chronic hypertensives with superimposed preeclampsia. Rates of stillbirth and SGA followed similar patterns to those noted for perinatal death. These results have been replicated in studies of chronic hypertensives and control pregnant women.[125,129] Rey and Couturier in Montreal enrolled 298 women who had a well-documented diagnosis of hypertension prior to pregnancy or who had hypertension (BP > 140/90) before 20 weeks' gestation and again after 6 weeks' postdelivery.[27] Perinatal deaths were substantially higher among chronic hypertensives with superimposed preeclampsia (101/1000) and modestly higher among chronic hypertensives without preeclampsia (29/1000) than among controls (12/1000).

Women with diabetes and superimposed preeclampsia are more likely to experience a perinatal death than are women with diabetes alone. Perinatal mortality was substantially higher in preeclamptic diabetic patients (60/1000) than normotensive diabetic patients (3/1000).[32] This was despite a lack of difference between preeclamptic and normotensive diabetic patients for age, parity, glucose control, blood urea nitrogen, and serum creatinine.

Thus, underlying maternal diabetes and hypertension adversely affect perinatal outcomes but preeclampsia superimposed on these maternal conditions has even greater adverse perinatal consequences. These findings are all the more impressive since the difficulty of diagnosing preeclampsia in the setting of hypertension or diabetes should have resulted in a diminution of the observed effect between superimposed preeclampsia and adverse perinatal outcomes.

CRITIQUE OF STUDIES

Methodological issues that cloud the interpretation of epidemiologic results include misclassification of diseased vs. nondiseased individuals, biased patient selection, differential loss to follow-up, lack of control for potential confounders, and difficulties in selecting controls. Classification of women into those with preeclampsia, those with transient hypertension of pregnancy, and controls has been inconsistent and difficult. Some of the differences in findings between studies may relate to misclassification and thereby combining women between these categories. For this reason it is appealing to rely on reports about women with more severe disease, such as eclampsia. However, because more severe disease may be more strongly associated with underlying maternal disease, such reports may result in inflated associations. Similarly, bias in subject selection may have overrepresented women with underlying maternal disease in some study populations. The reports reviewed generally did not indicate the proportion of subjects studied as a function of the underlying population affected. Thus, patients with early onset, severe, complicated, or confusing disease, perhaps indicative of a maternal etiology, may have been more likely to be included in these studies. In addition, only Chesley et al. carefully reported follow-up rates.[112] Mothers more familiar with the medical system, particularly those with underlying maternal disease, may have thus been overrepresented in maternal and perinatal morbidity statistics.

The problem of defining an appropriate control group is a difficult one in this literature. In prospective studies, the *a priori* likelihood of developing the outcome of interest should be a function of exposure (for example, maternal morbidity) status, and not some other factor(s). It has been argued that women with uncomplicated pregnancies have a lower rate of later cardiovascular disease than the general age- and race-matched population, and are therefore not appropriate controls. We argue that this is because women likely to develop later hypertension are also more likely to have hypertension during pregnancy. Therefore, women with uncomplicated pregnancies are reasonable controls as they differ in the likelihood of outcome by the exposure of interest and not some other factor. In addition, comparing the natural history among study participants to that in a general population survey disregards the problems of differential selection in exposed and unexposed.

CONCLUSION

Preeclampsia and transient hypertension in pregnancy continue to be relatively common, although preeclampsia appears to be much less commonly complicated by eclampsia than it was in the past. This likely represents improvement in medical care rather than change in the natural history of the disease. Risk factors for transient hypertension have rarely been studied separate from preeclampsia. However, it is clear that this syndrome is distinct from preeclampsia. The natural acute outcome for mother and baby from transient hypertension differs from preeclampsia in that it is uniformly benign. However, transient hypertension in pregnancy is strongly associated with later chronic hypertension in mothers.

Risk factors for the occurrence of preeclampsia include those associated with maternal cardiovascular risk as well as those that are unique to pregnancy and may represent an immunologic etiology. We propose that both maternal and placental causes converge to promote a pathologic cascade, resulting in the maternal and fetal syndrome. The natural history of preeclampsia also suggests a heterogeneity in long-term maternal effects as well as in perinatal outcomes depending upon the presence or absence of maternal predisposition to cardiovascular disease.

REFERENCES

1. Ness RB, Roberts JM: Heterogeneous causes constituting the single syndrome of preeclampsia: A hypothesis and its implications. *Am J Obstet Gynecol* 1996;175:1365–1370.
2. National High Blood Pressure Education Program Working Group Report on High Blood Pressure in Pregnancy. *Am J Obstet Gynecol* 1990;163:1689–1712.
3. Davey DA, MacGillivray I: The classification and definition of the hypertensive disorders of pregnancy. *Am J Obstet Gynecol* 1988;158:892–898.
4. Saftlas AF, Olson DR, Franks AL, et al: Epidemiology of preeclampsia and eclampsia in the United States, 1979–1986. *Am J Obstet Gynecol* 1990;163:460–465.
5. Douglas KA, Redman CWG: Eclampsia in the United Kingdom. *Br Med J* 1994; 309:1395–1400.
6. Eden TW: Eclampsia. *J Obstet Gynaecol Br Emp* 1922;29:386–401.
7. Corkill TF: Experience of toxaemia control in Australia and New Zealand. *Pathology and Microbiology* 1961;24:428–434.
8. Sibai BM, Caritis SN, Thom E, et al. and the National Institute of Child Health and Human Development Network of Maternal-Fetal Medicine Units: Prevention of preeclampsia with low-dose aspirin in healthy, nulliparous pregnant women. *N Engl J Med* 1993;329:1213–1218.
9. Kyle PM, Buckley D, Kissane J, et al: The angiotensin sensitivity test and low dose aspirin are ineffective methods to predict and prevent hypertensive disorders in nulliparous pregnancy. *Am J Obstet Gynecol* 1995;173:865–872.
10. Carroli G, Duley L, Belizán JM, et al: Calcium supplementation during pregnancy: A systematic review of randomized controlled trials. *Br J Obstet Gynaecol* 1994;101:753–758.
11. Hauth JC, Goldenberg RL, Parker CR Jr, et al: Low-aspirin therapy to prevent preeclampsia. *Am J Obstet Gynecol* 1993;168:1083–1093.
12. Ales KL, Charlson ME: Epidemiology of preeclampsia and eclampsia (letter). *Am J Obstet Gynecol* 1991;165(1):238.
13. Eskenazi B, Fenster L, Sidney S: A multivariate analysis of risk factors for preeclampsia. *JAMA* 1991;266:237–241.
14. MacGillivray J: Some observations on the incidence of preeclampsia. *Obstet Gyneaecol Br Emp* 1958;65:536–539.
15. Hansen JP: Older maternal age and pregnancy outcome: A review of the literature. *Obstet Gynecol Surv* 1986;41:726–742.
16. Zhang J, Zeisler J, Hatch MC, Berkowitz G: Epidemiology of pregnancy-induced hypertension. *Epidemiologic Rev* 1997;19(2):218–232.
17. Dekker GA, Sibai BM: Early detection of preeclampsia. *Am J Obstet Gynecol* 1991; 165:160–172.

18. Sibai BM, Gordon T, Thom E, et al and the National Institute of Child Health and Human Development Network of Maternal-Fetal Medicine Units: Risk factors for preeclampsia in healthy nulliparous women: A prospective multicenter study. *Am J Obstet Gynecol* 1995;172:642–648.

19. Tillman AJB: The effect of normal and toxemic pregnancy on blood pressure. *Am J Obstet Gynecol* 1955;70:589–603.

20. Fallis NE, Langford HG: Relation of second trimester blood pressure to toxemia of pregnancy in the primigravid patient. *Am J Obstet Gynecol* 1963;87:123–125.

21. Moutquin JM, Rainville C, Giroux L, et al: A prospective study of blood pressure in pregnancy: Prediction of preeclampsia. *Am J Obstet Gynecol* 1985;151:191–196.

22. Villar MA, Sibai BM: Clinical significance of elevated mean arterial blood pressure in second trimester threshold increase in systolic or diastolic blood pressure during third trimester. *Am J Obstet Gynecol* 1989;160:419–423.

23. Page EW, Christianson R: The impact of mean arterial blood pressure in the middle trimester upon the outcome of pregnancy. *Am J Obstet Gynecol* 1976;125:740–746.

24. Friedman EA, Neff RK: *Pregnancy Hypertension: A Systemic Evaluation of Clinical Diagnostic Criteria*. Littleton, MA: PSG; 1977:217.

25. Chesley LC: *Hypertension Disorders in Pregnancy*. New York: Appleton-Century-Crofts; 1978.

26. Roberts JM, Perloff DL: Hypertension and the obstetrician-gynecologist. *Am J Obstet Gynecol* 1977;127:316–325.

27. Rey E, Couturier A: The prognosis of pregnancy in women with chronic hypertension. *Am J Obstet Gynecol* 1994;171:410–416.

27a. Sibai BM, Lindheimer M, Hauth J, et al: Risk factors for preeclampsia, abruptio placentae, and adverse neonatal outcomes among women with chronic hypertension. *N Engl J Med* 1998;339:667–671.

28. Sibai BM, Mercer B, Sarinoglu C: Severe preeclampsia in the second trimester: Recurrence risk and long-term prognosis. *Am J Obstet Gynecol* 1991;165:1408–1412.

29. Sibai BM, El-Nazer A, Gonzalez-Ruiz A: Severe preeclampsia–eclampsia in young primigravid women: Subsequent pregnancy outcome and remote prognosis. *Am J Obstet Gynecol* 1986;155:1011–1016.

30. Mabie WC, Pernoll ML, Biswas MK: Chronic hypertension in pregnancy. *Obstet Gynecol* 1986;67:197–205.

31. Siddiqi T, Rosenn B, Mimouni F, et al: Hypertension during pregnancy in insulin-dependent diabetic women. *Obstet Gynecol* 1991;77:514–519.

32. Garner PR, D'Alton ME, Dudley DK, et al: Preeclampsia in diabetic pregnancies. *Am J Obstet Gynecol* 1990;163:505–508.

33. MacGillivray J: *Preeclampsia: The Hypertensive Disease of Pregnancy*. London: WB Saunders; 1983.

34. Smith CA: The effect of wartime starvation in Holland upon pregnancy and its product. *Am J Obstet Gynecol* 1947;53:599–606.

35. Chesley L (ed): Epidemiology of preeclampsia–eclampsia. In: *Hypertensive Disorders in Pregnancy*. New York: Appleton-Century-Crofts; 1978:35–55.

36. Stone JL, Lockwood CJ, Berkowitz GS, et al: Risk factors for severe preeclampsia. *Obstet Gynecol* 1994;83:357–361.

37. Wolfe HM, Zador I, Gross T, et al: The clinical utility of body mass index in pregnancy. *Am J Obstet Gynecol* 1991;164:1306–1309.

38. Sibai BM, Gordon T, Thom E, et al: Risk factors for preeclampsia in healthy nulliparous women: A prospective multicenter study. The National Institute of Child Health and Human Development Network of Maternal-Fetal Medicine Units. *Am J Obstet Gynecol* 1995;172:642–648.

39. Masse J, Forest J-C, Moutquin J-M, et al: A prospective study of several potential biologic markers for early prediction of the development of preeclampsia. *Am J Obstet Gynecol* 1993;169:501–508.

40. Nelson TR: A clinical study of preeclampsia. *J Obstet Gynaecol Br Emp* 1955;62:48–66.

41. Thomson AM, Billewicz WZ: Clinical significance of weight trends during pregnancy. *Br Med J* 1957;1:243–247.

42. Robertson EG: The natural history of oedema during pregnancy. *J Obstet Gynaecol Br Commonw* 1971;78:520–529.
43. Thomson AM, Hytten RE, Billewicz WZ: The epidemiology of oedema during pregnancy. *J Obstet Gynaecol Br Commonw* 1967;74:1–10.
44. Hamlin RHJ: The prevention of eclampsia and preeclampsia. *Lancet* 1952;1:64–69.
45. Adams EM, Finlayson A: Familial aspects of preeclampsia and hypertension in pregnancy. *Lancet* 1961;2:1357.
46. Chesley LC, Cooper DW: Genetics of hypertension in pregnancy: Possible single-gene control of pre-eclampsia and eclampsia in the descendants of eclamptic women. *Br J Obstet Gynaecol* 1986;93:898–908.
47. Roberts JM, Redman CWG: Preeclampsia: More than pregnancy-induced hypertension. *Lancet* 1993;341:1451–1454.
48. Kilpatrick DC, Gibson G, Livingston J, Liston WA: Preeclampsia is associated with HLA-DR4 sharing between mother and fetus. *Tissue Antigens* 1990;35:178–181.
49. Johnson N, Moodley J, Hammond MG: HLA status of the fetus born to African women with eclampsia. *Clin Exper Hyper in Preg* 1990;B9:311–316.
50. Redman CWG: Immunology of preeclampsia. *Semin Perinatol* 1991;15:257–262.
51. Robillard P, Hulsey TC, Alexander GR, et al: Paternity patterns and risk of preeclampsia in the last pregnancy in multiparae. *J Reprod Immunol* 1993;24:1–12.
52. Feeney JG, Scott JS: Pre-eclampsia and changed paternity. *Eur J Obstet Gynecol Reprod Biol* 1980;11:35–38.
53. Ikedife D: Eclampsia in multiparae. *Br Med J* 1980;280:985–986.
54. Chng PK: Occurrence of pre-eclampsia in pregnancies to three husbands. Case report. *Br J Obstet Gynaecol* 1982;89:862–863.
55. Robillard PY, Hulsey TC, Perianin J, et al: Association of pregnancy-induced hypertension with duration of sexual cohabitation before conception. *Lancet* 1994;344:973–975.
56. Strickland DM, Guzick DS, Cox K, et al: The relationship between abortion in the first pregnancy and development of pregnancy-induced hypertension in the subsequent pregnancy. *Am J Obstet Gynecol* 1986;154:146–148.
57. Seidman DS, Ever-Hadani P, Stevenson DK, et al: The effect of abortion on the incidence of pre-eclampsia. *Eur J Obstet Gynecol Reprod Biol* 1989;33:109–114.
58. Marti JJ, Herrman U: Immunogestosis. A new concept of "essential" EPH gestosis, with special consideration of the primigravid patient. *Am J Obstet Gynecol* 1977;128:489–493.
59. Klonoff-Cohen HS, Savitz DA, Cefalo RC, McCann MF: An epidemiologic study of contraception and preeclampsia. *JAMA* 1989;262:3143–3147.
60. Chng PK: Occurrence of pre-eclampsia in pregnancies to three husbands: Case report. *Br J Obstet Gynaecol* 1982;89:862–863.
61. Feeney JG, Scott JS: Pre-eclampsia and changed paternity. *Eur J Obstet Gynecol Reprod Biol* 1980;11:35–38.
62. Need JA, Bell B, Meffin E, et al: Pre-eclampsia in pregnancies from donor inseminations. *J Reprod Immunol* 1983;5:329–338.
63. Blanchette H: Obstetric performance of patients after oocyte donation. *Am J Obstet Gynecol* 1993;168:1803–1809.
64. Bulfin MJ, Lawler PE: Problems associated with toxemia in twin pregnancies. *Am J Obstet Gynecol* 1957;73:37.
65. Page EW: The relation between hydatid moles, relative ischemia of the gravid uterus, and placental origin of eclampsia. *Am J Obstet Gynecol* 1939;37:291.
66. Scott JS: Pregnancy toxaemia associated with hydrops foetalis, hydatidiform mole and hydramnios. *J Obstet Gynaecol Br Emp* 1958;65:689.
67. Klonoff-Cohen H, Edelstein S, Savitz D: Cigarette smoking and preeclampsia. *Obstet Gynecol* 1993;81:541–544.
68. Underwood P, Kesler K, O'Lane J, Callagan DA: Parental smoking empirically related to pregnancy outcome. *Obstet Gynecol* 1967;29:1–8.
69. Russell C, Taylor R, Law C: Smoking in pregnancy, maternal blood pressure, pregnancy outcome, baby weight and growth, and other related factors: A prospective study. *Br J Prev Soc Med* 1968;22:119–126.

70. Marcoux S, Brisson J, Fabia J: The effect of cigarette smoking on the risk of preeclampsia and gestational hypertension. *Am J Epidemiol* 1989;130:950–957.

71. Zabriskie J: Effect of cigarette smoking during pregnancy. Study of 2000 cases. *Am J Obstet Gynecol* 1963;21:405–411.

72. Duffus G, MacGillivray I: The incidence of preeclamptic toxaemia in smokers and non-smokers. *Lancet* 1968;i:994–995.

73. Roberts J: Possible dietary measures in the prevention of preeclampsia and eclampsia. *Clin Obstet Gynaecol* (Balliéres) (in press).

74. Zamudio S, Palmer SK, Dahms TE, et al: Blood volume expansion, preeclampsia, and infant birth weight at high altitude. *J Appl Physiol* 1993;75:1566–1573.

75. Mahfouz AA, el-Said MM, Alakija W, et al: Altitude and socio-biological determinants of pregnancy-associated hypertension. *Int J Gynaecol Obstet* 1994;44:135–138.

76. Moore LG, Hershey DW, Jahnigen D, et al: The incidence of pregnancy-induced hypertension is increased among Colorado residents at high altitude. *Am J Obstet Gynecol* 1982;144:423–429.

77. Degani S, Abinader E, Eibschitz I, et al: Isometric exercise test for predicting gestational hypertension. *Obstet Gynecol* 1985;65:652–654.

78. Gant NF, Chand S, Worley RJ, et al: A clinical test useful for predicting the development of acute hypertension in pregnancy. *Am J Obstet Gynecol* 1974;120:1–6.

79. Dekker GA, Makovitz JW, Wallenburg HCS: Comparison of prediction of pregnancy-induced hypertensive disease by angiotensin II sensitivity and supine pressor test. *Br J Obstet Gynecol* 1990;97:817–821.

80. Phelan JP, Everidge GJ, Wilder TJ, Newman C: Is the supine pressor test an adequate means of predicting acute hypertension in pregnancy? *Am J Obstet Gynecol* 1977;128:173–176.

81. Andersen GJ: The roll-over test as a screening procedure for gestational hypertension. *Aust NZ J Obstet Gynaecol* 1980;20:144–146.

82. Tunbridge RDG: Pregnancy-associated hypertension. A comparison of its prediction by "roll-over test" and plasma noradrenaline measurement in 100 primigravidae. *Br J Obstet Gynaecol* 1983;90:1027–1032.

83. Sibai BM, Anderson GD, McCubbin JH: Eclampsia II. Clinical significance of laboratory findings. *Obstet Gynecol* 1982;59:153–157.

84. Giles C, Inglis TCM: Thrombocytopenia and macrothrombocytosis in gestational hypertension. *Br J Obstet Gynaecol* 1981;88:1115–1119.

85. Redman CWG, Bonnar J, Beilin LJ: Early platelet consumption in preeclampsia. *Br Med J* 1978;1:467–469.

86. Weinstein L: Syndrome of hemolysis, elevated liver enzymes, and low platelet count: A severe consequence of hypertension in pregnancy. *Am J Obstet Gynecol* 1982;142:159–167.

87. Walker JJ, Cameron AD, Bjornsson S, et al: Can platelet volume predict progressive hypertensive disease in pregnancy? *Am J Obstet Gynecol* 1989;161:676–679.

88. Ahmed Y, Iddekinge BV, Paul C, et al: Retrospective analysis of platelet numbers and volumes in normal pregnancy and in pre-eclampsia. *Br J Obstet Gynaecol* 1993;1160:216–220.

89. Hutt R, Ogunniyi SO, Sullivan HF, Elder MG: Increased platelet volume and aggregation precede the onset of preeclampsia. *Obstet Gynecol* 1994;83:146–149.

90. Zemel MB, Zemel PC, Berry S, Norman G, et al: Altered platelet calcium metabolism as an early predictor of increased peripheral vascular resistance and preeclampsia in urban black women. *N Engl J Med* 1990;323:434–438.

91. Thornton CA: Factor VIII-related antigen and factor VIII coagulant activity in normal and preeclamptic pregnancy. *Br J Obstet Gynaecol* 1977;84:919–923.

92. Whigham KAE, Howie PW, Shah MM, Prentice CRM: Factor VIII related antigen/coagulant activity ratio as a predictor of fetal growth retardation: A comparison with hormone and uric acid measurements. *Br J Obstet Gynaecol* 1980;87:797–803.

93. Founie A, Monroziew M, Pontonnier G, et al: Factor VIII complex in normal pregnancy, preeclampsia and fetal growth retardation. *Br J Obstet Gynaecol* 1981;88:250–254.

94. Redman CWG, Denson KWE, Beilin LJ, et al: Factor VIII consumption in pre-eclampsia. *Lancet* 1977;1249–1252.

95. deBoer K, tenCate JW, Sturk A, et al: Enhanced thrombin generation in normal and hypertensive pregnancy. *Am J Obstet Gynecol* 1989;160:95–100.

96. Cadroy Y, Grandjean H, Pichon J, et al: Evaluation of six markers of aemostatic system in normal pregnancy and pregnancy complicated by hypertension or pre-eclampsia. *Br J Obstet Gynaecol* 1993;100:416–420.

97. Lieberman JR, Hagay ZJ, Mazor M, et al: Plasma antithrombin III levels in pre-eclampsia and chronic hypertension. *Int J Gynecol Obstet* 1988;27:21–24.

98. Graninger W, Tatra G, Pirich K, Nasz F: Low antithrombin III and high fibronectin in preeclampsia. *Eur J Obstet Gynecol Reprod Biol* 1985;19:223–229.

99. Saleh AA, Bottoms SF, Welch RA, et al: Preeclampsia, delivery and the hemostatic system. *Am J Obstet Gynecol* 1987;157:331–336.

100. Stubbs TM, Lazarchick J, Horger EO III: Plasma fibronectin levels in preeclampsia. A possible biochemical marker for vascular endothelial damage. *Am J Obstet Gynecol* 1984;150: 885–889.

101. Lazarchick J, Stubbs TM, Romein I, et al: Predictive value of fibronectin levels in normotensive gravid women destined to become preeclamptic. *Am J Obstet Gynecol* 1986;154: 1050–1052.

102. Ballegeer V, Spitz B, Kieckens L, et al: Predictive value of increased plasma levels of fibronectin in gestational hypertension. *Am J Obstet Gynecol* 1989;161:432–436.

103. Taylor RN, Casal DC, Jones LA, et al: Selective effects of preeclamptic sera on human endothelial cell procoagulant protein expression. *Am J Obstet Gynecol* 1991;165:1705–1710.

104. Taylor RN, Crombleholm WR, Friedman SA, et al: High plasma cellular fibronectin levels correlate with biochemical and clinical features of preeclampsia but cannot be attributed to hypertension alone. *Am J Obstet Gynecol* 1991;165:895–901.

105. Page EW, Christianson R: Influence of blood pressure changes with and without proteinuria upon outcome of pregnancy. *Am J Obstet Gynecol* 1976;126:821–833.

106. Sibai BM, Lipshitz J, Anderson GD, Dilts PV Jr: Reassessment of intravenous MgS04 therapy in preeclampsia–eclampsia. *Obstet Gynecol* 1981;57:199.

107. Pritchard JA, Pritchard SA: Standardized treatment of 154 consecutive cases of eclampsia. *Am J Obstet Gynecol* 1975;123:543.

108. Roberts JM: Pregnancy-related hypertension. In: Creasy RK, Resnick R: *Maternal Fetal Medicine Disorders, Part III*, Section 19, 804–843. Philadelphia: Saunders, 1994.

109. Adams EM, MacGillivray I: Long-term effect of preeclampsia on blood pressure. *Lancet* 1961;2:1373–1375.

110. Lindberg S, Axelsson O, Jorner O, et al: A prospective controlled five-year follow-up study of primiparas with gestational hypertension. *Acta Obstet Gynecol Scand* 1988;67:605–609.

111. Jonsdottir LS, Argrimsson R, Geirsson RT, et al: Death rates from ischemic heart disease in women with a history of hypertension in pregnancy. *Acta Obstet Gynecol Scand* 1995;74:772–776.

112. Chesley LC, Annitto JE, Cosgrove RA: The remote prognosis of preeclamptic women: Sixth periodic report. *Am J Obstet Gynecol* 1976;124:446–459.

113. Berman S: Observations in the toxemic clinic, Boston Lying-in Hospital, 1923–30. *N Engl J Med* 1930;203:361–365.

114. Herrick WW, Tillman AJB: The mild toxemias of late pregnancy. Their relation to cardiovascular and renal disease. *Am J Obstet Gynecol* 1936; 31:832–844.

115. Carleton H, Forsythe A, Flores R: Remote prognosis of preeclampsia in women 25 years old and younger. *Am J Obstet Gynecol* 1988;159:156–160.

116. Sibai BM, Sarinoglu C, Mercer BM: Eclampsia VII. Pregnancy outcome after eclampsia and long-term prognosis. *Am J Obstet Gynecol* 1992;166:1757–1763.

117. Fisher KA, Luger A, Spargo BH, Lindheimer MD: Hypertension in pregnancy: Clinical-pathological correlations and remote prognosis. *Medicine* 1981;60:267–276.

118. Adams E, MacGillivray I: Long-term effects of preeclampsia on blood pressure. *Lancet* 1961:1373–1378.

119. Pietrantoni M, O'Brien WF: The current impact of the hypertensive disorders of pregnancy. *Clin Exp Hypertens* 1994;16:479–492.

120. Eskenazi B, Fenster L, Sidney S, Elkin EP: Fetal growth retardation in infants of multiparous and nulliparous women with preeclampsia. *Am J Obstet Gynecol* 1993;169:1112–1118.
121. Suhonen L, Teramo K: Hypertension and preeclampsia in women with gestational glucose intolerance. *Acta Obstet Gynecol Scand* (Stockholm) 1993;72:269–272.
122. Lopez-Llera M, Horta JLH: Pregnancy after eclampsia. *Am J Obstet Gynecol* 1974;119:193–198.
123. Long PA, Abell DA, Beischer NA: Fetal growth retardation and preeclampsia. *Br J Obstet Gynaecol* 1980;87:13–18.
124. Moore MP, Redman CWG: Case-control study of severe pre-eclampsia of early onset. *Br Med J* 1983;27:580–583.
125. Sibai BM, Spinnato JA, Watson DL, et al: Pregnancy outcome in 303 cases with severe preeclampsia. *Obstet Gynecol* 1984;64:319–325.
126. Ferrazzani S, Caruso A, DeCarolis S, et al: Proteinuria and outcome of 444 pregnancies complicated by hypertension. *Am J Obstet Gynecol* 1990;162:366–371.
127. Plouin PF, Chatellier G, Breart G, et al: Frequency and perinatal consequences of hypertensive disease of pregnancy. *Adv Nephrol* 1986;57:69.
128. Naeye RL, Friedman EA: Causes of perinatal death associated with gestational hypertension and proteinuria. *Am J Obstet Gynecol* 1979;133:8.
129. Sibai BM, Abdella TN, Anderson GD: Pregnancy outcome in 211 patients with mild chronic hypertension. *Obstet Gynecol* 1983;61:571–576.

II

Cardiovascular Adaptation to Normal Pregnancy

3

Hemodynamic Changes

Margaret K. McLaughlin and James M. Roberts

In the first edition of this book published in 1978, Leon Chesley devoted one chapter, "Blood Pressure and Circulation," to the cardiovascular changes in both normal pregnancy and preeclampsia, the focus being studies performed on women with preeclampsia. Data relating to areas such as cardiac output were limited in number and scope, as development of reliable noninvasive technology was still in its infancy. Considerable progress has occurred since then, with many of the more recent studies focusing on cardiovascular adjustments to normal gestation. These will be the focus of this chapter, and studies related to abnormal pregnancies, particularly preeclampsia will be found in Chapters 5 and 6. Familiarity with, as well as accrual of, more knowledge of the factors influencing the control of blood pressure in normal pregnancy should help both in understanding the pathogenesis of hypertension in preeclampsia and in improved methods of studying and managing the disease.

HEMODYNAMIC CHANGES DURING PREGNANCY

The cardiovascular adaptation to pregnancy involves a complex physiological response by the maternal organism to the presence of the conceptus. The hemodynamic changes include, but are not restricted to, significant increases in cardiac output and blood volume, a decrease in perfusion pressure, and a marked reduction in total systemic vascular resistance.

In this chapter, the serial changes in indices of overall cardiovascular function are reviewed and discussed in relation to the major components contributing to the overall hemodynamic response to pregnancy. The goal of the hemodynamic response to pregnancy is to provide adequate uteroplacental perfusion for fetal development without compromising maternal function. Pregnancy-induced alterations in cardiovascular function are due to a complex interplay between the nervous system, circulating humoral factors, and functional and structural alter-

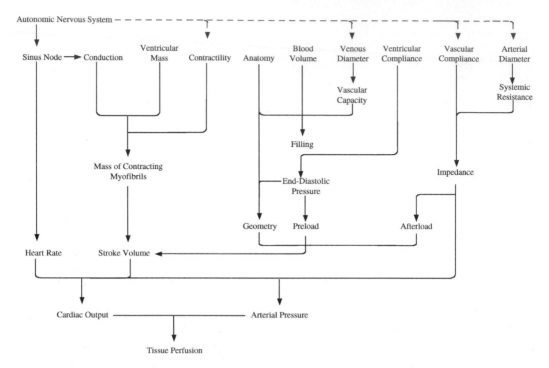

Figure 3–1. Schematic diagram integrating the various central and peripheral hemodynamic factors that regulate tissue perfusion.

ations that occur within the heart and vascular tissue (Fig. 3–1). Due to the highly dynamic nature of the cardiovascular system it has been difficult to determine the cause and effect relationships responsible for the hemodynamic profile observed during the course of pregnancy.

Serial Changes in Overall Cardiovascular Function

The optimal description of the serial hemodynamic changes during pregnancy includes measures obtained prior to pregnancy and throughout gestation in the same patient cohort. The need for this comparison is emphasized by a study that demonstrates persistent gestational effects on cardiovascular function in physically active women as long as one-year postpartum.[1]

Blood Pressure

In general, mean arterial pressure declines in the first trimester, reaching a nadir between 16 to 20 weeks' gestation with a return to control values near term.[1-11] Diastolic pressures decline to a greater extent than systolic pressures, the average mean change being about 10 mm Hg (Fig. 3–2). A careful assessment of hemodynamic changes during the menstrual cycle suggests that the early pregnancy decline in blood pressure is initiated in the luteal phase of the cycle.[12] A large cross-sectional study suggests an effect of parity on the magnitude of the diastolic pressure response[13] while a smaller longitudinal study did not observe any differ-

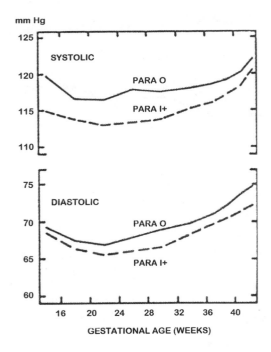

Figure 3–2. Mean blood pressure by gestational age in 6000 white women 25 to 34 years of age who delivered single-term infants. (*Reprinted, with permission, from Christianson R: Studies on blood pressure during pregnancy. 1. Influence of parity and age. Am J Obstet Gynecol 1976;125:509.*)

ence in either the time course or magnitude of the pregnancy-associated changes in arterial blood pressure.[1]

There is a significant difference in blood pressure as early as 9 weeks' gestation between women with a normal pregnancy outcome and those who later develop preeclampsia (Fig. 3–3). Depending upon the study, this difference was significant in diastolic and/or systolic pressures.[9,14,15] The methodology used to assess blood pressure during either normal or abnormal pregnancy (oscillometric or auscultatory) remains a subject of debate. In addition, differences in technique and lack of a prepregnancy measure are likely to account for some of the observed differences in absolute values reported.[16-21]

Diurnal blood pressure variation in normal pregnancy has been observed to follow a pattern in which there is a significant decline during sleep. This is of interest as this diurnal variation appears to be absent or shifted in women with preeclampsia.[22-29] The diurnal change in blood pressure has been observed using several different methods of blood pressure measurement. The magnitude varies between studies with systolic pressure changes ranging from 3 to 16 mm Hg systolic and up to 17 mm Hg diastolic pressure. In addition, it has been noted that gestational hypertensive women, as opposed to women with preeclampsia, demonstrate a similar or even greater fall in nocturnal systolic pressure as normal pregnant women.[25,26]

The diurnal variation in blood pressure during normotensive pregnancies and in gestational hypertension is apparent whether studied at bed rest or on 24-hour ambulatory monitoring.[25] It is of interest, however, that in an analysis of the longitudinal changes in the circadian blood pressure rhythm during pregnancy, 33% of the normal pregnancies studied did not demonstrate a significant circadian rhythm

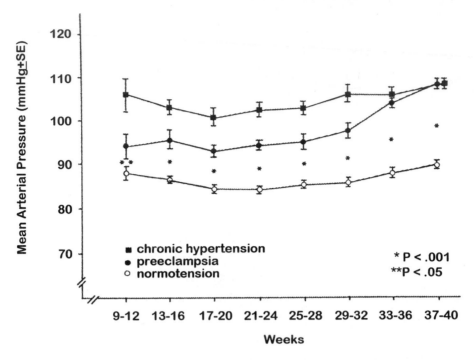

Figure 3–3. Averaged mean arterial blood pressures (± 1 SE) in women who remained normotensive throughout pregnancy (o—o), in women who developed preeclampsia (●—●), and in women who developed hypertension (■—■) by periods of 4 weeks. (*Reprinted, with permission, from Moutquin JM, et al: A prospective study of blood pressure in pregnancy: Prediction of preeclampsia. Am J Obstet Gynecol 1985;151:191–196.*)

in blood pressure.[25] Nocturnal position may be a confounding variable in the above studies.[30] Understanding the control mechanisms for the diurnal rhythm in blood pressure between normotensive and gestational hypertensive pregnancies and the loss of that diurnal regulation in women with preeclampsia should be of value.

Cardiac Function

The increased accuracy of noninvasive hemodynamic measures has resulted in several reports on alterations in cardiac function during pregnancy.[1,3,5,6,8,10,11,31-34] Similar to blood pressure, changes in cardiac output during gestation follow a very early onset being evident during the luteal phase of the menstrual cycle.[12] Cardiac output is significantly elevated by 5 weeks after the last menstrual period and reaches 125% of prepregnancy values by 8 weeks' gestation.[1,8] This peaks to approximately 50% above prepregnant levels by midgestation and in studies comparing to preconceptual values, plateaus or continues at a slight rise until term. Approximately 70% of the increase in cardiac output occurs by the 16th week of gestation[1] which is well before the marked increase in uterine blood flow. During twin gestation, there is a further increment of about 15% in cardiac output.[8] The pattern of change in one well designed serial study is shown in Figure 3–4.[8,11] These

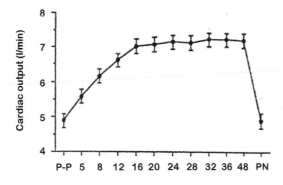

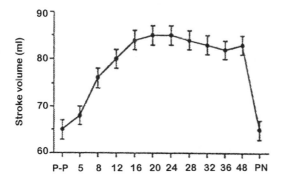

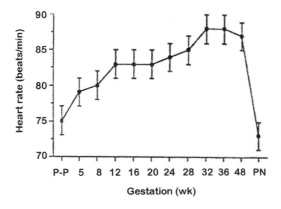

Figure 3–4. Longitudinal studies of cardiac output, stroke volume, and heart rate started before conception and continued through to the postnatal period. (*Reprinted from Hunter S, Robson SC: Adaptation of the maternal heart in pregnancy.* Br Heart J *1992;68: 540–543, with permission from the BMJ Publishing Group.*)

observations are consistent with those reported by Lees in 1967 in which values for cardiac output were obtained using the invasive indicator dye-dilution technique. A summary of studies that are longitudinal in design and include the first trimester is provided in Table 3–1.

There is considerable disparity as to the status of cardiac output in the last trimester of pregnancy. While the differences may be due to the variety of techniques used and the comparison to postpartum values, it also may be attributed to variation among subjects in the study population. The cardiac output pattern is typically expressed as a mean value; yet within a single study[35] cardiac output increased in some women, decreased in others, or remained unchanged in the third

TABLE 3-1. CARDIAC OUTPUT VALUES OBTAINED SERIALLY IN LONGITUDINAL STUDIES CONDUCTED DURING NORMAL PREGNANCY

Author	No.	1st Trimester	2nd Trimester	Change	3rd Trimester	Change	Technique
Lees (1967)[4a]	5	6.10 ± 0.82[a]	6.18 ± 0.69	—	6.26 ± 0.54	—	ID
Robson (1989)[8]	13	6.12 ± 0.11[b]	7.21 ± 0.11	↑	7.22 ± 0.11	—	DEC/M mode
Duvekot (1993)[5]	10	5.82 median	6.53 median	↑	5.78 median	→	DEC/M mode
Mabie (1994)[33]	18	6.7 ± 0.9[a]	7.5 ± 1.0	↑	8.2 ± 1.7	←	DEC
van Oppen (1996)[3]	50	7.26 ± 1.56[a]	7.60 ± 1.63	↑	7.38 ± 1.63	→	TEB
Geva (1996)[31]	34	5.8 ± 1.6[a]	7.85 ± 1.50	↑	7.35 ± 1.25	→	DEC
Mone (1996)[36]	38	5.9 ± 1.0[a]	6.6 ± 1.3	↑	6.2 ± 1.3	→	DEC
Clapp (1997)[1]	30	5.90 ± 0.26[b]	6.72 ± 0.29	↑	6.80 ± 0.28	—	M mode
Poppas (1997)[10]	14	6.8 ± 1.6[a]	7.6 ± 1.5	↑	7.9 ± 1.6	←	DEC
Gilson (1997)[4]	76	5.0 ± 0.2[a]	5.7 ± 0.2	↑	5.8 ± 0.2	—	M mode

Cardiac output values expressed in L/min

[a] Mean values ± SD
[b] Mean values ± SEM

ID = indicator dilution; DEC = Doppler echocardiography; TEB = thoracic electrical bioimpedance
Modified from van Oppen et al. *Obstet Gynecol* 1996;87:310–318.

trimester. Thus, the apparent discrepancy may simply represent a feature of physiologic variation in the adaptive response to pregnancy. It would be of interest to know if the pattern within an individual persisted in subsequent pregnancies.

The rate and magnitude of change in cardiac output appears to be a function of parity, with an earlier increment and greater magnitude of change observed in multiparous compared to nulliparous women.[1] This suggests that the initial pregnancy affects subsequent function in later pregnancies, which is of particular interest in preeclampsia, a disease that is predominant in nulliparous women.

Stroke Volume and Heart Rate

Cardiac output is the product of stroke volume and heart rate. As depicted in Figure 3–4, both stroke volume and heart rate increase during gestation, with stroke volume reaching a plateau by 16 weeks and heart rate continuing at a slight rise until about 32 weeks. In the studies that compare to prepregnancy values, both parameters were increased significantly by 5 or 8 weeks, respectively.[1,8] Heart rate and stroke volume are sensitive to changes in position and are highly variable between women.[1] Prior conditioning has a strong influence on baseline values at rest. The percent increase during pregnancy in these two parameters in a sedentary population tends to be more balanced, i.e., 21% in stroke volume and 22% in heart rate compared to 17% and 26% in a physically active group.[1] In spite of a significant increase in cardiac output during the luteal phase of the menstrual cycle, heart rate was not changed significantly,[12] suggesting a significant role for decreases in afterload during the luteal phase of the cycle contributing to increased cardiac output.[1,5,10,12] Parity increased both the magnitude and rate of change in stroke volume but did not affect the pattern of change in heart rate.[1]

Systemic Vascular Resistance

The marked increase in cardiac output coupled with a decline in mean arterial pressure indicates a marked reduction of systemic vascular resistance (see Fig. 3–4). The decline in systemic vascular resistance is significant at 5 weeks' gestation, and greater than 85% of this decline occurs by 16 weeks' gestation.[1,8] In the study of physically active women by Clapp and Capeless, 23% of the pregnancy-associated increase in cardiac output and 30% of the pregnancy-associated decrease in systemic vascular resistance were still present one-year postpartum.[1]

Properties of the Left Ventricle

Studies designed to identify the potential mechanisms responsible for the increase in cardiac output during pregnancy have focused on characterizing when preload, afterload, and contractility change at a particular point in gestation.[1,3,5,6,8,10,11,31-34,36] These investigational efforts include assessments of the properties of the left ventricle during pregnancy, including potential changes in geometry (dimension), and myocardial mass and the relationship of these parameters to myocardial function (see Fig. 3–1).

Myocardial contractility is the ability of the ventricles to eject blood against a given load. It is determined by the number of muscle cells activated (a function of ventricular mass and conduction) and the force of individual cell contraction. Under normal conditions, two major factors contribute to force of individual cell contraction. The first is the contractility of the myocardial myocytes themselves. Positive inotropic factors which include catecholamines or other hormones such as thyroxin can increase contractility by enhancing the interaction between calcium and the contractile proteins.[37] Little is known about the direct effects of the humoral changes in pregnancy on the inotropic regulation of the ventricle. The second determinant of force generation is length activation. An increase in ventricular filling (a function of ventricular compliance and blood volume) increases fiber length which in turn causes length activation (see Fig. 3–1). This is the basis of the Frank–Starling relationship. The preload determines the end-diastolic pressure and thus filling of the ventricle.

In theory, changes in end-diastolic dimension reflect changes in venous return and thus serve as an indicator of preload, i.e., increasing end-diastolic volume should lead to a concomitant increase in end-diastolic dimension thus lengthening myocardial fiber length. Whether this relationship holds true during pregnancy when compliance is also changing is not clear.

Ventricular Dimensions, Mass and Contractility

In most, but not all studies, the left ventricular end-diastolic dimension and left ventricular mass have been shown to increase during pregnancy, although absolute values obtained differ. In addition, there is an increase in the cross-sectional area of the left ventricle outflow tract.[1,3,8,10,11,31-34,36]

Attempts have been made to identify differences in time course between an increase in stroke volume and changes in ventricular dimensions in order to determine those factors that contribute to the increase in cardiac output. These data are summarized in Table 3–2. Interpretation of these results and their subsequent physiological significance are complicated by differences in methods used and whether control values are prepregnant or postpartum. Clapp and Capeless compared values in a physically active cohort to their prepregnancy values.[1] Left ventricular dimensions were estimated with M-mode ultrasound via a left parasternal long-axis view of the left atrium, left ventricle, and ascending aorta. Values obtained were used to calculate left ventricular end-diastolic and end-systolic volumes (the difference equals stroke volume). Both the end-diastolic volume and stroke volume were increased significantly at the earliest time point assessed which was 8 weeks' gestation.

In the study by Robson et al.[8] left ventricular end-diastolic dimension and left atrial dimension were significantly increased by week 12 of pregnancy and both parameters continued to increase throughout the second trimester (24–28 weeks). Increases in stroke volume in the same study preceded the increases in the end-diastolic dimension by about 4 weeks. The difficulty in assessing time course be-

TABLE 3–2. CHANGES IN PRELOAD AND AFTERLOAD THROUGHOUT PREGNANCY

Author	CO	SV	Preload (EDD)	Afterload (TPR)	(LV Mass)	Control
Robson (1989)[8]	↑5 weeks	↑8 weeks	LV ↑12 wk LA ↑12 wk	→	↑12 wk	1
Mabie (1994)[33]	↑a	↑16 wk	—	→	↑20 wk	3
Duvekot (1993)[5]	↑5–8 wk	↑8 wk	LV ↑25 wk LA ↓10 wk	→	↑25 wk	2
Mone (1996)[36]	↑a	↑9 wk	—	→	↑18 wk	3
Geva (1996)[31]	↑a	↑18 wk	—b	→	↑10 wk	3
Clapp (1997)[1]	↑8 wk	↑8 wk	—	→	—	1
Poppas (1997)[10]	↑12 wk	↑12 wk	No change	→	↑20 wk	3
Gilson (1997)[4]	↑15 wk	↑15 wk	—b	→	↑26 wk	3

a Early measurements not available.
b No change in LV EDD was observed; however, LV EDV was also used as an index of preload status and an increase was noted.
Control: 1 = pregnant; 2 = early pregnant; 3 = postpartum
CO = cardiac output; LV = left ventricle; SV = stroke volume; EDD = end-diastolic dimension; EDV = end diastolic volume; TPR = total peripheral resistance

tween studies is illustrated by Geva et al., who reported no change during pregnancy in left ventricular end-diastolic dimensions.[31] The 12-week values in the Geva study are nearly identical to those reported by Robson, the difference being that Geva compared pregnant to postpartum values while Robson compared to prepregnant values. This same problem exists in other studies of ventricular dimensional changes during pregnancy in which no gestational increases were reported.[10,36]

The fundamental question regarding the relationship between increasing stroke volume during pregnancy and its relationship to preload is discussed in more detail in Chapter 4.

Independent of changes in loading conditions, overt structural changes in the heart have been observed that may affect cardiac function in pregnancy. Increased left ventricular mass, often characterized by increased wall thickness, represents one adaptive response to pregnancy that is not contingent on the Starling mechanism. When left ventricular mass is increased, the heart functions on a new pressure–volume curve such that the filling pressure associated with a given volume may be shifted, increasing stroke volume. Left ventricular mass is calculated using values for chamber dimension and wall thickness. In all of the studies described, left ventricular mass increased throughout gestation, although there is some disagreement as to when the changes were initiated.[1,3,8,10,11,31-34,36]

Robson et al. reported that left ventricular mass was significantly increased by the 12th week of pregnancy and that it was 52% greater than prepregnant values by 38 weeks.[8] Echocardiographic data revealed marked hypertrophy of the left ventricle as evidenced by increases in posterior wall thickness as well as intraventricular septal thickness. These findings were corroborated by Geva et al., who also reported a marked hypertrophy of the left ventricle with increases in left ventricular mass and wall thickness noted by the 10th week.[31] These observed increases in left ventricular mass have been compared to the hypertrophic state that is commonly observed as a consequence of chronic exercise. Normalizing the left ventricular mass to body mass[36] removes the gestational effect while correcting to body surface area retains the significant increase.[31] However, either normalization is problematic as the former does not accurately reflect changes in lean body mass and the latter cannot be accurately estimated by conventional formulae during pregnancy.[1]

While the presence of ventricular hypertrophy suggests an increased ventricular performance due to an increase in the mass of myofibrils (see Fig. 3–1), other functional assessments are required to describe "contractility." Ventricular contractility during pregnancy has been assessed with both load-sensitive and load-adjusted indices of contractility.[8,10,31,32,36] The assessment of ventricular function using fractional shortening, ejection fraction, or velocity of circumferential shortening (all load-sensitive indices) demonstrated either enhanced function or no significant change.[31] Load-sensitive indices of contractility are difficult to interpret due to the difference in loading conditions and heart rate between nonpregnant and pregnant women.

The evaluation of ventricular performance using load-adjusted indices of contractility is in reasonable agreement to each other.[31,32,36]

The relationship between the velocity of shortening that is corrected to heart rate and end-systolic wall stress (termed stress-velocity index) was used to assess myocardial contractility in ten normal pregnant women during early labor, the early postpartum period, and at 4 weeks' postpartum.[32] This relationship, which is an afterload-adjusted and preload independent index of contractility, is graphed in Figure 3–5. These data points are superimposed on a "mean contractility line." This line and the shaded area surrounding it derive from studies of the stress–velocity index obtained in 78 normal subjects during baseline conditions and pharmacologic manipulation of afterload, preload, and contractility. The confidence limits (shaded area) define normal left ventricular contractility over the physiologic range in this nonpregnant population. In the time period of the study by Lang et al, there is a rightward and downward shift of the data points from visit 1 to visit 3 with the values remaining on the mean contractility line, indicating an increase in afterload without changes in contractility.

Mone et al. (1996) also compared the relationship between the stress–velocity index and heart rate corrected velocity of shortening in 33 women studied at six time points during and twice after normal gestation to the same "contractility line." The late gestation and early postpartum assessments of contractility are in agreement with Lang et al.[32,36]

Of interest in the study by Mone et al., the early pregnancy values are at the upper limits of normal (two SDs from the mean) such that there was a significant linear decline in the stress–velocity index throughout gestation reaching a nadir at the 2- to 4-week postpartum examination. These results were corroborated in a similar study conducted by Geva et al. in 1997.[31] Both groups speculated that this trend may be caused by hormonal factors or autonomic changes that influence cardiac

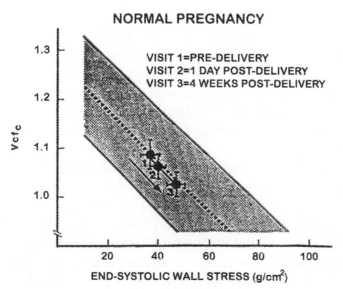

NORMAL PREGNANCY

VISIT 1=PRE-DELIVERY
VISIT 2=1 DAY POST-DELIVERY
VISIT 3=4 WEEKS POST-DELIVERY

END-SYSTOLIC WALL STRESS (g/cm²)

Figure 3–5. Average end-systolic wall stress (T_{es})-rate-corrected of fiber shortening (V_{cfc}) obtained in normotensive pregnant control subjects before delivery and 1 day and 4 weeks after delivery. From visit 1 to visit 3, data points shifted rightward and downward (arrow) but still fell on the mean contractility line, indicating increase in afterload without changes in contractility. (*Reprinted, with permission, from Lang RM, et al: Left ventricular mechanics in preeclampsia. Am Heart J 1991;121:1768–1775.*)

function independent of loading conditions. Taking all studies together, it may be concluded that systolic ventricular performance is preserved throughout pregnancy when assessed using load-independent indices. It would be of interest to compare the stress–velocity index during pregnancy to a population mean for this index that is obtained from female subjects studied during their reproductive years.

Systemic Arterial Parameters

A major conclusion drawn from all the above studies in pregnant women is that the gestational effect on afterload is a major contributor to ventricular performance and cardiac output changes during pregnancy. Afterload (or the arterial system load) is the mechanical opposition to the movement of blood out of the left ventricle. This arterial system load can be divided into a steady component, well known as the total or systemic vascular resistance and the pulsatile component. Systemic vascular resistance is determined primarily by the cross-sectional diameter of the resistance vasculature and as noted above, its marked decline during gestation is well characterized. Less easy to grasp is the concept of pulsatile load which is the load faced by the heart due to the response of the arterial tree to oscillations in pressure and flow.[38] It is possible that alterations in pulsatile load are responsible for maintaining the efficiency of ventricular–arterial coupling during pregnancy. In other words, understanding this component of the arterial tree should help us understand why cardiovascular performance remains intact despite the massive changes in volume and vascular tone occurring during pregnancy.[10,38]

Pulsatile load includes global arterial compliance (a measure of arterial-reservoir properties), aortic characteristic impedance (determined by local vessel wall stiffness and geometric properties), and indices of wave propagation and reflection (pulse wave velocity and global reflection coefficient).[10,38] These parameters were derived, in a study by Poppas et al., using noninvasive measures of instantaneous aortic pressure and flow velocities from 14 normal pregnant women during each trimester and again postpartum. A model-based analysis of instantaneous aortic pressure and flow velocities was performed to better understand changes in arterial compliance and wave propagation properties.[10] Global arterial compliance increased approximately 30% early in pregnancy and remained elevated thereafter. In this study, the change in compliance was temporally related to the decrease in systemic vascular resistance (Fig. 3–6). The observation of increased compliance during pregnancy is in keeping with other studies of vessel compliance in humans and animals during pregnancy.[39-45]

The increase in arterial compliance early in gestation suggests that an increase in vascular distensibility rather than the presence of the uteroplacental circulation is the major contributor to the change in compliance.[10] The two most likely contributors to increased vessel distensibility are vascular wall remodeling and reduced smooth muscle tone. The time course of vascular remodeling changes during pregnancy remains to be determined as most studies examined this parameter in late gestation. Reduced smooth muscle tone is one of the earliest detectable

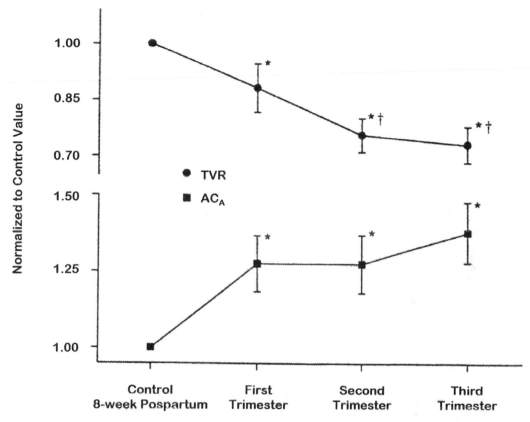

Figure 3–6. Temporal changes in AC_A and TVR during normal pregnancy. Data are normalized to 8-week postpartum control values (mean ± SEM; *P < 0.05, first, second, or third trimester vs. 8-week postpartum control; [†]P < 0.05, second or third vs. first trimester). (*Reprinted, with permission, from Poppas A, et al: Serial assessment of the cardiovascular system in normal pregnancy: Role of arterial compliance and pulsatile arterial load. Circulation 1997;95:2407–2415.*)

changes during gestation, supporting its contribution to the increase in arterial compliance.[1,7,8,46]

A fraction of the total power generated by the heart is consumed in maintaining the pulsatile nature of pressure and flow. This component of total power, termed oscillatory power, does not result in any net forward flow and therefore can be considered as wasted power. The ratio of the oscillatory power to the total power was used in this study as a measure of the inefficiency of LV–arterial coupling.[10] Total, steady, and oscillatory power were calculated from the instantaneous aortic pressure and flow velocity data. Total power increased significantly throughout pregnancy, attaining a peak value during the third trimester. Increments in both the steady and oscillatory components contributed to the increase in total power (Fig. 3–7). As a consequence, the ratio of oscillatory to total power, or the energy wasted in pulsations, was not significantly affected by pregnancy.[10]

In this same report the aortic characteristic impedance tended to decrease, but the changes were not significantly different.[10] A similar study using a larger cohort

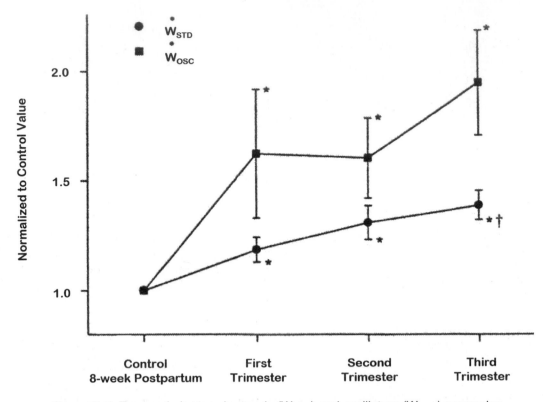

Figure 3–7. Temporal changes in steady (W_{STD}) and oscillatory (W_{OSC}) power during normal pregnancy. Data are normalized to 8-week postpartum control values (mean ± SEM; *$P < 0.05$, first, second, or third trimester vs. 8-week postpartum control; †$P < 0.05$, second or third vs. first trimester). (*Reprinted, with permission, from Poppas A, et al: Serial assessment of the cardiovascular system in normal pregnancy: Role of arterial compliance and pulsatile arterial load.* Circulation *1997; 95:2407–2415.*)

reported a significant decline in characteristic impedance during pregnancy.[36] The tendency for the aortic characteristic impedance to fall coupled with systemic vasodilation resulted in a reduction of the magnitude of arterial wave reflection. The model-based analysis performed on these data revealed that wave reflections at the aorta are delayed and arterial compliance increased for both conduit and systemic vessels. The results of the modeling are consistent with the concept that a generalized reduction in vascular tone is the factor most responsible for pulsatile arterial load changes during pregnancy. However, decreases in systemic vascular resistance alone are inadequate to explain the experimental observations; concomitant changes in wave propagation properties, including arterial compliance are necessary.[10]

The increased arterial compliance, coupled with changes in wave reflection and left ventricular properties described above, serves to counterbalance the effects of reduced systemic vascular resistance to maintain the efficiency of the left ventricle to arterial system energy transfer. Increased compliance also offsets the effect of reduced systemic vascular resistance on aortic diastolic pressure decay, thus preserving perfusion pressure to the coronary arteries and other vital organs.[10] The idea that without changes in pulsatile arterial load, reductions in systemic vascular resistance are actually deleterious to cardiovascular performance is a foreign concept to perinatal physiologists. It will be of great interest to examine whether women who develop preeclampsia fail to demonstrate a similar change in pulsatile arterial load. The idea is intriguing since it fully integrates the structural changes that pregnancy may induce in the vascular compartment with the regulation of vascular smooth muscle tone, addressing as depicted in Figure 3–1, the multifactorial components responsible for adequate tissue perfusion during pregnancy.

Systemic Venous Parameters

The lack of information regarding venous regulation during pregnancy greatly impairs our ability to evaluate this system during normal pregnancy and relate normal function to potential changes with preeclampsia. A Medline search of the literature through the middle of 1998 that used pregnancy as a focus and exploded the term "vein" resulted in 39 papers since 1965. The paucity of information during pregnancy explains the absence of any discussion of this critical contributor to cardiovascular performance in the first edition of Chesley's book.

The complex interactions between blood pressure, heart rate, end-diastolic filling and volume, ventricular contractility, and stroke volume, as well as the difficulty in accurately assessing vascular capacitance, impair our understanding of its role in cardiovascular homeostasis.[47] The volume expansion of pregnancy superimposed on potential intrinsic changes in venous regulation further clouds the issue.

Definitions. Terminology is often confused in the venous literature as a whole, and the pregnancy literature is no exception. Vascular capacity and vascular capacitance are often used interchangeably—but they are different parameters. Vascular capacity is the total blood volume contained at a specific distending pressure and is the sum of the unstressed volume and the stressed volume. The unstressed volume is the volume of the circulation at zero distending pressure while the stressed volume is the additional volume above the unstressed volume that is associated with a positive distending pressure. Vascular capacity is the volume at a specific pressure, whereas capacitance represents the entire volume/pressure relationship at a given level of venous smooth muscle tone. A change in venous smooth muscle activity leads to a new and different pressure–volume curve. Compliance (the ratio of the change in volume to a change in distending pressure), capacity, and stressed and unstressed volume are all subsets of vascular capacitance and the terms are not interchangeable. Furthermore, a true assessment of vascular capacitance in any physiologic or pathophysiologic condition requires an evaluation of all these component parts.[47,48]

Vascular capacitance is a major factor influencing the filling of the right heart and therefore has a critical effect on cardiac output in the intact circulatory system.[47,48] Any pregnancy-induced alteration of venomotor tone regulation will have a significant impact on cardiac output regulation.

Edema.   In addition to their role in the regulation of cardiac output, the proximal venules contribute to the exchange processes of tissues including the resorption of interstitial fluid and the transport of large molecules.[48] It is the instantaneous ratio of pre- to postcapillary resistance that determines the hydrostatic pressure of the blood in the exchange vessels and the filtration–resorption balance. The venules function as postcapillary flow resistors in controlling the transport processes between the intravascular and interstitial space.[49,50] As such, the normal edema formation of pregnancy and the abnormal patterns observed in preeclampsia are in part a function of veno-arterial regulatory mechanisms.[48,51] The marked change in precapillary arterial resistance during pregnancy would presumably require a similar adjustment in the postcapillary resistance regulation in order to maintain appropriate fluid dynamics in the capillary circulation.

Most of what we know about pregnancy-induced changes in venous regulation derives from animal studies, with only a few human studies on record.[15,41,42,51-64] The majority of literature during pregnancy focuses on three areas: the mean circulatory filling pressure, venous compliance and/or distensibility, and venomotor tone regulation. Venous distensibility is the change in volume with a change in pressure and its measured value will be affected by the amount of venous smooth muscle tone.

Mean Circulatory Filling Pressure.   The venous return to the right heart dynamically maintains the filling pressure, allowing adaptation to changing cardiac output requirements. A prerequisite for such regulation is that the vascular bed of appropriate tone should be adequately filled with blood. The mean circulatory filling pressure characterizes this steady state veno-cardiac coupling.[48] It is the pressure in the circulation after the heart has been arrested and the system has come into equilibrium.[65] The mean circulatory filling pressure provides an indication of the relationship between changes in blood volume compared to the size of the circulatory compartment and as such, it indicates to what extent the vascular compartment accommodates the gestational increase in blood volume.[41] Venous smooth muscle activation and changes in blood volume are mechanisms for changing the mean circulatory filling pressure.[47]

Data regarding the mean circulatory filling pressure during pregnancy derive from the animal literature, as arresting the heart in normal healthy pregnant women is experimentally problematic. Humphreys and Joels measured the mean circulatory filling pressure and related this measure to changes in unstressed volume, vascular compliance, and vascular capacity in pregnant rabbits.[41] The authors were careful to address potential technical limitations of this study. In spite of the noted limitations, it remains one of the better assessments of these parameters during pregnancy. The mean circulatory filling pressure following cardiac arrest was slightly, but significantly higher in the pregnant compared to nonpregnant rabbits

(7.2 ± 0.4 mm Hg vs. 6.1 ± 0.7 mm Hg, P < 0.01). The increase during pregnancy in mean circulatory filling pressure at control blood volume agrees with some earlier studies in other species.[42,53]

Figure 3–8 depicts the linear portion of the curves that Humphreys and Joels obtained relating the mean circulatory filling pressure to changes in blood volume. This curve is used to assess changes in compliance as well as unstressed volume. The slope of the regression line for these curves is significantly reduced in the pregnant rabbits, indicating an increase in vascular compliance, while extrapolation of the regression lines to the volume axis indicates no significant difference in unstressed vascular volumes. It is this increase in vascular compliance that allows for volume expansion during pregnancy with only a slight increase in mean circulatory filling pressure. Further support for this conclusion comes from the measure of vascular capacity. At a distending pressure of 6 mm Hg, the vascular capacity was

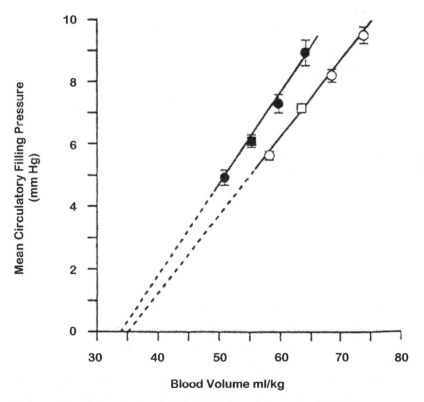

Figure 3–8. Mean circulatory filling pressure (MCFP) 0.5 minutes after reducing blood volume by 8% and increasing blood volume by 8 and 16% in 11 nonpregnant (•) and 10 pregnant rabbits (○). Changes are based on control blood volumes of 55.3 mL/kg in nonpregnant rabbits and 63.7 mL/kg in pregnant rabbits (see legend for Fig. 3–1). Lines are mean regression lines for each group, which have been extrapolated to volume axis. Vertical bars represent = 1 SE; square on each regression line indicates MCFP at control blood volume. (*Reprinted, with permission, from Humphreys PW, Joels N: Effect of pregnancy on pressure–volume relationships in circulation of rabbits. Am J Physiol 1994;267:R780–R785.*)

59.5 mL/kg in the pregnant rabbits and 54.5 mL/kg in the nonpregnant rabbits. This increase was sufficient to accommodate ≈60% of the 8.4 mL/kg increase in blood volume before incurring a change in mean circulatory filling pressure.[41] Davis et al. reported a larger increase in vascular capacity during pregnancy in the guinea pig, accounting for the smaller change in mean circulatory filling pressure in that study.[42] Increased compliance has also been observed in the pregnant dog with some disagreement between studies as to whether unstressed volume is also increased.[52,53] Factors that can contribute to changes in vascular capacitance include reduced sympathetic tone to capacitance vessels, stress relaxation in response to increased volume, and structural changes in the vessel walls.[41]

In reality, pressure–volume or stress–strain relationships of the venous wall cannot be accurately characterized either in vivo or in vitro without defining the contractile state of the vascular smooth muscle.[48] Measures of compliance or distensibility in vivo cannot distinguish between changes in wall structure from those caused by differences in venomotor tone. In the only known study in which the vascular smooth muscle was inactivated prior to assessing the stress–strain characteristics of mesenteric veins during pregnancy, the compliance of the mesenteric capacitance veins of Sprague–Dawley rats decreased by 40%, however, the unstressed volume doubled in comparison with nonpregnant females.[57] In the human, noninvasive measures suggest that venous distensibility increases with pregnancy[59-61,63] but this is not found in all studies[15,58,64] and could possibly be explained by differences in basal venomotor tone during the measurement period. This complicates the interpretation of the literature in venous distensibility measures during normal pregnancy or preeclampsia. Indeed authors use both the term "venous tone"[66] and "venous distensibility" when describing data obtained from venous plethysmography—a standard noninvasive technique for measuring venous distensibility. There are no longitudinal measures in human venous distensibility that include preconceptual values.

In the experiments by Humphreys and Joels, inhibiting sympathetic tone while making direct measures of vascular capacitance did not remove the difference in mean circulatory filling pressure between groups, indicating that the autonomic nervous system did not appear to be a major contributing factor to the observed changes in capacitance during pregnancy.[41] However, these studies were performed under anesthesia which might confound the results. While pressure–flow curves obtained in perfused vascular beds[67] as well as direct measures of stiffness in isolated arteries[45,68] support structural changes in the arterial system, there are too few data to make any such statement about venular structural changes during pregnancy.

Venomotor Tone Regulation.   In terms of cardiovascular homeostasis, the "active" regulation of capacitance remains a key question during pregnancy as this is one of the important mechanisms for influencing venous return to the heart. The systemic reflex capacitance reaction in humans is estimated to be ≈5 mL/kg.[48] The densely innervated, mesenteric venous microcirculation seems to have a key function in controlling the changes in vascular capacity. The majority of the blood volume shift in the intestinal vascular bed during activation of the baroreceptor reflex occurs in the intestinal venules.[48]

There is one study in which the effects of pregnancy on adrenergic regulation of capacitance veins was examined directly.[56] The response of capacitance-size mesenteric veins from cycling, early pregnant, and late pregnant rats transmural to nerve stimulation is depicted in Figure 3–9. The measured response to nerve stimulation at different frequencies was the percentage change in diameter compared with the diameter before each stimulation. There was a progressive decline in the sensitivity to sympathetic nerve stimulation from cycling to late gestation rats (Fig. 3–9). The frequency–response curves were repeated in the presence of the reuptake inhibitor, cocaine, which diminished the difference between the groups, suggesting that changes in neuronal reuptake mechanisms contributed in part to the observed responses. The reduced sympathetic nerve response was associated with a marked increase in sensitivity to exogenously applied norepinephrine during gestation, suggesting a possible denervation supersensitivity.[56] This decrease in sensitivity to nerve stimulation coupled with an increase in sensitivity to an exogenous adrenergic agonist indicates the potential complexity of the venular response to perturbations in cardiovascular homeostasis during pregnancy. In this same

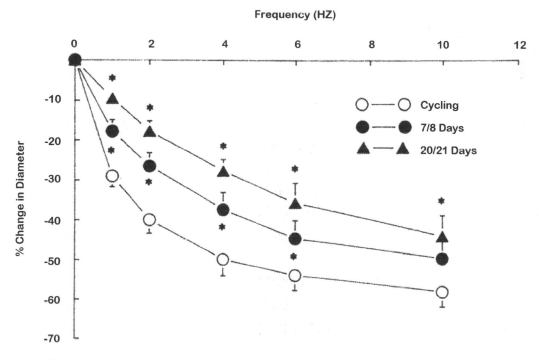

Figure 3–9. Response of mesenteric veins from nonpregnant cycling (N = 5), early-pregnant (N = 6), and late-pregnant (N = 5) rats to transmural nerve stimulation. Response is expressed as a percentage of change in diameter before contraction. Data are means ± SE. *P < 0.05 vs. control. (*Reprinted, with permission, from Hohmann M, et al: Norepinephrine sensitivity of mesenteric veins in pregnant rats. Am J Physiol 1990;259:R753–R759.*)

study, experiments performed on veins from pseudopregnant rats suggested that fetoplacental-dependent humoral effects initiated and reinforced the response to sympathetic nerve stimulation whereas differences in exogenous norepinephrine sensitivity seemed to be of maternal origin.

Summary.   In spite of the remarkable importance of venous function to cardiovascular homeostasis, we know little about pregnancy-induced changes in this system. In general, venous distensiblity/compliance increases during gestation although animal data would suggest that increased vascular capacitance does not quite accommodate the increase in blood volume. Whether mean circulatory filling pressure changes during human pregnancy is unknown. The sympathetic regulation of venous function both in terms of the regulation of venous return as well as fluid exchange in the capillary bed during pregnancy is of great interest, but little is known. Animal data suggest a reduction in the response to sympathetic activity. In summary, this is an area that requires a great deal of attention if we are to formulate a complete picture of the normal cardiovascular adaptation to pregnancy and subsequent changes during preeclampsia.

FACTORS RESPONSIBLE FOR CHANGES IN CARDIAC OR VASCULAR PROPERTIES

The regulation of cardiovascular function during pregnancy is dependent upon a complex interplay of systems as demonstrated in Figure 3–1. Blood pressure and its response to vasoactive stimuli have been the focus of many earlier studies in the search for mechanisms that cause the hemodynamic changes during pregnancy. This is because pressure is readily available and measurable at endpoint. However, the focus on blood pressure per se has probably inhibited our understanding of all the potential regulatory phenomena involved in the hemodynamic adaptation to pregnancy as it truly is an endpoint of all the factors noted in Figure 3–1. As each aspect of function is studied, it is apparent that many (if not all) of these parameters are affected by pregnancy. This caveat regarding blood pressure is true as well for studies pertaining to preeclampsia.[69]

Mechanisms for Overall Hemodynamic Response

Metabolic Control
Increases in systemic oxygen consumption provide a potent stimulus for increasing cardiac output as the goal of maintaining blood pressure is to provide sufficient tissue perfusion to meet metabolic needs (see Fig. 3–1). Due to the anabolic nature of gestation, it is reasonable to suggest that an increase in oxygen demand drives the cardiovascular response to pregnancy. In fact, there is a calculated increment of 51 mL O_2/min in basal oxygen consumption from preconceptual values during human pregnancy. This constitutes 20% of the total maternal oxygen uptake at term

and is a reflection of the metabolic demand of the pregnancy.[70] Most of the increased oxygen demand occurs in the heart, diaphragm, kidney, and the utero-placental unit.[70] The majority of the oxygen demand derives from the uterus and its contents in the last third of gestation.[70] However, the cardiovascular response to pregnancy peaks during the first half of gestation which is prior to this major increase in oxygen demand. Another indication that the cardiovascular response is greater than necessary to meet early metabolic needs is that the increase in systemic oxygen transport during pregnancy exceeds the increase in oxygen consumption. This is indicated by the narrowing of the arterial-mixed venous oxygen content.[71] Thus, the hemodynamic changes in pregnancy precede any significant increase in oxygen demand, and metabolic influences are not likely to constitute initiating signals to the increased cardiac output and reduced systemic vascular resistance.

Autonomic Nervous System

While the autonomic regulation of the cardiovascular system is a prime target for modification during pregnancy, its study is complicated by the baseline differences in heart rate, blood pressure, and blood volume occurring with pregnancy.[72]

Leon Chesley's chapter, "Blood Pressure and Circulation," in the previous edition of this text reviews the early work describing the effect of autonomic blockade on blood pressure maintenance in pregnant women. When supine, autonomic blockade resulted in a marked hypotensive effect that was alleviated by moving into the lateral recumbent position, suggesting that the predominant hypotensive effect of autonomic blockade was due to a loss of venomotor tone.

Pan et al., in an extensive study of blood pressure regulation in the pregnant rat, showed that blood pressure decreased profoundly and to a similar degree (40–50%) after either ganglionic or selective α-adrenoreceptor blockade in both gravid and nonpregnant rats, indicating that the adrenergic nervous system was of quantitatively similar importance in the maintenance of basal arterial pressure between the pregnant and nonpregnant condition.[73]

Assessing nervous activity directly is a better measure of the degree of sympathetic activity during pregnancy since the vascular smooth muscle response to sympathetic neurotransmitters may itself differ during pregnancy. O'Hagan and Casey evaluated renal sympathetic nerve activity in the chronically instrumented, pregnant rabbit, circumventing the difficulty of studying nervous activity under anesthesia during pregnancy. At rest, there was no effect of pregnancy on renal sympathetic nerve activity during late gestation.[74]

The differences in posture between rodents and humans might suggest that comparing the two is not prudent. Yet, in a carefully designed study in the human, Schobel and colleagues quantitated the level of sympathetic nerve activity to skeletal muscles' blood vessels using peroneal nerve microneurography. The measured basal sympathetic nervous activity did not differ between normal pregnant and age-matched, nonpregnant women (although it was increased in women with preeclampsia).[75] These human data support the animal literature that pregnancy does not affect the basal regulation of vascular tone by the sympathetic nervous system. However, the skeletal bed represents only one of the major regulators of systemic vascular resistance. The effect of pregnancy upon renal sympathetic nerve activity or splanchnic innervation in the human is unknown.

The largest body of literature regarding autonomic nervous system function during pregnancy concerns the regulation of pressure-mediated changes in heart rate and blood pressure. Studies conducted during early pregnancy examined reflex heart rate responses to pressure changes as an index of arterial baroreflex function.[72] Since the baroreflex regulation of heart rate is under both vagal and sympathetic influences, it is not necessarily reflective of the sympathetic control of vascular resistance and blood pressure. Newer studies directly measure sympathetic outflow in response to a variety of stimuli.[72,74] There is still no information about the effects of pregnancy on the afferent inputs to the central nervous system in response to pressure stimuli.

When studied in the awake state, the baroreflex-mediated heart rate response to increasing pressure stimuli is either enhanced, unchanged, or depressed during pregnancy.[72,76-81] These apparent discrepancies probably reside in the time of gestation studied and the differences in the control heart rate between pregnant and nonpregnant subjects. In experiments in which the normal gestational difference in resting heart rate exists prior to imposed pressure steps, the reflex bradycardia is accentuated by pregnancy.[72,77,81] This suggests that pregnancy augments sympathetic inhibitory activity to the heart in response to elevated blood pressures.

In the above studies pregnancy has little effect on the heart rate response to decreases in blood pressure.

Although the tachycardic response to hypotension appears unaffected by pregnancy, this does not reflect the overall sympathetic response to hypotension. Pregnant rats demonstrate an attenuated ability to increase renal sympathetic nerve outflow above baseline in response to hypotensive challenges.[78] The basal renal nerve outflow was increased during pregnancy in this same study, although data normalization for this measure is problematic. Pregnancy does not affect the basal postganglionic sympathetic nerve activity in skeletal blood vessels. In addition, there is no pregnancy effect upon the increase in sympathetic activity that occurs in response to a cold pressor test.[75] In general, systemic vasoconstriction in response to hypotension appears diminished by pregnancy while reflex tachycardia is maintained. The ability to increase cardiac output while buffering systemic vasoconstriction can serve to protect regional blood flows such as the uterine circulation during hypotensive challenges.[78]

There is remarkably little known about mechanisms responsible for pregnancy-induced changes in autonomic nervous system function. The progesterone metabolite 3α-hydroxy-dihydroprogesterone (3α-OH-DHP) that is elevated during pregnancy, has been shown to reduce renal sympathetic nerve activity through the activation of GABA receptors in the rostral ventrolateral medulla when administered acutely to the rat.[78] Interestingly, 3α-OH-DHP administration does not affect the baroreflex control of heart rate in nonpregnant rats in response to hypotension which is consistent with the lack of a pregnancy effect on reflex tachycardia.[78]

Cardiac Function

Various animal models have contributed to our understanding of potential mechanisms responsible for changes in cardiac function during pregnancy.[39,42,82,83] Similar to the vascular wall (discussed below), the heart responds directly to changes in load. Many of the alterations discussed above may reflect a response to both decreases in afterload and increases in preload. Nonetheless, several investigators have suggested that alterations in ventricular compliance and chamber size may be due to direct hormonal signals rather than load changes per se.[8,36,39,42,82,83]

Sex Steroids

As discussed in Chapter 8, the pseudopregnant rat has been a useful model in trying to separate the role of maternal from fetoplacental factors in initiating the physiologic response to pregnancy. Studies examining changes in cardiac output and stroke volume in pseudopregnant and pregnant rats suggest that the initial change in cardiac performance does not require the presence of the conceptus.[83] Because the hormonal environments of pregnancy and pseudopregnancy are very similar during the first 8 days following mating, it is likely that the initiating stimulus is hormonal in nature deriving from the maternal compartment.[83] This observation is in keeping with studies of Chapman et al. of the luteal phase of the menstrual cycle.[12] Progesterone, estrogen, and prolactin levels are all comparable in these models and may contribute, either separately or in combination, to the changes in cardiac function. Similar observations have been made from this model for renal hemodynamics (see Chap. 8).

While direct evidence for the involvement of sex steroids in cardiac function during human pregnancy is still lacking, studies in the guinea pig and sheep do provide supportive evidence.[40,42] Hart et al. characterized the pressure–volume curves following removal of hearts from pregnant guinea pigs and it was noted that left ventricular chamber size had increased. Consequently, left ventricular diastolic volume was increased at a given pressure, shifting the pressure–volume curve to the right and resulting in an increased stroke volume.[40]

In a parallel study conducted in virgin guinea pigs, the effects of chronic sex steroid exposure on cardiac function were examined.[42] After 28 days of estradiol treatment, cardiac output, stroke volume, and blood volume were all increased as in the pregnant animals at day 20 of gestation. A similar shift in the pressure–volume relationship was observed, with increased volume at a given filling pressure. This was again attributed to an increase in chamber size. While there was no change noted in left ventricular mass in the estrogen-treated animals, virgin guinea pigs dosed with progesterone exhibited a significantly increased left ventricular weight, characteristic of hypertrophy. Because the steroid hormone levels attained in these experiments were considerably higher than those measured during pregnancy, it is difficult to compare the models and to distinguish pharmacologic from physiologic behavior. Nonetheless the remarkable similarities between the two study groups allow the speculation that elevated estradiol and/or progesterone levels early in pregnancy may contribute to marked changes in cardiac structure and performance.

In a similar study in sheep, a single dose of estradiol also resulted in a shift in pressure–volume relationship of the heart. Similar to the guinea pig, left ventricular end-diastolic dimension was increased at any given filling pressure. In this study, the steroid regimen changed cardiac performance independent of any noted changes in preload or afterload.[82] These animal data support the suggestion from the human studies that there are load-independent humoral factors that contribute to the structural change of the heart during gestation.

Vascular Tone and Reactivity

The pregnancy reduction in systemic vascular resistance is accompanied by a decrease in vascular reactivity, the magnitude of which varies according to species, gestational age, and the vasoactive stimuli examined.[70,84-87] Systemic vascular resistance decreases through an increase in the cross-sectional diameter of the resistance circulation. Cross-sectional area increases as a result of increases in arterial diameter in individual resistance vessels or through the presence of new vessel growth. While both these processes occur during pregnancy, the predominate change in the first half of gestation appears to be increased vascular diameter through the loss of vascular tone.

While numerous mechanisms are postulated to explain the loss of vascular tone and reactivity during pregnancy, a unified theory remains to be determined. Furthermore, the mechanisms responsible for initiating the reduced vascular tone at the beginning of the pregnancy may be quite different than those that contribute to its maintenance throughout gestation. The vascular wall is very responsive to mechanical forces.[88-90] Early changes in blood pressure, blood flow, and wall stress due to active vascular smooth muscle relaxation can potentially induce further changes in endothelial cell and vascular smooth muscle structure and function that serve to maintain the initial vasodilation. Such changes would not then be the direct result of the mechanisms that cause the initial vasodilation. The mechanism(s) responsible for the initial relaxation would appear to be the key to understanding the regulation of systemic vascular resistance in general during pregnancy. The significant reduction in systemic vascular resistance that occurs during the luteal phase of the menstrual cycle is likely to be carried through into pregnancy.[12] This observation should focus our attention on study design for determining the mechanisms for the pregnancy-induced loss of vascular tone.

Structural Changes

Arterial diameter can increase with either relaxation of the vascular smooth muscle or through a structural remodeling of the vessel wall affecting diameter regulation.[90,91] Structural changes in the resistance vasculature can contribute to alterations in diameter regulation by affecting signal transduction through the vascular wall, i.e., the response to changes in pressure, flow, and shear stress.[91-94] Data from various species, including humans, would suggest that both structural changes and active vascular smooth muscle relaxation occur during pregnancy. Structural changes are evident by late gestation in the resistance arteries of the rat[45] and also occur in conduit arteries such as the aorta of the human[39] and the main uterine artery of all species studied. These changes include changes in geometry, decreased stiffness (or increased compliance), and associated changes in matrix protein content.[39-45,95]

Autonomic Nervous System

As discussed above, a reduction in afferent sympathetic outflow to the resistance vasculature could readily explain the reduction in systemic vascular resistance. However, the alterations in autonomic nervous system activity during pregnancy appear to be more involved in an organism's ability to respond to pressure stimuli rather than changing the basal tone maintenance per se. Evaluation of the regulatory role of the autonomic nervous system however, is a bit complex, as there is evidence that vascular reactivity to neurotransmitters is reduced during normal pregnancy.[70,84,96]

One of the best studies available to assess adrenergic vascular reactivity during pregnancy in humans was performed by Nisell et al.[96] The study combined measuring blood levels of the administered agonists, calf blood flow, and cardiac output in both pregnant and nonpregnant subjects. This verified that both groups received an equivalent experimental stimuli and allowed evaluation of the components of the pressor response. The absolute blood pressure response to norepinephrine, the primary sympathetic neurotransmitter, did not differ between groups. Of importance, however, the pressor response in the pregnant women was due solely to an increase in cardiac output, while in the nonpregnant women it was caused by systemic vasoconstriction. This is an elegant example of the difficulty in examining blood pressure alone as a measure of systemic vascular reactivity. The identical blood pressure response between groups suggested no pregnancy effect. Based upon the cardiac output data however, the correct conclusion to be drawn was that normal pregnancy blunted the systemic vasoconstrictor response to norepinephrine.

Although basal sympathetic outflow does not decrease during pregnancy in humans (at least to the skeletal bed),[75] the vascular response to vasoconstrictor neurotransmitters is probably reduced. Thus, a given level of nervous acitvity may result in a different vascular response. It is very likely that there are local mechanisms within the arterial wall itself that account for the pregnancy relaxation and these in turn are initiated by humoral signals deriving from the ovary, the placenta, or possibly the pituitary.

Steroids

Steroid hormones, particularly estrogen and progesterone, are likely candidates for initiating the early vasodilation.[86,97,98] However, the evidence for their role is strongest with regard to volume homeostasis, cardiac remodeling, and uterine blood flow regulation.[42,84,86,99] Steroid hormone treatment of the nonpregnant rat does not duplicate the reduction of systemic vascular resistance nor the changes in renal hemodynamics with pregnancy.[98] Nonetheless, the initial rise in glomerular filtration rate, the increased cardiac output, and the reduction in systemic vascular resistance in the rat are due to signals maternal in origin, as these changes occur in pseudopregnant animals in which the hormonal profile mimics the first 8 to 10 days of rat gestation in the absence of any fetoplacental contribution.[83,99,100] Placental factors, as yet undetermined, contribute to the maintenance of glomerular filtration rate later in pregnancy in the rat.

Endothelial Factors

Vasoactive molecules derived from the endothelium are likely candidates for modifying vascular smooth muscle tone during gestation.[84,85,87] As noted above, this is the subject of several reviews which are only briefly summarized here.[70,84-87]

Prostaglandins are highly vasoactive molecules produced in the endothelium as well as the vascular smooth muscle and platelets. Under normal conditions, vasodilatory prostaglandins do not appear to participate in the pregnancy-induced vasodilation with perhaps the exception of the uterine vasculature.[84,101-103] Prostaglandins can compensate when other important vascular mediators such as nitric oxide, a molecule produced by nitric oxide synthase in the endothelium, is inhibited.[104] There are several other studies in the rat that suggest that the nitric oxide synthase and cyclooxygenase systems are quite responsive to perturbations in the animal. For example, mild vitamin E deprivation has a fairly profound effect on the balance between these two systems in the functional behavior of resistance-size mesenteric arteries from the rat. The nature of the cyclooxygenase products produced in this model is altered by pregnancy.[105-107] This is of interest in preeclampsia as one of several theories involves the role of oxidative stress in the disease process.

Experiments to demonstrate a greater modification of vascular behavior by any class of molecules require that the removal of their influence should cause a greater loss of tone or potentiation in response to vasoactive stimuli in the pregnant vs. nonpregnant groups. Nitric oxide synthase inhibition in most studies during late gestation in the rat causes a greater potentiation of pressure responsiveness to angiotensin II and norepinephrine than in nonpregnant controls. Whether this is true for total systemic resistance requires measures of the cardiac output in order to calculate effects on vascular resistance and hence, specific vessel effects[85] (see "Autonomic Nervous System" above).

Two interesting studies used venous plethysmography women to isolate vascular responses to a particular bed. The data suggest a role for nitric oxide in the control of hand and forearm blood flow and the vascular reactivity to angiotensin II during normal human pregnancy.[108,109]

The second messenger for nitric oxide, cyclic GMP, increases in plasma and urinary excretion of nitrite, and nitrate parallels this rise in animals on a low nitrite diet. This demonstrates that endogenous nitric oxide production increases in rats (also reported in ewes), although the source of production remains to be identified. Whether it occurs in humans still awaits longitudinal analysis of 24-hour urine samples before, during, and after pregnancy while on controlled diets.[85,87]

In the renal circulation, nitric oxide synthase inhibition at midgestation equalizes glomerular filtration, renal plasma flow, and renal vascular resistance between pregnant and nonpregnant animals.[110] This is supported by in vitro differences in myogenic reactivity which are normalized between groups with nitric oxide synthase inhibition during midgestation in the rat.[111] However, in late gestation where myogenic reactivity is likewise reduced, nitric oxide synthase inhibition does not cause an increase in reactivity normalizing the responses between groups.[112] Chapter 8 provides a comprehensive discussion of the role of sex steroids, peptide hormones, and endothelium-derived relaxing factors in mediating the renal vasodilation.

In blood vessels from humans, a large component of the relaxation response to acetylcholine is mediated by non-nitric oxide synthase mechanisms.[113,114] While there is evidence for an increase in mRNA transcripts in the aorta from the pregnant rat there is no convincing evidence that basal nitric oxide synthase activity has increased during pregnancy either through measures of cyclic GMP in large vessels such as the aorta or measures of arginine to citrulline conversion in other vascular beds.[85,87] The signal transduction pathway distal to nitric oxide is unchanged during pregnancy, a remarkably consistent finding among the numerous reported studies. Since the complete time course and the systemic generality of the endothelial changes occurring in pregnancy are unknown, the initiating signals for the early vasodilation remain to be determined.

Vascular Smooth Muscle

Remarkably little is known about vascular smooth muscle regulation during pregnancy. Observations have included: (1) reductions in vascular smooth muscle contractility and/or reactivity; (2) hyperpolarization of vascular smooth muscle resting membrane potential;[115] and (3) numerous potential alterations in receptor function and endothelial modification of one or all of the above.[70,84-87] Little is known about postmembrane signal transduction. Observations are limited to describing the organ or cellular response to pregnancy and the initiating mechanisms require further examination. Based upon the data available, it appears that we have a more comprehensive understanding of the potential mechanisms involved in the regulation of renal and uterine hemodynamics during pregnancy than the rest of the circulation.

Organ Blood Flow

Individual organ blood flows help serve to identify the major contributors to the reduced systemic resistance. Leon Chesley in his first edition chapter, "Blood Pressure and Circulation," provides a comprehensive analysis of the earlier work in humans that characterizes blood flow changes during gestation, summarized in

Tables 1 through 7. A 1994 review by Stock and Metcalfe covers the animal as well as the human literature.[70]

Flow increases to the renal, uterine, coronary, mammary, skin, diaphragm, and skeletal beds, although the gestational pattern of change differs between species. The increase in uterine blood flow becomes more pronounced as gestation advances, mirroring the increase in fetal growth. In sheep, this marked increase in uterine blood flow does not keep pace with the growth of the fetus and placenta, resulting in an increase in uterine oxygen extraction as pregnancy proceeds.[70] Whether this is true for humans is not known.

The most profound circulatory change in nonreproductive tissues is that which occurs in renal hemodynamics as discussed in detail in Chapter 8. There is an increase in glomerular filtration rate due to an increase in renal plasma flow that appears to coincide with the very early rise in heart rate and cardiac output. This represents the earliest significant change in organ blood flow associated with pregnancy.

Of particular interest to the study of preeclampsia are potential changes occurring during pregnancy in cerebral blood flow regulation. The study quoted in Leon Chesley's first edition chapter suggests that normal pregnancy has no effect on cerebral blood flow. However, the pregnancy data were compared to "nonpregnant" controls who happened to be men. In addition, total blood flow was measured using the nitrous oxide method; potential regional changes in flow would not be detected by this method.

Ikeda at al. studied 10 women at 7 to 19 weeks' gestation and again 50 days postmedical pregnancy termination using the xenon 133 washout technique by means of single-photon emission computed tomography.[116] There were 8 to 13% decreases in flow in the frontal, temporal, and parietal lobes with no significant difference in the occipital lobe following the termination. This suggested that pregnancy resulted in early increases in maternal regional cerebral blood flow. These data contrast somewhat with an earlier study by the same group, although subject selection, gestational age, measurement techniques (Doppler), and the sites of measurement differed between the two studies.[117] The authors note a small literature suggesting gender differences in cerebral blood flow with women in their reproductive years having a higher cerebral blood flow than men of the same age. A study by Belfort et al. showed a reduced resistance index in small-diameter cerebral vessels in late-gestation women compared to a nonpregnant control group. In the same study, estradiol treatment of postmenopausal women also reduced the resistance index, lending support to the idea of a hormonal effect on cerebral blood flow regulation.[118] Whether such effects are direct or not is unknown. The important question as to the status of cerebral blood flow in women who will develop preeclampsia–eclampsia, or those who already have the disease, remains unanswered as current studies are in remarkable conflict with each other.[119-122]

Noninvasive measures of uterine blood flow in women have contributed some additional information to Chesley's original review. Diameter and mean flow velocity measurements obtained by Doppler and imaging ultrasound were combined to yield volumetric flow in the common iliac and uterine arteries in a nonpregnant control group and 18 pregnant women. The uterine artery diameter doubled by 21 weeks' gestation, with peak diastolic velocity measures occurring at 36 weeks' gestation. The estimated unilateral uterine artery blood flow at week 36 was 312 mL/min. The authors noted a decrease in external iliac artery flow, suggesting a redistribution of pelvic flow to favor the uterus.[123] Their calculated uterine artery flow is in remarkable agreement with a similar study performed by Thaler et al. who report a unilateral flow of 95 mL/min before pregnancy increasing to a mean of 342 mL/min in late gestation.[124]

CONCLUSION

Based on the responses described here, it is apparent that the most important changes in cardiac function occur in the first 8 weeks of pregnancy. The temporal relationships between the hemodynamic parameters that define cardiac function may be summarized as follows (as depicted in Fig. 3–1). Cardiac output is increased as early as the 5th week of pregnancy and this initial increase is a function of reduced systemic vascular resistance and an increase in heart rate. Between weeks 10 and 20, notable increases in plasma volume occur such that preload is increased. Ventricular performance during pregnancy is influenced by both the decrease in systemic vascular resistance and changes in pulsatile arterial load. Our knowledge of the regulation of venous capacitance during pregnancy is limited. Vascular capacity increases due, in part, to an increase in vascular compliance. Multiple factors contribute to these changes in overall hemodynamic function allowing the cardiovascular system to adjust to the physiologic demands of the fetus while maintaining maternal cardiovascular performance.

ACKNOWLEDGMENTS
The authors thank Susan Davis and Michelle Misiak Reed for expert secretarial support, the library staff, and Tracy Keith, PhD for her thoughtful comments. This work was supported by US Public Health Service research grants R01 HD30325 and 2 PO1 HD30367.

REFERENCES

1. Clapp JF, Capeless E: Cardiovascular function before, during, and after the first and subsequent pregnancies. *Am J Cardiol* 1997;80(11):1469–1473.
2. Moutquin JM, et al: A prospective study of blood pressure in pregnancy: Prediction of preeclampsia. *Am J Obstet Gynecol* 1985;151:191–196.
3. VanOppen ACC, et al: A longitudinal study of maternal hemodynamics during normal pregnancy. *Obstet Gynecol* 1996;88:40–46.
4. Gilson GJ, et al: Changes in hemodynamic, ventricular remodelling, and ventricular contractility during normal pregnancy: A longitudinal study. *Obstet Gynecol* 1997;89:957–962.
4a. Lees MM, et al: A study of cardiac output at rest throughout pregnancy. *J Obstet Gynaecol Br Commonw* 1967;74:319–328.

5. Duvekot JJ, et al: Early pregnancy changes in hemodynamics and volume homeostasis are consecutive adjustments triggered by a primary fall in systemic vascular tone. *Am J Obstet Gynecol* 1993;169:1382–1392.
6. Duvekot JJ, Peeters LLH: Maternal cardiovascular hemodynamic adaptation to pregnancy. *Obstet Gynecol Surv* 1994;49:S1–S14.
7. Capeless EL, Clapp JF: Cardiovascular changes in early phase of pregnancy. *Am J Obstet Gynecol* 1989;161:1449–1453, pt 1.
8. Robson SC, et al: Serial study of factors influencing changes in cardiac output during human pregnancy. *Am J Physiol* 1989;256:H1060–H1065.
9. Page EW, Christianson R: The impact of mean arterial pressure in the middle trimester upon the outcome of pregnancy. *Am J Obstet Gynecol* 1976;125:740–746.
10. Poppas A, et al: Serial assessment of the cardiovascular system in normal pregnancy: Role of arterial compliance and pulsatile arterial load. *Circulation* 1997;95:2407–2415.
11. Hunter S, Robson SC: Adaptation of the maternal heart in pregnancy. *Br Heart J* 1992;68: 540–543.
12. Chapman AB, et al: Systemic and renal hemodynamic changes in the luteal phase of the menstrual cycle mimic early pregnancy. *Am J Physiol* 1997;273:F777–F782.
13. Christianson R: Studies on blood pressure during pregnancy. 1. Influence of parity and age. *Am J Obstet Gynecol* 1976;125:509.
14. Reiss RE, et al: Retrospective comparison of blood pressure course during preeclamptic and matched control pregnancies. *Am J Obstet Gynecol* 1987;156:894–898.
15. Smith AJ, et al: Hypertensive and normal pregnancy: A longitudinal study of blood pressure, distensibility of dorsal hand veins and the ratio of the stable metabolites of thromboxane A_2 and prostacyclin in plasma. *Br J Obstet Gynaecol* 1995;102:900–906.
16. Quinn M: Automated blood pressure measurement devices: A potential source of morbidity in preeclampsia. *Am J Obstet Gynecol* 1994;170:1303–1307.
17. Halligan A, O'Brien E: Ambulatory blood pressure monitoring during pregnancy: Establishment of standards of normalcy. *Am J Hypertens* 1996;9:1240–1241.
18. Higgins JR, et al: Can 24-hour ambulatory blood pressure measurement predict the development of hypertension in primigravidae? *Br J Obstet Gynaecol* 1997;104:356–362.
19. Gupta M, et al: Accuracy of oscillometric blood pressure monitoring in pregnancy and preeclampsia. *Br J Obstet Gynaecol* 1997;104:350–355.
20. Brown MA, et al: Ambulatory blood pressure monitoring during pregnancy. Comparison with mercury sphygmomanometry. *Am J Hyperten* 1993;6(9):745–749.
21. Churchill D, Beevers DG: Differences between office and 24-hour ambulatory blood pressure measurement during pregnancy. *Obstet Gynecol* 1996;88:455–461.
22. Öney T, Meyer-Sabellek W: Variability of arterial blood pressure in normal and hypertensive pregnancy. *J Hyperten* 1990;8:S77–S81.
23. Beilin LJ, et al: Circadian rhythms of blood pressure and pressor hormones in normal and hypertensive pregnancy. *Clin Exp Pharmacol Physiol* 1982;9:321–326.
24. Sawyer MM, et al: Diurnal and short-term variation of blood pressure: Comparison of preeclamptic, chronic hypertensive, and normotensive patients. *Obstet Gynecol* 1981;58: 291–296.
25. Benedetto C, et al: Blood pressure patterns in normal pregnancy and in pregnancy-induced hypertension, preeclampsia, and chronic hypertension. *Obstet Gynecol* 1996;88:503–510.
26. Seligman SA: Diurnal blood-pressure variation in pregnancy. *J Obstet Gynecol* 1971;78: 417–422.
27. Redman CWG, Beilin LJ, Bonnar J: Reversed diurnal blood pressure rhythm in hypertensive pregnancies. *Clin Sci Mol Med* 1976;51:687s–689s.
28. Halligan A, et al: Diurnal blood pressure difference in the assessment of preeclampsia. *Obstet Gynecol* 1996;87:205–208.
29. Ayala DE, et al: Heart rate and blood pressure chronomes during and after pregnancy. *Chronobiologia* 1994;21(3–4):215–225.
30. Uttendorfsky OT, et al: Blood pressure measurements during pregnancy: Circadian rhythm? *Am J Obstet Gynecol* 1983;146(2):222–225.
31. Geva T, et al: Effects of physiologic load of pregnancy on left ventricular contractility and remodeling. *Am Heart J* 1997;133:53–59.

32. Lang RM, et al: Left ventricular mechanics in preeclampsia. *Am Heart J* 1991;121:1768–1775.
33. Mabie WC, et al: A longitudinal study of cardiac output in normal human pregnancy. *Am J Obstet Gynecol* 1994;170:849–856.
34. Robson SC, et al: Combined doppler and echocardiographic measurement of cardiac output: Theory and application in pregnancy. *Br J Obstet Gynaecol* 1987;94:1014–1027.
35. Bader RA, et al: Hemodynamics at rest and during exercise in normal pregnancy as studied by cardiac catheterization. *J Clin Invest* 1955;34:1524–1536.
36. Mone SM, Sanders SP, Colan SD: Control mechanisms for physiological hypertrophy of pregnancy. *Circulation* 1996;94:667–672.
37. Opie LH: Mechanisms of cardiac contraction and relaxation. In: Braunwald E, ed. *Heart Disease: A Textbook of Cardiovascular Medicine*, 5th ed, vol 1. Philadelphia: WB Saunders; 1997; 360–393.
38. Shroff SG: Pulsatile arterial load and cardiovascular function—facts, fiction, and wishful thinking. *Therapeutic Res* 1998;19(2):59–66.
39. Hart MV, et al: Aortic function during normal human pregnancy. *Am J Obstet Gynecol* 1986;154:887–891.
40. Hart MV, et al: Hemodynamics during pregnancy and sex steroid administration in guinea pigs. *Am J Physiol* 1985;249:R179–R185.
41. Humphreys PW, Joels N: Effect of pregnancy on pressure–volume relationships in circulation of rabbits. *Am J Physiol* 1994;267:R780–R785.
42. Davis LE, et al: Vascular pressure–volume relationships in pregnant and estrogen-treated guinea pigs. *Am J Physiol* 1989;257:R1205.
43. Slangen BFM, et al: Aortic distensibility and compliance in conscious pregnant rats. *Am J Physiol* 1997;272:H1260–H1265.
44. Danforth DN, Manalo-Estrella P, Buckingham JC: The effect of pregnancy and of Enovid on the rabbit vasculature. *Am J Obstet Gynecol* 1964;88:952–959.
45. Mackey K, et al: Composition and mechanics of mesenteric resistance arteries from pregnant rats. *Am J Physiol* 1992;263:R2–R8.
46. Robson SC, et al: Serial changes in pulmonary haemodynamics during human pregnancy: A non-invasive study using Doppler echocardiography. *Clin Sci* 1991;80:113–117.
47. Rothe CF: Physiology of venous return: An unappreciated boost to the heart. *Arch Intern Med* 1986;146:977–982.
48. Monos E, Bérczi V, Nádasy G: Local control of veins: Biomechanical, metabolic, and humoral aspects. *Physiol Rev* 1995;75(3):611–666.
49. Mellander S, Björnberg J: Regulation of vascular smooth muscle tone and capillary pressure. *NIPS* 1992;7:113–124.
50. Mellander S, et al: Autoregulation of capillary pressure and filtration in cat skeletal muscle in states of normal and reduced vascular tone. *Acta Physiol Scand* 1987;129:337–351.
51. Rosén L, et al: Mechanisms for edema formation in normal pregnancy and preeclampsia evaluated by skin capillary dynamics. *Int J Microcirc* 1990;9:257–266.
52. Cha SC: Influence of pregnancy on mean systemic filling pressure and cardiac function in guinea pigs. *Can J Physiol Pharmacol* 1992;70:669–674.
53. Douglas BH: Effect of hypervolemia and elevated arterial pressure on circulatory dynamics in pregnant animals. *Am J Obstet Gynecol* 1967;98:889–894.
54. Goodlin RC: Mean circulatory filling pressure in pregnant rabbits. *Am J Obstet Gynecol* 1984;148:224.
55. MacCausland AM, et al: Venous distensibility during pregnancy. *Am J Obstet Gynecol* 1961;81:472–479.
56. Hohmann M, et al: Norepinephrine sensitivity of mesenteric veins in pregnant rats. *Am J Physiol* 1990;259:R753–R759.
57. Hohmann M, et al: Venous remodeling in the pregnant rat. *Clin & Exp Hypertension Preg B* 1991;10:307–321.
58. Duncan SLB, Bernard AG: Venous tone in pregnancy. *J Obstet Gynaecol Br Commonw* 1968;75:142–150.
59. Fawer R, et al: Effect of the menstrual cycle, oral contraception and pregnancy on forearm blood flow, venous distensibility and clotting factors. *Eur J Clin Pharmacol* 1978;13:251–257.

60. Goodrich SM, Wood JE: Peripheral venous distensibility and velocity of venous blood flow during pregnancy or during oral contraceptive therapy. *Am J Obstet Gynecol* 1964;90:740–744.
61. Pickles CJ, et al: Changes in peripheral venous tone before the onset of hypertension in women with gestational hypertension. *Am J Obstet Gynecol* 1989;160:678–680.
62. Skudder PA, Farrington DT: Venous conditions associated with pregnancy. *Semin Dermatol* 1993;12:72–77.
63. Sakai K, et al: Venous distensibility during pregnancy: Comparisons between normal pregnancy and preeclampsia. *Hypertension* 1994;24:461–466.
64. Edouard DA, et al: Venous and arterial behavior during normal pregnancy. *Am J Physiol* 1998;274:H1605–H1612.
65. Guyton AC, Polizio D, Armstrong GC: Mean circulatory filling pressure measured immediately after cessation of heart pumping. *Am J Physiol* 1954;179:261–272.
66. Stainer K, et al: Abnormalities of peripheral venous tone in women with pregnancy-induced hypertension. *Clinical Science* 1986;70:155–157.
67. Humphreys PW, Joels N: The response of the hind-limb vascular bed of the rabbit to sympathetic stimulation and its modification by pregnancy. *J Physiol* 1982;330:475–488.
68. McLaughlin MK, Keve TM: Pregnancy-induced changes in resistance blood vessels. *Am J Obstet Gynecol* 1986;155:1296–1299.
69. Roberts JM, Redman CWG: Pre-eclampsia: More than pregnancy-induced hypertension. *Lancet* 1993;341:1447–1452.
70. Stock MK, Metcalfe J: Maternal physiology during gestation. In: *The Physiology of Reproduction*, ed 2. New York: Raven Press; 1994:947–973.
71. Gilson GJ, Mosher MD, Conrad KP: Systemic hemodynamics and oxygen transport during pregnancy in chronically instrumented, conscious rats. *Am J Physiol* 1992;263:H1911–H1918.
72. Heesch CM, Rogers RC: Effects of pregnancy and progesterone metabolites on regulation of sympathetic outflow. *Clin Exp Pharmacol Physiol* 1995;22:136–142.
73. Pan Z-R, et al: Regulation of blood pressure in pregnancy: Pressor system blockade and stimulation. *Am J Physiol* 1990;258:H1559–H1572.
74. O'Hagan KP, Casey SM: Arterial baroreflex during pregnancy and renal sympathetic nerve activity during parturition in rabbits. *Am J Physiol* 1998;274:H1635–H1642.
75. Schobel HP, et al: Preeclampsia—A state of sympathetic overactivity. *N Engl J Med* 1996;335:1480–1485.
76. Ekholm EMK, et al: Cardiovascular autonomic reflexes in mid-pregnancy. *Br J Obstet Gynaecol* 1993;100:177–182.
77. Leduc L, et al: Baroreflex function in normal pregnancy. *Am J Obstet Gynecol* 1991;165(4):886–890, pt 1.
78. Masilamani S, Heesch CM: Effects of pregnancy and progesterone metabolites on arterial baroreflex in conscious rats. *Am J Physiol* 1997;272:R924–R934.
79. Brooks VL, Keil LC: Changes in the baroreflex during pregnancy in conscious dogs: Heart rate and hormonal responses. *Endocrinology* 1994;135:1894–1901.
80. Ekholm EMK, Erkkola RU: Autonomic cardiovascular control in pregnancy. *Eur J Obstet Gynecol Reprod Biol* 1996;64:29–36.
81. Conrad KP, Russ RD: Augmentation of baroreflex-mediated bradycardia in conscious pregnant rats. *Am J Physiol* 1992;262:R472–R477.
82. Giraud GD, et al: Estrogen-induced left ventricular chamber enlargement in ewes. *Am J Physiol* 1993;264:E490–E496.
83. Slangen BFM, et al: Hemodynamic changes in pseudopregnancy in chronically instrumented conscious rats. *Am J Physiol* 1997;272:H695–H700.
84. Poston L, McCarthy AL, Ritter JM: Control of vascular resistance in the maternal and fetoplacental arterial beds. *Pharmacol Ther* 1995;65:215–239.
85. Sladek SM, Magness RR, Conrad KP: Nitric oxide and pregnancy. *Am J Physiol* 1997;272:R441–R463.
86. Magness RR, Gant NF: Control of vascular reactivity in pregnancy: The basis for therapeutic approaches to prevent pregnancy-induced hypertension. *Semin Perinatol* 1994;18:45–69.
87. McLaughlin MK, Conrad KP: Nitric oxide biosynthesis during pregnancy: Implications for circulatory changes. *Clin Exp Pharmacol Physiol* 1995;22:164–171.

88. Davies PF, et al: Spatial relationships in early signaling events of flow-mediated endothelial mechanotransduction. *Annual Rev Physiol* 1997;59:527–549.

89. Mulvany MJ, Aalkjaer C: Structure and function of small arteries. *Physiolog Rev* 1990; 70(4):921–961.

90. Gibbons GH, Dzau VJ: The emerging concept of vascular remodeling. *N Engl J Med* 1994;330(20):1431–1438.

91. Gandley RE, et al: Contribution of chondroitin-dermatan sulfate-containing proteoglycans to the function of rat mesenteric arteries. *Am J Physiol* 1997;273:H952–H960.

92. Johnson P: The myogenic response. In: Greiger SR (ed.): *Handbook of Physiology. The Cardiovascular System. Vascular Smooth Muscle*. Bethesda, MD: American Physiological Society;1980:409–442.

93. Johnson P: Autoregulation of blood flow. *Circ Res* 1986;59:483–496.

94. Brayden JE, Halpern W, Brann LR: Biochemical and mechanical properties of resistance arteries from normotensive and hypertensive rats. *Hypertension* 1983;5:17–25.

95. Griendling KK, Fuller EO, and Cox RH: Pregnancy-induced changes in sheep uterine and carotid arteries. *Am J Physiol* 1985;248:H658–H665.

96. Nisell H, Hjerndahl P, Linde B: Cardiovascular responses to circulating catecholamines in normal pregnancy and in pregnancy-induced hypertension. *Clin Physiol* 1985;5:479–493.

97. Pepe GJ, Albrecht ED: Actions of placental and fetal adrenal steroid hormones in primate pregnancy. *Endocrine Rev* 1995;16(5):608–648.

98. Conrad KP, et al: Effects of 17β-estradiol and progesterone on pressor responses in conscious ovariectomized rats. *Am J Physiol* 1994;266:R1267–R1272.

99. Baylis C: Glomerular filtration and volume regulation in gravid animal models. *Bailliére's Clin Obstet Gynaecol* 1994;8:235–264.

100. Buttrick PM, et al: Effects of pregnancy on cardiac function and myosin enzymology in the rat. *Am J Physiol* 1987;252:H846–H850.

101. Conrad KP, Dunn MJ: Renal synthesis and urinary excretion of eicosanoids during pregnancy in rats. *Am J Physiol* 1987;253:F1197–F1205.

102. Conrad KP: Possible mechanisms for changes in renal hemodynamics during pregnancy: Studies from animal models. *Am J Kidney Dis* 1987;IX:253–259.

103. Magness RR, et al: Endothelial vasodilator production by uterine and systemic arteries. I. Effects of ANG II on PGI_2 and NO in pregnancy. *Am J Physiol* 1996;270:H1914–H1923.

104. Danielson LA, Conrad KP: Prostaglandins maintain renal vasodilation and hyperfiltration during chronic nitric oxide synthase blockade in conscious pregnant rats. *Circ Res* 1996; 79:1161–1166.

105. Davidge ST, et al: Pregnancy and lipid peroxide-induced alterations of eicosanoid-metabolizing enzymes in the aorta of the rat. *Am J Obstet Gynecol* 1993;169:1338–1344.

106. Davidge ST, Hubel CA, McLaughlin MK: Cyclooxygenase-dependent vasoconstrictor alters vascular function in the vitamin E-deprived rat. *Circ Res* 1993;73:79–88.

107. Davidge S, Hubel C, McLaughlin M: Lipid peroxidation increases arterial cyclooxygenase activity during pregnancy. *Am J Obstet & Gynecol* 1994;170:215–222.

108. Williams DJ, et al: Nitric oxide-mediated vasodilation in human pregnancy. *Am J Physiol* 1997;272:H748–H752.

109. Anumba D, et al: The role of nitric oxide in the modulation of vascular tone in normal pregnancy. *Br J Obstet Gynaecol* 1996;103:1169–1170.

110. Danielson LA, Conrad KP: Nitric oxide mediates renal vasodilation and hyperfiltration during pregnancy in chronically instrumented, conscious rats. *J Clin Invest* 1995;96:482–490.

111. Gandley RE, Conrad KP, McLaughlin MK: Nitric oxide regulates myogenic behavior in the renal resistance vasculature at mid-pregnancy in the rat. *J Soc Gynecol Invest* 1996; 3(2)(suppl):100A.

112. Gandley RE, et al: Intrinsic tone and passive mechanics of isolated renal arteries from virgin and late pregnant rats. *Am J Physiol* 1996;1997:R22–R27.

113. Pascoal IF, Umans JG: Effect of pregnancy on mechanisms of relaxation in human omental microvessels. *Hypertension* 1996;28:183–187.

114. Pascoal IF, et al: Contraction and endothelium-dependent relaxation in mesenteric microvessels from pregnant rats. *Am J Physiol* 1995;269:H1899–H1904.

115. Meyer MC, Brayden JE, McLaughlin MK: Characteristics of the vascular smooth muscle in the maternal resistance circulation during pregnancy. *Am J Obset & Gynecol* 1994;169: 1510–1516.

116. Ikeda T, et al: Effect of early pregnancy on maternal regional cerebral blood flow. *Am J Obstet Gynecol* 1993;168:1303–1308.

117. Ikeda T, Mori N: Assessment of cerebral hemodynamics in pregnant women by internal carotid artery pulsed Doppler velocimetry. *Am J Obstet Gynecol* 1990;163:494–498.

118. Belfort MA, et al: Effects of estradiol-17β and progesterone on isolated human omental artery from premenopausal nonpregnant women and from normotensive and preeclamptic pregnant women. *Am J Obstet Gynecol* 1996;174:246–253.

119. Williams KP, Wilson S: Maternal cerebral blood flow changes associated with eclampsia. *Am J Perinatol* 1995;12:189–191.

120. Demarin V, Rundek T, Hodek B: Maternal cerebral circulation in normal and abnormal pregnancies. *Acta Obstet Gynecol* (Scand) 1997;76:619–624.

121. Morriss MC, et al: Cerebral blood flow and cranial magnetic resonance imaging in eclampsia and severe preeclampsia. *Obstet & Gynecol* 1997;89:561–568.

122. Ohno Y, et al: Transcranial assessment of maternal cerebral blood flow velocity in patients with pre-eclampsia. *Acta Obstet Gynecol* (Scand) 1997;76:928–932.

123. Palmer SK, et al: Quantitative estimation of human uterine artery blood flow and pelvic blood flow redistribution in pregnancy. *Obstet Gynecol* 1992;80(6):1000–1006.

124. Thaler I, et al: Changes in uterine blood flow during pregnancy. *Am J Obstet Gynecol* 1990;162:121–125.

4

Control of Volume and Body Tonicity

Jacques A. Dürr and Marshall D. Lindheimer

Editors' Comment

Chesley, in this text's first edition, took a standard approach to volume and tonicity. Chapter 8, "Fluid and Electrolytes," summarized the literature, documenting increases in plasma and red cell volumes in normal pregnancy and the lower values observed in preeclamptic gestations. There was a detailed analysis of the methodology and results of studies designed to determine interstitial fluid content, as well as total body and intracellular water. His review, and a number of tables citing the older literature bear rereading, and reflect the positions on these subjects in contemporaneous texts, the more recent reports being mainly confirmatory in nature. Chesley also discussed the significance of "gestational hypervolemia" focusing on the effect of the "dilutional anemia" on viscosity, and considering the increase in volume as a reservoir defense against hemorrhage, though he did suggest it helped fill the dilated vasculature!

The topic of volume and tonicity during pregnancy remained descriptive through most of the decade which followed this text's first edition, when suddenly controversy arose concerning interpretation of the observed volume changes. To some, the physiologic hypervolemia of pregnancy was seen as a suboptimal response to the general arterial vasodilation characteristic of gestation, the so-called "underfill" and "primary arterial vasodilation" theories. Others espoused views that the hypervolemia is absolute ("overfill"), an epiphenomenon to other changes such as increased levels of circulating mineralocorticoids; and still others believed that a series of changes ("resetting") in volume control during gestation lead to a state where the increased absolute volume is "sensed" as normal ("normalfill"). (See references 1 through 8 to appreciate these controversies.)

In the late 1990s, led by the reports from Schrier and Peeters and their colleagues,[1,2,4,5,7,8] respectively, the "underfill" theory has gained momentum to a point where theory is being hailed by some as dogma. The importance of settling these disputes is not trivial, as the view that prevails will have broad influences both in our understanding and management of preeclampsia. Thus, the chapter which follows, while noting the changes in volume and tonicity in normal pregnancy, devotes considerable discussion to the controversy described above. In addition, an essay containing an historical review of concepts such as "effective" volume and osmolality, written by the first author, has been added as an appendix. The editors believe that these topics have extreme relevance, not only to the research scientist but to the clinician managing patients with edematous and hypertensive disorders.

INTRODUCTION

Marked alterations in the volume, as well as the composition and dynamics of body fluids take place during gestation. All fluid compartments enlarge and cardiac output increases. There is a proportionally larger increase in plasma volume than red cell mass, producing the "physiologic anemia of pregnancy," and similarly, the cumulative gain of water in excess of sodium and other solutes results in the "gestational hyponatremia." Also of interest is that the control mechanisms which determine homeostasis "conspire" to preserve these changes around their *new steady states* as if they were the norm for pregnancy. Thus, effective plasma osmolality (P_{osm}) (or its surrogate, plasma sodium, P_{Na}) is maintained some 10 mOsm/kg/H_2O (or ~5 mEq/L) below nonpregnant values by the simultaneous downward resetting of the osmolality thresholds for thirst sensation and vasopressin release.[3,9] Similarly, any change in blood volume to values above or below the new steady state are corrected appropriately, as if the absolute increase in volume during pregnancy were "sensed" as normal.[3]

The significance of these changes in the *milieu interieur* is debated. Some interpret these as a physiologic adaptation to the metabolic demands of pregnancy, while for others these changes are but reflex hemodynamic responses to the stress of pregnancy. The teleologically meaningful views that the cumulative gains in salt and water shield the pregnant woman and her fetus from potentially deleterious accidents such as bleeding from a *placenta previa*, or that the decreased P_{osm} facilitates volume expansion when salt is unavailable, are seductive. Thus, as recalled by Chesley,[10] by the end of the 18th century, physicians had noted the extraordinary tolerance of pregnant women for hemorrhage, and "the plethora of pregnancy" was a common concept that kept alive the Galenic tradition of phlebotomy for any complication of gestation. This notion contrasts sharply with that of some reviewers who suggest that these changes, rather than desirable, are mere manifestations of the organism's attempts to restore a decreased "effective circulating blood volume." They argue that activation of the renin–aldosterone axis, salt and water retention, decreased blood pressure, tachycardia, and hyponatremia are all findings of pregnancy that can be seen as suggestive of vascular "underfill." Disciples of this dogma[2,3,5] see in pregnant subjects the characteristic state of "arterial underfill" first described by Frank Epstein and colleagues[11-13] in patients with traumatic systemic arteriovenous (AV) fistulae and Sheila Sherlock and her group in patients with cirrhosis of the liver,[14,15] respectively. Thus, as recounted by Dame Sherlock, the typical findings of palmar erythema, warm skin, bounding pulse wave, and bright red pulsating spider angiomata, prompted their demonstration of peripheral arterial vasodilation in patients with decompensated cirrhosis of the liver. They compared the circulatory state of their patients to that of the patients with systemic AV fistulae, studied by Epstein and colleagues,[11] and to that seen in the "generalized vasodilation of acute beriberi."[15] Peripheral arterial vasodilation in cirrhosis is now well accepted.[16]

As recalled by de Wardener,[17] Starling considered that renal salt and water retention was caused by a hemorrhage because, with the failing heart, "the vascular bed is bled into the veins and cardiac cavities." Thus, Starling recognized that salt and water excretion by the kidneys was controlled by changes in the volume of blood contained in the arteries and capillaries, rather than the total volume of blood. Epstein revived this notion by stressing that his patients with systemic AV fistulae are literally "bleeding into their own veins."[12] In retrospect, however, this cliché may have been unfortunate as it overdramatizes the "underfill," i.e., the hemorrhagic aspects of AV shunts, but neglects their associated counterpart, namely the "overflow" or increased venous return associated with the decreased resistance. Indeed, as will be discussed, in the case where the lowered vascular resistance occurs to the regions of the vascular bed where the flow becomes laminar and where exchanges of fluid and nutrients take place, i.e., in the setting of peripheral arteriolar vasodilation, the decrease in peripheral vascular resistance (PVR) may be viewed as a bonus rather than a handicap for overall cardiovascular performance. Thus, if by the end of the 18th century, the barber–surgeons and old-time physicians, who resorted to bloodletting, were familiar with the extraordinary tolerance of pregnant women for hemorrhage,[10] modern physiologists have realized their phenomenal cardiac competence as well. To best illustrate this point, it will suffice to recall that out of 26 female Soviet medal winners at the 1956 Olympic Games, 10 were pregnant at the time.[18]

Finally, in addition to the diverse views which assimilate pregnancy to a state of vascular overflow (plethora), underfill (peripheral vasodilation, placental AV shunting), or enhanced cardiovascular performance, there is a fourth opinion which simply assumes that volume homeostasis and renal salt and water handling are essentially normal during gestation, only occurring around different setpoints of cardiac output, blood volume, and body fluid tonicity.[19] Since, according to this last view, the hypertensive complications of gestation would be approached and treated in the same way as in the nonpregnant state,[20] it becomes obvious that these diverse theories, rather than of mere academic interest, have therapeutic implications. History shows that the management and therapy are greatly affected by the prevailing dogma. The controversy concerning salt restriction or the use of diuretics (today's version of phlebotomy) in the treatment of hypertension in gestation reflects our poor understanding of volume homeostasis in pregnancy. Thus, a clear knowledge of the physiology of body fluid regulation in pregnancy is essential for the comprehensive approach to preeclampsia, undoubtedly the most dramatic and still the most debated cardiovascular complication of gestation.

As discussed elsewhere,[3] for years dispute existed among obstetricians regarding the correct gestational values for blood volume, blood pressure, heart rate, cardiac output, glomerular filtration rate (GFR), effective renal plasma flow (ERPF), urine flow rate, urinary concentrating and diluting capacity, and renal handling of water, sodium, and other solutes. The notion that posture affects these parameters[21-23] eventually prevailed.[24,25] Indeed, it is now clear that during supine recumbency the gravid uterus hinders normal venous return.[25] The hemodynamic correlate, occasionally spectacular, is the supine hypotensive syndrome,[26,27] also referred to as the *vena cava inferior syndrome* demonstrable in 11% of pregnant women near term.[26] Thus, all the parameters of "effective blood volume" listed above are likely to be affected profoundly by posture. Eventually, lateral recumbency, proposed as early as 1933,[22,23] has emerged as the standard position for most renal function studies during gestation[27,28] (see Chap. 8). The measurement of static parameters such as blood volume is also markedly affected by posture, as venous pooling promotes transudation of fluid and retards the equilibrium of the dyes. The reader, therefore, must keep in mind these many methodologic pitfalls when reviewing the literature on volume regulation during gestation.

This chapter focuses on the functional aspects of osmoregulation and volume homeostasis. Wherever possible, we will complement the purely descriptive aspects of maternal body fluid homeostasis with a more comprehensive physiologic and historical analysis. Finally, some of these topics are quite controversial and depending on the bias one entertains, the same change in pregnancy may evoke either evolution, compensation, or merely accommodation. In such instances we will try to describe the evidence in a manner that permits the readers to draw their own conclusions.

BODY FLUID DISTRIBUTION

Weight Gain and Water Space

The weight gain of primigravidas averages 12.5 kg,[30,31] with the bulk occurring during the second half of gestation. At term, fetus, amniotic fluid, and placenta account for nearly 5 kg. The accumulation of fat accounts for another 3.5 to 4 kg over the first two-thirds of pregnancy.[32] The nonfat portion of the weight gain is best estimated by the volume of distribution of water. In studies using deuterium oxide (D_2O) as marker, the increase in total body water averaged 7.5 L[30,31,33] by 38 weeks' gestation. Extrapolated to term, the average gain in total water is 8.5 L.[30,33] In a subset of mothers with generalized edema but otherwise healthy, the mean increase in total body water was 10.8 kg.[30,33] Similar results have been confirmed by authors using water labeled with the sable isotope of oxygen (^{18}O), or by the less accurate but clinically more applicable method of bioelectrical impedance.[34-36]

The precise extracellular portion of the increase in water space is debated and ranges from 4 to 7 L. Extracellular markers such as Na-thiocyanate, mannitol, bromide, sodium, etc., may be inadequate in pregnancy since their protein binding (thiocyanate) or distribution between extra- and intracellular compartment changes and since, with few exceptions,[3] little is known about their penetration into the uterine contents.[37] Moreover, while the change in the intravascular portion of the extracellular fluid may follow a predictable course in pregnant women, the extravascular fraction which participates in the "edema of pregnancy" is extremely variable among subjects. Thus, the *average* gain of 6.5-kg based on a review of an extensive literature,[30] must be accepted with caution.

Intravascular Volume

In most studies only one component of the intravascular volume, either the plasma or red blood cell volume is measured directly. The other component is then calculated from the hematocrit. This may be inadequate[10] since the "peripheral vein" and "whole body" hematocrits are markedly different. Ideally, both volumes should be measured separately. Thus, the total blood volume, estimated with tagged red blood cells alone, was 11% smaller than when a dye was used simultaneously to measure plasma volume.[38] Of interest, in spite of all the hemodynamic alterations, including systemic vasodilation and decrease in hematocrit and blood viscosity, the "whole body hematocrit" may be 89% of the peripheral vein hematocrit, just like in the nonpregnant state. If plasma markers such as tagged albumin or Evans blue escape the intravascular compartment more promptly in late gestation, vascular volume may be overestimated. Conversely, the improper mixing of the tagged red cell or plasma marker due to pooling of blood in the lower extremities, may underestimate vascular volume. Taking all these potential pitfalls into consideration, Chesley's review of the literature suggests an average increase in blood volume of ~1.3 L.[10]

Plasma Volume

The increase in plasma volume starts in the first trimester, accelerates in midgestation, and stabilizes after the 34th week.[39-41] Compilation of individual measurements from 31 disparate studies performed on populations with diverse social, economic, and ethnic backgrounds, revealed a mean plasma volume of 2580 and 3655 mL for nonpregnant (N = 440) and pregnant (N = 955) women, respectively.[10] This represents, on average, a one liter or 42% increase in plasma volume.[10] The two curves in Figure 4–1 are from two studies performed in Aberdeen 10 years apart. Note that the typical decrease in plasma volume in late pregnancy disappeared when the pregnant subjects were studied in lateral recumbency.[41] Thus, 1200 mL may reflect more closely the true physiologic increase in plasma volume during pregnancy[3] (see also Table 9–1 in Chap. 9).

In most studies the weight of the baby at term correlates with the plasma volume expansion during gestation. This finding led to the assumption that maternal volume expansion is somehow beneficial to the baby, since the greater the expansion, the larger the baby. This theory seems further supported by the finding that hypertensive patients who fail to demonstrate normal plasma volume expansion also deliver babies who are smaller for their gestational age. However, this hypothesis may not be correct, and the converse may be true, i.e., larger babies, and hence placentae, may trigger larger increases in blood volume. Indeed, the increase in plasma volume does correlate with placental mass.[42] Thus, the determinant of

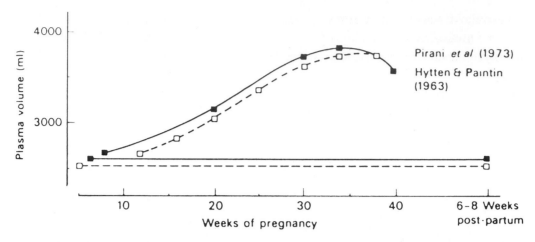

Figure 4–1. Changes in plasma volume during gestation. Results of two studies in primigravidae performed in Aberdeen, 10 years apart. In the 1973 study,[41] the subjects were placed in left lateral recumbency and the late pregnancy decrease in plasma volume is not apparent. (*Reprinted, with permission, from Letsky E: The haematological system. In: Hytten F, Chamberlain G, eds.* Clinical Physiology in Obstetrics. *Oxford: Blackwell Scientific Publications; 1980:43–78.*)

plasma volume expansion, in last analysis, may be the size of the product of conception. This alternative explanation also accounts for the larger changes in plasma volume observed in multiple pregnancies.

Note however that this last correlation has also been advanced as supporting the *shunt factor* in the etiology of plasma volume expansion. Thus, according to this other popular theory, the maternal volume expansion represents a compensatory salt and water retention triggered by a decrease in the *effective blood volume.*[1] However, since, as discussed, larger maternal blood volume expansion is associated with healthier babies, this last theory has to deal with a strange conclusion, one that predicts that a larger maternal hemodynamic stress results in a healthier baby. From the viewpoint of blood volume control, physiologists generally believe that *the increased blood volume in response to greater metabolic demands is a two-step operation in which the dimensions of the heart and vascular bed are first increased, while the ensuing demand for greater filling is satisfied in a second step.*[43]

This physiological sequence of events, however, may also occur in response to the opening of an AV shunt,[3] where the ensuing renal salt and water retention are aimed at satisfying the demand for better filling of the vascular tree. The cardiovascular implications of plasma volume expansion during pregnancy can therefore be viewed either as a normal physiologic response to increased metabolic demand or rather, the physiologic response to a pathologic process. The seemingly parallel relationship between the increasing blood volume and cardiac output described in the older literature is incorrect,[10,38] as are reports of preterm decreases in blood volume and cardiac output both being artifacts. Chesley[10] commented on the incidence of cardiac decompensation in heart disease patients which peaks in the 4th month of gestation. As expected, this corresponds to the time of maximum increase in cardiac output. Maximum plasma volume expansion, however, occurs later, reaching its maximum only during the 8th month. It has to be pointed out, nevertheless, that the peak incidence of cardiac decompensation seems to coincide temporally with the phase of accelerated plasma volume expansion and thus, one could argue that the increase in blood volume does burden the heart.

The alternative view that plasma volume expansion follows a deteriorating *effective blood volume* due to AV shunting has already been noted.[1] Systemic vasodilation and/or placental AV shunting could trigger a series of events which lead to volume expansion. The activation of the renin–angiotensin–aldosterone axis during gestation is often presented as evidence for such a mechanism. Indeed, the inexorable consequences of activation of this system are salt and water retention and volume expansion. However, this explanation may be too simplistic since, unlike in other states of vascular "underfill" with high plasma renin activity and stimulation of aldosterone, pregnancy is associated with an enhanced rather than depressed ability to excrete salt and water loads. This will be discussed further in the light of the overall regulation of "effective blood volume."

Finally, other nonhemodynamically mediated humoral mechanisms may also increase the blood volume. These may come from the placenta and/or the fetus. The idea of an embryo or fetus taking over and controlling maternal physiologic functions has occasionally captivated the imagination of an investigator dealing with one or another parameter in pregnancy.[44] Indeed, the placenta is a hormone factory and as a result it may be more appropriate to liken it to a gland rather than to a hollow AV shunt.[3] Thus, human placental lactogen (HPL), a hormone of trophoblastic origin, markedly potentiates the anabolic effect of growth hormone in hypophysectomized rats.[45] This hormonal synergism in itself may explain the cardiovascular and renal changes as well as the associated increase in plasma volume. On the other hand, molar pregnancy, a disorder characterized by a relative deficiency in HPL, is also associated with plasma volume expansion.[46] Finally, while in molar pregnancy, a cystic material of trophoblastic origin replaces the fetus in the uterine cavity, in pseudopregnancy (at least in rodents) the uterus is empty, yet plasma volume expansion occurs just like in normal pregnancy.[47,48] Thus, while it appears that the gestational increase in plasma volume cannot be accounted for by one single hemodynamic or endocrine mechanism, the presence of the product of conception is not required for the early changes to occur.

It becomes apparent, therefore, that plasma volume expansion may not be explained entirely by a normal physiologic response to an increased metabolic demand or a reduced *effective blood volume*. Thus, rather than guessing the causes of volume expansion in gestation, it may be more fruitful to assess its consequences. Besides favoring tissue perfusion, the increased blood volume can be viewed as a buffer in case of a massive hemorrhage such as occasionally occurs at delivery. Indeed, while a blood loss of 2 L would result in irreversible cardiovascular shock in a nonpregnant patient, it is tolerated remarkably well at delivery.[38] Thus, viewed from a teleologic perspective, the hypervolemia of pregnancy appears to be the provision set by nature which *allowed the human race to survive, especially prior to the advent of blood banks.*[38] Other important consequences of volume expansion will be discussed in relation to cardiovascular physiology.

Red Blood Cell Volume

While the plasma volume increases by ~1.2 L, the red blood cell mass increases by only 250 to 500 cc, depending on iron supplementation.[10,40,49] This leads to a relative hemodilution with a decrease in the hematocrit from an average of 40 to 33%. Thus, the physiologic anemia of pregnancy is merely dilutional and hides, in fact, an increase in red blood cell mass. In the rat, a species extensively used to study the physiology of pregnancy, increases in plasma volume and hemodilution are also consistent findings. However, in the rat, half of the increase in blood volume occurs over the last quarter of gestation and averages ~60%, a value somewhat larger than the ~45% increase observed in human gestation.[50]

Relevant to pregnancy may be the notion that red blood cells behave like passive osmometers and as a result should swell during dilutional hyponatremia. Thus, this prediction has been used advantageously in patients with sickle-cell disease, as an iatrogenic hyponatremia induced by dDAVP, resulted in a proportional dilution in the mean corpuscular hemoglobin concentration (MCHC), and hence in the frequency of sickle-cell crises.[51] Whether normal red blood cells like those from patients with sickle-cell anemia fail to regulate their own volume actively in vivo is not known. However, if this were the case, then changes in the MCHC induced by a decrease in plasma sodium concentration could be predicted by the formula $MCHC = (1 - \delta Na) \cdot MCHC_{nl}$, where δNa is the fractional change in plasma Na, and $MCHC_{nl}$, the normal MCHC. In spite of a significant decreased effective body tonicity, i.e., in spite of "total body dilution," no changes in MCHC or red cell mean corpuscular volume (MCV) seems to exist in normal pregnancy.[37,49] Therefore, the absence of any red cell swelling in the hypotonic environment of pregnancy implies a decrease in red blood cell solute content, and direct measurements of red cell electrolyte or solute content in both early[52] and late[53] gestation are consistent with such predictions.

A corollary of unchanged MCV is that the 250 to 400 mL increase in red blood cell mass during gestation is not merely the result of erythrocyte swelling. Thus, based on available evidence, one has to postulate that the red blood cell adapts to pregnancy by decreasing its solute content. As will be discussed further below, when extended to the entire body, the notion of a primary decrease in intracellular solute content could explain the decreased plasma sodium and the apparent reset osmostat of gestation.[3]

Interstitial Volume

The extravascular portion of the extracellular fluid increases by 1.7 L, but this increment is highly variable. The bulk of this volume (~95%) accumulates during the last quarter of gestation, at a time when the blood volume has reached a plateau, and hence may represent some "overflow." Acceptance of some edema as "physiological" in pregnancy comes from a retrospective review of a total of 24,079 medical records of women who delivered at the Aberdeen Maternity Hospital from the period of 1950 to 1959. Edema was reported in 40% of the charts and, furthermore, babies born to edematous mothers were less likely to be premature and were heavier than those born to nonedematous mothers.[54] In a prospective study, clinical evidence of edema was found at some stage in pregnancy in 80% of normal women.[55] The women who were free of clinical evidence of edema, nevertheless, had a progressive increase in leg volume and finger circumference similar to the rest of the subjects.

Although the association of an increased capillary hydrostatic pressure in the legs and a decreased colloid osmotic pressure due to the decrement in plasma albumin should increasingly favor accumulation of pedal edema as pregnancy advances, there is no correlation between leg edema and the level of oncotic pressure.[56] The accumulation of interstitial fluid during gestation does not appear to obey the classic Starling forces as fluid in ordinary pitting ankle edema would. Rather, an explanation for the accumulation of interstitial fluid in pregnancy may be found in the hormonal-induced changes of the mucopolysaccharide-rich ground substance.[31,56] The oncotic pressure exerted by proteins varies linearly with pH within physiological limits.[57] Of interest and of relevance to gestation, is that this pH dependency is more marked for the hyaluronate-rich protein constituents of the interstitium.[57] For example, the oncotic pressure exerted by Warton's jelly from the umbilical cord, a "model of the interstitium," is 16 times more sensitive to pH changes than plasma proteins.[57] This observation has obvious implications in body fluid distribution during gestation since, in addition to the changes in the ground substance, there is a decrease in pCO_2 and hence a tendency for respiratory alkalosis.[32] However, as noted by Chesley,[58] "although the question has been controversial for more than 40 years, the pH of the blood does not change significantly" (i.e., pH 7.44 vs 7.40), little is known of the pH of the interstitial space.

During pregnancy, the increased imbibition of the ground substance, to some extent an "interstitial sponge," may superficially mimic pitting edema. Its nature, however is different. The diffusion rate of low-molecular-weight solutes in this type of interstitial "gel" averages at least 95% of their diffusion rate in free fluid, yet the bulk flow of free interstitial fluid from one area to another is reduced more than 10,000-fold.[59] Thus, the function of this bound gel may be to prevent large shifts of free fluid to dependent locations, without preventing diffusion.[59] Yet another function of this space is to facilitate intercellular diffusion by maintaining cells apart.[59] Because this interstitial fluid is tightly bound to the connective tissue, it cannot be mobilized and hence the cosmetic use of diuretics in gestation is not merely pointless, but may actually be dangerous.[31]

The hydrostatic and colloid osmotic pressures of the interstitium were measured in an attempt to gain further insight into the transcapillary fluid dynamics which take place during gestation.[60] Surprisingly, while the colloid osmotic pressure of plasma decreased during gestation, the colloid osmotic pressure of the interstitium decreased even more. This suggests an increased capillary ultrafiltration and a higher capillary hydrostatic pressure since the capillary ultrafiltration coefficient seems unaltered during pregnancy.[60] An increased capillary hydrostatic pressure is anticipated by the decreased precapillary resistance associated with the systemic vasodilation and expanded blood volume. However, for an increased transcapillary colloid osmotic pressure difference to be maintained in the steady state, an enhanced rate of interstitial protein removal must also occur, otherwise diffusion would reestablish equilibrium. Enhanced lymphatic drainage must therefore be postulated. Since lymphatic drainage and reduction in interstitial colloid osmotic pressure are important "safety factors against edema,"[59,61] pregnancy has been characterized as a state of reduced "safety margin" against edema formation.[60] This may explain the propensity of pregnant women to rapidly develop edema once hydrostatic pressures have reached a threshold value.

From a different point of view, however, a reduced safety margin against edema formation signifies an enhanced safety margin against vascular engorgement. Indeed, the interstitial fluid spaces can be assimilated to a high capacity overflow reservoir for the circulatory system.[59] This particular arrangement of the capillary hydraulics and oncotic pressure differences makes it possible for pregnant women to rapidly shift large volumes of fluid back and forth between the intravascular and the interstitial compartments. By making this provision, nature has endowed the mother-to-be with an extra small bank account were she can instantaneously tap or deposit extra fluid on demand.

During pregnancy, circulatory efficiency takes precedence over body aesthetics. Perhaps this explains the legendary tolerance of pregnant women to large blood losses at delivery, allowing them to draw rapidly from an extra pool of interstitial fluid. Appropriate studies to test this hypothesis are needed. If indeed the mother is equipped with mechanisms allowing her to tap more rapidly from a larger interstitial reservoir, then a rapid loss of intravascular volume such as in hemorrhage would be corrected rapidly by "autotransfusion" of interstitial fluid. However, the hematocrit and plasma protein decreased at similar rates after hemorrhage in control and pregnant goats, suggesting that in this species such a protective mechanism does not exist.[62] Conversely, acute infusions of "isotonic" saline in rats suggested that during gestation the intravenous fluid was retained longer in the vascular compartment.[63] Unfortunately, anesthesia and catheterization may have affected the labile transcapillary balance of the pregnant rats. Moreover, it has been argued elsewhere that changes in hematocrit cannot be used to assess hemodilution if the "isotonic" fluid used in saline shrinks the red blood cells of hyponatremic pregnant rats.[3] These approaches, as discussed, may be further complicated by errors in the hematocrit when it is derived from the MCV and the cell count obtained in the Coulter counter with the red cells suspended in Isoton.[64] This problem may have been overlooked even in some of the most carefully conducted studies in gestation.

Of special interest is the pattern and distribution of the interstitial hydrostatic pressures recorded during human gestation.[60] First, the interstitial hydrostatic pressure has also been found to be negative during pregnancy.[59,61] However, while the negativity of the interstitial hydrostatic pressure is preserved in the nondependent areas as pregnancy advances, it rises progressively in the dependent areas. These findings suggest that during late gestation a transcapillary pool of fluid develops that may be available for rapid mobilization.[3] Thus, in the context of body fluid regulation, this possibility deserves further attention. Indeed, such considerations lead us to envision the maternal circulating blood volume as extending into a virtual space beyond the strict boundaries of the vascular bed. The exact size of this "underground river" is unknown, but since capillary ultrafiltration is markedly enhanced and extravascular volume increased, its presence has to be suspected. What fraction of this fluid transits back to the blood through the lymphatics and what fraction returns through the end-capillary network is unknown. While studies based on deuterium oxide (D_2O) as the marker of body water revealed that in pregnant women without generalized edema, the gain in water between the 10th and 30th weeks of gestation could be accounted for by the gains in the products of conception, maternal blood volume, and new tissues in the uterus and breasts, the gains in water between the 30th and 38th weeks exceeded such calculated gains by 1.5 to 2 L.[33] This extra water accumulating during the last stages of gestation is thought to represent expansion of the interstitial fluid.[3,33] As discussed, under normal conditions the interstitial compartment is "dry" (negative pressure) and as a result offers a very high resistance to bulk flow. However, once edema prevails, the interstitial fluid becomes freely movable. Of interest in this context is to recall that the compliance of the interstitial space is identical to that of the intravascular bed.[43] Thus, in view of the tight coupling of the mechanics of the interstitial space and blood volume, it seems legitimate to conclude that control of blood volume and control of extracellular fluid space are indistinguishable.[43] This notion is reminiscent of an idea entertained by Maurice B. Strauss, now in vogue again, that the receptors for the "effective blood volume" may be located in the interstitial compartment.[65] The rapid transcapillary shift of potentially significant volumes of plasma ultrafiltrate explains why in late gestation posture has such a pronounced effect on the measurement of blood volume and, like in other edematous states, explains the discrepancies when corpuscular elements or dyes are used to measure "blood volume."

BODY FLUID COMPOSITION

The profound changes in the volumes and distribution of the extracellular fluid compartments that were reviewed above are also associated with early changes in body fluid composition. Although the physiologic feedback systems that control the composition of body fluids deal with a parameter that is of a different physical dimension than those involved in the control of the extracellular volume, both functions are intimately interrelated as one affects the other by necessity. Thus, any transient change in the tonicity of one compartment (intra- or extracellular), will affect the volume of the other, and vice versa. The additional necessity to maintain constant the composition and/or volume of the intracellular compartment, implies that the control of body fluid composition and volume are reciprocal functions. Still there are views that in the overall scheme of volume regulation, the kidney first retains or loses salt, and only then does the body correct its composition, i.e., tonicity, by appropriate gains or losses of water.[43] Alternatively, one reads that the need for volume control may be directly met by the regulation of water metabolism, i.e., regulation of the composition of body fluids, regardless of whether the resulting changes in the composition of fluids are transient or permanent. Thus, it has been argued that the *slightest impingement on the working capacity of the heart will result in retention of the needed amount of water regardless of any minor osmotic pressure changes that may be involved.*[43] Finally, as both systems are intimately integrated, the control of volume and tonicity probably operate simultaneously. The two "feedback systems" which regulate the tonicity of body fluids, i.e., which are involved in osmoregulation are the "osmolality-thirst-water intake" loop and the "osmolality-vasopressin-antidiuresis" loop, respectively.

Osmoregulation during Gestation

The decrement in body fluid tonicity is perhaps one of the most intriguing changes characteristic of pregnancy. Indeed, the $\sim$10 mOsm/kg H_2O decrease in plasma osmolality represents a true lowering in "effective" tonicity since the nonpermeable solutes, sodium and its anions, account for the largest fraction of this decrease.[3] The lowering in plasma urea, a solute which diffuses freely through plasma membranes, and hence "osmotically" an "ineffective" solute,[3] is only minimally responsible for the lower plasma osmolality.[9,66,67] This true decrease in "effective" plasma osmolality starts during the luteal phase of the menstrual cycle, continues over conception, and reaches its nadir around the 10th week of gestation[28] (Fig. 4–2) after which these low values are maintained until term. Body tonicity falls similarly during rat gestation.[67]

The physiological significance of this decrease is not yet understood, it cannot merely be explained by stimulation of the nonosmotic pathway of vasopressin (AVP) release[1,3] and thirst that occur in response to a decreased "effective blood volume" and often invoked to explain the hyponatremia of edematous disorders.[1,2] Rather, the normal osmotic control of AVP release appears to be reset around this new steady-state osmolality which is defended as if it were the norm for gestation.[9,66] Thus, the baseline plasma AVP levels are not suppressed in spite of the decreased body fluid tonicity. If tonicity were to be further decreased or increased above the new steady state, however, the plasma AVP levels change in a predictable manner[24,66] along a line that is displaced to the left of that observed in the nonpregnant state (Fig. 4–3). Hence the term "reset osmostat" for AVP release, coined to describe such a reset relationship between plasma AVP and plasma osmolality (P_{osm}) has been adopted by us and others, as it stresses that the apparent threshold for AVP secretion and the steady-state P_{osm} are both significantly reset (decreased) during gestation, yet the "basal" plasma AVP levels remain unchanged.[9,66]

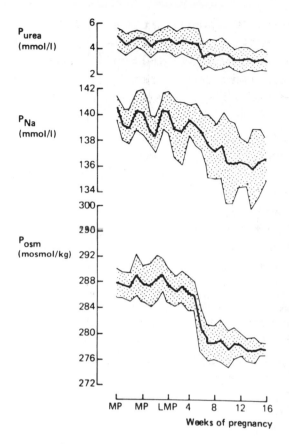

Figure 4–2. The time course for changes in plasma osmolality, sodium, and urea levels during human gestation. (*Reprinted, with permission, from Davison JM, Vallotton MB, Lindheimer MD: Plasma osmolality and urinary concentration and dilution during and after pregnancy: Evidence that lateral recumbency inhibits maximal urinary concentrating ability.* Br J Obstet Gynaecol *1981;88: 472–479.*)

It is important to note that the osmostat for thirst and drinking must also be reset by the same magnitude for the decreased steady-state plasma tonicity to be maintained.[9,66,68] Indeed, if the threshold P_{osm} for thirst and water intake were not altered, the P_{osm} would eventually drift back toward that found in the nonpregnant state, and plasma AVP would increase above the normal baseline levels along the line defining its new relationship with osmolality. This explains why exogenous AVP alone fails to induce hyponatremia in rats unless water intake is induced by adding either sugar to the water (J.A.D, personal observation) or by feeding a liquid diet.[69] The pregnant woman experiences and verbalizes thirst sensation at plasma osmolalities that are significantly below nonpregnant subjects.[3,9,32] Furthermore, Brattleboro rats that are genetically deficient in AVP, and hence have diabetes insipidus (DI), nevertheless demonstrate a similar decrease in their steady-state plasma tonicity during gestation, in spite of their inability to concentrate their urine.[68] As can be seen in Table 4–1, the pregnant DI rat achieves this by a prodigious increase in her daily water intake. Moreover, during gestation, the apparent threshold for AVP secretion is identical in Long–Evans controls and in heterozygous Brattleboro rats.[68] The only difference that could be found was a decrease in the slope for AVP secretion in the heterozygous animals, consistent with their decreased pituitary content of AVP[68] (Fig. 4–4).

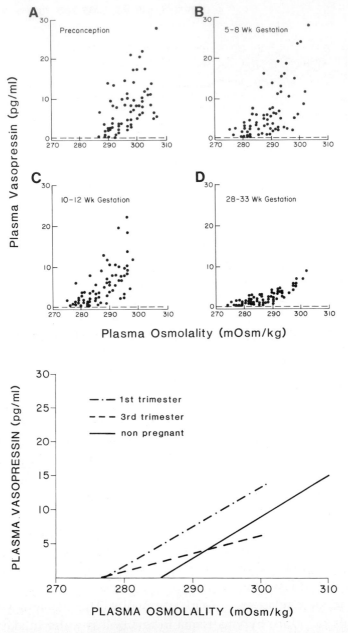

Figure 4–3. Relationship between plasma vasopressin (ordinate) and osmolality (absicca) during serial hypertonic saline infusion in eight women starting before conception and completed postpartum (graphs in upper panel). Each point represents an individual plasma determination. The graph at the bottom contains the highly significant mean regression lines which demonstrate the marked decrease in the osmotic threshold for AVP release during pregnancy defined by the absiccal intercept. (Note, the preconception [panel A] and postpartum [not shown] were combined in the graph as "nonpregnant.") Of interest is the decreased slope of the regression line (the gain of plasma vasopressin per unit rise in osmolality, which led to studies demonstrating that the metabolic clearance of vasopressin was increased in late pregnancy. (*Modified from Davison JM, Shills EA, Philips PR, Lindheimer MD: Serial evaluation of vasopressin release and thirst in human pregnancy. Role of human chorionic gonadotrophin in the osmoregulatory changes of gestation. J Clin Invest 1988;81:798–806; reprinted, with permission, from Lindheimer MD, Katz AI: The normal and diseased kidney in pregnancy. In: Schrier RW, Gottschalk CW, eds. Diseases of the Kidney,* ed 6. Boston: Little, Brown and Co.; 1997:2063–2097.)

TABLE 4–1. BASAL VALUES OF PLASMA OSMOLALITY AND WATER BALANCE IN NEAR-TERM HOMOZYGOUS BRATTLEBORO GRAVID AND VIRGIN RATS

	Virgin	Pregnant	P
Plasma Osm (mOsm/kg)	310 ± 6.0^a $(13)^b$	292 ± 3.5 (11)	< 0.001
Hematocrit (%)	40.3 ± 2.2 (13)	33 ± 1.8 (11)	< 0.001
Plasma urea N (mg/100 mL)	21.9 ± 5.2 (6)	19.5 ± 5.6 (6)	NS
Plasma Na (mEq/L)	146 ± 1.5 (6)	139 ± 1.1 (6)	< 0.001
Water intake (mL/24 h)	169 ± 23 (6)	375 ± 49 (6)	< 0.001
Urine volume (mL/24 h)	138 ± 18 (6)	$336 + 46$ (6)	< 0.001
Urinary Osm (mOsm/kg)	145 ± 45 (6)	135 ± 41 (6)	NS

^{a} ± SD
^{b} N
NS = not significant.
Reprinted from Dürr JA, Stamoutsos B, Lindheimer MD: Osmoregulation during pregnancy in the rat—evidence for resetting of the threshold for vasopressin secretion during gestation. J Clin Invest 1981;68:337–346 by copyright permission of the American Society for Clinical Investigation.

Potential Mechanisms Responsible for the Reset Osmostat

Decreased "Effective Blood Volume"

The two mechanisms which contribute to maintaining a lower plasma sodium in edematous states with decreased "effective blood volume" are the nonosmotic release of AVP and the impaired delivery of fluid to the diluting segments of the nephron. The "nonosmotic" pathway of AVP release is baroreceptor-mediated. Any decrease in "effective blood volume" may stimulate AVP release and result in body fluid dilution by promoting renal water reabsorption.[70] The normal renal diluting capacity may be further impaired by the increased proximal tubular fluid and solute reabsorption seen in the salt-avid states with decreased "effective blood volume." However, as discussed, pregnancy can hardly be equated with a state of "vascular underfill."[1,2] First, not only do pregnant rats suppress AVP and dilute their urine normally in response to a water load,[66] but extensive studies in the pregnant DI rat further demonstrate that AVP is not required for the plasma osmolality to be decreased.[68] Rather, AVP merely facilitates the maintenance of the new lower steady-state body fluid tonicity. Moreover, decreased delivery of tubular fluid to the distal nephron as an alternative explanation for the hyponatremia mediated by "ineffective blood volume"[1,2] cannot be invoked either, as the fractional renal clearance of lithium, a marker of proximal sodium handling, is unchanged by pregnancy in the rat.[71] Furthermore, the combination of a high salt diet with continuous deoxycorticosterone acetate (DOCA) administration together with norepinephrine infusion that resulted in a significant increase in arterial pressure, suppression of the renin–aldosterone system, and renal escape from the effects of mineralocorticoids that resulted presumably in an "effective volume expansion," failed to correct the decreased P_{osm} of the pregnant rats. Indeed, both the baseline P_{osm} and the osmotic threshold for AVP release remained 7 to 10 mmOsm/kg H_2O below those observed in virgin controls.[71]

The development of a highly sensitive electrothermal atomic absorption method for the determination of trace lithium levels in biological fluids[72] makes it

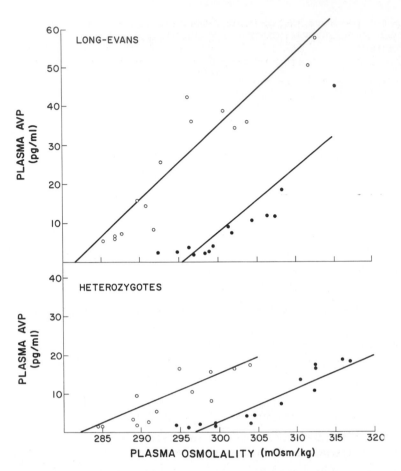

Figure 4–4. Relationship of plasma vasopressin to plasma osmolality in virgin (closed circles) and near term (open circles) Long–Evans (panel A) and heterozygote Brattleboro rats, in which tonicity was altered by intraperitoneal injections of saline solutions ranging from 200 to 1200 mOsmol. Note the reduced slope in animals heterozygote for diabetes insipidus, but in both groups the slopes of the regression lines in gravid and virgin animals were parallel. (*Reprinted, with permission, from Barron WM, Durr JA, Stamoutsos BA, Lindheimer MD: Osmoregulation during pregnancy in homozygous and heterozygous Brattleboro rats.* Am J Physiol *1985;248: R229–237.*)

possible to measure the fractional renal clearances from the natural trace blood and urine lithium levels in pregnant women without administration of exogenous lithium.[73] There was no change in the fractional renal clearance of lithium in human pregnancy; observations were similar to those in rodent gestation described above.[73,74] Since the fractional clearance of lithium is normal, yet the glomerular filtration rate (GFR) is increased during gestation, the absolute delivery of fluid to the diluting segment is also increased; a finding that may explain the tendency of pregnant rats to eliminate a water load better than their virgin controls.[66] Thus, the two common mechanisms invoked to explain the hyponatremia of edematous states with decreased effective blood volume cannot be incriminated in pregnancy.

Finally, balance studies performed over a ten-fold range in sodium intake[75] during gestation were associated, essentially, with stable plasma sodium levels and only minimal changes in the extracellular fluid volume. At one extreme of salt intake one should have observed worsening, while at the other improvement, of hyponatremia or alternatively one would have observed a marked change in the extracellular fluid volume if the hyponatremia were due to a "decreased effective blood volume."[3]

The rise in GFR (see below) and the increased delivery of fluid from the proximal tubule, together with normal AVP levels that are suppressible with water loading, confer a fatal blow to the theories that attempt to explain the reset osmostat of gestation as a consequence of a decreased "effective blood volume."[1,2] Indeed, at no stage during rat pregnancy can one detect enhanced or nonsuppressible AVP levels. Rather, early pregnancy is even associated with a tendency to polyuria and probably suppression of AVP secondary to volume expansion, a postulate that was advanced to explain the decrease in peripheral vascular resistance.[32] The nonosmotic, i.e., volume-mediated pathway of AVP release, has been assessed in rats during gestation.[76] These studies show that AVP responds similarly to a fractional decrease in blood volume during gestation (Fig. 4–5). Furthermore, as discussed, chronic volume expansion with salt and DOCA does not alter the baseline P_{osm} or the osmotic threshold for AVP secretion in pregnant rats.[71] Moreover, since addition

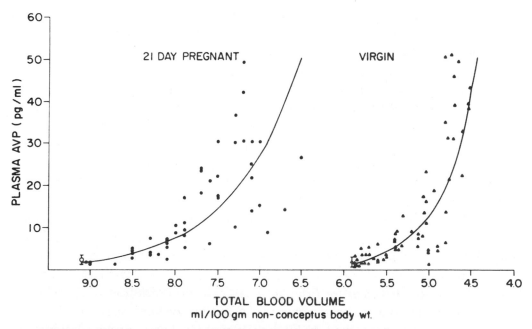

Figure 4–5. Plasma vasopressin (AVP) response to an isosmotic decrease in blood volume in the pregnant rat. Results demonstrate that pregnant animals, with increased absolute blood volume, respond to fractional changes in blood volumes in a manner similar to the virgin controls. (*Reprinted from Barron WM, Stamoutsos BA, Lindheimer MD: Role of volume in the regulation of vasopressin secretion during pregnancy in the rat. J Clin Invest 1984;73:923–932 by copyright permission of the American Society for Clinical Investigation.*)

of norepinephrine designed to prevent the decrease in blood pressure during gestation also failed to affect the lower P_{osm} in pregnant rats,[71] neither the low pressure atrial, nor the high pressure arterial baroreceptors are involved in resetting the osmotic control for AVP secretion.[3]

Furthermore, pseudopregnancy also fails to reproduce the decrease in P_{osm}[77] in spite of all the associated hemodynamic alterations that mimic gestation and hence should also result in a decreased effective blood volume.[47,78] Finally, as discussed, estrogen, progesterone, or a combination thereof can mimic the hemodynamic alterations of pregnancy[79] yet in our hands, these steroids failed to reproduce the hyponatremia of pregnancy.[67,68] Thus, circulatory factors alone are unlikely to explain the early decrease in body fluid tonicity in the gravid mother, and other factors related to the product of conception may be involved. Of note, however, is the observation that P_{osm} does decrease slightly in the second half of the menstrual cycle.[80]

Other Humoral Mechanisms

The mechanism by which the osmostat is reset during gestation is still unclear. Hormones such as prostaglandins, progesterone, estrogen, and angiotensin II which are known to affect either renal functions and/or thirst, do not seem to be involved in the reset osmostat.[68,81] As reviewed elsewhere, prolactin, opioid antagonists, and placental extracts also failed to produce changes in P_{osm} in the rat.[77] Human chorionic gonadotrophin (hCG), however, may be one of the humoral factors involved in the reset osmostat since it tends to decrease the osmotic threshold for AVP release during chronic administration in premenopausal women (but not in male volunteers) and since an apparently persistent reset osmostat could be documented in a patient with a molar pregnancy with high circulating hCG levels.[82] The osmotic threshold for AVP eventually normalized in this patient as plasma hCG immunoreactivity disappeared within 6 weeks after evacuation. However, the rat, an animal species where the reset osmostat of pregnancy was first described,[66] lacks a humoral equivalent of hCG (although administration of hCG to virgin rats may decrease their P_{osm}).[82] Most recently some have implicated the ovarian peptide relaxin,[83,84] but more studies are needed in this respect. Still it is tempting to speculate that the action of hCG may be manifested by stimulating the ovaries to secrete relaxin, explaining its effect on premenopausal women, and its ineffectiveness in men.

Respiratory and Thirst Center Effects on AVP Osmoregulation

Although accepting the notion of a true reset osmostat, Hytten[32] has also attempted to explain part of the reset osmostat by the ~10 mm Hg decrease in pCO_2 which occurs during pregnancy. Thus, the downward resetting of the respiratory center controlling pCO_2 during gestation has to be associated with a commensurate decrease in plasma bicarbonate if a normal plasma pH is to be maintained, as seems to be the case in pregnancy.[58] Therefore, if the compensatory renal losses of bicarbonate were to be associated with equivalent losses of sodium, this could result in a decreased

P_{osm}. Hence, according to this explanation, the renal compensation for the respiratory alkalosis may be responsible for the 10 mOsm/kg H_2O drop in P_{osm} observed early in gestation.[32] Such a decrease would be of sufficient magnitude to suppress AVP secretion and create a state of continuous diuresis, a phenomenon that could further explain the polyuria common in early gestation.[32] It may well be that the hypothalamic center that controls pCO_2 resets at a faster rate than the centers which regulate AVP and thirst. Progesterone is the hormone responsible for resetting the pCO_2-dependent respiratory drive.[32,58] This effect of progesterone has been used to treat hypopneic syndromes. However, as discussed, different regimens of progesterone[68] aimed at simulating the blood levels during gestation, even when administered in rats with pseudopregnancy[77] have failed to decrease their P_{osm}.

Moreover, as mentioned earlier, the decrease in plasma bicarbonate in compensated respiratory alkalosis is usually balanced in the nonpregnant state by a commensurate increase in the plasma chloride (Cl^-). Therefore, in order to accommodate this postulate, one would have to invoke some intracellular events that lead to a resetting of both the respiratory and osmotic thresholds. The possibility that some subtle alterations in the chemical makeup of the intracellular milieu may occur during gestation cannot be discarded.

Intracellular Mechanisms

The "almost universal complaint of excessive thirst in early pregnancy" advanced by Hytten as a further evidence for an early and transient DI syndrome,[32] rather suggests that resetting of the osmotic threshold for thirst sensation precedes the resetting of the osmotic threshold for AVP release. Indeed, if thirst is still perceived at plasma osmolalities that are below the nonpregnant values, then thirst rather than AVP may be the driving force which tends to decrease the tonicity, since decreasing body tonicity should suppress rather than stimulate thirst.[9,66,85] A faster resetting of the osmotic threshold for drinking will produce a situation akin to primary polydipsia. There is some evidence that this occurs.[82]

Since, in last analysis, it must be the intracellular tonicity that determines the osmolality of body fluids, a primary decrease in intracellular solute content may be responsible for the reset osmostat observed in pregnancy. For instance hyponatremia may be explained by a "sick-cell syndrome" in which intracellular solutes such as potassium decrease along with nondiffusible organic anions in chronically debilitated patients[86-88] that could result in a typical reset osmostat.[89] Similarly, total body potassium depletion associated with the chronic use of diuretics can be linked with refractory hyponatremia that responds to potassium repletion.[90] However, disagreement persists regarding the definition and/or even the existence of the clinical entity called "sick-cell" syndrome.[86,87,88,91] Still, the discovery that cachexins or cytokines are elevated in all the chronic debilitating diseases associated with a high incidence of hyponatremia, such as tuberculosis, HIV infection, and even congestive heart failure, among many others,[92-94] may revive the old idea of sick-cell syndrome, by providing the missing link. The major role of cytokines in the immunologic alterations of pregnancy is well known.[95,96] Thus, besides playing a major role in the tolerance to the implanted embryo, cytokines may also explain both the *nausea gravidarum* and reset osmostat of gestation. Further research in this field is needed.

As discussed, pertinent to pregnancy is the notion that hyponatremia could result from a primary decrease in intracellular solute. This mechanism may best be understood by considering the relation between serum sodium (Na_s) and the quotient between total exchangeable sodium and potassium ($Na_e + K_e$) and total body water (TBW). This equation (Na_s) = ($Na_e + K_e$)/TBW, derived from a large number of experiments[97] predicts that, everything else being equal, hyponatremia could result from a primary depletion in total exchangeable potassium (K_e), the major intracellular solute.[97] Thus, total body potassium (Edelman et al.),[97,98] rather than total body sodium (Peters)[99,100] appears to be the primary determinant of body fluid tonicity and intracellular volume. A decrease in total intracellular solutes may explain a number of hypotonic states with a reset osmostat.[89] These include even cases of congestive heart failure and cirrhosis of the liver,[97,101,102] clinical states in which the hyponatremia has traditionally been explained by the "nonosmotic" release of AVP triggered by an "ineffective blood volume."[2] Similarly, in the caval dog, a classic model of decreased "effective blood volume," the negative cumulative potassium balance[103] is such that it could alone explain the persistent hyponatremia and the "inappropriate" drinking. If the cell swelling associated with the "water intoxication" induced by the nonosmotic release of AVP is "corrected" by potassium losses (cell volume regulation), then a "reset osmostat" will ensue. This possibility deserves further consideration.

During gestation, the tonicity of body fluids decreases by 3% (8–10 mOsm/kg) on average.[9,66] Since total exchangeable potassium is in the order of 2000 to 2500 mEq in the nonpregnant state,[37,97] it was argued that a depletion or "relocation" of less than 70 mEq of exchangeable potassium (K_e) could account entirely for the reset osmostat.[3] This hypothesis stresses the potential importance intracellular fluid volume and composition may have in the overall regulation of body fluids, an aspect of physiology traditionally neglected in the clinical sciences.[3,104] It has been argued further that such a small change in total body potassium can not be detected by balance studies, especially if it occurs over the first few weeks of gestation[3] given the fact that the "normal" daily intake of potassium is within this range. Thus, direct measurements are therefore required to test this alternative explanation for the reset osmostat of pregnancy.[3] This notion has recently received consideration, as investigators find a decreased total amount of potassium, chloride, and other solutes in red blood cells very early in pregnancy.[52,53,105]

When multiple regression rather than simple correlation analysis is used to analyze the raw data used by Edelman et al. to demonstrate their classic equivalence between serum sodium (Na_s) and total exchangeable sodium, potassium, and total body water: (Na_s) = ($Na_e + K_e$)/TBW,[37,38] a slightly different but more accurate equation is obtained: (Na_s) = ($Na_e + p \cdot K_e$)/TBW (Durr JA, Lopez-dell Valle R, unpublished observation), in which the regression coefficient p is ~0.94. This equation suggests that the intracellular salts of potassium, unlike those of sodium in the extracellular space are not strictly of the monovalent species. Indeed, as discussed in the appendix at the end of this chapter, the osmolality of a solution of a salt of a monovalent cation K_nX, i.e., potassium in the present example, can be expressed as a function of the concentration of that cation by the formula $[Osm] = ((n + 1)/n) \times [K]$, provided that the salt is totally dissociated at that concentration and at that pH. Although neither the nature nor the exact concentrations of the individual intracellular anions (mainly phosphates) are known, our regression analysis suggests that the salts of potassium are on average not strictly monovalent, since $p < 1.0$. The classic correlation of Edelman suggests that hyponatremia can be explained either by excess total body water relative to total exchangeable sodium plus potassium, or by a relative decrease in one and/or the other of these anions.[97] Our analysis suggests further that, everything else being equal, a decrease in serum sodium (Na_s) can also be explained by an alteration in p, which is an averaged index of the speciation of potassium salts in the intracellular compartment. This coefficient may be altered in a number of different ways during gestation. Thus, as discussed, an altered makeup of intracellular anions may be invoked. Alternatively, the ratio of the mono- to the dibasic phosphates of potassium K_2HPO_4/KH_2PO_4 may be altered by changes in intracellular pH. Thus, a slight change in the intracellular pH resulting from the mild respiratory alkalosis could account for the reset osmostat of gestation. This alternative hypothesis deserves further evaluation with, perhaps, nuclear magnetic resonance analysis.

Finally, as reviewed by Chesley, some have suggested that sodium may move out of the cells and return after delivery.[58] Thus, since all living cells contain some low level of intracellular sodium, it is theoretically possible that the "apparent" reflection coefficient σ of cell membranes for sodium, given by the ratio of the *tonicity* of sodium (as perceived by living cells) to its *osmolality* (as measured by an osmometer), is less than unity ($\sigma < 1$), since in the ratio Na_{ton}/Na_{osm}, Na_{ton} may be smaller than Na_{osm}. Indeed, in last analysis, what sets the osmostat is not the osmolality per se, as read by the osmometer, but rather the tonicity, i.e., the "effective osmolality," as sensed by the cells.[106] Thus, it may be possible that the apparent reflection coefficient σ increases during pregnancy, presumably because of more efficient extrusion mechanisms brought about by the new hormonal environment.[3] Increased red cell sodium–lithium countertransport has been documented[107] as well as increased red cell sodium pump activity during pregnancy.[108,109] The sodium–lithium exchanger has many similarities with the sodium–hydrogen ion exchanger that, according to some, may play a role in essential hypertension,[110] as its activity in red blood cells correlates inversely with renal lithium clearance. Although pregnant women do have a normal fractional clearance of lithium (Li_{cl}/GFR), since their glomerular filtration rate (GFR) is significantly increased, the increased sodium–lithium contertransport observed in their erythrocytes must also occur in their kidneys, and may be ubiquitous. In the rat, at least, the renal microsomal Na/K ATPase activity is also enhanced during gestation.[111] Thus, as postulated earlier,[3] a global increase in the activity of multiple cellular sodium transport and extrusion systems may result in a net increase in the effective reflection coefficient for sodium and thereby mediate the reset osmostat.

However, it has been established that the "apparent reflection coefficient" σ for sodium already approximates unity in the nonpregnant state,[106] i.e., for "effective osmotic" purposes, sodium is totally impervious to normal living cells. Thus, a presumed enhancement in the extrusion rate of sodium from cells cannot further improve its apparent reflection coefficient σ, and hence another explanation must be found. One may postulate that because the cell membranes are completely impermeable to sodium,[106] the persistent lower steady-state intracellular sodium concentrations may also explain the reset osmostat. Indeed, if the intracellular concentration of any "effective" solute were to be decreased by whatever mechanism, the initially higher "effective" osmolality of the extracellular fluid will cause the cells to shrink, and thirst will be perceived and AVP will be released until the amount of water ingested and retained, together with the renal losses of salts, will decrease the tonicity of the extracellular fluid and again match the tonicity that, given the total amount of "effective" intracellular solutes, results in a normal or near normal cell volume.

Chesley calculated that since the sucrose and sodium spaces each decreased by 2.15 L during the first week of puerperium, the net loss of sodium must have been 300 mEq (2.15 × 142 = 301).[58] However, since the actual loss of sodium fell short of the expected loss by about 50%, he postulated that some sodium must have either returned to the bone or to an intracellular location. Such estimates, however, assume that the plasma sodium concentration (~140 mEq/L) is the same during pregnancy and the puerperium, and therefore ignore that a substantial fraction of the calculated loss may have been virtual. Indeed, after delivery the concentration of plasma sodium, i.e., the amount of sodium that is packed in one liter of extracellular space, is significantly higher and this may account, to a large extent, for the apparently "lost" sodium.

Water Channels and Urea Transporters

The rapid movement of water and urea down their activity gradients across cell membranes is due to the presence of a variety of water channels and/or urea transporters.[112] Without such channels, living cells would be totally impermeable to water and urea and hence osmotically isolated from their surrounding fluid. At the limit, such cells could be maintained in hypotonic media at room temperature without any deleterious effects just like Xenopus oocytes. Medical students are familiar with the typical cumulative pattern of the hemolysis curves that are obtained for red cells when the osmolality of the medium is decreased progressively. In fact, acquisition of osmotic water permeability in Xenopus oocytes following transient expression of water channels has allowed investigators to clone and characterize these channels. All the water channels from the aquaporin family have a molecular mass of ~30 kDa in their unglycosylated form, and have six transmembrane-spanning domains. Most water channels are inactivated by mercurial compounds.

The channel-forming integral protein (CHIP) represents the archetype of the aquaporin family of water channels.[113] Ontogeny of these channels during fetal development has received recent attention as at birth, water is rapidly reabsorbed from the distal lung in preparation for alveolar gas exchanges[114,115] and the renal concentrating ability appears at that time.[116-119] It has been suggested that the acquisition of CHIP by red cells during fetal development "may confer red cells with the ability to rehydrate rapidly after traversing the renal medulla, which becomes hypertonic after birth."[116] Although we have learned more about the ontogeny of these proteins during fetal development in recent years, *virtually nothing is known of the expression of these genes in pregnancy* . . . .[112]

Aquaporin 2 (AQP2), also named WCH-CD, the water channel of the renal collecting duct, unlike the other members of the CHIP family of water channels, is not "constitutively" expressed and inserted in cell membranes, but rather its expression and insertion/retrieval from the apical membrane of the principal cells of the collecting duct is controlled by vasopressin.[120] Mutations that abolish the water channel function of AQP2, and hence cause congenital nephrogenic diabetes insipidus resistant to vasopressin are increasingly recognized.[121] The close correlation between renal expression of AQP2 and the state of antidiuresis in physiologic as well as pathologic settings, has led to a new paradigm in which antidiuresis is equated with AQP2 channel function. The recent finding of an increased AQP2 expression and increased insertion of AQP2 in the apical membranes of the collecting tubule during pregnancy in the rat[122] is very interesting as it challenges this emerging dogma. Indeed, in the light of our current knowledge of the central role played by AQP2 water channels in renal water retention, and the notion that pregnant rats have a similar or even less negative free water clearance in the basal state, and have an enhanced ability to rapidly increase renal free water clearance and eliminate an acute water load much faster than controls,[66] makes the significance of this intriguing observation is unclear. Thus, since the urine of pregnant rats is not more concentrated than that of virgin controls,[66,122] it would appear that the AQP2 system is less efficient during gestation. This would be anticipated in the light of the markedly increased delivery of tubular fluid to the distal nephron discussed above. Therefore, it seems doubtful that increased AQP2 expression during gestation could be responsible for the sustained decrease in plasma osmolality. Moreover, a vasopressin antagonist that decreased the expression of AQP2 in pregnant animals to levels of control rats receiving the same antagonist, failed to "correct" the hyponatremia of pregnancy,[122] a finding reminiscent of the decrease in plasma osmolality observed in the pregnant, vasopressin-deficient Brattleboro rat.[68] As was alluded to, any increased expression of renal AQP2, if functional, should be associated with an inability to eliminate a water load and result in water intoxication. Pregnancy does not mimic the syndrome of inappropriate antidiuretic hormone secretion (SIADH) that would be predicted if the increased expression of AQP2 were functional. Thus, further characterization of AQP2 as well as other water and urea channels during pregnancy are awaited for a better understanding of the reset osmostat of gestation.

The answer to the enigma of the decreased effective osmolality and reset osmostat of gestation may not reside in the vasopressin-regulated renal AQP2, but rather in AQP4, which may play a major role in the mechanism of central osmoreception.[123] Indeed, this aquaporin is found in a number of brain regions associated with the osmoregulation of thirst and vasopressin secretion. Further studies in pregnancy are awaited.

The Diabetes Insipidus Syndrome of Late Gestation

The plasma of pregnant women contains an enzyme, or iso-enzymes, of placental origin which rapidly inactivate(s) vasopressin in vitro and presumably also in vivo.[124] Plasma enzymatic activity increases with advancing gestation so that by midgestation, vasopressin levels cannot be detected if the enzyme is not inhibited at the time blood is drawn. The circulating vasopressinase is an exopeptidase that has slight predilection for cystine-aminopeptides such as vasopressin and oxytocin, an observation that explains why it has also been named pitocinase and oxytocinase. Of interest, this enzyme is only detected in the plasma of pregnant human and nonhuman primates, and appears to be absent from the blood of other gravid mammals.[124] This enzyme increases the metabolic clearance rate (MCR) of vasopressin by up to four times in late gestation.[125] Enhanced degradation of vasopressin may explain, in part, why the slope of the line depicting the relationship between vasopressin and plasma osmolality is decreased in the third trimester[125] (see Fig. 4–3). Note that since there is a quadrupling of the MCR of circulating vasopressin during late gestation in humans, and since the plasma levels of vasopressin remain normal, there must also be a quadrupling of the secretion rate of vasopressin.[3]

A syndrome of transient diabetes insipidus (DI) of late gestation, that is resistant to vasopressin, but responsive to dDAVP, a vasopressinase-resistant synthetic vasopressin analog, has been described in 1987,[126] and now appears to be the major form of transient DI associated with pregnancy.[124] Thus, the *diabetes insipidus gravidarum* appears to be due to excessively high quantities of circulating vasopressinase.[124] A review of the literature on this syndrome reveals that this syndrome is consistently associated with liver dysfunction, occurring in the setting of either preeclampsia, and/or its HELLP syndrome equivalent, or in association with the fatty liver disease of pregnancy.[124]

RENAL FUNCTION

The enhanced expression of AQP2 illustrates only one among the many profound changes that take place in the kidney during gestation. Indeed, given the key role played by the kidney not only in the maintenance of body fluid composition, but also in volume homeostasis in general, the reader may wonder whether other changes may occur in the kidneys during pregnancy. At first glance, one may assume that Borst's purely mechanistic "willingness" of the normal kidney to excrete salt and water[127] under a given perfusion pressure could explain the retention of salt and water during gestation since, as reviewed below, pregnancy is characterized by a decreased mean arterial pressure.[3] Indeed, the notion that a purely mechanistic "pressure-volume output" relationship of the kidney[3] could be involved in the long-term regulation of blood pressure and/or volume homeostasis has caught the imagination of many physiologists and clinicians.[127-130] In fact, the fundamental relationship between renal perfusion pressure and volume output (Fig. 4–6), also known as pressure natriuresis or diuresis, has been identified by Guyton and colleagues as the parameter which has the ultimate influence in the long-term control of blood pressure.[131,132] In this modern view of fluid homeostasis, the role of hormones is merely to modulate the kidney's basic "willingness" to excrete sodium and water at a given perfusion pressure.[70,129] The intrinsic "willingness" of the kidney to mount a certain rate of salt and water output at a given perfusion pressure, may be controlled by the renal interstitial hydrostatic pressure[133-135] which, in contrast to most other tissues, is positive. Many believe that in essential hypertension, this curve is shifted to the right so that volume output comes into equilibrium with volume intake at a higher renal perfusion pressure. During gestation the kidneys are more inclined to eliminate salt and water as the renal function curve is shifted to the left, at least in pregnant sheep[136] (Fig. 4–6). This finding was predictable[3] since clinical experience suggests that pregnant women always come into salt and water balance at a lower mean arterial blood pressure, regardless of intake. The resetting to the left of the renal pressure–volume output relationship shows that the hemodynamics of pregnancy can hardly be equated with a putative vascular "un-

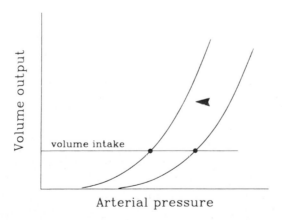

Figure 4–6. Schematic "arterial pressure–volume output" curve or renal function curve, the pressure natriuresis or diuresis, i.e., the "willingness" of the kidneys to excrete salt and water as a function of their perfusion pressure. The average blood pressure at any given steady "volume" intake (horizontal line) is given by the intersection of the renal function curve (output) and the horizontal intake line. Pregnancy is characterized by a shifting of the renal function curve to the left, i.e., during pregnancy, and volume intake and volume output (salt and water balance) are achieved at a lower mean arterial pressure.[3] (*Reprinted, with permission, from Durr JA: Maternal fluid adaptation to pregnancy. In: Brace RA, Ross MG, Robillard JE, eds. Reproductive and Perinatal Medicine. Vol. XI. Fetal and Neonatal Body Fluids. Ithaca, NY: Perinatal Press; 1989:227–270.*)

derfill,"[1] as such a state would merely be associated with a decrease in renal output of salt and water below the intake (horizontal line) on the right hand curve and below the equilibrium point set by intake at a lower mean arterial pressure, rather than on a new curve with higher "volume output" (left hand curve) (Fig. 4–6). Note also the prediction that the gain in the renal function curves may also be enhanced during gestation,[3] and indeed pregnant rodents and women tend to excrete loads of salt and water proportionally better than controls,[20,66,75,137] which does not appear to be the case in sheep.[136]

However, as will be seen, while marked changes in renal function occur during pregnancy, nothing is known about these fundamental hydraulic renal variables. Nitric oxide seems to play a major role in the pressure natriuresis mechanism since it increases the renal interstitial pressure for each given value of renal perfusion pressure, and thus shifts the renal function curve to the left.[138] The role of nitric oxide in the cardiovascular and renal adaptations to pregnancy are discussed in Chapter 8.

The evidence currently available which suggests that the renal perfusion pressure is better coupled to the renal interstitial hydraulic pressure during pregnancy, and hence may account for the resetting of the renal function curve,[136] is only conjectural. Much more information is available concerning the effects of pregnancy on the conventional parameters of renal function, i.e., renal hemodynamics (glomerular filtration rate and effective renal plasma flow) and tubular functions. Here again, rather than offering a purely descriptive review of all the changes in renal functions which occur during gestation, we will present this review from a functional perspective as this approach will help the reader grasp the implications of such changes on maternal adaptations to gestation.

Renal Plasma Flow and Glomerular Filtration Rate

The postulate that there must be an even increase in deep and superficial single nephron glomerular filtration rate (SNGFR) during gestation, suggested by the finding that SNGFR measured by micropuncture studies in accessible superficial nephrons increases in the same proportion than whole kidney GFR,[48,78] indicates that there must be a balanced vasodilation of both pre- and postglomerular resistance vessels. Indeed, effective renal plasma flow (ERPF) increases in proportion to the increased glomerular plasma flow rate,[48] and there is no increase in glomerular capillary pressure[139] (Fig. 4–7). The potential mechanisms[140] that may be responsible for the decrease in "effective renal vascular resistance," which mirrors the increase in ERPF, as documented in undisturbed, chronically instrumented rats, is discussed in Chapter 8.

In the rat with filtration pressure equilibrium, i.e., where ultrafiltration ceases before blood reaches the glomerular end-capillary network due to the balancing of oncotic and hydrostatic pressures, the increased GFR can be entirely accounted for by an increased glomerular plasma flow rate[48,78] (see Fig. 4–7). There is no need to postulate increased glomerular hydrostatic pressure or an alteration in K_f, the glomerular capillary ultrafiltration coefficient.

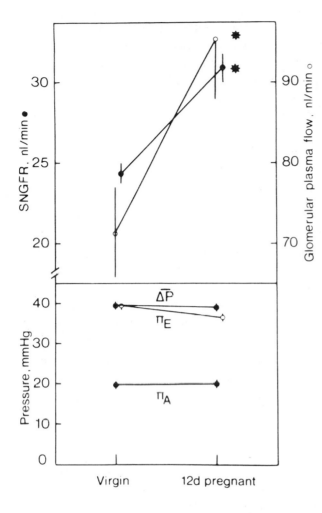

Figure 4–7. Comparison of glomerular hemodynamics in midterm pregnant and virgin Munich–Wistar rats. Data obtained by micropuncture demonstrate an increase in single nephron glomerular filtration rate (SNGFR) is accounted for by an increase in glomerular plasma flow rate (upper panel). Neither changes in glomerular hydrostatic pressures (middle panel) nor changes in glomerular capillary ultrafiltration coefficients (K_f) (lower panel) need to be invoked to explain the increased GFR. (*Reprinted, with permission, from Baylis C: Renal hemodynamics and volume control during pregnancy in the rat. Semin Nephrol 1984;4:208–220.*)

The ERPF, measured by p-aminohippurate (PAH) clearance, an index of renal blood flow, rises markedly during human gestation. Midpregnancy increments of 60 to 80% are normal.[141,142] The decrease in ERPF in late gestation is not related to position;[143] GFR increases early in pregnancy, averaging a 50% increase from the 16th week until term. Since the changes in GFR and ERPF are not exactly parallel in human gestation, the filtration fraction (FF = GFR/ERPF) decreases initially and then increases in the third trimester. The changes in the hematocrit and plasma oncotic pressure certainly contribute to the increased GFR in human pregnancy and may partially explain the change in filtration fraction.[3] The exact mechanism(s) responsible for the increased renal perfusion in normal pregnancy is/are unknown.[139] There are probably many humoral factors that play important roles as discussed in detail in Chapter 8.

Tubular Functions

Although a variety of humoral factors that may act via the nitric oxide-cGMP system and have significant vasodilating effects on the glomerulus, the enhanced GFR of pregnancy may result alternatively from a primary increase in the proximal or ascending limb solute reabsorption. Indeed, this would, via decreased delivery of the glomerular ultrafiltrate to the macula densa, i.e., via the tubuloglomerular feed-back mechanism, lead to a secondary increase in GFR. This explanation would be consistent with the enhanced renal microsomal Na/K-ATPase activity[111] that par-allels the increased tubular load, i.e., the GFR. Thus, rather than a consequence,[143] one could see in the enhanced Na/K-ATPase activity a cause for the increased GFR and tubular load of sodium.

The ~30% volume expansion which takes place in pregnant rats at 12 days' gestation is not associated with suppression of the normal tubuloglomerular feed-back (TGF) activity as would normally be observed in volume expanded states.[144] Besides being consistent with the view that the kidney "does not sense its status as volume expanded,"[144] this observation would also be consistent with the postulate of a primary-enhanced solute reabsorption at tubular sites prior to the sensing sites involved in the TGF mechanism. The TGF mechanism ensures that the delivery of NaCl to the low-capacity transport systems of the distal nephron remains within narrow limits.[145] For instance, a primary-enhanced reabsorption of sodium and chloride in the ascending limb could indirectly increase GFR through the normal TGF mechanism.[145,146] Increased GFR mediated by a primary increase in solute re-absorption at sites prior to the macula densa have been described with protein loading and with vasopressin.[145]

As discussed, when the trace lithium clearance method is used as an index of proximal tubular fluid and solute reabsorption,[147,148] normal fractional proximal fluid and solute reabsorption are reported (Li_{Cl}/GFR, see p. 123) during third trimester human pregnancy.[73] Thus, trace lithium levels decrease by 58% in the ex-act inverse proportion to the increase in GFR. Therefore, an unchanged proximal fractional reabsorption, associated with an increased tubular load (GFR), signifies an enhanced absolute proximal solute reabsorption, which could be the "primum movens" for the increased GFR. Similar results were observed with the exogenous lithium method[71,74] in rats as well as in humans.[74]

Renal Salt and Water Handling

Salt Handling (Also See Chapter 9)

In spite of a decreased arterial pressure, sodium excretion in pregnant subjects matches intake with high precision. Thus, conventional balance studies performed at "normal" levels of sodium intake would be inadequate to detect a cumulative gain in sodium of 900 mEq which occurs over the entire period of human gestation since this would represent at most only 2 to 3 mEq/day of extra sodium retained, a fraction far too small to be accounted for in a 24-hour urine collection. When salt is drastically restricted to 10 mEq/day, pregnant women decrease their urinary sodium to values that are similar to those observed in nonpregnant controls sub-jected to such diets.[19] This, observation, however, may suggest a subtle salt leak,[143] because when intake is so low the few milliequivalents of sodium that a pregnant woman retains become a proportionately larger fraction of the intake, and thus a difference in urinary sodium excretion between pregnant and nonpregnant subjects should be observed.[3] The small amount of extra salt that needs to be retained daily during pregnancy is so trivial compared to the "normal" daily intake that at any time during pregnancy the mother can be considered to be in "salt balance." Indeed, at no stages during gestation can one detect indices of salt depletion, such as low fractional excretion of sodium (FE_{Na}), low urine Na concentration, or a low fractional excretion of lithium (FE_{Li}), or the inability to excrete a salt load. Thus, the outcome in weight gain, edema, and blood pressure was identical in a study where more than 2000 pregnant women were asked either to reduce their salt intake as much as possible or to select salty foods and add salt to the diet.[149] Although strict balance studies were not performed on this large cohort, it appears that in all likelihood, pregnant subjects handle near extremes of salt intake normally.

Late gestation in humans[20,75,150] or rats[137] is characterized by a preserved or even improved ability to excrete acute sodium loads provided the loads are expressed in percent of the extracellular volume. Short-term balance studies performed in second and third trimester pregnant women have demonstrated that salt intakes over a ten-fold range (27–240 mEq/24 h Na excretion), are associated with unchanged blood pressures and only minimally altered blood volume, changes qualitatively similar to those expected in nonpregnant subjects.[75]

With chronic salt loading, the fractional excretion of lithium increases in pregnant rats in a manner similar to virgin controls.[71] Moreover, pregnant rats decrease their proximal fractional sodium reabsorption appropriately when chronically expanded with deoxycorticosterone acetate (DOCA) and a high salt diet, and hence demonstrate a normal renal escape phenomenon to mineralocorticoids.[71] This observation, when taken together with the other observations reviewed here, is difficult to reconcile with the "underfill" theory of pregnancy.[1] Indeed, as discussed, the cardinal feature encountered in all hyponatremic edematous states with decreased "effective blood volume" and an activated renin–aldosterone system with enhanced sympathetic output, is the basic inability to maintain adequate sodium balance and to escape from the chronic renal effects of mineralocorticoids.

Water Handling

Renal water handling is of particular interest in gestation in view of the significant decrease in plasma osmolality documented in humans as well as in rats[9,66] (see above). As reviewed elsewhere, the control of posture is an important factor in the correct evaluation of urinary diluting and concentrating capacity during gestation.[29] Supine recumbency impairs maximum diluting ability,[24,25] while lateral recumbency impairs maximum concentrating ability.[28,77] These postural factors are only partially dependent on AVP.[29] Pregnancy in humans and rats is associated with a preserved or improved ability to dilute the urine and excrete a water load.[9,66] Similarly, there is no difference in the renal concentrating ability during pregnancy in humans[9] or rats[66] and most human studies, even in the absence of strict control of posture, detect only trivial, if any, impairments in the maximum concentrating ability.[20,77] As with salt handling, an apparently normal ability of the kidney to handle water is difficult to reconcile with the proposal that the hyponatremia of pregnancy is due to vascular underfill. Indeed, such states are characterized by the inability to dilute the urine and excrete a water load.

HEMODYNAMICS

The ultimate teleologic significance of the alterations in volume and tonicity regulation during pregnancy requires consideration of their hemodynamic implications. Thus, a brief review of gestational hemodynamic changes will follow, a more detailed discussion having taken place in the preceding chapter.

Cardiac Performance

Cardiac output increases 40% in pregnancy, rising rapidly in the first trimester, after which values are sustained until term, the older descriptions of a preterm decrease are spurious due to positioning the subjects in supine recumbency for their tests.[151-153] Pregnant women also experience profound alterations in the mechanical, elastic, and dynamic properties of the entire vascular tree. The changes in the left ventricular (LV) mechanical properties are such that the efficiency of the LV to systemic energy transfer is maintained in the face of increasing compliance of the aorta and a global decrease in peripheral resistance.[151] Although the increased compliances of the aorta and the large arteries through their effect on the "pulsatile arterial load" have important hemodynamic effects,[151] it may be naive to assume that this represents one of the body's adaptive mechanisms to "accommodate the increased intravascular volume" without increasing mean arterial pressure.[151] Indeed, even if the compliance of the entire arterial tree were to double, it would have only minimal effects, if any, on the amount of blood that can be stored in the vascular bed, given the fact that the compliance of the low pressure system is several orders of magnitude lower. Rather, characterization of the serial changes in the pulsatile arterial load and their physiologic role in ventricular-systemic coupling during normal pregnancy, may ultimately provide the key to understanding hypertensive complications of pregnancy. Therefore, the establishment of "a reference for comparison"[151] by studying the normal pattern may be the first step to understanding the cause of preeclampsia.

Of particular interest are observations that cardiac output increases normally in pregnancy.[18,153] This suggests that a normal or even supranormal "cardiac reserve" may be maintained on top of the increased basal cardiac output. An increased cardiac reserve has now been documented during gestation in guinea pigs.[154] Structural, i.e., vessel remodeling with better elastic properties, and functional, i.e., decreased smooth muscle tone, confer much better outflow impedance characteristics in the face of a generalized vasodilation, which alone would only reduce the resistance to the steady flow, but bear no effect on the pulsatile afterload. At the extreme, a marked decrease in peripheral vascular resistance (PVR) without the associated increase in arterial compliance, which permits rapid absorption of the LV energy delivered during the systolic phase and subsequently release it over the diastolic phase, may result in an intermittent venous return that could considerably impede the cardiac output. It has been argued[3] that the anatomic correlate of the clinical impression of a "hyperkinetic heart" may be due more to the increased aortic compliance observed by noninvasive methods[155] than to the actual decrease in systemic arterial resistance. The increase in size and compliance of the aortic root and/or size in cardiac chambers may[151] or may not[155,156] revert back totally to the values before conception.

Arterial Blood Pressure

As detailed in Chapter 3, in spite of the progressive increase in blood volume and cardiac output, the mean arterial pressure actually decreases during gestation due to a concomitant and marked decrease in peripheral vascular resistance. Most studies show a larger decrease in diastolic than in systolic blood pressure,[18] so that there is a tendency, at least in the earlier stages of pregnancy, for an increased pulse pressure. A frequent clinical correlate is the presence of capillary pulsations[63] that may not be dampened completely by the increased aortic compliance; the implications of which have been poorly investigated.[3] The traditional explanation of a placental AV shunt[157,158] to account for the increased cardiac output and decreased systemic resistance fails to account for the early changes that can best be explained by systemic vasodilation.[153,159]

Baroreceptor Function

The profound changes in pregnancy have been studied and documented for over 40 years, yet few studies on baroreceptor function during pregnancy have been performed.[3] Obstetricians are well aware of the labile, capricious nature of the hypertension in preeclamptic patients with a reversed pattern of decreased blood pressure at night,[160] observations compatible with a deranged baroreceptor function. The minute to minute regulation of the circulation is ensured by receptors at strategic locations within the cardiovascular circuit, those studied most being the sinoaortic and atrial baroreceptors.[70] Others, such as the juxtaglomerular apparatus, may also be relevant to gestation.

Baroreceptors which are located in the high pressure, arterial side of the circulation, appear to play the predominant role in cardiovascular adjustments in humans.[70] In quadrupeds, where large volume shifts are less likely to occur on rising, the role of the baroreceptors located within the low pressure side of the circulation, i.e., the atria, is much more important.[70]

Slowing of the heart rate in response to elevations in blood pressure is a simple baroreflex which can be studied in humans. Seligman[161] assessed the baroreceptor-mediated slowing of the heart rate during elevations in blood pressure induced by angiotensin II or phenylephrine. The "gain" appeared to be normal or even enhanced, since with a similar rise in blood pressure, pulse interval increased more during gestation. Thus, the baroreceptors of the pregnant woman do not sense the arterial filling or "effective blood volume" as being depressed, otherwise the gain would have been decreased. The baroreceptors, therefore, must have reset to the hemodynamic conditions characteristic of gestation. Resetting of baroreceptor function over time, however, can be a general characteristic of any system that does not have an "infinite gain," without a significant role in the long-term control of blood pressure.

The ongoing debate whether the vascular tree in pregnancy is functionally "underfilled," "overfilled," or merely "normal"[1] has prompted a number of experiments in which surrogate parameters of baroreceptor activation were assessed, such as AVP, plasma–renin activity (PRA), and catecholamines, as well as a multiplicity of renal function studies. Interpretation of these indirect studies is still a subject of controversy. A simpler approach would have been to examine directly how the pregnant woman perceives her own circulation.[3]

Some information is now available on the efferent loop of the baroreceptor pathway in rats and rabbits. In these species the relation between renal sympathetic nerve activity (RSNA) and blood pressure appears to be reset to a lower operating blood pressure during pregnancy.[162-164] Careful studies on heart rate response to changes in blood pressure performed in chronically instrumented awake rats[165] do not suggest increased sympathetic outflow during gestation either. Of interest, while the dose response curves to the pressor effect of methoxamine were shifted to the right during pregnancy (less sensitivity), the depressor responses to sodium nitroprusside were unaltered. Similar studies in conscious dogs do not suggest an increased hypotension-induced tachycardia either, as would be anticipated if pregnant dogs sensed their circulatory system as "underfilled."[166] In fact, the hypotension-induced increase in heart rate was blunted during gestation, as was the "nonosmotic" release of AVP, yet the reflex increase in PRA was augmented.[166] This finding supports the notion that the humoral indices of baroreceptor activation may not be reliable.[3]

Of particular relevance to pregnancy, one which may mimic a state of systemic shunting, is the activation of a vasovagal, cardioacceleratory reflex when an AV shunt is opened in the dog. Indeed, it has been demonstrated that opening of a non-hypotensive AV shunt causes a significant increase in type B atrial receptor discharge. Furthermore, a high correlation between receptor activity and shunt flow suggests that the receptor discharge is due to the increased, pulsatile venous return.[167] Indeed, rather than absolute pressure, the relevant stimulus for both the sinoaortic and the atrial receptors are the pulsatile changes in pressure; pulse pressure for the sinoaortic receptors[70] and an increase in V-wave amplitude for the atrial receptors.[167] The activity of both receptors tends to increase with mean pressure but not if the pulsatile stimulus falls simultaneously. In both, the frequency of discharge varies with the rate of rise of the stimulus. Thus, while the opening of an AV shunt results only in a minimal increase in mean right atrial pressure, the amplitude of the V wave is larger, its peak higher, and its rate of rise steeper and, in addition, the frequency is increased.[167] This may stimulate the low pressure barore-ceptor more than simple volume expansion.[3] Similarly, because of the low periph-eral resistance, enhanced systolic function,[151] and aortic compliance, the pulsatile changes in the pressures sensed by the sino-aortic receptor are also enhanced; hence this receptor also will "sense" the blood pressure as being higher. The result will be the resetting of the mean arterial blood pressure to lower values.

If as postulated, pulsatile venous return and increased aortic compliance re-set both high and low pressure baroreceptors, and the nonosmotic release of va-sopressin is under tonic inhibition by baroreceptor fibers which transit in the va-gus,[70] then the increased discharge due to the pulsatile flow is also likely to reset the nonosmotic control of vasopressin secretion. This means that vasopressin, and in more general terms, all vasoactive hormones under baroreceptor control will be modulated around a new setpoint of "effective" blood volume. Thus, baseline AVP and catecholamine levels are not elevated during gestation in spite of the de-creased blood pressure,[9,66,77] and the baroreceptor control of AVP appears to be reset around the new hemodynamic variables typical for gestation.[76] Similarly, the renin–aldosterone system, although enhanced, appears to change appropri-ately with salt loading.[50] Although, as eloquently argued by Frank Epstein, pos-tulating a *resetting of central baroreceptors* to explain that the circulatory and renal changes of cirrhosis are a *formulation that comes perilously close to being the seman-tic equivalent of "diminished effective blood volume,"*[168] this is exactly what distin-guishes the physiology of pregnancy from the pathology of cirrhosis.[3] These con-siderations clearly stress that more detailed studies on baroreceptor function during pregnancy may elucidate not only the mechanisms of the normal cardio-vascular adaptations to pregnancy, but may furnish valuable clues for the under-standing of preeclampsia.[3]

It took the human race a fair number of generations to acquire, along with orthostasis, a predominance of the high pressure baroreceptor control over receptors in the low pressure circulation, the latter characteristic in quadrupeds.[3] During pregnancy, however, the baroreceptor control system may revert back to its original low pressure predomi-nance, momentarily taking the woman back the genealogic tree, to stages prior to *Homo erectus.*[3] Thus, the question as to whether preeclampsia (a disease for which there is as yet no animal model) could result from an abnormal cross-talk between the two baroreceptor control systems, is a legitimate one. Indeed, preeclampsia could result from a suboptimal compliance of the aorta. As discussed, in support of this postulate is the notion that the aortic root is larger and more compliant during gestation[151,155] and that these changes may not revert back to normal.[155,156] Such a hysteresis of the aortic root may be the anatomic correlate which accounts for the observation that preeclampsia is mainly a disease of the primigravida and is less likely to recur in subsequent pregnancies.[3] Thus, the experimental manipulations of the aortic root or the sino-aortic baroreceptor may be the key to an animal model of preeclampsia. The sino-aortic baroreflex dysfunction in severe preeclampsia has very important therapeutic implications.[169]

CIRCULATORY ADEQUACY

Another question relevant to volume homeostasis in pregnancy is whether the circulatory adaptations, in a teleologic sense, represent a preparation for increased cardiac performance or rather, if they are merely compensatory. Answers to these questions, too, have therapeutic implications; this section reviews the physiology of AV shunts, the "effective blood volume," and mean circulatory filling pressure (MCFP) as hemodynamic determinants of maternal circulatory performance which may affect the volume and distribution of body fluid during gestation.

Hemodynamic Implications of Arteriovenous Shunts

There is a view[157,158] that the hemodynamic changes of pregnancy can be accounted for primarily by the placental AV shunt. Clinical observations which support this include the increased cardiac output, heart rate, and pulse pressure, as well as increments in mixed venous oxygen saturation and total blood volume. Furthermore, there is a rise in venous pressure in the territories sharing the same drainage as the uterus and a continuous bruit with systolic accentuation audible over the placenta[3,157] (Table 4–2).

While the concordance with an AV fistula appears perfect[3,157,158,170] (see Table 4–2), the timing of the maternal circulatory changes and placental blood flow are strikingly different.[3] Thus, the increased cardiac output and decreased peripheral resistance are early events, clearly established in the initial weeks of gestation, well before uterine blood flow reaches its highest levels. In addition, the increment in cardiac output exceeds the total uterine blood flow. Upon acute opening of a large AV shunt, there is normally vasoconstriction in the vascular bed outside the fistula with decreased venous return from these areas.[171] During pregnancy, on the contrary, there is an enhanced systemic tissue perfusion.[18] Also, whereas the slightest decrease in "effective blood volume," such as occurs with the opening of the shunt

TABLE 4–2. COMPARISON OF THE HEMODYNAMICS OF PREGNANCY WITH THE CIRCULATORY CHARACTERISTICS OF ARTERIOVENOUS SHUNTS[a]

	AV Shunt	Pregnancy
Heart rate	↑	↑
Blood pressure	↓	↓
Pulse pressure	↑	↑
Cardiac output	↑	↑
Central AV O_2 difference	↓	↓
Blood volume	↑	↑
Bruit at auscultation	+	+
Proximal arteriolar dilatation	+	+
Absent capillaries	+	+

[a] The last three characteristics refer to the placental circulation. The other characteristics may be unrelated to the placenta and be the result of systemic vasodilation rather than placental shunting.
Adapted from Dürr JA: Maternal fluid adaptation to pregnancy: In: Brace RA, Ross MG, Robillard JE, eds. Reproductive and Perinatal Medicine. Vol XI. Fetal and Neonatal Body Fluids. Ithaca, NY: Perinatal Press; 1989:227–270.

results in renal vasoconstriction (with exquisite sensitivity), in pregnancy one notes a markedly enhanced effective renal plasma flow (ERPF). Converting ERPF into total renal blood flow may better convey the overwhelming increase in renal perfusion which may also exceed the entire uterine circulation during pregnancy.

Given that the *area of diminished vascular resistance is being generalized rather than localized in the uterus*,[170] it may be tempting to assimilate the entire systemic circulation to a transient AV shunt during gestation.[3] In this respect temporary occlusion of the uterine circulation of pregnant dogs results in only minimal hemodynamic alterations, suggesting that compared to the rest of the systemic flow, the placental shunt is of minor hemodynamic significance.[172] Nevertheless, whether or not placental circulation can be incriminated, there are numerous other aspects of the maternal circulation which mimic a large systemic shunt,[172] and a review of the hemodynamic and cardiovascular repercussions should help us understand the circulatory adaptations in pregnancy.

Statements such as "the subject with an arteriovenous fistula is literally bleeding into his large veins"[12] may have been unfortunate, and in general, too much emphasis has been devoted to the hemorrhagic aspect of AV fistulae with too little thought given to their necessary counterpart, namely the enhanced venous return. The most straightforward consequence of "bleeding into the large veins" is an enhanced venous return which leads to enhanced cardiac filling and hence, increased cardiac output. To paraphrase Epstein's quote, one could propose that "the subject with an AV fistula is literally transfusing blood into his large veins." With this semantic swap, the reader may start to wonder which aspect of the fistula predominates in the circulatory physiology of pregnancy, the bleeding or the transfusion?

Under normal circumstances cardiac reserve is enormous and the only limit to the cardiac output compensation for an AV shunt is an adequate venous return.[173,174] This simply restates Starling's observation that the cardiac output "may be increased or diminished within very wide limits according to the inflow."[175] In "areflex" dogs, i.e., animals with total ablation of cardiovascular reflexes, opening an AV fistula which accommodates as much as 82% of the baseline cardiac output was associated with an instantaneous increase in cardiac output and only a minimal (10%) decrease in the nonshunt systemic blood flow.[176] Such healthy reflex compensation in the "areflex" dog is purely mechanical, driven by the enhanced venous return. Moreover, simultaneous transfusion of a modest volume of blood or saline drastically elevates the nonshunt, systemic perfusion[171] to values that can exceed preshunt control[173,176] (Fig. 4–8). Such a hemodynamic "overcompensation" in systemic perfusion obtained with an additional small transfusion occurred because volume expansion further increased an already enhanced venous return. Indeed, as was discussed in Chapter 3 and will be further detailed below, the MCFP, which determines the gradient for venous return, is increased by volume expansion. In this context, the blood volume expansion that develops in association with chronic AV fistulae[177,178] should be seen as a beneficial hemodynamic adjustment.[173]

The influence of blood viscosity on cardiac work and venous return has been recognized for some time.[179-182] Of importance in the rheology of circulation,[179] is the cru-

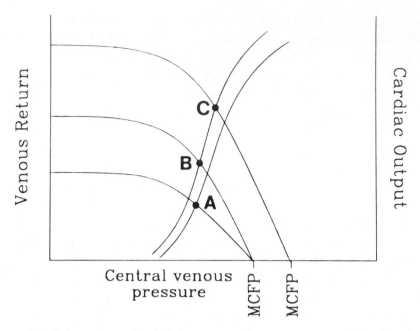

Figure 4–8. Schematic cardiac function curves. The venous return (left ordinate) and cardiac output (right ordinate) are represented as a function of the central venous pressure. The baseline venous return and cardiac output curves intersect at point A, at a given central venous pressure characteristic of the baseline hemodynamic state. The acute opening of an AV shunt results in an increased venous return and a steeper cardiac function curve due to afterload reduction. In the areflex dog, mean circulatory filling pressure (MCFP) is not affected by the opening of an AV fistula and thus venous return and cardiac output equate at B, a new equilibrium point of enhanced cardiac output characteristic of the new hemodynamic state with open fistula. With volume expansion the venous return curve is shifted to the right and intersects the cardiac output curve at C, at a markedly enhanced cardiac output. This is the circulatory state characteristic of pregnancy.[3] Note that the central venous pressure is affected only minimally, if at all, by these two maneuvers. (*Reprinted, with permission, from Durr JA: Maternal fluid adaptation to pregnancy. In: Brace RA, Ross MG, Robillard JE, eds.* Reproductive and Perinatal Medicine. Vol XI. Fetal and Neonatal Body Fluids. *Ithaca, NY: Perinatal Press; 1989:227–270.*)

cial role played by viscosity in the particular setting of an AV shunt. Thus, in the absence of a systemic shunt, the total systemic resistance is given by the sum of the individual resistances which are distributed in series along the vascular tree [$R_s = (R_1 + R_2 + \ldots)$]. The point of highest resistance along this circuit is encountered in the small vessels. At this level, the flow (Q) has become laminar and thus obeys Poiseuille's law: $Q = \delta P \cdot (\pi r^4/8\eta L)$. This equation, when rearranged to $\delta P = Q \cdot (8\eta L/\pi r^4)$, conforms to the familiar formula $\delta P = Q \cdot R$, where δP is the pressure change and R the resistance. Neglecting for a moment the other parameters, one sees that total peripheral resistance is directly proportional to the viscosity (η), a prediction that has been documented experimentally.[180-183] The presence of AV shunts introduces an interesting situation since now the resistances in the circuit are in parallel rather than in series and thus the total systemic resistance is related to the individual resistances by the equation $1/R_s = (1/R_{f-} + 1/R_{f+})$, where R_{f-} and R_{f+} represent the blood flow outside and through the AV fistula, respectively. Thus, in this case, one would anticipate that a decrease in viscosity will allow the systemic circulation to literally steal flow from the fistula. Indeed, a drop in viscosity will reduce resistance drastically in the systemic circulation where the laminar flow obeys Poiseuille's law ($R = 8\eta L/\pi r^4$) while affecting minimally, if at all, the resistance in the shunt where the vessel radius is larger and hence, turbulent flow occurs. Thus like volume expansion,[173,176] decreases in viscosity may affect systemic flow more than fistula flow.

This nuance on viscosity, in regard to shunt situations, may not be trivial. Indeed, its fundamental implications go beyond maternal adaptation to gestation and certainly deserve further investigation. Thus, if the circulatory effects of viscosity[179] were studied in the absence of concomitant acute anemia by performing exchange transfusion with hemoglobin or fluorinated polymers rather than with dextrans, different conclusions on cardiac output responses may have been reached. Indeed, in this particular study, acute anemia was found to decrease peripheral resistance presumably by causing "the small arteries and veins to participate in multiple microscopic shunts,"[179] a situation that mimics pregnancy. Such hemodynamic consequences support the prediction that viscosity has differential effects on flow in the nonshunt areas of the peripheral systemic circulation.

A sophisticated computerized simulation of the circulatory system[181] could predict the overall cardiovascular effects of altered blood viscosity when associated with varying degrees of systemic shunting. Unfortunately, Guyton and associates[181] did not make provisions for a block labeled "pregnancy" when building their monumental computerized analog model of the circulatory system with 354 blocks and nearly 500 equations. Conceivably, the elements for a pregnancy block are present, distributed in virtual form among the other 354 elements which compose this exhaustive model of circulation. Modest attempts at understanding circulatory homeostasis of pregnancy in terms of the Guytonian model have in fact been undertaken, but information is still too scant to permit such an exhaustive systems analysis of the circulatory adaptation to pregnancy.[44,184] Furthermore, since simulation cannot substitute for experimentation, questions such as those under discussion ultimately will need to be taken to the laboratory. A clue to preeclampsia may be lurking somewhere in these rheologic aspects of the maternal circulation.

To summarize; increased systemic perfusion is possible in the setting of an AV shunt provided it is associated with both a decreased blood viscosity and an expanded blood volume. Furthermore, anemia will potentiate this effect. Nature took advantage of this ideal constellation of hemodynamic and rheologic parameters by endowing the pregnant woman with the attributes of a decreased systemic resistance, an increased blood volume, and a decreased blood viscosity and hematocrit. This explains how an AV fistula is better tolerated by an already hypotensive, systemically vasodilated subject with a dilutional "anemia." One tempting explanation is that systemic vasodilation, blood volume expansion, and decreased blood viscosity are necessary changes most suited to prepare the pregnant woman to withstand the anticipated development of a uterine AV fistula. However, the recurrent question as to whether these changes are "deliberate" choices of nature or an adaptive response to a hemodynamic stress remains open. An ultimate answer to this question may be deeply rooted in the concept of mean circulatory filling pressure (MCFP), which will be discussed here.

The Role of the Mean Circulatory Filling Pressure

As alluded to, the striking increase in cardiac output and systemic perfusion obtained with expansion of the blood volume results from an increase in MCFP. The MCFP (see Fig. 4–8) may be the most important extracardiac parameter of circulatory competence[180-183] (see also Chap. 3). In mathematical or hydrodynamic terms, it represents the hydraulic pressure, i.e., the average pressure, obtained upon summation of all the individual pressures recorded simultaneously in each infinitesimal segment of the cardiovascular system. In practical terms, MCFP is the pressure recorded in the vascular tree at equilibrium in the absence of blood flow.[185] It has also been recognized as the "static blood pressure" by Starr,[186-188] who measured it in humans in the immediate postmortem period. Everything else being equal, the MCFP is the major determinant of cardiac performance.[183]

One of the great contributions of Guyton to circulatory physiology was to plot simultaneously on the same graph Starling's most simple "Law of the Heart"[175] expressing cardiac output (CO) as a function of the central venous pressure (CVP) [CO = f(CVP)] and the curve expressing venous return (VR) also as a function of the CVP or the right atrial pressure [VR = f(CVP)] (Fig. 4–8). Equating venous return with cardiac output (VR = CO) provides the CVP at which both curves intersect (point A).[180,183] This point constitutes the graphical solution of Guyton's circuit analysis of the circulation (see Fig. 4–8). Thus, the key to circulatory physiology which resides in the seemingly redundant statement that cardiac output equals venous return, represents the algebraic solution of a system of two simultaneous equations. Note that the difference between right atrial pressure (CVP) and MCFP represents the pressure gradient for venous return. Note also that in turn, and in keeping with the "Law of the Heart," VR determines CO.[175] In essence, both VR and CO are a function of the right atrial pressure (CVP) and the MCFP.

When analyzed in these terms, one realizes graphically that the acute opening of an AV fistula magnifies the slope of the venous return curve without affecting the MCFP. This may also be associated with a simultaneous increase in the gain of the cardiac function curve due to decreased afterload resistance. The result is the intercept (B) at a higher CO (see Fig. 4–8). Furthermore, if there is a simultaneous volume expansion, as observed in chronic AV fistulae, or as was simulated by transfusion in Guyton's "areflexic" dogs,[176] the MCFP is increased and thus the venous return curve is shifted to the right. In this case the venous return and cardiac function curve intersect at a new equilibrium point C, of further enhanced cardiac output (see Fig. 4–8). This equilibrium point C, which could be obtained by a simultaneous systemic vasodilation (A to B) and volume expansion (MCFP), (B to C), is characteristic of the circulatory state in gestation. As can be seen, because of the "gain" of the cardiac function curve, central venous pressure will be affected only minimally with opening of an AV fistula in competent hearts. The minimal effect of AV fistulae on right-sided heart chamber end-diastolic pressures has been illustrated in patients with traumatic AV fistula.[12] Thus, the increased cardiac performance and associated cardiac enlargement in gestation[79,189] should be viewed as a result of a decreased afterload and a primary increase in cardiac size rather than the result of an increased venous return and the Frank–Starling mechanism.[99] The effect of a shunt-like venous return on the low pressure baroreceptor and its implications have been discussed above.[167]

The MCFP is significantly elevated in pregnant dogs, rabbits, sheep, and guinea pigs.[154,184,190-192] In the only study in which this pressure was reported to be normal, the authors calculated that an increase of only 1 mm Hg ("that might not be detected") was required to increase the cardiac output of the nonpregnant guinea pigs.[193] Furthermore, pregnant dogs respond to epinephrine infusions with an increase in the MCFP in a manner similar to nonpregnant animals (BP/MCFP), suggesting that they are able to increase their vascular tone normally. In addition, the slope relating MCFP to changes in blood volume is not altered by pregnancy,[154,184,192,193] rather the blood volume–MCFP relationship is merely shifted to the right. Thus, since the MCFP is increased, not only the "unstressed" (i.e., capacitance) but also the "stressed" (i.e., distending) components of the intravascular volume are elevated during gestation. The higher MCFP has led some to suggest that the increased cardiac output may be secondary to "a relative overfilling of the circulatory system" during pregnancy.[154,184] Since the blood volume–MCFP relationship represents a measure of total circulatory compliance,[194] and for practical purpose total body venous compliance,[195] one is led to conclude that the venous tone was not altered in pregnancy, a finding which again would support relative vascular overfill as the sole cause for the increased MCFP in the pregnant animals. However, a hyperkinetic heart pumping against a very low systemic resistance may "handle" a large venous return and maintain normal filling pressures in spite of increased blood volume, provided that there is an enhanced venous capacitance. Rather than "relative overfilling," this may be the prevailing condition in pregnancy. In this situation, a relatively larger volume of blood is pooled within the venous system at pressures below the MCFP (see below). Experiments in both pregnant dogs[184] and sheep[192] also demonstrated a preserved cardiac reserve. Thus, in spite of an enhanced output at rest, the heart had not "used up" its reserves and moved to the flat part of the Starling curve. This observation is therefore also consistent with a primary increase in cardiac size independent of the Frank–Starling mechanism.

Cardiac output increases normally with exercise in humans and there appears to be a normal Frank–Starling curve relationship throughout gestation. As pregnancy advances, end-diastolic volume and stroke volume increase and the heart appears to move up its Starling curve.[189] This observation would imply that there is no change in the inotropic state of the heart during human gestation, a conclusion that militates against "underfill" and sympathetic system activation. Furthermore, according to Katz et al., the mechanism of cardiac adaptation would be similar to that observed in chronic volume overload.[189] These adaptive responses which may be mediated by increased lengths and number of sarcomeres that develop both in series and in parallel, would account[189] for the unimpaired shortening characteristics of the left ventricle despite progressive enlargement during pregnancy.

Physiologists record the MCFP or "static pressure" to gain further insight into the dynamic conditions under which the circulatory system operates.[184] In this light, the circulatory physiology of pregnancy can hardly be assimilated to a mere vascular underfill. However, since in practice the determination of MCFP requires interruption of cardiac output and ablation of all cardiovascular reflexes, this ultimate vital sign is unlikely to figure on the bedside chart next to the patient's blood pressure and heart rate. Neither the arterial nor the central venous pressures can predict the MCFP. As the difference between the MCFP and the central venous pressure (CVP) represents the pressure gradient for venous return, the MCFP constitutes the upper limit for the CVP above which the venous return ceases.[183] It is also important to understand that when taken alone, the MCFP provides little information on circulatory adequacy. Indeed, while the older concept of "backward" heart failure has been assimilated with "diastolic dysfunction,"[196] the increased CVP in heart failure can only be due to an increase in the MCFP and not to a postulated "back pressure" secondary to pump failure or diastolic dysfunction. Thus, congestive heart failure (CHF), which was viewed by Peters as the prototype of a clinical state with "ineffective blood volume,"[99,100] is also associated with an increased MCFP, and hence the MCFP alone is not sufficient to gauge circulatory competence.

It has been argued that pregnancy mimics the hyperdynamic state observed in patients with cirrhosis of the liver,[1-3] another "edematous state" characterized by a decreased "effective blood volume." However, measurements performed in a rat model of liver cirrhosis have clearly demonstrated that, unlike in pregnancy, the MCFP was not elevated.[197] Thus, the increased blood volume in liver cirrhosis, unlike in pregnancy, is mainly stored as "unstressed" volume that does not distend the vascular bed beyond its increased capacity.

The concept of MCFP is rarely used in clinical discussions. Another traditional description such as the heart as a pump emptying a dam fed by a river is an unfortunate cliché, and is inadequate to predict the increase in CVP associated with heart failure since the source of the river feeding the dam is the pump itself,[186-188] i.e., one is dealing with a closed circuit. Since the increased CVP in CHF is due to an increase in MCFP, a more accurate analogy would call either for an additional river that feeds the closed circuit and/or an enhanced vasoconstriction to account for the increased MCFP. The additional river leaves the system on the high pressure side of the circuit, i.e., at the kidneys, and represents input and output. Vasoconstriction of the circuit is mediated by the autonomic nervous system and humoral mechanisms under the control of the baroreceptor. With these extra provisions, however, the simple analogy of the circulatory system turns into a circuit analysis.

The Role of "Effective Blood Volume"

"Effective blood volume" is another historic concept with relevance to the current debate regarding body fluid physiology during gestation,[1] but unlike the MCFP, the notion of "effective blood volume" surfaces frequently on medical rounds.[1,3] Thus, a review of the hemodynamics of pregnancy in light of this concept is in order.

In Peters' view, the "effective blood volume" is that dynamic part of the circulation or a function thereof which informs the body on the adequacy of the cardiac or hemodynamic performance. As discussed, in humans the most important sensors or "volumeters"[99,100] are those located within the arterial side of the circulation.[12,70,168] These baroreceptors are thought to "sense" the "effective blood volume" or a function thereof. However, while the MCFP is very difficult to measure, the "effective blood volume" has no measure at all. Indeed, it is only a mental image, a functional concept that may be understood, yet that escapes any clear definition. Nevertheless, generations of physicians have been seduced by this concept probably because of its operational aspect rich in finalistic implications. Indeed, in the overall scheme of cardiovascular and body fluid physiology, autonomic, humoral, and renal responses seem designed for the ultimate defense of the "effective blood volume." Hence, because of these provisions selected by evolution, as vague as this concept may be, it may have at one time or another proven useful in managing a patient, and thus, in spite of its elusiveness, this concept has dominated the US medical literature for the past 50 years.[70]

Referring to the notion of "effective blood volume," one of Peters's most clairvoyant disciples subsequently noted that "the intellectual appeal of this explanation lies in its adherence to the principle that [quoting Peters]: '*the disorders encountered in disease may be regarded as normal physiologic responses to unusual conditions produced by pathologic processes.*'[168] However, of particular significance was Epstein's caution that "the weakness of the theory is the uncertain (and sometimes circular) definition of 'effective blood volume.'"[168] The temptation for physicians is great to see in many of the maternal body fluid and cardiovascular adaptations to pregnancy "normal physiologic responses to unusual conditions produced by pathological processes . . . ."[168] Indeed, most of the parameters of body fluid homeostasis that are "reset" in pregnancy and can be reduced to "normal physiological responses . . . " according to the principle set forward by Peters.[1,3] Thus, for example, the hyponatremia of pregnancy, rather than representing a true reset osmostat[66] may be explained by the activation of thirst and AVP secretion in response to a decreased "effective blood volume,"[1] while the clinical similarities between pregnancy and cirrhosis have already been discussed. Furthermore, in addition to hyponatremia and absolute increments in blood volume, both cirrhosis and pregnancy are characterized by a low blood pressure, a bouncing pulse pressure, tachycardia, and edema. However, as noted in contrast to cirrhotic rats, the MCFP is elevated during pregnancy.[154,184,190,191,192,197] Thus, rather than considering gestation as a pathological process, it may be more appropriate to approach the physiology of pregnancy with other premises. The more cautious approach adopted here forces one to reject the *a priori* of the traditional formalism of Peters.[1] Indeed, genuine resetting of the circulatory dynamics may take place. Thus, reducing the physiology of gestation to the nonpregnant state may not be justified. As reviewed here, when all the known hemodynamic and body fluid changes of pregnancy are analyzed carefully, the circulatory state prevailing in pregnancy cannot be reduced unequivocally either to a state of "underfill" nor to a state of "overflow."[1,67,77]

Of interest is a catheterization study in minimally anesthetized pregnant baboons, often cited as an example of decreased "effective blood volume."[198] If, cardiac filling pressures are the parameters arbitrarily selected[198] in the "circular definition" of effective blood volume, then the underfill seems to disappear in midgestation, at a time when the uterine circulation develops and thus an AV shunt appears. The explanation for the improved cardiac filling pressures after the second half of gestation is the late change in blood volume in the pregnant baboon. In spite of elevations in plasma renin activity and aldosterone and an adequate sodium diet, expansion of blood volume in this species seems to occur only in the second half of gestation. In human gestation, however, plasma volume starts to increase in the first trimester. Thus, transient maladaptation to the circulatory changes of pregnancy may be argued in the baboon, at least when lightly anesthetized, and when cardiac filling pressures are chosen as the "measure" of effective blood volume.[201] Note however that such a conclusion is based on the premises that the norm for cardiac filling pressures during pregnancy are those recorded in the nonpregnant state, and that the elusive "effective blood volume" is given by the central venous pressure (CVP). It may be appropriate to recall that in primates, the predominant baroreceptor is not located in the low pressure system but rather in the high pressure side of the circulation[70] and, as discussed previously, the "gain" of this baroreceptor appears to be increased during gestation. Although no balance studies were performed, a 50 mmol/day sodium diet should have been adequate to correct the underfill of the low pressure system. Thus, the *Papio hamadryas*, the baboon species studied in this report, may be a subtle salt waster, at least in the earlier stages of gestation. A trend for salt wasting has been suggested in human gestation as well.[20] However, since natriuresis is also the characteristic of volume expansion, the question becomes as to whether it is the often overused Swan–Ganz catheter[199,200,201] or the baroreceptor, which is the more appropriate way to appraise the "effective blood volume."

To summarize then, at first glance the hemodynamic alterations associated with gestation in the baboon may be explained by "underfill" complicated by primary renal salt wasting. The latter may be further complicated by the increased glomerular filtration rate, or may be due to humoral factors, such as progesterone, prostaglandins, and the nitric oxide–cGMP system. The resulting decrease in "effective blood volume" may then be viewed as activating the renin–aldosterone axis. This example conforms to the approach based on the premise of Peters that the physiologic changes of pregnancy may be regarded as "normal physiologic responses to unusual conditions."[168]

Global Assessment of Circulatory Adequacy During Gestation

The review on the physiologic implications of AV fistulae, blood viscosity, blood volume, MCFP, and "effective blood volume" was necessary, as these are highly relevant to pregnancy. Indeed, given the ongoing changes characteristic of pregnancy, one can see that an increase in the MCFP represents a bonus in terms of cardiovascular adequacy. Figure 4–9 compares schematically the circulatory system in the pregnant and the nonpregnant state. On the ordinate are recorded the individual pressures along the vascular tree, starting from the left ventricle in systole and extending all the way to the right atrium. The dotted curve depicts the intravascular

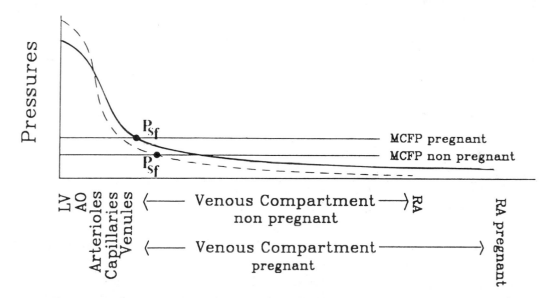

Figure 4–9. Schematic representation of the intravascular pressures along the vascular bed in the absence of circulation (horizontal MCFP-lines) and when the heart is beating (solid and dotted curves) in the pregnant (solid) and the nonpregnant state (dotted lines). To the left, the highest pressures are recorded in the left ventricle (LV) and the aorta (AO). The intravascular pressures decrease sharply as blood transits through the resistance vessels and the rate of decrease falls as blood transits through the low-resistance venous system until it reaches the right atrium (RA). The scale on the abscissa is proportional to the volumes of blood in the respective vascular compartments. In the absence of flow, all pressures equalize along a horizontal line of MCFP. Each curve intersects its respective line of MCFP at an indifferent point P_{sf}. This point is located somewhere in the venous compartment. Note that the MCFP is higher during gestation and that the volume of blood pooled at pressures lower than that of the MCFP is also larger during gestation. (*Reprinted, with permission, from Durr JA: Maternal fluid adaptation to pregnancy. In: Brace RA, Ross MG, Robillard JE, eds. Reproductive and Perinatal Medicine. Vol XI. Fetal and Neonatal Body Fluids. Ithaca, NY: Perinatal Press; 1989:227–270.*)

pressures recorded in the nonpregnant state and the solid line, the pressures recorded during gestation. The individual segments of the circulatory system, i.e., arterial, capillary, and venous compartments are depicted on the abscissa, in a scale proportional to their respective volumes. As discussed, in the absence of circulation, all the pressures equalize along a horizontal line which represents the MCFP. From the present review we learned that pregnancy is associated with decreased mean arterial pressure, increased capillary pressures, increased blood volume (venous compartment), increased MCFP, and a normal to decreased CVP. This leads to the graph of Figure 4–9. As can be seen, the pressure curves intersect their respective MCFP lines somewhere in the venous compartment at points labeled P_{sf}. When the heart is pumping, all pressures recorded to the left of this point are higher than the MCFP and all pressures to the right of this point are lower than the MCFP.

The total amount of blood "stored" at pressures lower than the MCFP is larger during pregnancy. Guyton's theory implying a linear relationship between venous return (VR) and the difference between MCFP and the CVP, i.e., the "gradient for venous return": $VR = (CVP - MCFP)/R_{sf}$,[182,183] has been confirmed by others.[202] Moreover, the position of the "indifferent point" P_{sf}[202] is defined since the ratio $(CVP - MCFP)/VR$ which represents the flow resistance (R_{sf}) between this point (P_{fs}) and the right atrium is constant (slope of venous return).[183] Since the value of R_{sf} is consistently less than 20% of the total systemic resistance,[202] the indifferent point P_{sf} must lie within the venous compartment. When extrapolated to the parallel circuits of the circulatory system, this model helps explain how changes in CVP will influence local capillary pressures. If the capillary pressures of a given vascular bed are located upstream from P_{sf}, a rise in CVP will be associated with a fall in capillary pressure. Conversely, in the territories where the capillary pressures are below P_{sf}, intracapillary pressures will rise. During these differential changes, therefore, blood may shift to temporary intravascular reservoirs and/or extracellular fluid may shift in either direction across the vascular bed.

Thus, when considered in the setting of a decreased capillary "safety factor" for edema and an expanded venous reservoir, both characteristics of pregnancy, this model may account for important functional aspects of maternal circulatory adaptation to gestation. Although values for capillary pressures in many vascular beds are lacking, one may speculate that alterations in the maternal circulatory system are such that maximum hemodynamic stability is ensured. A number of studies remain to be done to elucidate this aspect of circulatory physiology during gestation. Such studies are complex and require the simultaneous determination of interrelated variables such as capillary and interstitial hydrostatic pressures, capillary and interstitial colloid osmotic pressures, central venous pressure, MCFP, cardiac output, and transcapillary fluxes in different regions of the maternal circulation. Only once these complex interactions are elucidated, can a better model of maternal adaptation to gestation be envisioned.[44]

Finally, the kidney assumes a central role in this system since it has the last word in the overall vascular filling. If it fails to retain sodium and water adequately, circulatory underfill occurs, as illustrated perhaps by the example of the pregnant baboon.[201] If however, it achieves its task, maternal circulatory performance may be far superior than would be expected, if the changes, like in the rat with liver cirrhosis,[197] were mere responses to systemic arterial "underfill." Considered in light of the principles discussed in the preceding sections, it would make sense that the kidney is the sole organ in the body where interstitial hydrostatic pressures are positive rather than negative,[59,133] and where capillary pressures are higher than average. Clearly, a mass of interesting information is awaiting to be discovered when physiologists approach pregnancy with these principles in mind.

CONCLUSION

To the casual observer, pregnancy is characterized by relatively slow and gradual changes as exemplified in the gradual increase in abdominal girth. Thus, as noted by Hytten, research has been guided by the subjective principle that for any change in pregnancy, the more advanced the pregnancy, the greater the change.[32] In this context the third trimester was the preferred stage for studies, and investigators have recurrently attempted to compare the circulatory physiology of late gestation to the nonpregnant state arbitrarily selected as the norm.[201] This chapter stressed the notion that the circulatory and body fluid physiology of pregnancy may not be reducible to the nonpregnant state. Comparisons with the nonpregnant state for other purposes than to show difference may be meaningless, since for pregnancy the norm is pregnancy. Pregnancy, by strict definition, is a binary function, and a subject is either pregnant or not. Thus, for once semantics and physiology agree, and concepts such as "more pregnant" do not bear any physiologic meaning as would the notion of "more underfilled." Hytten[32] remarked further that "recently our views have changed and we now realize that most of the really dramatic physiological happenings of pregnancy take place in the earliest stages. In this respect, the changes associated with pregnancy differ radically from most physiological adaptations in which the body reacts to a situation by trying to restore homeostasis. In pregnancy the 'adaptation' precedes the need, that is to say, the mother makes prior arrangements, often months in advance, to meet situations some of which may never arise." This view is diametrically opposed to the traditional view on body fluid regulation in which, as Epstein recalled, one looks for "normal physiologic responses to unusual conditions produced by pathologic processes."[99,100,168]

One of the aims of this chapter was to point out the diverse philosophies hidden behind the studies of maternal body fluid "adaptation" to pregnancy. The reader should resist the seduction of doctrines based on teleologic premises and keep an open mind when approaching the physiology of gestation. Pregnancy should be approached as a physiologic entity with an extra dimension. "Fetomaternal" physiology can neither be reduced to the physiology of the mother alone nor to the physiology of the fetus separately without the danger of losing its dimension.

APPENDIX
(By J.A. Dürr)

On What is "Effective" in "Effective Blood Volume"

A Historical Review and Reappraisal of an Old Paradigm

The acquisition and maintenance of body fluids have long been recognized as among the most primeval conditions required to sustain life. Thus, as retraced by Strauss,[203] the original observation by Claude Bernard (1859) that the cells of higher organisms, unlike the unicellular aquatic organisms, do not come into direct contact with the external environment, but rather live in their own internal sea, led to the postulate that stability in the composition of this *milieu intérieur* constitutes the *sine qua non* condition for "freedom and independence of existence." As recalled by Strauss half a century later, Starling (1909) went one step further by stressing that, for survival, stability in volume of body fluids was as important as the stability in their composition. Finally, yet another half century later, Strauss,[203] paraphrasing Starling, wrote that: "Man is provided with distinct mechanisms for the regulation of the amount as well as the composition of the body fluids. Thirst and appetite under the regulation of the central nervous system and the kidneys under the influence of circulatory, humoral, and possibly neurologic factors subserve this office." Strauss further noted, echoing Smith,[204] that "this stability is determined largely by what the kidneys retain—provided that thirst and appetite furnish a surplus: the kidneys cannot supply deficits. Freedom requires adequate intakes as well as the overflow of excesses."[203] The stability in composition and volume of body fluids, key to survival, therefore, hinges more on the fine tuning of renal excretions (i.e., on the maintenance), than on the *acquisition*, i.e., the precise "metering" of the intakes of solutes and water, and hence, the kidneys have the final word in body fluid homeostasis.

The extraordinary range over which the kidneys independently modulate the rates of excretion of salts and water, and thereby guarantee volume and fluid composition stability, has baffled clinicians and physiologists for the last 50 years.[13,65,99,100] Although attention has focused on the role of the kidney in regulation of extracellular fluid composition and volume, its effects on the intracellular compartment should not be ignored. Thus, basing his arguments on the laws of osmosis that govern the distribution of water across cell membranes, Strauss noted that "since the major solutes in the extracellular fluid (sodium, chloride, and bicarbonate) are largely excluded from the cells, the renal control of these ions is in considerable measure responsible for changes in intra- and extracellular fluid volumes. Accordingly the kidney, through its regulation of the composition of the extracellular fluid, may affect not only extracellular, but also intracellular, volume."[203] Similar reasoning had led Peters to propose that "sodium is therefore the instrument by which the distribution of water in the body is regulated."[100]

Since Peters also knew that "the most potent stimulus to thirst appears to be the effective osmotic pressure of the extracellular fluid; that is, the sum of the partial osmotic pressures of those solutes that cannot diffuse freely across cellular membranes, of which the most important ordinarily are sodium salts,"[100] he concluded that "since these determine the distribution of water between cells and extracellular fluid, it may be the state of hydration of the cells that controls thirst."[100] As exactly the same can be said for the osmoregulation of vasopressin, which mediates renal water retention, both fluid intake and output are controlled by the cells. Moreover, antidiuretic hormone, through its antidiuretic (V2) and vascular (V1) isoreceptors, has profound effects on both the composition and volume of the extracellular fluid.[70] Therefore, the question arises as to which one of the parameters—composition or volume of the intra- or extracellular fluids—is primarily involved in the acquisition and maintenance of body fluids.

It is reasonable to assume that the *milieu intérieur* that needs to be preserved to best ensure Claude Bernard's "freedom and independence of existence" is the *intracellular* compartment. Indeed, for the living cells, the *milieu intérieur* is the intracellular fluid. However, one may argue that delivery of oxygen and nutrients to, and removal of waste products from the living cells, are contingent on circulatory adequacy. Given the pivotal reciprocity imposed by the laws of osmosis on the volume and tonicity of both compartments, the *primum mobile* of osmotic and volume regulation cannot be resolved by neatly prioritizing functions. This reciprocity may have been forgotten as osmoregulation now evokes nearly exclusively the regulation of plasma sodium, i.e., of the *composition* of extracellular fluid (ECF). Thus, the near perfect correlation that exists between plasma vasopressin (AVP) and plasma sodium (see Figures 4–3 and 4–4 in the text) reflects the correlation that exists between AVP and the intracellular potassium or relative cell volume. Although it is reasonable to assume that normally the intracellular makeup sets the osmostat, clinical experience reveals that the edematous disorders with decreased "effective blood volume," are almost consistently associated with a lower plasma osmolality. Indeed, AVP and thirst are not only controlled by tonicity but also by volume,[70] thereby closing a physiologic feedback loop. Hyponatremia may therefore result from a trade-off between the need to satisfy simultaneously the osmotic imperatives of the intracellular fluid and the volume demands of the extracellular fluid. Such a trade-off has been incriminated in the *pathogenesis* of the hyponatremia of gestation,[1] though implicit to such reasoning is that pregnancy is a state of vascular underfill. However, as detailed in the text, the evidence required to reduce the hyponatremia and volume expansion of pregnancy to mere manifestations of a diseased state is still lacking.

When clinicians first explored volume and osmotic regulation, the measurement of sodium as recounted by Peters, was a "protracted, meticulous procedure for which few laboratories are equipped, and which is ill adapted to the regulation of therapy in clinic."[99] Peters (1887–1955) nevertheless guessed that the "measurement of sodium should be more generally practiced as soon as simple and practical flame photometers become available."[99] The flame photometer has been replaced with the more practical ion-selective electrodes. Although the concept of "effective blood volume" coined by Peters[99,100] to "explain" a variety of clinical disorders associated with avid renal salt and water retention has resulted in the practice of measuring sodium in clinical settings, Peters may not have foreseen that hyponatremia would eventually surface as the most frequent laboratory abnormality encountered in hospitalized patients.[205,206] Indeed, in the 1940s, when clinician–scientists began to focus on volume regulation in edematous disorders in earnest, the concentration of sodium in the serum of patients with congestive heart failure was far "more discussed than investigated."[99]

In order to place the historical debate on the role played by sodium in osmotic and volume regulation, some quantitative considerations are required. Osmolality exerted by a sodium salt Na_nX in solution can be expressed as a function of the concentration of its sodium ions (Na^+) by the formula $Osm = [(n + 1)/n] \times [Na^+]$, provided the salt fully dissociates into ($n \times Na^+$) and X^{-n}. Indeed, since the osmolality is produced by the sum total of all the solutes, $Osm = [Na^+] + [X^-] + [Na_nX]$, when the salt is totally dissociated into ($n \times Na^+$) and X^{-n}, and hence when $[Na_nX] = 0$ and $[X^-] = [Na^+]/n$, then $Osm = [Na^+] + [Na^+]/n = [(n + 1)/n] \times [Na^+]$. Second, since the salts of Na in the extracellular fluid (ECF) account for over 96% of all the solutes that are *osmotically active* in regard to cell membranes, and since the overwhelming species are monovalent salts (Cl^- and HCO_3^-), i.e., $n = 1$, the equation reduces to $Osm \simeq 2 \times [Na^+]$, and hence the "effective osmolality" of the ECF can be accounted for entirely by the salts of Na. Moreover, since the total exchangeable sodium (Na_e) in the body is confined to the extracellular compartment,[97] the plasma sodium concentration P_{Na} will be provided by the equation $P_{Na} = Na_e/ECF$, and hence, for a given P_{Na}, the ECF is entirely dependent on Na_e. Thus, sodium represents the "hard currency" by which the organism buys its extracellular volume. Note that the equation $ECF = Na_e/P_{Na}$ predicts that if plasma sodium were to be reset from its normal value of $P_{Na} = 142$ mEq/L to the lower value of 132, the same total body sodium would now allow the body to "buy" ~7.5% more ECF. Thus resetting the P_{Na}, i.e., the osmostat, is equivalent to reevaluating or devaluating sodium, the currency of volume. Hence, by resetting the pregnant woman's P_{Na} to a lower value,[9,68] she gets a discount on her extracellular volume. This, however, does not mean that her hyponatremia is the manifestation of a diseased-volume homeostasis.

This example serves to illustrate that osmotic and volume regulations, although concerned with physiologic parameters of different physical dimensions, are functions that are, by necessity, intimately interrelated.[43] Thus, while Smith recognized that "the antidiuretic and the antinatriuretic systems may apparently be excited and inhibited wholly independently of each other," he also noted that "at any specific level of antinatriuretic activity, the antidiuretic system operates rapidly to promote the conservation or excretion of water in such a manner as to maintain the osmotic concentration of the body fluids at a fixed constant value (about 283 ± 11 mOsm/L), regardless of body fluid volume."[65] His observation that the coefficient of variation of the osmotic pressure of plasma "is only 1.2%, possibly the smallest coefficient of variation among all known physiological variables,"[207] led him to propose that "in consequence of this final integration, the osmotic pressure of the body fluids is one of the most closely regulated of all homeostatic states and tends to take precedence over volume regulation."[65] For Smith, "the steady state, the physiological desideratum, around which water balance is co-ordinated is the osmotic pressure of the plasma."[207] This view was shared by Strauss, and by Peters, who felt that, among the major osmotically active components to which cell membranes are impervious, namely the sodium and potassium salts, "the chief variable among these is the sodium of the extracellular fluid, which is, therefore, the principal determinant of the relative volume of the intracellular fluid. When the concentration of sodium falls, the cells take up water and swell, when the concentration of sodium rises, the cells give up water and contract."[99] However, given the extraordinary speed with which water diffuses across cell membranes and continually matches intra- and extracellular osmolalities to claim that the ultimate target of osmoregulation is the *osmotic pressure of the plasma*[207] or the *sodium of the extracellular fluid*,[99] rather than the osmotic pressure of the cytosol or the potassium of the intracellular fluid, is tautological and hence, becomes a mere matter of taste. Sodium and potassium are both the targets as well as the instruments of osmoregulation.

Because osmoregulation, through sodium, leads to "price fixing" of the ECF volume, it necessarily affects volume homeostasis. Conversely, if the renal retention or losses of sodium and water occur in disproportionate ways, they will necessarily affect tonicity. Smith traced the remarkable constancy of the osmotic pressure of the plasma he marveled so much about back to the fresh water and marine teleosts and beyond.[203] This constancy, as Strauss remarked, "almost as much as the presence of a backbone, speaks for the common ancestry of all members, and suggests that the composition of the fluid was fixed early in vertebrate evolution, possibly in some common provertebrate ancestor."[204] The value of the tonicity of body fluids is located midway between fresh water and the estimated salinity of the sea at the time the first vertebrate appeared. This led him to suggest that the vertebrate progenitors had already left the sea for brackish or fresh water when they ultimately moved on land,[203] "taking with them a bit of the primeval ocean in their extracellular fluid."[13] This means, in last analysis, that the prize of the ECF has remained unchanged at roughly 140 mEq Na/L literally since antediluvian times.

The cell probably functions best when its milieu meets a given set of physicochemical conditions of temperature, pH, and ionic strength. Indeed, no one contests the effects of pH and temperature on enzymatic functions, but that of ionic strength is just as important. Thus, the "salting out" phenomenon, in which a given protein is unfolded and precipitated when the medium reaches a threshold ionic strength, can be put to advantage to obtain after renaturation, the "salt-poor albumin" fraction used in clinical practice. The salts of sodium and potassium, the major extra- and intracellular solutes, are both highly caotropic, and hence "incompatible" when it comes to preserve the structure and function of proteins.[208] The discovery of "compatible solutes," i.e., solutes that stabilize the structure of proteins and prevent them from denaturation in high salt environments, has renewed interest in the intracellular events that participate in osmoregulation.[208] Indeed, these intracellular "compatible" solutes with typical "antifreeze" functions, also called "idiogenic osmoles,"[209] should more properly be labeled "osmolytes," and play a crucial role in osmoregulation.[208] The brain is enclosed and attached to the walls of the rigid skull. It can neither afford to swell nor shrink, hence mechanisms to protect brain cells from swelling or shrinking in response to changes in the ECF osmolality are of utmost importance. The intracranial location of the osmoreceptors for both thirst and AVP release, together with the brain osmolyte system subserve this vital function. Teleologically, therefore, enclosing the brain with its billions of delicate intercellular synaptic connections in a rigid box and providing the means of ensuring volume constancy, protects the organism from losing its acquired information. A decrement in plasma sodium from 142 to 135, not uncommon in gestation, if unbalanced, would increase brain volume by 5%, a change resulting perhaps in a marked increase in intracranial pressure. Whether such changes explain the nausea of early gestation is unknown.

Among the most significant contributions of Peters was his introduction into the clinical practice of assessing electrolytes and the kidney, in a context such as the disorders encountered in disease are "regarded as normal physiologic responses to unusual conditions produced by pathologic processes."[99] This was illustrated best by his profound interest in the "edematous states." The vivid clinical picture of avid renal sodium and water retention in the face of a grotesquely expanded ECF compartment in patients with the nephrotic syndrome, congestive heart failure, or cirrhosis of the liver with ascites, clearly suggested to him that what was sensed and ultimately regulated at the renal level could not have been the total extracellular volume, but rather must have been some fraction or function thereof. By coining this elusive fraction of the blood volume as the "effective blood volume" (EBV), Peters revived the suggestion first made by Starling[17] that sodium excretion might be related to a function of the volume of the circulating blood. The persistent fascination with this concept resides probably less in the fact that the EBV cannot be measured, than in the fact that no one agrees on its units. Thus, the question remains, should the EBV simply be expressed in units of volume, or should it be expressed in units of volume per time, so as to account for the vague notion of some flow? Others will argue that the EBV should also contain units of pressure so as to account for the notion of "fullness" alluded to by Peters and those who invoke it in their own research. As it has neither units nor can be measured, the EBV is of little scientific interest.

The notion of EBV is a purely *operational concept* historically meant to stimulate thinking in the emerging field of volume homeostasis.[99,100] Although just a concept, the notion of "effective blood volume" has prompted clinicians to distinguish diuresis from natriuresis,[13,65,70] stimulated the quest for the volume receptors[13,65] or "volumeters" (another term coined by Peters), and conferred to the kidneys a *raison d'être* that hitherto only a few had appreciated. Therefore, and in spite of the fact that half a century later[99] one still cannot "quantify the will-o'-the-wisp of effective blood volume,"[168] this legacy of Peters[210] deserves its current place in the history of medicine, although this concept did not prevent Papper, reflecting on the future of our understanding of volume regulation in cirrhosis from stating, that "in the distant future this subject may, at most, be discussed after sherry at an occasional meeting of a History of Medicine Society."[211]

The ensuing search for the putative volume receptors has been an exciting one. At the time of Smith's historic "apologetic" review,[65] there were two major candidates, the low pressure (atrial) and the high pressure (sino-aortic) intrathoracic baroreceptors.[70] Space travel has stimulated a renewed interest in the well-known "atrial reflex" diuresis observed when, in the absence of the gravitational pull, blood redistributes centrally and distends the atria. The immersion of subjects up to the neck in "thermoneutral" baths became a common technique used to mimic this translocation of blood into the low pressure intrathoracic vascular bed.[212] This procedure results in a natriuresis and diuresis associated with inhibition of plasma–renin activity, aldosterone production, AVP and catecholamine release,[212] and an increase in the release of the atrial natriuretic peptide (ANP), among many other changes characteristic of volume expansion.

Gauer et al.[43] believed that "since changes of pressure within the low-pressure system directly result from changes in blood volume, stretch receptors incorporated in the walls could signal changes of blood volume to the central nervous system and thereby evoke adaptive reflexes." The idea of a receptor that stretches as a linear function of the blood volume, and that is strategically located at the atrium, where filling of the heart, and hence cardiac output is controlled, is very appealing. However, although the low-pressure atrial baroreceptors which mediate the "Henry–Gauer" diuretic reflex are important in quadrupeds, the high-pressure sino-aortic baroreceptors may play the more prominent role of volumeters in "erect" humans.[70] Indeed, if the low-pressure receptors were as predominant in humans as they are in the dog, the antidiuretic response to quit standing[213] would be magnified so immensely that humans would be plagued by persistent nocturia. This is because an upright position leads to pooling of ~500 mL of blood in the dependent vessels, unassociated with any increase in the tone of the vascular bed.[43] This observation has led to the conclusion that, "in the reciprocal adjustments of vascular capacity and blood volume to achieve a normal measure of J.P. Peters's 'fullness of the blood stream,' blood volume must be considered as the prime variable."[43]

The "predominant" receptors for the control of EBV in humans are not located in the low-pressure venous compartment, but rather are located in the arterial tree. This view, pioneered by Frank Epstein, was based on his studies of cardiovascular and renal responses to acute compressions of traumatic arteriovenous fistulae in young male Korean War veterans.[11,12] He showed that natriuresis or antinatriuresis (and to some extent also a diuresis or antidiuresis) depended on compressing or releasing the compression of the AV fistula. Epstein felt that "when an arteriovenous shunt is occluded, the arterial tree is emptied more slowly and less completely." He further noted that the "pressures in the great veins, the right atrium, and the pulmonary vessels tend to fall as these regions become less distended with blood." In this seminal study, Epstein also listed the known circulatory states, chronic as well as acute, in which the kidneys tend to retain sodium, and noted that in some of these conditions the volume of blood in the central veins is reduced, while in others these vessels are engorged, but "in all, however, there exists a tendency towards inadequate filling of the systemic arterial tree" and hence, he concluded that "renal excretion or retention of sodium is conditioned by the degree of filling of some portion of the arterial tree."[12] The predominance of the high-pressure baroreceptor in humans[70] is highly relevant to pregnancy, and is characterized by a resetting of the baroreceptor to a lower mean arterial blood pressure (MAP).

The MAP, a surrogate for renal perfusion pressure, evokes yet another parameter that influences volume homeostasis. Indeed, if any neural or humoral factor is to play any significant role in the overall regulation of volume, then it must ultimately affect the fundamental "renal perfusion pressure–volume output" relationship[129] (see Fig. 4–6 in the text), i.e., the intrinsic "willingness" of the kidney to mount a diuresis and natriuresis (volume output) at any given perfusion pressure, as foreseen by Borst.[127] This mechanism, referred to as the "pressure natriuresis" is best demonstrated in the isolated perfused kidney (removed from external humoral or neural influences).[214] As noted by Gauer et al.,[43] given the first law of the heart in which cardiac output and hence, MAP are functions of the cardiac filling pressure of the heart (CVP) (see Fig. 4–8 in the text), if one further assumes that "the arterial pressure directly affects the excretory function of the kidney, then, it is possible to construct an analog model of the circulation in which cardiac output is regulated through a change in extracellular volume without the help of any neural or humoral mechanisms." Such an analog model was first constructed by Guyton et al.,[181] the salient aspect of this computerized systems analysis being assumption of a close relationship between the arterial blood pressure and the excretory function of the kidney. Epstein had also considered this basic mechanism before, because in all his subjects "the increase in sodium excretion produced by closing a fistula was accompanied by an elevation of the calculated mean arterial pressure." Although not dismissing this basic mechanism, clinical evidence led Epstein to favor the existence of some reflex humoral or neural mechanism, since "the increase in pressure was always much smaller than that required in Selkurt's experiments to bring about the change in sodium excretion," and since "the change in sodium excretion from patient to patient could not be correlated with the magnitude of the response of the blood pressure."[12] Hence, in his view, "renal retention of salt and water would fall into the same category as a variety of vascular reactions (e.g., the carotid sinus and aortic reflexes) designed to maintain the integrity of the circulation."

Therefore, provided that the appropriate "blocks" required to account for the neural and humoral reflexes affecting Borst's "willingness"[127] of the kidney to excrete sodium and water at a given perfusion pressure are included, the various components of the hydraulic system proposed by Guyton et al. not only "mesh remarkably well,"[43] but their entire circuit analysis provides the framework ultimately required to fully understand volume regulation. Thus, Epstein's prediction that "the experimental creation of a large arteriovenous fistula might be expected to promote the renal retention of salt, at least until a new equilibrium is established,"[12] is now understood by the circuit analysis of Guyton et al.[181]

Gauer et al. had stressed that "the existence of a quantitative relationship between the pressures in the low-pressure system and total blood volume lies at the basis of the generally considered possibilities for the control of plasma volume, i.e., control either by physical or by neuroendocrine regulatory mechanisms, respectively."[43] Our review points to an integration of both mechanisms, whereby the baroreceptors, through neuroendocrine mediations, merely modulate the fundamental renal "perfusion pressure–volume output" relationship (see Fig. 4–6).

While the degree of fullness of a rigid-walled container can be expressed as percent of total capacity, the most expedient way to define fullness for a container with elastic walls, is to establish its pressure–volume diagram first and then measure the filling pressure.[43] However, while this gauges the "fullness" of an elastic container when its liquid content is at rest, one encounters difficulties in applying this approach to the dynamic state of the circulatory system. One would be required to momentarily stop the circulation and let all the pressures throughout the vascular tree equalize and then take measurements. As an intern, Starr was called to the bedside of a patient to "pronounce" him dead, with congestive heart failure (CHF) as the probable cause of death. He was puzzled by the persistence of jugular vein distension even after the patient's heart had stopped beating, and hence presumably after the pressures throughout the entire vascular compartment must have equalized.[187] Indeed, the analogy, still invoked today to "explain" jugular vein distension in patients with CHF, is that of "backward heart failure,"[196] whereby the blood is assumed to be pooled upstream of the failing heart. The persistence of jugular distension after the heart had stopped beating, convinced Starr that it could not have resulted from a build-up of blood or "*Blutstauung*" upstream of the failing heart.[187] He eventually measured this "static blood pressure" in patients who had recently expired from different causes.[186,187] This rather simple experiment of postmortem "static blood pressure" recording produced one of the most revolutionary findings of modern cardiology, namely that the subgroup of patients who expired with CHF had significantly higher pressures in their vascular tree after the heart had stopped.[187]

The gist of "static blood pressure" will escape understanding as long as it is only considered under the static, i.e., purely Pascalian conditions of hydraulics that prevail at autopsy, when the heart has ceased to beat. Under those conditions, the static pressure is a function of the total blood volume and the capacity and compliance of the vascular bed and offers little interest to the pathologist who rarely goes to the bedside. It may be of interest to recall that *since the volume elasticity of the arterial system is about 200 times higher than that of the total circulation, the compliance of the vascular bed is practically identical with the compliance of the low-pressure system which holds approximately 80% of the total blood volume.*[43] Thus, when the heart starts to beat again, only a minimal amount of blood is transferred from the low-pressure, high capacity venous system into the high-pressure, low capacity arterial tree, because of the marked differences in compliance of the two systems (normally 30- to 60-fold rather than the 200-fold quoted). However, there will be a marked rise in the arterial blood pressure but only a modest fall in the pressures in the great veins.

It is also important to note that although the compliance of the low-pressure system is practically identical with the total vascular compliance, the "static blood pressure" and the CVP are two different cardiovascular parameters. Thus, once the heart starts to beat again, the CVP, equal to the "static blood pressure" in the absence of blood flow, will decrease and the arterial blood pressure will increase. Therefore, the "static blood pressure," called the "mean circulatory filling pressure" (MCFP),[180,182,185] the "mean vascular pressure,"[215] the "mean systemic pressure,"[216] or the "hydrostatic mean pressure,"[216] should not be confused with the CVP. Under steady-state conditions, where the heart handles all the blood it receives from the low resistance venous compartment, i.e., the total venous return (VR), this VR depends on the overall resistance (R) and the difference between the MCFP and the CVP, VR = (MCFP − CVP)/R, (see Fig. 4–8 in text). As "shown" in Figure 4–8 and by this equation, VR, for a given MCFP and R, is a linear function of the CVP, and the MCFP represents the upper limit of the CVP at which VR vanishes. The concepts of *vis a tergo* and *vis a fronte* from the older cardiovascular physiology treatises, can be substituted by a familiar equation in which flow is expressed as a function of a resistance and the pressure differences across that resistance.

One of the many contributions made by Guyton to our understanding of the circulatory system, is to have plotted on the same graph the familiar curve depicting the cardiac output (CO) as a nonlinear function of the CVP (i.e., the law of the heart), along with the curve depicting the VR as another function of the CVP (see Fig. 4–8 in the text). That CVP at which the two curves intersect, i.e., where VR = CO, represents the graphic solution of the circuit under analysis,[180] as it is the CVP that is characteristic of that system. The intuitive Gaussian concept that in the steady state, CO and VR are equal, is graphically evident. Note that graphic extrapolation of the venous return curve to the abscissa provides the MCFP (see Fig. 4–8 in the text), and the difference between this pressure and the CVP represents the "pressure gradient for venous return."

Starr, who had fully grasped the crucial role of the MCFP in cardiovascular physiology, has constructed an analog model of the circulatory system[186] to better demonstrate his ideas. Unfortunately, however, neither his analog model nor his postmortem measurements in humans,[186,188] both published in 1940, received much interest. Lack of enthusiasm cannot be attributed to World War II, as in 1949, Starr still did not get a wide audience when he tried to revive this subject.[187] The same fate occurred to the works of Weber and Starling, who where the first to introduce such concepts, and who also felt compelled to construct analog models to get their ideas accepted.[215] Resistance to this idea may come from the fact that given the dynamic nature of the cardiovascular system, one tends to lose track of the role of the MCFP, that can only be measured postmortem, yet that exerts its effect only once the heart beats. To make matters worse, once the heart is in motion, only one point along the circulatory tree will have a pressure that is equal to the

MCFP (see Fig. 4–9 in the text). Thus, while a purely static hydraulic system can be visualized in a simple graph, the dynamic cardiovascular system cannot be analyzed that way. Short of taking the reader to an actual dog laboratory, the composite plots devised by Guyton[180] remain the best tools for conveying this paradigm of cardiovascular dynamics. In essence, the intersection between the line of venous return and that of cardiac output constitutes the graphic solution for the two simultaneous equations that describe the cardiovascular dynamics. The difficulty in grasping the meaning of the MCFP may explain why yet another clinician–scientist, who, when realizing the central role of MCFP in cardiovascular dynamics, felt compelled both to building his own version of an analog model,[217] and to producing a videotape of his model.

The invitation made by Starr to "look on heart failure as a physiological process gone wrong,"[188] complements the teachings of Peters. In fact all the analog models of the circulation proposed since the initial "heart–lung" preparation of Starling,[216] were prompted by the need to help clinicians understand the normal physiologic processes that are required for understanding the "disorders encountered in diseases."[99] It was again up to the clinician–scientists to improve on these basic anephric models[182,215,217] of the circulatory system by adding the kidneys,[127,181] as their effect on the major determinants of cardiac output such as the CVP and MCFP were inescapable. Inclusion of output and intake has taken the original, isolated model that obeys thermodynamically reversible processes into the realm of a complex circuit governed by thermodynamically irreversible processes, thereby giving it the elements required for the long-term control of osmolality and volume in living organisms. Integration with the environment satisfies the views expressed by Ludwig, Claude Bernard, and Starling.[17,203]

Since the rate limiting factor is related to the solutes (salts) rather than the solvent (water) in the thermodynamic exchange with the environment, it has been felt that "the need for volume control may be directly met by the regulation of water metabolism."[43] Thus, although the low inertia of water may make it the ideal vector for the rapid control of volume, the proposal that "the slightest impingement on the working capacity of the heart will result in retention of the needed amount of water regardless of any minor osmotic pressure changes that may be involved,"[43] when extended to the chronic hyponatremic states, may be at odds with the views of Smith and his contemporaries. Indeed, according to their view, once the needed amount of water has been retained, the initial volume stimulus should leave way to the "physiologic *desideratum*" which is ultimately, in the opinion of Smith, the defense of tonicity. Thus, as long as hyponatremia persists, one must assume that the decrease in "effective blood volume" has not been corrected, and hence, neither a salt nor a water load can be excreted. This is a common experience in patients with congestive heart failure or cirrhosis of the liver.[2] Pregnant women, on the other hand, have an increased ability to excrete salt and water loads. Invoking a primary increase in renal hemodynamics to account for their preserved ability to achieve sodium balance and escape from mineralocorticoids and eliminate a water load,[2] contradicts the very observation that started the circular argument of "underfill,"[1] namely the hyponatremia and volume expansion. Indeed, if the pregnant woman has a preserved, or even an enhanced ability to excrete independently salt and water, then why does she have hyponatremia and an expanded extracellular fluid volume in the first place?

The ongoing debate as to whether the characteristic changes in body fluid volume and tonicity of pregnancy should merely be reduced to *normal physiologic responses to unusual conditions produced by pathologic processes,*[99] or whether these changes have implications which go far beyond mere compensations, has obvious therapeutic implications. The key elements required for integrating and, ultimately, understanding the regulation of composition and dynamics of body fluids reviewed in the context of pregnancy have been retraced in this brief history of the concepts of "effective osmolality," "effective blood volume," "mean circulatory filling pressure," and "volume receptors." Based on these paradigms it may be fruitful now to compare again the changes in the composition, distribution, and dymamics of body fluids seen in the pregnant women with those observed in patients with "decompensated" liver cirrhosis,[2] perhaps the most dramatic clinical examples of decreased "effective blood volume." The similarities go beyond the mere first clinical impression of two subjects with a distended belly, low blood pressure, warm skin, and dependent edema. Indeed, both also have an expanded blood volume, a decreased peripheral vascular resistance, and hyponatremia.[1] However, the two clinical entities differ markedly not only when tested against the traditional surrogate indices of "effective blood volume" such as renal salt and water handling as well as baroreceptor functions, but also when analyzed in the light of modern cardiovascular hemodynamics. Thus, the unique combination of peripheral arteriolar vasodilation, with the decreased blood viscosity due to "physiologic anemia," and the increased MCFP secondary to volume expansion, confer to the pregnant woman a state of cardiovascular competence that is superior to the nonpregnant state (see Figs. 4–8 and 4–9). From this point of view, the question as to whether pregnancy itself may be considered as a doping measure for high performance sport[218] becomes a legitimate one.

REFERENCES

1. Schrier RW, Dürr JA: Pregnancy: An overfill or underfill state. *Am J Kidney Dis* 1987; 4:284–289.
2. Schrier RW: Pathogenesis of sodium and water retention in high-output and low-output cardiac failure, nephrotic syndrome, cirrhosis, and pregnancy. *N Engl J Med* 1988;319:1065–1072, 1127–1134.
3. Dürr JA: Maternal fluid adaptation to pregnancy. In: Brace RA, Ross MG, Robillard JE, eds. *Reproductive and Perinatal Medicine. Vol XI: Fetal and Neonatal Body Fluids.* Ithaca, NY: Perinatal Press; 1989:227–270.
4. Duvekot JJ, Cheriex EC, Pieters FAA, et al: Early-pregnancy changes in hemodynamics and volume homeostasis are consecutive adjustments triggered by a primary fall in systemic vascular tone. *Am J Obstet Gynecol* 1993;169:1382–1392.
5. Schrier RW, Briner VA: Peripheral arterial vasodilation hypothesis of sodium and water re-

tention in pregnancy: Implications for the pathogenesis of preeclampsia. *Obstet Gynecol* 1991;77:632–639.
6. Brown MA, Gallery EDM: Volume homeostasis in normal pregnancy and preeclampsia: Physiology and clinical implications. *Clin Obstet Gynaecol* (Baillière) 1994;8:287–310.
7. Lindheimer MD, Katz AI: The normal and diseased kidney in pregnancy. In: Schrier RW, Gottschalk CW, eds. *Diseases of the Kidney*, ed 6. Boston: Little Brown and Co; 1997:2063–2097.
8. Duvekot JJ, Peters LL: Renal hemodynamics and volume homeostasis in pregnancy. *Obstet Gynecol Surv* 1994;49:830–839.
9. Davison JM, Gilmore EA, Durr JA: Altered osmotic thresholds for vasopressin secretion and thirst in human pregnancy. *Am J Physiol* 1984;246:F105–F109.
10. Chesley LC: Plasma and red cell volumes during pregnancy. *Am J Obstet Gynecol* 1972;112:440–450.
11. Epstein FH, Shadle OW, Ferguson TB, McDowell ME: Cardiac output and intracardiac pressures in patients with arteriovenous fistulas. *J Clin Invest* 1953;32:543–547.
12. Epstein FH, Post RS, McDowell M: The effect of an arteriovenous fistula on renal hemodynamics and electrolyte excretion. *J Clin Invest* 1953;32:233–241.
13. Epstein FM: Renal excretion of sodium and the concept of a volume receptor. *Yale J Biol Med* 1956;29:282–298.
14. Hecker R, Sherlock S: Electrolyte and circulatory changes in terminal liver failure. *Lancet* 1956;2:1121–1125.
15. Murray JF, Dawson AM, Sherlock S: Circulatory changes in chronic liver disease. *Am J Med* 1958;358–367.
16. Schrier RW, Arroyo V, Bernardi M, et al: Peripheral arterial vasodilation hypothesis: A proposal for the initiation of renal sodium and water retention in cirrhosis. *Hepatology* 1988;8:1151–1157.
17. de Wardener HE: Control of sodium excretion. In: Gottschalk CW, Berliner RW, Giebisch GH, eds. *Renal Physiology—People and Ideas*. American Physiological Society. Baltimore: Waverly Press, Inc; 1988:217–246, chap VII.
18. de Swiet M: The cardiovascular system. In: Hytten F, Chamberlain G, eds. *Clinical Physiology in Obstetrics*. Oxford: Blackwell Scientific Publications; 1980:3–42.
19. Bay WH, Ferris TF: Factors controlling plasma renin and aldosterone in pregnancy. *Hypertension* 1979;1:410–415.
20. Lindheimer MD, Katz AI: Renal physiology and disease in pregnancy. In: Selden DW, Giebisch G (eds.): *The Kidney: Physiology and Pathophysiology*, 2nd ed. New York, Raven 1992:3371–3433.
21. Hendricks CH, Barnes AC: Effects of supine position on urinary output in pregnancy. *Am J Obstet Gynecol* 1955;69:1225–1232.
22. Janney JC, Riley G, Walker EW: Studies in kidney function. II. Effect of posture on diuresis. *Proc Soc Exp Biol Med* 1933;32:398–402.
23. Walker EW, McManus M, Janney JC: Kidney function in pregnancy. II. Effects of posture on diuresis. *Proc Soc Exp Biol Med* 1933;31:392–397.
24. Lindheimer MD, Weston PV: Effect of hypotonic expansion on sodium, water, and urea excretion in late pregnancy: The influence of posture on these results. *J Clin Invest* 1969;48:947–956.
25. Pritchard JA, Barnes AC, Bright RH: The effect of the supine position on renal function in the near-term pregnant woman. *J Clin Invest* 1955;34:777–781.
26. Howard BK, Goodson JH, Mengeret WF: Supine hypotensive syndrome in late pregnancy. *Obstet Gynecol* 1953;1:371–377.
27. Kinsella SM, Lohmann G: Supine hypotensive syndrome. *Obstet Gynecol* 1994;83:774–788.
28. Davison JM, Vallotton MB, Lindheimer MD: Plasma osmolality and urinary concentration and dilution during and after pregnancy: Evidence that lateral recumbency inhibits maximal urinary concentrating ability. *Br J Obstet Gynaecol* 1981;88:472–479.
29. Durr JA: Diabetes insipidus in pregnancy. *Am J Kidney Dis* 1987;9:276–283.
30. Hytten FE: Weight gain in pregnancy. In: Hytten F, Chamberlain G, eds. *Clinical Physiology in Obstetrics*. Oxford: Blackwell Scientific Publications; 1980:193–233.
31. Hytten FE, Thomson AM: Weight gain in pregnancy. In: Lindheimer MD, Katz AI, Zuspan

FP, eds. *Hypertension in Pregnancy. Perspectives in Nephrology and Hypertension.* New York: John Wiley & Sons; 1976:179–187.

32. Hytten FE: Physiological changes in early pregnancy. *J Obstet Gynaec Br Commonw* 1968; 75:1193–1197.

33. Hytten FE, Thomson AM, Taggart N: Total body water in normal pregnancy. *J Obstet Gynaec Br Commonw* 1966;73:553–561.

34. Forsum E, Sadurskis A, Wagner J: Resting metabolic rate and body composition of healthy Swedish women during pregnancy. *Am J Clin Nutr* 1988;47:942–947.

35. Catalano PM, Wong WW, Drago NM, Amini SB: Estimating body composition in late gestation: A new hydration constant for body density and body water. *Am J Physiol* 1995;268: E153–E158.

36. Lukaski HC, Siders WA, Nielsen EJ, Hall CB: Total body water in pregnancy: Assessment by using bioelectrical impedence. *Am J Clin Nutr* 1994;59:578–585.

37. Hytten FE, Leicht I, eds: *The Physiology of Human Pregnancy*, ed 2. Oxford: Blackwell Scientific Publications; 1971.

38. Pritchard JA: Changes in the blood volume during pregnancy and delivery. *Anesthesiol* 1965;26:393–399.

39. Hytten FE, Paintin DB: Increase in plasma volume during normal pregnancy. *J Obstet Gynaec Br Commonw* 1963;70:402–407.

40. Letsky E: The haematological system. In: Hytten F, Chamberlain G, eds. *Clinical Physiology in Obstetrics*. Oxford: Blackwell Scientific Publications; 1980:43–78.

41. Pirani BB, Campbell DM, MacGillivray I: Plasma volume in normal first pregnancy. *J Obstet Gynaec Br Commonw* 1973;80:884–887.

42. Rovinsky JJ, Jaffin H: Cardiovascular hemodynamics in pregnancy. I. Blood and plasma volumes in multiple pregnancy. *Am J Obstet Gynecol* 1965;93:1–15.

43. Gauer OH, Henry JP, Behn C: The regulation of extracellular fluid volume. *Ann Rev Physiol* 1970;32:547–595.

44. Longo LD: Maternal blood volume and cardiac output during pregnancy: A hypothesis of endocrinologic control. *Am J Physiol*. 1983;245:R720–R729.

45. Josimovich JB, Atwood BL: Human placental lactogen (HPL), a trophoblastic hormone synergising with chorionic gonadotropin and potentiating the anabolic effects of pituitary growth hormone. *Am J Obstet Gynec* 1964;88:867–879.

46. Pritchard JA: Blood volume changes in pregnancy and the puerperium. IV. Anemia associated with hydatidiform mole. *Am J Obstet Gynecol* 1965;91:621–629.

47. Baylis C: Glomerular ultrafiltration in the pseudopregnant rat. *Am J Physiol* 1982;234: F300–F305.

48. Baylis C: Glomerular filtration and volume regulation in gravid animal models. *Clin Obstet Gynecol* (Baillière) 1994;8:235–264.

49. Hytten FE, Lind T, eds: Diagnostic indices in pregnancy. In: *Documenta Geigy*. Basel: Ciba-Geigy; 1973.

50. Barron WM: Volume homeostasis during pregnancy in the rat. *Am J Kidney Dis* 1987;9:296–302.

51. Rosa RM, Bierer BE, Thomas R, et al: A study of induced hyponatremia in the prevention and treatment of sickle-cell crisis. *N Engl J Med* 1980;303:1138–1143.

52. MacPhail S, Thomas TH, Wilkinson R, et al: Erythrocyte hydration in normal human pregnancy. *Br J Obstet Gynaecol* 1991;98:1205–1211.

53. Herbinger W, Wichmann H: Die extrazellulären und intraerythrozytären Elektrolyte wärend der zweiten Schwangerschaftshälfte. *Gynecologia* 1967;163:1–13.

54. Thomson AM, Hytten FE, Billewicz WZ: The epidemiology of oedema during pregnancy. *J Obstet Gynaec Br Commonw* 1967;74:1–10.

55. Robertson EG: The natural history of oedema during pregnancy. *J Obstet Gynaec Br Commonw* 1971;78:520–529.

56. Robertson EG: Oedema in normal pregnancy. *J Reprod Fert Suppl* 1969;9:27–36.

57. Will BR, Brace RA: Physiological effects of pH changes on colloid osmotic pressures. *Am J Physiol* 1985;248:H890–H893.

58. Chesley LC: Fluids and Electrolytes. In: *Hypertensive Disorders in Pregnancy.* New York: Appleton-Century-Crofts, 1978:199–228.
59. Guyton AC, Granger HJ, Taylor AE: Interstitial fluid pressure. *Physiol Rev* 1971;51:527–563.
60. Øian P, Maltau JM, Noodeland H, Fadnes HO: Oedema-preventing mechanisms in subcutaneous tissue of normal pregnant women. *Br J Obstet Gynaecol* 1985;92:1113–1119.
61. Guyton AC: A concept of negative interstitial pressure based on pressures in implanted perforated capsules. *Circ Res* 1963;12:399–414.
62. Olsson K, Anden NE, Johansson K, Thornstrom U: Effects of acute haemorrhagic hypotension during pregnancy and lactation in conscious goats. *Acta Physiol Scand.* 1987;129:479–487.
63. Douglas BH, Coleman TG: Circulatory dynamics of pregancy. I. Fluid shifts following saline infusion. *Am J Obstet Gynecol* 1970;107:551–559.
64. Beautyman W, Bills T: Osmotic error in erythrocyte volume determinations. *Am J Hematol* 1982;12:383–389.
65. Smith HW: Salt and water volume receptors. An exercise in physiologic apologetics. *Am J Med* 1957;23;623–652.
66. Durr JA, Stamoutsos B, Lindheimer MD: Osmoregulation during pregnancy in the rat—evidence for resetting of the threshold for vasopressin secretion during gestation. *J Clin Invest* 1981;68:337–346.
67. Lindheimer MD, Barron WM: Water metabolism and vasopressin secretion during pregnancy. *Clin Obstet Gynaecol* (Baillière) 1994;311–331.
68. Barron WM, Durr JA, Stamoutsos BA, Lindheimer MD: Osmoregulation during pregnancy in homozygous and heterozygous Brattleboro rats. *Am J Physiol* 1985;248:R229–R237.
69. Verbalis JG: Pathogenesis of hyponatremia in an experimental model of the syndrome of inappropriate antidiuresis. *Am J Physiol* 1994;267:R1617–R1625.
70. Dürr JA, Schrier RW: Cardiovascular and hemodynamic effects of arginine vasopressin. In: Brenner BM, Stein JH, eds. *Body Fluid Homeostasis. Contemporary Issues in Nephrology Series.* New York: Churchill Livingstone; 1987:131–161.
71. Barron WN, Dürr JA, Schrier RW, Lindheimer MD: Role of hemodynamic factors in osmoregulatory alterations of rat pregnancy. *Am J Physiol* 1989;257:R909–R916.
72. Miller NL, Dürr JA, Alfrey AC: Measurement of endogenous lithium levels in serum and urine by electrothermal atomic absorption spectometry: A method with potential clinical applications. *Anal Biochem* 1989;182:245–249.
73. Dürr JA, Miller NL, Alfrey AC: Lithium clearance derived from the natural trace blood and urine lithium levels. *Kidney Int Suppl* 1990;28:S58–S62.
74. Atherton JC, Bielinska A, Davison JM, et al: Sodium and water reabsorption in the proximal and distal nephron in conscious pregnant rats and third trimester women. *J Physiol* (Lond) 1988;396:457–470.
75. Brown MA, Gallery EDM: Volume homeostasis in normal pregnancy and preeclampsia: Clinical implications. *Clin Obstet Gynecol* (Baillière) 1994;8:287–310.
76. Barron WM, Stamoutsos BA, Lindheimer MD: Role of volume in the regulation of vasopressin secretion during pregnancy in the rat. *J Clin Invest* 1984;73:923–932.
77. Lindheimer MD, Barron WM, Dürr JA, Davison JM: Water homeostasis and vasopressin release during rodent and human gestation. *Am J Kidney Dis* 1987;9:270–275.
78. Baylis C: The determinants of renal hemodynamics in pregnancy. *Am J Kidney Dis* 1987;9:260–264.
79. Hart MV, Hosenpud JD, Hohimer AR, Morton MJ: Hemodynamics during pregnancy and sex steroid administration in guinea pigs. *Am J Physiol* 1985;249:R179–R185.
80. Chapman AB, Zamudio S, Woodmansee W, et al: Systemic and renal hemodynamic changes in the luteal phase of the menstrual cycle mimic early pregnancy. *Am J Physiol* 1997;273:F777–F782.
81. Dürr JA, Stamoutsos BA, Lindheimer MD: Plasma osmolality (P_{osm}) in pregnant rats in the absence of vasopressin (AVP) and during angiotensin blockade. *Kidney Int* 1981;19:238 (abstr).
82. Davison JM, Shills EA, Philips PR, Lindheimer MD: Serial evaluation of vasopressin release and thirst in human pregnancy. Role of human chorionic gonadotropin in the osmoregulatory changes of gestation. *J Clin Invest* 1988;81:798–806.

83. Wilson BC, Summerlee AJ: Effects of exogenous relaxin on oxytocin and vasopressin release and the intramammary pressure response to central hyperosmotic challenge. *J Endocrinol* 1994;141:75–80.

84. Johnson MR, Brooks AA, Steer PJ: The role of relaxin in the pregnancy associated reduction in plasma osmolality. *Hum Reprod* 1996;11:1105–1108.

85. Robertson GL: Abnormalities of thirst regulation. Nephrology forum. *Kidney Int* 1984;25: 460–469.

86. Flear CTG, Singh CM: Hyponatraemia and sick cells. *Br J Anaesth* 1973;45:976–994.

87. Flear CTG: Hyponatremia. *Lancet* 1974;ii:164–166.

88. Sick cells and hyponatraemia (editorial). *Lancet* 1974;i:342–343.

89. DeFronzo RA, Goldberg M, Agus ZS: Normal diluting capacity in hyponatremic patients. Reset osmostat or a variant of inappropriate antidiuretic hormone secretion. *Ann Int Med* 1976;84:538–542.

90. Fichman MP, Vorherr H, Kleeman CR, Tefler N: Diuretic-induced hyponatremia. *Ann Int Med* 1971;75:853–863.

91. Leaf A: Hyponatraemia. *Lancet* 1974;ii:1119–1120.

92. Champsi JH, Bermudez LE, Young LS: The role of cytokines in mycobaterial infection. *Biotherapy* 1994;7:187–193.

93. Moldawer LL, Sattler FR: Human immunodeficient virus-associated wasting and mechanisms of cachexia associated with inflammation. *Semin Oncol* 1998;25:73–81.

94. Levine B, Kalman J, Mayer L, et al: Elevated circulating levels of tumor necrosis factor in severe chronic heart failure. *N Engl J Med* 1990;323:236–241.

95. Argiles JM, Carbo N, Lopez-Soriano FJ: TNF and pregnancy: The paradigm of a complex interaction. *Cytokine Growth Factor Rev* 1997;8:181–188.

96. Vinatier D, Dufour P, Tordjeman-Rizzi N, et al: Immunological aspects of ovarian function: Role of the cytokines. *Eur J Obstet Gynecol Reprod Biol* 1995;63:155–168.

97. Edelman IS, Leibman J, O'Meara MP, Birkenfeld LW: Interrelations between serum sodium concentration, serum osmolality and total exchangeable sodium, total exchangeable potassium and total body water. *J Clin Invest* 1958;37:1236–1256.

98. Edelman IS: The pathogenesis of hyponatremia: Physiologic and therapeutic implications. *Metab* 1956;5:500–507.

99. Peters JP: The role of sodium in the production of edema. *N Engl J Med* 1948;239:353–362.

100. Peters JP: The problem of cardiac edema. *Am J Med* 1952;12:66–76.

101. Earley LE, Sanders CA: The effect of changing serum osmolality on the release of antidiuretic hormone in certain patients with decompensated cirrhosis of the liver and low serum osmolality. *J Clin Invest* 1959;38:545–550.

102. Maffly RH, Edelman IS: The role of sodium, potassium and water in the hypo-osmotic states of heart failure. *Prog Cardiovasc Dis* 1961;4:88–104.

103. Thrassher TN, Moor-Gillon M, Wade CE, et al: Inappropriate drinking and secretion of vasopressin after caval constriction in dogs. *Am J Physiol* 1983;244:R850–R856.

104. Leaf A: Regulation of intracellular fluid volume and disease. *Am J Med* 1970;49:291–295.

105. Bolton LM, Thomas TH, Macphail S, et al: Alterations in erythrocyte chloride content accompanying the changes in erythrocyte hydration and potassium content in normal human pregnancy: A comparison with pregnancy induced hypertension. *Br J Obstet Gynaecol* 1993;100:679–683.

106. Dürr JA, Hoffman WH, Hensen J, et al: Osmoregulation of vasopressin in diabetic ketoacidosis. *Am J Physiol* 1990;259:E723–E728.

107. Worley RJ, Hentschel W, Cormier C, et al: Increased sodium–lithium countertransport in erythrocytes of pregnant women. *New Engl J Med* 1982;307:412–416.

108. MacPhail S, Thomas TH, Wilkinson R, et al: A serial study of erythrocyte sodium content and sodium pump kinetics in pregnancy. *Clin Sci* 1990;79:631–638.

109. Bolton LM, Thomas TH, Macphail S, Dunlop W: A serial study of erythrocyte sodium pump kinetics and sodium content in the puerperium. *Am J Obstet Gynecol* 1994;170:693–698.

110. Weder AB: Red-cell lithium-sodium countertransport and renal lithium clearance in hypertension. *New Engl J Med* 1986;314:198–201.

111. Lindheimer MD, Katz AI: Kidney function in the pregnant rat. *J Lab Clin Med* 1971;78: 633–641.
112. Wintour EM: Water channels and urea transporters. *Clin Exp Pharmacol Physiol* 1997;24:1–9.
113. Agre P, Preston GM, Smith BL, et al: Aquaporin CHIP: The archetypal molecular water channel. *Am J Physiol* 1993;265:F463–F476.
114. King LS, Nielsen S, Agre P: Aquaporin-1 water channel protein in lung: Ontogeny, steroid-induced expression, and distribution in rat. *J Clin Invest* 1996;97:2183–2191.
115. Umenishi F, Carter EP, Yang B, et al: Sharp increase in rat lung water channel expression in the perinatal period. *Am J Respir Cell Biol* 1996;15:673–679.
116. Smith BL, Baumgarten R, Nielsen S, et al: Concurrent expression of erythroid and renal aquaporin CHIP and apperance of water channel activity in perinatal rats. *J Clin Invest* 1993;92:2035–2041.
117. Agre P, Smith BL, Baumgarten R, et al: Human red cell aquaporin CHIP. II. Expression during normal fetal development and in a novel form of congenital dyserythropoietic anemia. *J Clin Invest* 1994;94:1050–1058.
118. Yamamoto T, Sasaki S, Fushimi K, et al: Expression of AQP family in rat kidneys during development and maturation. *Am J Physiol* 1997;272:F198–F204.
119. Butkus A, Alcorn D, Earest L, et al: Expression of aquaporin-1 (AQP-1) in the adult and developing sheep kidney. *Biol Cell* 1997;89:313–320.
120. Knepper MA: Molecular physiology of urinary concentrating mechanisms: Regulation of aquaporin water channels by vasopressin. *Am J Physiol* 1997;272:F3–F12.
121. Oksche A, Rosenthal W: The molecular basis of nephrogenic diabetes insipidus. *J Mol Med* 1998;76:326–337.
122. Ohara M, Martin PY, Xu DL, et al: Upregulation of aquaporin-2 water channel expression in pregnant rats. *J Clin Invest* 1998;101:1076–1083.
123. Wells T: Vesicular osmometers, vasopressin secretion and aquaporin 4: A new mechanism for osmoreception? *Mol Cell Endocrinol* 1998;136:103–107.
124. Dürr JA, Lindheimer MD: Diagnosis and management of diabetes insipidus during pregnancy. *Endocr Pract* 1996;2:353–361.
125. Lindheimer MD, Davison JM: Osmoregulation, the secretion of arginine vasopressin and its metabolsism during pregnancy. *Eur J Endocrinol* 1995;132:133–143.
126. Dürr JA, Hoggard JG, Hunt JM, Schrier RW: Diabetes insipidus in pregnancy associated with abnormally high vasopressinase activity. *New Engl J Med* 1987;316:1070–1074.
127. Borst JGG: Hypertension explained by Starling's theory of circulatory homeostasis. *Lancet* 1963;I:677–682.
128. Leaf A, Kerr WS, Wrong O, Chatillon JY: Effect of graded compression of the renal artery on water and solute excretion. *Am J Physiol* 1954;179:191–200.
129. Guyton AC, Manning RD, Hall JE, et al: The pathogenic role of the kidney. *J Cardiovasc Pharmacol* 1984;6:S151–S161.
130. Guyton AC, Coleman TG: Quantitative analysis of the pathophysiology of hypertension. *Circ Res* 1969;24(suppl I):I1– I19.
131. Hall JE: Symposium: Arterial pressure and body fluid homeostasis. Introductory comments. *Federation Proc* 1986;45;2862–2863.
132. Hall JE, Guyton AC, Coleman TG, et al: Regulation of arterial pressure: Role of pressure natriuresis and diuresis. *Federation Proc* 1986;45:2897–2903.
133. Granger JP: Regulation of sodium excretion by renal interstitial hydrostatic pressure. *Federation Proc* 1986;45:2892–2896.
134. Granger JP, Scott JW: Effects of renal artery pressure on interstitial pressure and Na excretion during renal vasodilation. *Am J Physiol* 1988;255:F828–833.
135. Granger JP: Pressure natriuresis. Role of renal interstitial hydrostatic pressure. *Hypertension* 1992;19(suppl 1):I9–I17.
136. Quillen EW Jr, Nuwayhid BS: Steady-state arterial pressure-urinary output relationships during ovine pregnancy. *Am J Physiol* 1992;263:R1141–R1146.
137. Katz AI, Lindheimer MD: Renal handling of acute sodium loads in pregnancy. *Am J Physiol* 1973;225:696–699.

138. Guarasci GR, Kline RL: Pressure natriuresis following acute and chronic inhibition of nitric oxide synthase in rats. *Am J Physiol* 1996;270:R469–478.

139. Baylis C: Glomerular filtration and volume regulation in gravid animal models. *Clin Obstet Gynecol* (Baillières) 1994;8:235–264.

140. Conrad KP: Possible mechanisms for changes in renal hemodynamics during pregnancy: Studies from animal models. *Am J Kidney Dis* 1987;9:253–259.

141. Sturgiss SN, Dunlop W, Davison JM: Renal haemodynamics and tubular function in human pregnancy. *Clin Obstet Gynaecol* (Baillière) 1994;8:209–234.

142. Chapman AB, Abraham WT, Zamudio S, et al: Temporal relationships between hormonal and hemodynamic changes in early human pregnancy. *Kidney Int* (Dec. 1998).

143. Roberts M, Lindheimer MD, Davison JM: Altered glomerular permselectivity to neutral dextrans and heteroporous membrane modeling in human pregnancy. *Am J Physiol* 1996;270: F338–F343.

144. Baylis C, Blantz RC: Tubuloglomerular feedback activity in virgin and 12-day pregnant rats. *Am J Physiol* 1985;249:F169–F173.

145. Briggs JP, Schermann J: The tubuloglomerular feedback mechanism: Functional and biochemical aspects. *Ann Rev Physiol* 1987;49:251–273.

146. Navar LG, Ploth DW, Bell PD: Distal tubular feedback control of renal hemodynamics and autoregulation. *Ann Rev Physiol* 1980;42:557–571.

147. Thomsen K: Lithium clearance: A new method for determining proximal and distal tubular reabsorption of sodium and water. *Nephron* 1984;37:217–223.

148. Thomsen K, Olsen OK: Renal lithium clearance as a measure of the delivery of water and sodium from the proximal tubule in humans. *Am J Med Sci* 1984;288:158–161.

149. Robinson M: Salt in pregnancy. *Lancet* 1958;i:178–181.

150. Chesley LC, Valenti C, Rein H: Excretion of sodium loads by nonpregnant and pregnant normal, hypertensive and pre-eclamptic women. *Metabolism* 1958;7:575–588.

151. Poppas A, Shroff SG, Korcarz CE, et al: Serial assessment of the cardiovascular system in normal pregnancy. Role of arterial compliance and pulsatile arterial load. *Circulation* 1997; 95:2407–2415.

152. Lees MM, Taylor SH, Scott DB, Kerr MG: A study of cardiac output at rest throughout pregnancy. *J Obstet Gynaec Br Commonw* 1967;74:319–328.

153. Bader RA, Bader ME, Rose DJ, Braunwald E: Hemodynamics at rest and during exercise in normal pregnancy as studied by cardiac catheterization. *J Clin Invest* 1955;34:1524–1536.

154. Cha SC, Aberdeen GW, Nuwayhid BS, Quillen EW Jr: Influence of pregnancy on mean systemic filling pressure and the cardiac function curve in guinea pigs. *Can J Physiol Pharmacol* 1992;70:669–674.

155. Hart MV, Morton MJ, Hosenpud JD, Metcalfe J: Aortic function during normal human pregnancy. *Am J Obstet Gynecol* 1986;154:887–891.

156. Clapp JF III, Capeless E: Cardiovascular function before, during, and after the first and subsequent pregnancies. *Am J Cardiol* 1997;80:1469–1473.

157. Burwell CS: The placenta as a modified arteriovenous fistula, considered in relation to the circulatory adjustments to pregnancy. *Am J Med Sci* 1938;195:1–7.

158. Burwell CS, Strayhorn WD, Flickinger D, et al: Circulation during pregnancy. *Arch Int Med* 1938;62:979–1003.

159. Robson SC, Hunter S, Boys RJ, Dunlop W: Serial study of factors influencing changes in cardiac output during human pregnancy. *Am J Physiol* 1989;256:H1060–H1065.

160. Redman CWG, Beilin LJ, Bonnar J: Variability of blood pressure in normal and abnormal pregnancy. In: Lindheimer MD, Katz AI, Zuspan FP, eds. *Hypertension in Pregnancy. Perspectives in Nephrology and Hypertension.* New York: J. Wiley & Sons; 1976:53–60.

161. Seligman SA: Baroreceptor reflex function in pre-eclampsia. *J Obstet Gynaecol Br Commonw* 1971;78:413–416.

162. Crandall ME, Heesch CM: Baroreflex control of sympathetic outflow in pregnant rats: Effects of captopril. *Am J Physiol* 1990;258:R1147–R1423.

163. Heesch CM, Rogers RC: Effects of pregnancy and progesterone metabolites on regulation of sympathetic outflow. *Clin Exp Pharmacol Physiol* 1995;22:136–142.

164. O'Hagan KP, Casey SM: Arterial baroreflex during pregnancy and renal sympathetic nerve activity during parturition in rabbits. *Am J Physiol* 1998;274:H1635–H1642.
165. Conrad KP, Russ RD: Augmentation of baroreflex-mediated bradycardia in conscious pregnant rats. *Am J Physiol* 1992;262:R472–477.
166. Brooks VL, Keil LC: Changes in the baroreflex during pregnancy in conscious dogs: Heart rate and hormonal responses. *Endocrinology* 1994;135:1894–1901.
167. Tripathi A, Singh M: Type B atrial receptor discharge increases on opening a nonhypotensive arteriovenous shunt in the dog. *Proc Soc Exper Biol Med* 1985;78:426–431.
168. Epstein FH: Underfilling versus overflow in hepatic ascites. *N Engl J Med* 1982;307:1577–1578.
169. Wasserman N, Kirshorn B, Rossavik IK, et al: Implications of sino-aortic baroreceptor reflex dysfunction in severe preeclampsia. *Obstet Gynecol* 1989;74:34–39.
170. Winner W: The role of the placenta in the systemic circulation; a reappraisal. *Obstet Gynecol Surg* 1965;20:545–554.
171. Judson WE: Cardiovascular renal regulation in the hyperkinetic states. *Prog Cardiovasc Dis* 1961;4:65–87.
172. Claviano VV: Evidence for an arteriovenous fistula in the gravid uterus. *Surg Gynecol Obstet* 1963;117:301–304.
173. Frank CW, Wang HH, Lammerant J, et al: An experimental study of the immediate hemodynamic adjustments to acute arteriovenous fistulae of various sizes. *J Clin Invest* 1955;34:722–736.
174. Van Loo A, Heringman EC: Circulatory changes in the dog produced by acute arteriovenous fistula. *Am J Physiol* 1949;158:103–113.
175. Patterson SW, Starling EH: On the mechanical factors which determine the output of the ventricles. *J Physiol* 1914;48:357–379.
176. Guyton AC, Sagawa K: Compensations of cardiac output and other circulatory functions in areflex dogs with large A-V fistulas. *Am J Physiol* 1961;200:1157–1163.
177. Hilton JG, Kanter DM, Hays DR, et al: The effect of acute arteriovenous fistula on renal functions. *J Clin Invest* 1955;34:732–736.
178. Warren JV, Elkin DC, Nickerson JL: The blood volume in patients with arteriovenous fistulas. *J Clin Invest* 1951;30:220–226.
179. Fowler NO, Holmes JC: Blood viscosity and cardiac output in acute experimental anemia. *J Appl Physiol* 1975;39:453–456.
180. Guyton AC: Determination of cardiac output by equating venous return curves with cardiac response curves. *Physiol Rev* 1955;35:123–129.
181. Guyton AC, Coleman TG, Granger HJ: Circulation: Overall regulation. In: Comroe JH, Giese AC, Sonnenschein RR, eds. *Annual Review of Physiology*. Palo Alto: Annual Reviews, Inc; 1972:13–46.
182. Guyton AC, Lindsey AW, Kaufman BN: Effect of mean circulatory filling pressure and other peripheral circulatory factors on cardiac output. *Am J Physiol* 1955;180:463–468.
183. Guyton AC: Venous return. In: Hamilton WF, Dow P, eds. *Circulation. Handbook of Physiology Series*. Washington, DC: American Physiological Society; 1963:1099–1133.
184. Douglas BH, Harlan JC, Langford HG, Richardson TQ: Effect of hypervolemia and elevated arterial pressure on circulatory dynamics of pregnant animals. *Am J Obstet Gynecol* 1967;98:889–894.
185. Guyton AC, Polizo D, Armstrong GG: Mean circulatory filling pressure measured immediately after cessation of heart pumping. *Am J Physiol* 1954;179:261–267.
186. Starr I: Role of the "static blood pressure" in abnormal increments of venous pressure, especially in heart failure. II. Clinical and experimental studies. *Am J Med Sci* 1940;199:40–55.
187. Starr I: Our changing viewpoint about conjective failure. *Ann Int Med* 1949;30:1–23.
188. Starr I, Rawson AJ: Role of the "static blood pressure" in abnormal increments of venous pressure, especially in heart failure. I. Theoretical studies on an improved circulation schema whose pumps obey Starling's Law of the Heart. *Am J Med Sci* 1940;199:27–39.
189. Katz R, Karlinger JS, Resnik R: Effects of a natural volume overload state (pregnancy) on left ventricular performance in normal human subjects. *Circulation* 1978;58:434–441.

190. Goodlin RC, Niebauer MJ, Holmberg MJ, Zucker IM: Mean circulatory filling pressure in pregnant rabbits. *Am J Obstet Gynecol* 1984;148:224–225.
191. Humphreys PW, Joels N: Effect of pregnancy on pressure–volume relationships in circulation of rabbits. *Am J Physiol* 1994:267:R780–R785.
192. Tabsh K, Monson R, Nuwayhid B: Regulation of cardiac output in ovine pregnancy. *Soc Gynecol Invest* 1985;32nd meeting, 53P (abstr).
193. Davis LE, Hohimer AR, Giraud GD, et al: Vascular pressure–volume relationships in pregnant and estrogen-treated guinea pigs. *Am J Physiol* 1989;257:R1205–R1211.
194. Richardson TQ, Stallings JO, Guyton AC: Pressure–volume curves in live, intact dogs. *Am J Physiol* 1961;201:471–474.
195. Yamamoto J, Trippodo NC, Ishise S, Frohlich ED: Total vascular pressure–volume relationship in the conscious rat. *Am J Physiol* 1980;238:H823–H828.
196. Andreoli TA: Edematous states: An overview. *Kidney Int* 1997;51(suppl 59):S2–S10.
197. Ingles AC, Hernandez I, Garca-Estan J, et al: Increased total vascular capacity in conscious cirrhotic rats. *Gastrenterol* 1992;103:275–281.
198. Phippard AF, Horvath JS, Glynn EM, et al: Circulatory adaptation to pregnancy—Serial studies of haemodynamics, blood volume, renin and aldosterone in the baboon (Papio hamadryas). *J Hypertension* 1986;4:773–779.
199. Robin ED: The cult of the Swan–Ganz catheter. Overuse and abuse of pulmonary flow catheters. *Ann Intern Med* 1985;103:445–449.
200. Robin ED: Overuse and abuse of Swan–Ganz catheters. *Int J Clin Monit Comput* 1987;4:5–9.
201. Shoemaker WC: Use and abuse of the balloon tip pulmonary artery (Swan–Ganz) catheter: Are patients getting their money's worth? *Crit Care Med* 1990;18:1294–1296.
202. Vesprille A, Jansen JC: Mean systemic filling pressure as a characteristic pressure for venous return. *Pfluegers Arch* 1985;405:226–233.
203. Strauss MB: *Body Water in Man: The Acquisition and Maintenance of Body Fluids.* Boston: Little, Brown and Co; 1957.
204. Smith HW: *From Fish to Philosopher.* Boston: Brown and Co; 1953.
205. Anderson RJ, Chung HM, Kluge R, Schrier RW: Hyponatremia: A prospective analysis of its epidemiology and the pathogenetic role of vasopressin. *Ann Intern Med* 1985;102:164–168.
206. Natkunma A, Shek CC, Swaminathan R: Hyponatremia in a hospital population. *J Med* 1991;22:83–96.
207. Smith H: *Principles of Renal Physiology.* New York: Oxford University Press; 1956.
208. Burg M: Molecular basis of osmotic regulation. *Am J Physiol* 1995;268:F983–F996.
209. McDowell ME, Wolf AV, Steer A: Osmotic volumes of distribution—Idiogenic changes in osmotic pressure associated with administration of hypertonic solutions. *Am J Physiol* 1955;180:545–558.
210. Peters JP: *Body Water: The Exchange of Fluids in Man.* Springfield, IL: Charles C Thomas; 1935.
211. Papper S: Liver–kidney interrelationships—A personal perspective. In: Epstein M (ed.): *The Kidney in Liver Disease,* ed 2. New York: Elsevier 1983:3–10.
212. Epstein M: Renal effects of head-out water immersion in man: Implications for an understanding of volume homeostasis. *Physiol Rev* 1978;58:529–581.
213. Epstein FH, Goodyear AVN, Lawrason FD, Relman AS: Studies of the antidiuresis of quiet standing: The importance of changes in plasma volume and glomerular filtration rate. *J Clin Invest* 1951;30:63–72.
214. Selkurt EE, Hall PW, Spencer MP: Influence of graded arterial pressure decrement on renal clearance, p-aminohippurate and sodium. *Am J Physiol* 1949;159:369–378.
215. Anderson RM, Fritz JM, O'Hare JE, Ariz T: The mechanical nature of the heart as a pump. *Am Heart J* 1967;73:92–105.
216. Starling EH: Arris and Dale Lectures on some points in the pathology of heart disease. *Lancet* (London) 1897i;569–572.
217. Anderson RM, Larson DF, Lundell DC: The interrelationship of factors controlling cardiac output. *Med Hypoth* 1983;10:77–95.
218. Strobel E: Pregnancy as a doping measure? Dangerous development in high performance sports. *Fortschr Med* 1988;106:14.

III

Clinical Spectrum
of Preeclampsia

5

Preeclampsia–Eclampsia

John C. Hauth and F. Gary Cunningham

Leon Chesley was a PhD, and thus did not practice medicine. In his single-authored first edition of this text, descriptions of the clinical presentation of preeclampsia–eclampsia were divided among at least seven chapters, where he reviewed both the historical literature as well as many pertinent studies published in the 1960s and 1970s. As usual, these reviews are scholarly and perceptive, and bear rereading. Our purpose here is to describe the clinical spectrum of preeclampsia–eclampsia in a single chapter combining a review of recent publications with the hands-on experience of two maternal–fetal medicine subspecialists at two tertiary care institutions in which over 15,000 women with preeclampsia have been managed over the past decade.

Preeclampsia is characterized by the onset of hypertension and proteinuria in women after 20 weeks' gestation (see Chap. 1). The distinguishing features of women with preeclampsia are arteriolar spasm and increased vascular reactivity. At initial presentation, the clinical spectrum of preeclampsia is highly variable and is usually related to the severity of the disease, particularly vasospasm and endothelial damage. These in turn may disparately involve some or all target organs and thus, clinical and laboratory findings are related to the degree of organ system involvement with subsequent ischemia and necrosis.

Equally important are the adverse maternal consequences that develop or that are created by events subsequent to those apparent at initial presentation. Included at the severe end of this clinical spectrum are maternal consequences of management interventions such as the use of aggressive intravascular volume expansion with colloid and/or crystalloid solutions. Also, inappropriate response to appreciable blood loss from placental abruption, cesarean delivery, or postpartum hemorrhage from trauma or uterine atony may result in severe maternal morbidity such as acute pulmonary injury (adult respiratory distress syndrome), pulmonary edema, acute renal failure, and death. Thus, following the initial presentation of the woman with severe preeclampsia or eclampsia and a decision to effect delivery, the potential exists to create immense adverse maternal decompensation of many organ systems as a direct consequence of management decisions.

In most women in whom good prenatal care is provided, the diagnosis of preeclampsia is suspected by new-onset hypertension, oftentimes before development of proteinuria. In its earliest stages few, if any, clinical symptoms are manifest. With progression of disease, proteinuria worsens and other evidence of endothelial dysfunction may become apparent.

HYPERTENSION

As discussed in Chapter 1, Korotkoff phase V (K_5) is used to define diastolic blood pressure in pregnancy. Indeed, arguments by others to use K_4 seem to have ceased, especially since Shennan et al.[1] confirmed that K_4 cannot be accurately reproduced. Brown et al.[1a] provided clinical data to support the use of K_5. Currently in the United States, a diagnosis of hypertension during gestation is defined as a sustained blood pressure increase to levels of 140 mm Hg systolic or 90 mm Hg diastolic. Technically, blood pressure may depend greatly on maternal position and contractions during labor. Ideally, measurements should be taken in a uniform manner at each prenatal visit or in labor with a proper cuff size while the woman is sitting.[2] Additionally, there is the well-known circadian oscillation of blood pressure in normal pregnancy. This diurnal rhythm is blunted and even reversed with pregnancy-induced hypertension and preeclampsia, but persists in women with uncomplicated chronic hypertension.[3,4] Also noted in Chapter 1, hypertension in pregnancy is diagnosed only if there are at least two abnormal values 6 hours apart.

PROTEINURIA

Proteinuria is an important sign for the diagnosis and severity of preeclampsia, and Chesley[5] rightfully concluded that the diagnosis is questionable in its absence. It may develop late in the course of the disease. As discussed in Chapter 1, in the United States, proteinuria is defined by most as 300 mg or more per 24 hours, or 100 mg/dL or more in at least two random urine specimens collected 6 or more hours apart.[2] The degree of proteinuria may fluctuate widely over any 24-hour period, even in severe cases. Therefore, a single random sample may fail to demonstrate significant proteinuria.

PREECLAMPSIA

The diagnosis of preeclampsia has traditionally required the identification of gestational hypertension plus proteinuria. This combination markedly increases the risk of perinatal mortality and morbidity. For example, in their classic study, Friedman and Neff[6] showed that hypertension alone, defined by a diastolic blood pres-

TABLE 5–1. PREECLAMPSIA: INDICATIONS OF SEVERITY

Abnormality	Mild	Severe
Maternal		
Systolic blood pressure	< 160 mm Hg	> 160–180 mm Hg
Diastolic blood pressure	< 100 mm Hg	110 mm Hg or higher
Proteinuria		
Dipstick	1–2 +	3–4 +
24-h collection	≥ 300 mg	≥ 5 g
Headache	Absent	Present
Visual disturbances	Absent	Present
Upper abdominal pain	Absent	Present
Oliguria (< 500 mL/24 h)	Absent	Present
Convulsions	Absent	Present
Serum creatinine	Normal	Elevated
Thrombocytopenia	Absent	Present
Hyperbilirubinemia	Absent	Present
Liver enzyme elevation	Minimal	Marked
Pulmonary edema	Absent	Present
Fetal		
Growth restriction	Absent	Present
Oligohydramnios	Absent	Present

Modified, with permission, from Cunningham FG, et al., Williams Obstetrics, 20 ed. Stamford, CT: Appleton &Lange, 1997: 695.

sure of 95 mm Hg or greater, was associated with a threefold increase in the fetal death rate (see also Chap. 2). In this same group, i.e., diastolic pressure greater than 95 mm Hg, perinatal mortality was increased another six- to sevenfold if there was 3+ or 4+ proteinemia. The absolute level of proteinuria, however, and/or the rate of increase once proteinuria is established has little predictive value for maternal or fetal outcomes.

Severity of Preeclampsia

The severity of preeclampsia is assessed by the frequency and intensity of the abnormalities listed in Table 5–1. The more profound the frequency and intensity of these aberrations, the more likely is the need for pregnancy termination. It is important to note that *the differentiation between mild and severe preeclampsia cannot be rigidly pursued, because apparently mild disease may progress rapidly to severe disease.*

EFFECTS OF PREECLAMPSIA ON ORGAN SYSTEMS

Deterioration of function in a number of organs and systems, presumably as a consequence of vasospasm and endothelial dysfunction, have been identified in severe preeclampsia. For descriptive purposes, these effects are separated into maternal and fetal consequences, however, these aberrations usually are encountered simultaneously. Although there are many possible maternal consequences of severe preeclampsia, for simplicity these effects are considered by analysis of the maternal blood volume, and cardiovascular, renal, hepatic, cerebral, hematologic, endocrine, and regional blood flow changes with subsequent end-organ derangements. The major cause of fetal compromise occurs as a consequence of reduced uteroplacental perfusion.

Extracellular Fluid Shifts and Blood Volume

Extracellular Fluid

Alterations in volume homeostasis in preeclamptic women are discussed in detail in Chapter 9. The volume of *extracellular fluid* in women with severe preeclampsia–eclampsia is usually markedly expanded. The etiology of the expanded extracellular fluid (edema) beyond the normally increased volume that characterizes pregnancy may be due to several factors, also discussed in Chapters 9 and 12, including the role of endothelial damage in small vessels with subsequent capillary leakage into the extracellular space. Hypertension contributes to extravasation of intravascular fluid as does the lower plasma colloid oncotic pressure associated with the disease. Øian et al.[8] have shown that in severe preeclampsia capillary hydrostatic pressure was decreased by 40% compared with normotensive third-trimester control women. They attributed this to increased interstitial colloid osmotic pressure from protein extravasation.

All of these factors favor excessive accumulation of extracellular fluid. Edema is evident at a time when, paradoxically, aldosterone levels are reduced compared with the remarkably elevated levels for normal pregnancy. Electrolyte concentrations do not differ appreciably from those of normal pregnancy unless there has been vigorous diuretic therapy, sodium restriction, or administration of water with sufficient oxytocin to produce antidiuresis. Edema does not ensure a poor prognosis, and absence of edema does not ensure a favorable outcome.

Wheeler et al.[9] have provided data to show that vasospasm and capillary leakage with diminished blood flow may be associated with diminished oxygen delivery and increasing acidosis. Acute acidemia, primarily of metabolic origin, usually follows an eclamptic convulsion. Serum lactic acid levels increase and the *bicarbonate* concentration falls. The intensity of acidosis relates to the rate of lactate production and its failure to be metabolized to bicarbonate.

Blood Volume

At the same time that interstitial volume increases, intravascular space deficits occur as fluid is inappropriately distributed into the extracellular space. Thus women with eclampsia become hemoconcentrated, a fact emphasized by Dieckmann[10] over 45 years ago. Women of average size should have a blood volume of nearly 5000 mL during the last several weeks of a normal pregnancy, compared with about 3500 mL when nonpregnant. On the other hand, many women who subsequently develop eclampsia or severe preeclampsia, commonly do not achieve this degree of volume expansion. In preeclamptic women, peripheral resistance is much higher than in normal pregnancy. Though there is debate in the literature, the diminished intravascular system should not be perceived as underfilled as evidenced by appropriately lower renin, angiotensin II, and aldosterone levels compared with those in normal pregnant women. Pritchard et al.[11] described five women with eclampsia in whom much or all of the anticipated additional 1500 mL of blood normally present late in pregnancy was absent when measured with erythrocytes tagged with [51]chromium. Subsequently, in a normotensive pregnancy, these five women expanded their blood volume by a mean of 47%. In most women with severe preeclampsia and multiorgan effects, these differences are similar to those in women with eclampsia, however, they usually are not as marked with mild preeclampsia or gestational hypertension.[12]

The clinical consequences of failure of normal pregnancy blood volume expansion can be devastating. Prior to delivery in women with severe preeclampsia, treatment with marked water and salt restriction or with diuretics is contraindicated. Such treatment may place these women at an especially high risk for complications because it may appreciably deplete their intravascular volume further and impair major organ perfusion. This may well aggravate the metabolic acidemia as inadequate cellular perfusion results in diversion from aerobic to anaerobic metabolism, namely the pyruvate–lactic acid anaerobic pathway.

In the absence of hemorrhage, the intravascular compartment in eclamptic women usually is not (as some claim) underfilled "compared with the nonpregnant state." The more likely explanation is that arteriolar vasospasm and endothelial leakage has contracted the intravascular space and this reduction persists until after delivery when the vascular system typically dilates, blood volume increases, and the hematocrit falls. *The woman with eclampsia is unduly sensitive to vigorous fluid therapy administered in an attempt to expand the contracted blood volume to normal pregnancy levels.* Benedetti et al.[13,14] have appropriately criticized attempts of investigators in the 1980s to "improve" eclampsia or severe preeclampsia by aggressive intravascular volume expansion. They reported that women with severe preeclampsia who develop pulmonary or cerebral edema usually do so postpartum and that aggressive intrapartum fluid is often followed by a progressive postpartum rise in cardiac filling pressures. Despite this sensitivity to volume overload, women with severe preeclampsia are sensitive to even normal blood loss at delivery and management of excessive blood loss in these women should be early and aggressive.

In clinical practice, we have frequently encountered appreciable derangement of various organ systems—for example, acute renal failure and adult respiratory distress syndrome—which appeared related to a failure to appreciate the need for, and rapidly replace, appreciable blood loss. These recommendations, however, have not been addressed in formal trials, and to do so would be quite difficult.

Cardiovascular Changes

Normal Hemodynamic Changes in Late Pregnancy

The cardiovascular changes in both normal and hypertensive pregnancy are discussed in detail in Chapters 3 and 8. Those chapters focus on many of the interpretive and technical problems that surround the study of the cardiovascular system in pregnancy, and reviewing these will help the reader to understand why many of the reports of cardiovascular alterations in pregnant hypertensive women are so disparate. Here, the primary focus is on a series of invasive hemodynamic studies, most performed near delivery in women with severe preeclampsia.

Clark et al.[15] reported their findings from studies in which pulmonary arterial catheterization was used to study normal pregnant women at term. They found that women in normal late pregnancy have a marked decrease in systemic vascular resistance (21%), pulmonary vascular resistance (34%), and the colloid oncotic pressure/pulmonary capillary wedge pressure (COP/PCWP) gradient. The pulse is increased as well as the cardiac output (43%). As shown in Figure 5–1, although cardiac output was increased, the left ventricular stroke work index is close to the normal range for such values in nonpregnant women.

Hemodynamic Changes with Severe Preeclampsia–Eclampsia

In contrast to healthy pregnant women, those with severe preeclampsia or eclampsia show markedly increased pulmonary and systemic vascular resistance. Along with diminished intravascular volume, these resistances may have marked hemodynamic effects. Hemodynamic data obtained prior to active treatment of severe preeclampsia and eclampsia identified low to normal left ventricular filling pressures, high systemic vascular resistances, and hyperdynamic left ventricular function (Table 5–2). A critique of this literature will be found in Chapter 8, including discussion of the careful study of Visser and Wallenburg.[17] These investigators compared central hemodynamic findings in 87 severe untreated preeclamptic women, 47 preeclamptics who received vasodilators and colloid expanding infusions, and 10 normotensive controls.

At Parkland Hospital, Hankins et al.[19] studied eight women with eclampsia

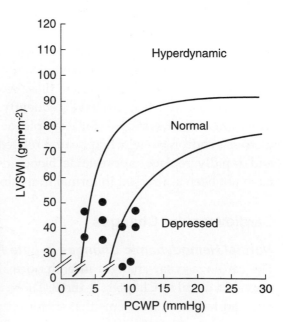

Figure 5–1. Relationship between left ventricular stroke work index (LVSWI) (cardiac output) and pulmonary capillary wedge pressure (PCWP) in ten normal pregnant women in the third trimester. (*Data from Clark SL, Cotton DB, Wesley L, et al: Central hemodynamic assessment of normal term pregnancy. Am J Obstet Gynecol 1989;161:1439–1442*).

TABLE 5–2. SEVERE PREECLAMPSIA AND ECLAMPSIA: ASSOCIATED HEMODYNAMIC MEASUREMENTS

Therapy	No.	Cardiac Output (L/min)	Pulmonary Capillary Wedge Pressure (mm Hg)	Left Ventricular Stroke Work Index (g/m/m^{-2})	Systemic Vascular Resistance (dynes/sec/cm^{-5})
Before therapy					
Groenendijk et al. (1984)[16]	10	4.66	3.3	44	1943
Visser and Wallenburg (1991)[17]	87	(3.3)[a]	7	NA[b]	3003
Magnesium, hydralazine, and fluid restriction					
Benedetti et al. (1980)[18]	10	7.4	6.0	82	1332
Hankins et al. (1984)[19]	8	6.7	3.9	66	1357
Magnesium, hydralazine, and volume expansion					
Rafferty and Berkowitz (1982)[20]	3	11.0	7.0	89	780
Phelan and Yurth (1982)[21]	10	9.3	16.0	89	1042

Values are those reported soon after pulmonary artery catheterization was performed, and are the means for each study.
[a] Reported as cardiac index (CI = L/min^{-1}/m^{-2}).
[b] Not available.

175

who had been given magnesium sulfate but in whom volume expansion was avoided. They found that initial central venous pressure ranged from zero to 3 mm Hg and PCWP was 1 to 5 mm Hg. Predictably, cardiac response to this—including increased peripheral vascular resistance—is to work harder, which is reflected by a higher left ventricular stroke work index (LVSWI), as shown in Figure 5–2. This index is almost double that of healthy pregnant women, as depicted in Figure 5–1.

Women treated with magnesium sulfate and hydralazine *plus aggressive intravenous fluid therapy or volume expansion* had the highest cardiac outputs. A comparison of volume-restricted women with those hydrated aggressively shows hyperdynamic ventricular function in both groups, but two markedly different responses with respect to PCWPs (Fig. 5–3). Fluid restriction resulted in PCWP < 10 mm Hg and most were < 5 mm Hg compared with much higher PCWPs in women given aggressive intravenous fluid therapy. Of important note, in either case with these otherwise young, healthy women, cardiac function is hyperdynamic.

Pulmonary Edema

Severe hypertension raises left-sided filling pressures.[22] Moreover, aggressive fluid administration with severe preeclampsia causes normal left-sided filling pressures to become substantively elevated, while increasing an already normal cardiac output to supranormal levels (see Chap. 8). This is illustrated in Figure 5–4 which is a literature composite of LVSWI plotted against PCWP in 49 women with severe preeclampsia managed with aggressive fluid administration. The eight women who developed pulmonary edema had a markedly elevated LVSWI and the highest left ventricular filling pressures.

As discussed in Chapter 8, there is no evidence that *cardiac contractility* is impaired in the otherwise healthy woman with severe preeclampsia. Thus, and not

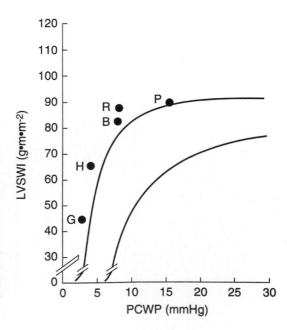

Figure 5–2. Ventricular function in severe preeclampsia–eclampsia. Data plotted represent mean values obtained in each of six studies cited in Table 5–2. Left ventricular stroke work index (LVSWI) and pulmonary capillary wedge pressure (PCWP) are plotted on a standard ventricular function curve. Points falling within the two solid lines represent normal function, while those below represent depressed function. Points above the solid lines represent hyperdynamic ventricular function. Each letter adjacent to the data points is the first initial of the last name of the investigator cited in Table 5–2.

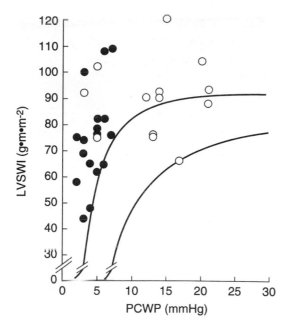

Figure 5–3. Ventricular function in women with severe preeclampsia–eclampsia. Left ventricular stroke work index (LVSWI) and pulmonary capillary wedge pressure (PCWP) are plotted. Closed circles represent women with restricted intravenous fluids (Benedetti et al.,[18] Hankins et al.,[19]). Solid circles represent women given aggressive fluid therapy (Rafferty and Berkowitz,[20] Phelan and Yurth[21]). (*Reprinted, with permission, from Hankins GDV, Wendel GW Jr, Cunningham FG, Leveno KJ: Longitudinal evaluation of hemodynamic changes in eclampsia.* Am J Obstet Gynecol *1984;150:506–512.*)

surprisingly, it is the older, usually chronically hypertensive and obese woman who develops pulmonary edema with superimposed preeclampsia.[23,24] This is commonly due to a combination of increased pulmonary capillary permeability and severe hypertension, usually longstanding (Fig. 5–5). Sibai et al.[24] reported that during a 9-year period, 37 women with severe preeclampsia developed pulmonary edema (2.9%). The majority of these women were given excessive colloid and crystalloid infusions. Dexamethasone given to enhance fetal lung maturity has also been implicated as a possible cofactor.[25] Lehmann et al.[26] described 89 maternal deaths

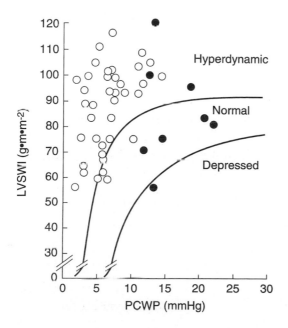

Figure 5–4. Literature summary of the relationship between left ventricular stroke work index (LVSWI) and pulmonary capillary wedge pressure (PCWP) in 49 women with severe preeclampsia managed with aggressive fluid administration to expand their intravascular volume. The eight women depicted with solid circles developed clinical pulmonary edema.

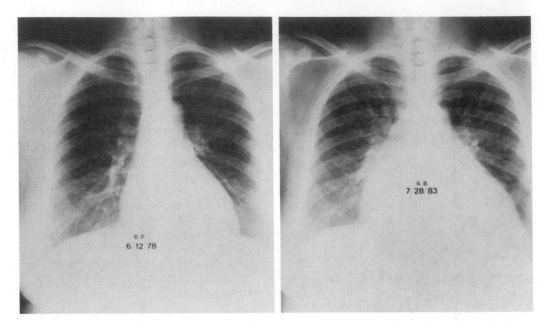

Figure 5–5. At age 37, this chronically hypertensive woman developed heart failure postpartum. Six months later (6–12–78), the cardiac silhouette had returned to upper limits of normal size. Despite antihypertensive medication, this patient's blood pressure was not controlled and 5 years postpartum (7–28–83) she now has obvious cardiomegaly. Patient died 2 years later of hypertensive heart failure.

at Charity Hospital of Louisiana in New Orleans between 1965 and 1984, with the single most common cause of death at autopsy being pulmonary edema. They concluded that potentially preventable pulmonary edema was responsible for one-third of obstetric deaths from hypertension and hemorrhage.

Depending upon maternal age and other factors, persisting tachycardia after delivery may be due to a number of factors (Table 5–3). In most cases, especially in otherwise healthy young women, the hyperdynamic circulation combined with hemorrhage and anemia accounts for persistent tachycardia.

Renal Changes

Renal changes in preeclampsia are the focus of Chapter 8. During normal pregnancy, renal blood flow and glomerular filtration are briefly increased appreciably, but with development of preeclampsia, both perfusion and filtration are substantially re-

TABLE 5–3. DIFFERENTIAL DIAGNOSIS OF SEVERE TACHYCARDIA FOLLOWING DELIVERY IN A WOMAN WITH SEVERE PREECLAMPSIA

Hyperdynamic heart
Anemia and hemorrhage
Primary heart disease
Pulmonary embolism
Myocardial infarction

duced yet usually remain above nonpregnant values. Levels that are much below those in normal nonpregnant women are the consequence of severe disease. Plasma uric acid concentration is typically elevated, especially in women with severe disease. The elevation proceeds and exceeds that expected for the reduction in glomerular filtration rate alone that accompanies preeclampsia.[27] Serum uric acid measurement for clinical classification of pregnancy was recently shown to be limited.[27a]

The reasons for decreased renal function in women with preeclampsia are incompletely understood but may relate to altered hemodynamics as well as changes in glomerular morphology (see Chap. 8). Although most preeclamptic women experience only moderate decrements in function, on occasion dysfunction is severe and leads to acute renal failure, usually tubular necrosis, and rarely, cortical necrosis.[11] Preeclampsia is often associated with reduced and/or concentrated urine volumes, but the decrease is rarely associated with a vasopressin-resistant type of transient diabetes insipidus. There is anecdotal evidence that dopamine—a renal vasodilator—when infused into oliguric preeclamptic women, increases urine output, fractional sodium excretion, and free water clearance.[28] We caution against *intensive intravenous fluid therapy in women with preeclampsia and with oliguria.*

Taufield et al.[29] reported that preeclampsia is associated with diminished urinary excretion of calcium because of increased tubular reabsorption. This mechanism would explain the decreased calcium excretion in hypertensive and future hypertensive pregnant women.

Acute Renal Failure

After delivery, in the absence of underlying chronic renovascular disease, complete recovery of renal function in the immediate puerperium usually can be anticipated. Women with severe preeclampsia or eclampsia, especially those manifesting hemolysis, elevated liver enzymes, and low platelets—or the *"HELLP" syndrome*—may, however, be at increased risk for acute tubular necrosis, and may have a guarded remote prognosis.[30] Renal insufficiency from *tubular necrosis* is more common in neglected cases and is invariably associated with hypovolemic shock, commonly resulting from hemorrhage at delivery, for which timely and adequate blood replacement is not given. Severe preeclampsia complicated by placental abruption further increases the risk for acute renal failure. Indeed, these two entities accounted for 40% of 75 cases of pregnancy-associated renal failure as well as irreversible acute cortical necrosis.[31,32]

Sibai et al.,[30] from the University of Tennessee, reported observations from 31 women with acute renal failure complicating hypertensive disorders of pregnancy. Eighteen had "pure" preeclampsia, and the remainder had antecedent chronic hypertension, parenchymal renal disease, or both. Half required dialysis and three of these women died as a direct cause of renal failure. About half of these 18 women had suffered placental abruption and almost 90% had postpartum hemorrhage. Frangieh et al.[33] later reported that 3.8% of eclamptic women from the same institution had acute renal failure. This same group[34] also reported that 3% of 67 women with HELLP syndrome developed renal failure. Early identification and proper management of renal failure in women with pure preeclampsia can prevent residual renal damage. It should be noted, however, that these cited series may be selective of tertiary centers, as the incidence of acute renal failure in pregnancy severe enough to require dialysis is uncommon.

Hepatic Changes

Epigastric or *right upper quadrant pain* likely results from hepatocellular necrosis, edema, and ischemia that stretches the Glisson capsule. The characteristic pain is frequently accompanied by elevated serum liver enzymes. *Periportal hemorrhagic necrosis* (Fig. 5–6) in the periphery of the liver lobule is the most likely reason for increased serum liver enzymes.[35,36] In the past, this lesion was often identified at autopsy and was long considered to be a characteristic lesion of eclampsia. Such extensive lesions are seldom identified in nonfatal cases with liver biopsy.[37]

Bleeding from these necrotic lesions may cause *hepatic rupture* or they may extend to form a *subcapsular hematoma*. Such hemorrhages without rupture may be more common than previously suspected. Using computed tomography, Manas et al.[38] showed that five of seven women with preeclampsia and upper abdominal pain had hepatic hemorrhage such as that shown in Figure 5–7. Surgical repair was not necessary in any of these women, but six required blood transfusions. Subcapsular hemorrhage may be extensive enough to rupture the capsule, resulting in fatal intraabdominal hemorrhage.[38a] Prompt surgical intervention may save the patient's life. Smith et al.[39] reviewed 28 cases of spontaneous hepatic rupture associated with preeclampsia and added seven cases of their own. The mortality rate was 30%, and they concluded that packing and drainage was superior to lobectomy. Stain et al.[40] used hepatic artery occlusion, either by ligation or embolization, in eight women.

Rinehart et al.[41] recently reviewed the English medical literature from 1960 to 1997. They found 141 patients with preeclampsia-associated hepatic hemorrhage and rupture during this 38-year interval. Maternal survival was highest with arterial embolization (90%), next with laparotomy with hepatic resection or arterial ligation (80%), and then with laparotomy with hepatic resection (68%). These cases can be extremely complex and one such woman at Parkland Hospital survived after receiving blood and blood products from more than 200 donors during six surgical procedures in 48 hours. Hunter et al.[42] described a similar woman who required a liver transplant in order to survive.

Oosterhof et al.[43] described increased hepatic artery resistance using Doppler sonography in 37 women with preeclampsia (Fig. 5–8). Of interest, they found no significant differences in women with uncomplicated preeclampsia compared with those with HELLP syndrome. Thus, increased resistance to hepatic blood flow may play a role in development of these lesions.

HELLP Syndrome

Liver involvement in preeclampsia–eclampsia is serious and is frequently accompanied by evidence of other organ involvement, especially the kidney and brain,

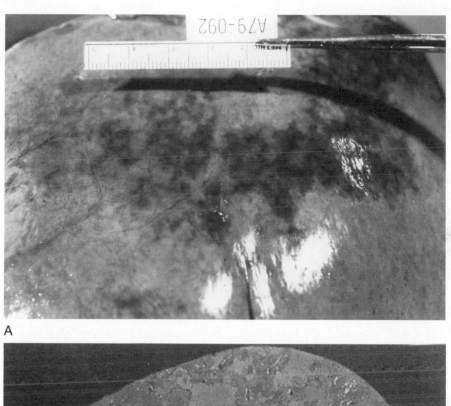

A

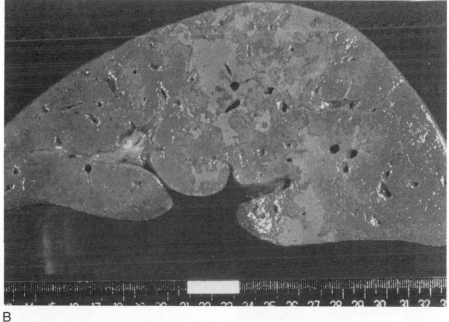

B

Figure 5–6. A. Liver from a woman who died from eclampsia. Dark mottled surface is from numerous large hepatic infarctions similar to those seen in Figure B. **B.** Liver of a second woman who died from eclampsia. There are multiple regions of hepatic infarction seen as serpinginous pale zones. (*Reprinted, with permission, from Knox TA, Olans LB: Liver disease in pregnancy.* N Engl J Med *1996;335: 568–576. Copyright © 1996 Massachusetts Medical Society. All rights reserved.*)

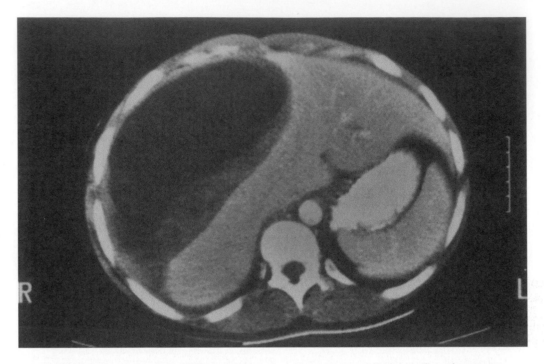

Figure 5–7. Abdominal CT scan after oral and intravenous administration of contrast medium. There is acute hepatic hemorrhage of the right lobe with a subcapsular hematoma. (*Reprinted, with permission, from Knox TA, Olans LB: Liver disease in pregnancy.* N Engl J Med *1996;335:569–576. Copyright © 1996 Massachusetts Medical Society. All rights reserved.*)

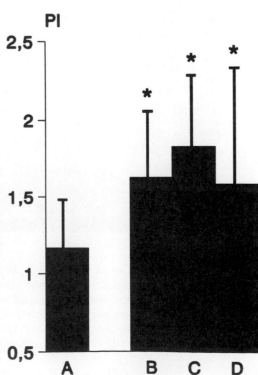

Figure 5–8. Mean (± SD) pulsatility index (PI) of the common hepatic artery in (A) 37 uncomplicated pregnancies; (B) 11 pregnancies complicated by preeclampsia; (C) 13 pregnancies with HELLP syndrome and proteinuria; and (D) 7 with HELLP syndrome and without proteinuria. Asterisk (*) signifies a significant difference from uncomplicated pregnancies ($P < 0.02$). (*Reprinted, with permission, from Oosterhof H, Voorhoeve PG, Aarnoudse JG: Enhancement of hepatic artery resistance to blood flow in preeclampsia in presence or absence of HELLP syndrome (hemolysis, elevated liver enzymes, and low platelets).* Am J Obstet Gynecol *1994;171:526–530.*)

along with hemolysis and thrombocytopenia.[44,45] Weinstein[46] named this the *HELLP syndrome*—Hemolysis, *E*levated liver enzymes, and *L*ow *P*latelets—and this term is now widely used. Sibai et al.[47] identified this constellation in almost 20% of women with severe preeclampsia or eclampsia that they managed in their tertiary care center at the University of Tennessee. Five of the 437 women died. This same group[34] cited other complications including placental abruption (9%), acute renal failure (3%), pulmonary edema (8%), and subcapsular liver hematoma (1%). They also reported that one-fourth of these women delivered by cesarean section had wound hematomas and/or infections.[48]

In addition to immediate morbidity, subsequent adverse pregnancy outcomes are increased in women with HELLP syndrome. Sibai et al.[49] observed a 3% incidence of recurrence of HELLP syndrome in 192 subsequent pregnancies, while Sullivan et al.[50] noted this to be 27%. Both groups confirmed a high incidence of recurrent preeclampsia, preterm delivery, fetal growth restriction, placental abruption, and cesarean delivery.

Central Nervous System Changes

In neglected or, less often, fulminant cases of preeclampsia, eclampsia may develop. The seizures are of the grand mal variety and may appear before, during, or after labor. Seizures that develop more than 48 hours postpartum, however, especially in primiparas, may be encountered up to 10 days postpartum.[51,52]

It is not known precisely what effects preeclampsia has on cerebral blood flow. Belfort et al.[53] used transcranial Doppler ultrasound and found that preeclamptic women with headache are significantly more likely to have abnormal cerebral perfusion than women without headache. Evidence is consistent with vasospasm or with impairment of autoregulation with passive overdistension of cerebral arterioles. These changes persist for at least 24 hours.[53a] Morriss et al.[54] used *magnetic resonance angiography* to measure cerebral artery flow in severely preeclamptic and eclamptic women. Although cerebral blood flow was not altered, these women had been given magnesium sulfate after their eclamptic seizures and before angiography was performed. In similar circumstances, Belfort et al.[55] have shown that a 6-g loading dose of magnesium sulfate reversed middle cerebral artery vasoconstriction.

Nonspecific *electroencephalographic* abnormalities can usually be demonstrated for some time after eclamptic convulsions. Sibai et al.[56] observed that 75% of 65 eclamptic women had abnormal electroencephalograms within 48 hours of seizures. Half of these abnormalities persisted past one week, but most were normal by 3 months. An increased incidence of electroencephalographic abnormalities has been described in family members of eclamptic women, a finding suggestive that some eclamptic women who convulse have an inherited predisposition to do so.[57]

The principal postmortem cerebral lesions described in Chapter 7 are edema, hyperemia, focal anemia, thrombosis, and hemorrhage. Sheehan[58] examined the brains of 48 eclamptic women very soon after death, and hemorrhages, ranging from petechiae to gross bleeding, were found in 56%. According to Sheehan, if the brain is examined within an hour after death, most often it is as firm as normal, and there is no obvious edema. Of 76 types of lesions in these 48 women, the most common are shown in Figure 5–9[59] and were pia-arachnoid hemorrhages (8), cortical petechiae (17), subcortical petechiae (6), and multiple small focal softenings or petechiae in white matter or midbrain (17).

Massive *intracranial hemorrhage* from a ruptured intracerebral vessel, an arteriovenous malformation, or a berry aneurysm may cause coma or death. An example of intracerebral hypertensive hemorrhage in a young woman with untreated severe preeclampsia is shown in Figure 5–10. Sheehan and Lynch[59] reported that 6 of 76 women with fatal eclampsia had massive white matter hemorrhage that caused coma and death. They also reported a high mortality rate with bleeding into the basal ganglia or pons. These latter lesions are common in women with underlying chronic hypertension and superimposed preeclampsia. Hemorrhage in deep areas of the brain may result from rupture of *Charcot–Bouchard microaneurysms* that occur as a result of hypertension and aging.[60] Treatment of cerebrovascular hemorrhage is the same as for any nonpregnant woman.

Govan[61] investigated the cause of death in 110 fatal cases of eclampsia and

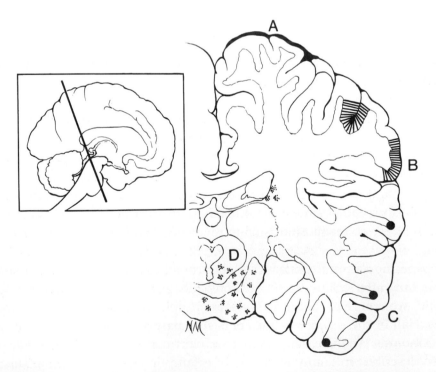

Figure 5–9. Composite illustration showing location of cerebral hemorrhages and petechiae in women with eclampsia: (A) pia-arachnoid hemorrhage; (B) cortical petechiae; (C) subcortical petechiae; and (D) focal softenings or petechiae in midbrain or white matter. (*Data from Sheehan HL, Lynch JB, eds: Cerebral lesions. In:* Pathology of Toxaemia of Pregnancy. *Baltimore: Williams & Wilkins; 1973.*)

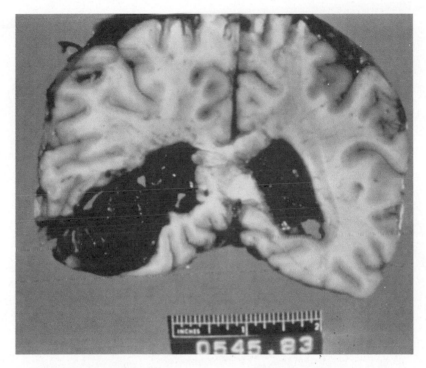

Figure 5–10. Hypertensive hemorrhage with eclampsia. (*Reprinted, with permission, from Cunningham FG, et al: Williams Obstetrics, ed 20. Stamford, CT: Appleton & Lange; 1997.*)

concluded that cerebral hemorrhage was responsible in 39 (35%). Small cerebral hemorrhagic lesions were also found in 85% of the 47 women who died of cardiorespiratory failure. A regular finding was fibrinoid changes in the walls of cerebral vessels. The lesions sometimes appeared to have been present for some time, as judged from the surrounding leukocytic response and hemosiderin-pigmented macrophages. These findings are consistent with the view that prodromal neurologic symptoms and convulsions may be related to these lesions.

Using cranial computed tomography scanning, Brown et al.[62] found that nearly half of eclamptic women studied had abnormal findings such as those shown in Figure 5–11. The most common findings were hypodense cortical areas, which corresponded in location to petechial hemorrhage and infarction sites reported at autopsy by Sheehan and Lynch[59] and shown in Figure 5–9. Using magnetic resonance imaging, Morriss et al.[54] confirmed remarkable changes, especially in the area of the posterior cerebral artery (Fig. 5–12). These findings may provide an explanation of why some women with preeclampsia convulse but others do not. The brain, like the liver and kidney, seems to be more involved in some women than in others. Thus, the extent of ischemic and petechial subcortical lesions, further altered by an inherent seizure threshold, probably influences the incidence of eclampsia.

Witlin et al.,[63] in a retrospective review at the University of Tennessee from 1985 to 1995, reported 24 women with a variety of cerebrovascular disorders and

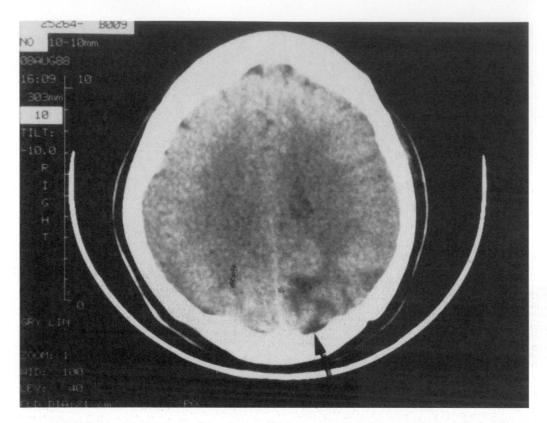

Figure 5–11. Cranial CT of a woman with eclampsia. Radiographic low density areas (arrow) are seen in the left occipital lobe. (*Photograph courtesy of Diane Twickler, MD.*)

seizures. Presumption of eclampsia delayed the definitive diagnosis in ten women. The authors concluded that suspected eclampsia unresponsive to magnesium sulfate therapy warrants an immediate neuroimaging study. Of interest, in the women with an intracranial hemorrhage, severe hypertension was not an associated predictive factor.

Blindness

Compared with normotensive women, preeclamptic women have increased intraocular pressure in the peripartum period.[64] Although visual disturbances are common with severe preeclampsia, blindness, either alone or accompanying convulsions, is not. Women with varying degrees of blindness usually are found to have radiographic—either CT or MR imaging—evidence of extensive occipital lobe hypodensities; this is likely an exaggeration of the lesions described above. Herzog et al.[65] reported that MR imaging was superior to CT in identifying specific brain lesions responsible for this type of blindness. Over a 14-year period at Parkland Hospital, Cunningham et al.[66] described 15 women with severe preeclampsia or eclampsia who also had blindness. This persisted for 4 hours to 8 days, but in all it resolved completely. There is, however, anecdotal evidence of incomplete healing,

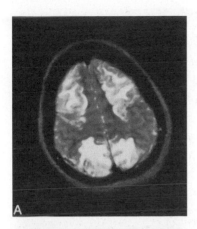

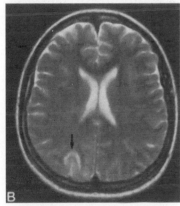

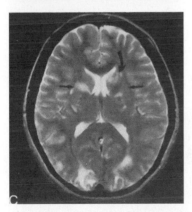

Figure 5–12. Axial T$_2$-weighted magnetic resonance images in three women with eclampsia. **A.** Patient with extensive bilateral areas of white matter edema in the frontoparietal regions. **B.** Patient with focal area of abnormal signal at the gray-white matter junction (*arrow*). **C.** Patient with lesions in the basal ganglia, internal capsule, and right external capsule (*straight arrows*); left caudate nucleus (*curved arrow*); and occipital subcortical white matter. (*Reprinted from Morriss MD, Twickler DM, Hatab MR, et al: Cerebral blood flow and cranial magnetic resonance imaging in eclampsia and severe preeclampsia.* Obstet Gynecol *1997; 89: 561–568. Reprinted with permission from the American College of Obstetricians and Gynecologists.*)

perhaps due to retinal thrombosis (M. Lindheimer, personal communication). Retinal artery vasospasm may be associated with visual disturbances. Belfort et al.[55] found that a 6-g bolus of magnesium sulfate caused retinal artery vasodilation. *Retinal detachment* may also cause altered vision, although it is usually one-sided and seldom causes total visual loss as in some women with cortical blindness. Surgical treatment is seldom indicated, the prognosis is good, and vision usually returns to normal within a week.

Lövestam-Adrian et al.[67] reported that in type 1 diabetic patients deterioration of retinopathy occurred during pregnancy in 4 of 8 women who developed preeclampsia compared with only 5 of 65 who did not (P = 0.005).

Coma

It is rare for a woman with eclampsia not to awaken after a seizure. It is also rare for a woman with severe preeclampsia to become comatose without an antecedent seizure. Prognosis for these women is guarded. In some women, cerebral hemorrhage as described previously and depicted in Figure 5–10, causes coma. Equally ominous is coma caused by generalized cerebral edema. In two eclamptic women with coma managed at Parkland Hospital, extensive cerebral edema was documented by CT. More likely, there are less extensive and multifocal areas of edema on CT that are widespread. Women with those findings may appear lethargic rather than frankly comatose (G. Cunningham and D. Twicker, unpublished observations). Because coma usually follows sudden and severe blood pressure elevations, it is more likely that this phenomenon represents an inability to autoregulate cerebral blood flow with severe acute hypertension; the result being generalized cerebral edema.[68] Figure 5–13 shows CT scans which demonstrate cerebral edema in a preeclamptic woman with acute exacerbation of severe hypertension postpartum. She became comatose immediately following the hypertensive episode, but this lasted only for several hours. Follow-up scans showed eventual resolution.

Hematologic Changes

Hematologic abnormalities develop in some, but certainly not all women who develop preeclampsia. These include thrombocytopenia, which at times may become

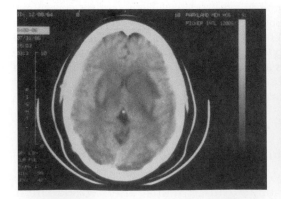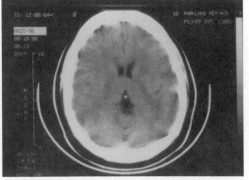

Figure 5–13. Computed tomographs in a woman with cerebral edema following acutely exacerbated severe hypertension. Radiograph on left shows slit-like effaced ventricles as well as sharply demarcated gray-white interface, both indicating parenchymal swelling. The radiograph on the right taken 10 days later shows diminished edema manifest by larger ventricles and loss of gray-white interface demarcation.

so severe as to be life-threatening; the decreased level of some plasma clotting factors; and traumatization of erythrocytes that may display bizarre shapes and undergo rapid hemolysis.

Coagulation

Alterations in coagulation and platelet abnormalities are discussed in detail in Chapter 10. Hematologic changes consistent with intravascular coagulation, and less often erythrocyte destruction, may complicate preeclampsia and especially eclampsia. Since the early description by Pritchard et al.[69] of an eclamptic coagulopathy, there has been little evidence that it is so commonly encountered to be clinically worrisome. Table 5–4 lists data from 91 women with *eclampsia* who would be presumed to have the worst changes of the spectrum of preeclampsia. Thrombocytopenia, infrequently severe, was the most common finding. Serum fibrin degradation products were elevated only occasionally. Nolan et al.[70] found significant elevations of D-dimer fragments of fibrin degradation with preeclampsia, however, these were clinically insignificant. Unless some degree of placental abruption develops, plasma fibrinogen does not differ remarkably from levels found late in normal pregnancy. The same is true for *prothrombin* and *partial thromboplastin times*. The *thrombin time* was somewhat prolonged in one-third of the cases of eclampsia even when elevated levels of fibrin degradation products were not identified. The reason

TABLE 5–4. EVIDENCE FOR DISSEMINATED INTRAVASCULAR COAGULATION IN 91 WOMEN WITH ECLAMPSIA

	Normal Intrapartum Nulliparas	Most Abnormal Value for Each Case of Eclampsia
Platelets[a]		
Mean (per μL)	278,000	206,000
−2 standard deviations	150,000	—
< 150,000	0/20	24/91
< 100,000	0/20	14/91
< 50,000	0/20	3/91
Fibrin degradation products[b]		
8 μg/mL or less	17/20	51/59
16 μg/mL	3/20	6/59
> 16 μg/mL	0/20	2/59
Plasma fibrinogen[a]		
Mean (mg/dL)	415	413
−2 standard deviations	285	—
< 285 mg/dL	0/20	7/89
Fibrin monomer		
Positive	1/20	1/14

[a] Lowest value identified for each case of eclampsia.
[b] Highest value identified for each case of eclampsia.
Reprinted, with permission, from Pritchard JA, Cunningham FG, Mason RA: Coagulation changes in eclampsia: Their frequency and pathogenesis. *Am J Obstet Gynecol* 1976;124:855–864.

for this elevation is not known, but it has been attributed to hepatic derangements discussed below.

The coagulation changes just described are also identified in women with severe preeclampsia, but certainly are no more common. These observations in eclampsia, are most consistent with the concept that coagulation changes are the consequence of preeclampsia–eclampsia, rather than the cause.

Thrombocytopenia

The frequency and intensity of maternal thrombocytopenia are dependent upon the intensity of the disease process, the length of delay between the onset of preeclampsia and delivery, and the frequency with which platelet counts are performed. After delivery, the platelet count will increase progressively to reach a normal level within a few days.[71,72] Overt thrombocytopenia defined by a platelet count less than 100,000/μL is an ominous sign. It signifies severe disease and delivery is usually indicated because the platelet count most often will continue to decrease, although very rarely to levels below 25,000/μL. These observations, however, do not warrant immediate cesarean delivery.

Leduc et al.[73] conducted a retrospective study of 100 women with preeclampsia severe enough to warrant admission to the obstetric intensive care unit at the Baylor College of Medicine. Half of these women had thrombocytopenia defined as less than 150,000/μL. Of these 50, in 14 the count was 100,000 to 150,000/μL, in 22 it was 50,000 to 100,000/μL, and in 14 it was below 50,000/μL. About half of the 50 women with thrombocytopenia had other criteria for HELLP syndrome. Despite these findings, only two women had evidence of consumptive coagulopathy with prolonged coagulation times and decreased plasma fibrinogen levels. Terrone et al.[73a] recently confirmed this, and these findings show that thrombocytopenia is a marker for adverse maternal–fetal outcomes (Table 5–5).

TABLE 5–5. MATERNAL-FETAL COMPLICATIONS IN 100 WOMEN WITH PREECLAMPSIA SEVERE ENOUGH TO WARRANT ADMISSION TO AN OBSTETRIC ICU

Platelet Count	Maternal Complications	Fetal Complications
> 150,000/μL (N = 50)	Cortical blindness (1) Parietal infarct (1) Pulmonary edema (1) Abruptio placentae (1)	Growth restriction (3)
100,000–150,000/μL (N = 14)	Abruptio placentae (2) Cortical blindness (1)	Growth restriction (4) Death (1)
50,000–100,000/μL (N = 22)	Abruptio placentae (2) Coagulopathy (2) Pulmonary edema (1) Aspiration pneumonia (1)	Growth restriction (11) Death (2)
< 50,000/μL (N = 14)	Coagulopathy (2) Cerebral hemorrhage (1) Death (1)	Growth restriction (3) Death (2)

Reprinted from Leduc L, Wheeler JM, Kirshon B, et al: Coagulation profile in severe preeclampsia. *Obstet Gynecol* 1992;79:14–18. Reprinted with permission from the American College of Obstetricians and Gynecologists.

The exact cause(s) of thrombocytopenia is not clear. Possible mechanisms are discussed in detail in Chapter 10 and undoubtedly increased platelet aggregation plays a role in preeclamptic women.[74] Immunologic processes or simply platelet deposition at sites of endothelial damage may be the cause.[69] Alternatively, Samuels et al.[75] suggested that platelet surfaces are altered. Burrows et al.[76] reported that platelets from preeclamptic women were more likely to have platelet-associated IgG, even if thrombocytopenia did not develop. While they believed this mechanism implied an autoimmune process, IgG frequently binds to platelets damaged by any mechanism.

Of clinical relevance, Kelton et al.[77] showed that thrombocytopenia with preeclampsia was frequently associated with a prolonged bleeding time. This was true even with normal platelet levels.

Neonatal Thrombocytopenia

Thiagarajah et al.,[78] and Weinstein[46] reported thrombocytopenia in neonates whose mothers had preeclampsia. Conversely, Pritchard et al.,[79] in a large clinical study, did *not* observe severe thrombocytopenia in the fetus or infant at or very soon after delivery. No cases of fetal or neonatal thrombocytopenia were identified, despite severe maternal thrombocytopenia. Thrombocytopenia did develop later in some of these infants after hypoxia, acidosis, and sepsis occurred. *Hence, maternal thrombocytopenia in hypertensive women is not a fetal indication for cesarean delivery.*

Fragmentation Hemolysis

Thrombocytopenia that accompanies severe preeclampsia and eclampsia may be accompanied by evidence of erythrocyte destruction characterized by hemolysis, schizocytosis, spherocytosis, reticulocytosis, hemoglobinuria, and occasionally hemoglobinemia.[45,69] An example of changes seen in a peripheral blood smear is shown in Figure 5–14. These derangements result in part from microangiopathic hemolysis, and human and animal studies are suggestive that intense vasospasm causes endothelial disruption, with platelet adherence and fibrin deposition. Cunningham et al.[80] described erythrocyte morphologic characteristics using scanning electron microscopy. Women with eclampsia, and to a lesser degree those with severe preeclampsia, demonstrated schizocytosis and echinocytosis but not spherocytosis when compared with healthy pregnant women. Sanchez-Ramos et al.[81] described increased erythrocyte membrane fluidity in women with HELLP syndrome and postulated that these changes predispose to hemolysis. Finally, Grisaru et al.[82] have demonstrated that erythrocytic membrane changes in preeclamptic women may facilitate the hypercoagulable state.

Other Clotting Factors

A severe deficiency of any of the soluble coagulation factors is very uncommon in severe preeclampsia–eclampsia unless another event coexists that predisposes to consumptive coagulopathy, such as placental abruption, fatty liver, or hepatic infarction. There are a number of subtle alterations of the coagulation cascade in-

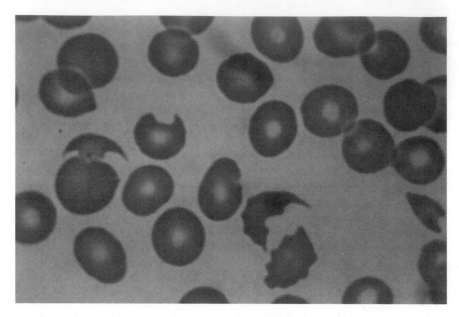

Figure 5–14. Peripheral blood smear showing multiple schizocytes characteristic of microangiopathic hemolysis.

duced by severe preeclampsia that are of questionable clinical significance. These include changes in antithrombin III, fibronectin, thrombomodulin, thrombin, and protein C, as well as many others. These are discussed in detail in Chapter 10.

A number of mutations that affect coagulation may predispose women to an appreciably increased risk for preeclampsia and/or thromboembolic complications. One well-known example is the *lupus anticoagulant* or other forms of *antiphospholipid antibodies*. One more recently discovered is the *factor V Leiden mutation*. Hastings et al.[83] extracted DNA from 3005 predominantly Caucasian women and 166 (5.5%) were heterozygous and 4 (0.13%) were homozygous for this mutation. Medical record reviews of 116 of these women revealed an incidence of preeclampsia of 22%, thromboembolic complications in 7.8%, and pulmonary embolism in 2.6%. Dizon-Townson et al.[84,85] have also reported significant associations in women heterozygous for the factor V Leiden mutation with deep vein thrombosis and severe preeclampsia.

Uteroplacental Perfusion

Compromised placental perfusion from vasospasm is almost certainly a major culprit in the genesis of increased perinatal morbidity and mortality associated with preeclampsia.

Measurements of Placental Perfusion

Attempts to measure human maternal placental blood flow have been hampered by several obstacles, including inaccessibility of the placenta, the complexity of its venous effluent, and the unsuitability of certain investigative techniques for humans. Despite formidable problems, Assali et al.[86] and Metcalfe et al.[87] measured uterine blood flow in pregnant women and obtained reasonably consistent results. Both groups used a nitrous oxide Fick principle method that required cannulation of a uterine vein. Total uterine perfusion was measured, rather than maternal placental blood flow. Uterine blood flow in normal-term pregnant women was approximately 500 to 700 mL/min.

Browne and Veall[88] estimated changes in maternal placental flow through the use of a ^{24}Na– clearance technique. This method required needle insertion into the intervillous space. They, as well as Weis et al.[89] observed that ^{24}Na was cleared two to three times more rapidly in normotensive pregnant women than in preeclamptic women. This implied a two- to threefold decrease in uteroplacental perfusion in hypertensive women compared with normotensive controls.

Indirect Methods

The consistent results and conclusions obtained from these early studies continue to be supported by other methods of investigation. For instance, Brosens et al.[90] reported that the mean diameter of myometrial spiral arterioles of 50 normal pregnant women was 500 μm. The same measurement in 36 women with preeclampsia was 200 μm. Implications of this are discussed in detail in Chapter 11.

Everett et al.[91] presented evidence that the *dehydroisoandrosterone sulfate clearance rate* through placental conversion to estradiol-17β reflected maternal placental perfusion. Fritz et al.[92] reported that the technique paralleled uteroplacental perfusion in primates. Normally, as pregnancy advances, this measurement increases greatly. The placental clearance rate decreases before the onset of overt hypertension.[93] Finally, placental clearance is decreased in women given diuretics or hydralazine.[94]

Doppler velocimetry measurement of uterine artery blood flow has been used to estimate changes in uteroplacental perfusion. Vascular resistance is estimated by comparing arterial systolic and diastolic velocity waveforms. Fleischer et al.,[95] Trudinger and Cook[96], and Irion et al.[96a] reported increased systolic–diastolic ratio in uterine arteries of women with preeclampsia. Others have not confirmed this.[97] Absent end-diastolic flow or reversal of flow is associated with increased fetal morbidity and mortality in hypertensive women.[98,99] Thaler et al.[100] reported that the presence of a systolic or diastolic notch or a combination of both is associated with elevated resistance indices in the uterine and umbilical vessels. Nifedipine therapy and epidural analgesia have been reported to decrease abnormally elevated systolic–diastolic ratios.[101-103]

Ducey et al.[104] described systolic–diastolic velocity ratios from both uterine and umbilical arteries in 136 pregnancies complicated by hypertension. Among 51 women considered to have preeclampsia, 20% had normal umbilical artery velocity ratios; 15% had normal umbilical but abnormal uterine artery ratios; and in 40% both ratios were abnormal. Atkinson et al.[105] showed that elevated umbilical artery systolic–diastolic ratio is not a clinically useful predictor for preeclampsia in a low-risk population. This was also confirmed by Zimmerman et al.[106] and Irion et al.[96a]

In our experiences, diminished uterine artery flow velocities are seldom encountered with *uncomplicated* preeclampsia. This is true even with severely elevated blood pressures. With associated fetal growth restriction, however, aberrant flow velocities are often seen in both umbilical and aortic vessels.[107] In some reports, women were studied *because* of growth restriction. Thus, it appears that preeclampsia alone may not be associated with significant changes in the uterine artery systolic–diastolic ratio. Aberrations in fetal blood flow velocities detected in hypertensive pregnancies are much more likely if there is restricted fetal growth.[108,109]

Finally, *magnetic resonance imaging* was recently described by Francis et al.[110] to hold promise for measuring placental perfusion. The Nottingham group used perfusion-sensitive echoplanar imaging (EPI) and showed that pregnancies complicated by fetal growth restriction had significantly decreased placental perfusion rates compared with normal pregnancies. These preliminary data, while exciting, need to be verified and refined.

CONCLUSION

Preeclampsia is a fascinating clinical syndrome unique to pregnant women. Unlike chronic essential hypertension, it is characterized primarily by arteriolar vasospasm, markedly increased peripheral vascular resistance as compared with normal pregnancy, varying aspects of endothelial damage, and it almost always promptly reverses following delivery. Because virtually every organ system can be affected, preeclampsia is a true "systemic disease." Thus, in addition to hypertension and proteinuria, there is varying organ system involvement. The wide clinical spectrum of adverse maternal effects associated with preeclampsia frequently are further confounded by adverse maternal consequences created by clinical management events subsequent to those apparent at initial clinical presentation.

REFERENCES

1. Shennan A, Gupta M, Halligan A, et al: Lack of reproducibility in pregnancy of Korotkoff phase IV as measured by mercury sphygmomanometry. *Lancet* 1996;347:139–142.
1a. Brown MA, Buddle ML, Farrell T, et al: Randomized trial of management of hypertensive pregnancies by Korotkoff phase IV or phase V. *Lancet* 1998;352:777–781.
2. National High Blood Pressure Education Program Working Group: Report on high blood pressure in pregnancy. *Am J Obstet Gynecol* 1990;163:1689–1712.
3. Redman CWG, Beilin LS, Bonnar J: Variability of blood pressure in normal and abnormal pregnancy. In: Lindhimer MD, Katz AL, Zuspan FP, eds. *Hypertension in Pregnancy*. New York: John Wiley & Son; 1976:53–59.
4. Benedetto C, Zonca M, Marozio L, et al: Blood pressure patterns in normal pregnancy and in pregnancy-induced hypertension, preeclampsia, and chronic hypertension. *Obstet Gynecol* 1996;88:503–510.
5. Chesley LC: Diagnosis of preeclampsia. *Obstet Gynecol* 1985;65:423–425.
6. Friedman EA, Neff RK: Pregnancy outcome as related to hypertension, edema, and protein-

uria. In: Lindheimer MD, Katz AI, Zuspan FP, eds. *Hypertension in Pregnancy*. New York: John Wiley & Sons; 1976:13.

7. Cunningham FG, MacDonald PC, Gant NF, et al, eds: Hypertensive disorders in pregnancy. In: *Williams Obstetrics*, ed 20. Stamford, CT: Appleton & Lange; 1997:695, chap 31.

8. Øian P, Maltau JM: Calculated capillar hydrostatic pressure in normal pregnancy and preeclampsia. *Am J Obstet Gynecol* 1987;157:102–106.

9. Wheeler TC, Graves CR, Troiano NH, Reed GW: Base deficit and oxygen transport in severe preeclampsia. *Obstet Gynecol* 1996;87:375–379.

10. Dieckmann WJ: *The Toxemias of Pregnancy*, ed 2. St. Louis: Mosby; 1952.

11. Pritchard JA, Cunningham FG, Pritchard SA: The Parkland Memorial Hospital protocol for treatment of eclampsia: Evaluation of 245 cases. *Am J Obstet Gynecol* 1984;148:951–963.

12. Silver H, Seebeck M: Comparison of methods of blood volume measurement in normotensive and preeclamptic pregnancies. *Am J Obstet Gynecol* 1996;174:452.

13. Benedetti TJ, Quilligan EJ: Cerebral edema in severe pregnancy-induced hypertension. *Am J Obstet Gynecol* 1980b;137:860–862.

14. Benedetti TJ, Kates R, Williams V: Hemodynamic observations in severe preeclampsia complicated by pulmonary edema. *Am J Obstet Gynecol* 1985;152:330–334.

15. Clark SL, Cotton DB, Wesley L, et al: Central hemodynamic assessment of normal term pregnancy. *Am J Obstet Gynecol* 1989;161:1439–1442.

16. Groenendijk R, Trimbros JBM, Wallenburg HCS: Hemodynamic measurements in preeclampsia: Preliminary observations. *Am J Obstet Gynecol* 1984;150:232–236.

17. Visser W, Wallenburg HCS: Central hemodynamic observations in untreated preeclamptic patients. *Hypertension* 1991;17:1072–1077.

18. Benedetti TJ, Cotton DB, Read JC, Miller FC: Hemodynamic observations in severe preeclampsia with a flow-directed pulmonary artery catheter. *Am J Obstet Gynecol* 1980a; 136:465–470.

19. Hankins GDV, Wendel GW Jr, Cunningham FG, Leveno KJ: Longitudinal evaluation of hemodynamic changes in eclampsia. *Am J Obstet Gynecol* 1984;150:506–512.

20. Rafferty TD, Berkowitz RL: Hemodynamics in patients with severe toxemia during labor and delivery. *Am J Obstet Gynecol* 1980;138:263–270.

21. Phelan JP, Yurth DA: Severe preeclampsia. I. Peripartum hemodynamic observations. *Am J Obstet Gynecol* 1982;144:17–22.

22. Cotton DB, Gonik B, Dorman KF: Cardiovascular alterations in severe pregnancy-induced hypertension: Acute effects of intravenous magnesium sulfate. *Am J Obstet Gynecol* 1984; 148:162–165.

23. Cunningham FG, Pritchard JA, Hankins GCV, et al: Idiopathic cardiomyopathy or compounding cardiovascular events? *Obstet Gynecol* 1986;67:157–168.

24. Sibai BM, Mabie BC, Harvey CJ, Gonzalez AR: Pulmonary edema in severe preeclampsia–eclampsia: Analysis of thirty-seven consecutive cases. *Am J Obstet Gynecol* 1987;156: 1174–1179.

25. Desai DK, Moodley J, Naidoo DP, Bhorat I: Cardiac abnormalities in pulmonary oedema associated with hypertensive crises in pregnancy. *Br J Obstet Gynaecol* 1996;103:523–528.

26. Lehmann DK, Mabie WC, Miller JM, Pernoll ML: The epidemiology and pathology of maternal mortality: Charity Hospital of Louisiana in New Orleans, 1965–1984. *Obstet Gynecol* 1987;69:833–840.

27. Chesley LC, Williams LO: Renal glomerular and tubular function in relation to the hyperuricemia of preeclampsia and eclampsia. *Am J Obstet Gynecol* 1945;50:367–375.

27a. Lim K-H, Friedman SA, Ecker JL, et al: The clinical utility of serum uric acid measurements in hypertensive diseases of pregnancy. *Am J Obstet Gynecol* 1998;178:1067–1071.

28. Kirshon B, Lee W, Mauer MB, Cotton DB: Effects of low-dose dopamine therapy in the oliguric patient with preeclampsia. *Am J Obstet Gynecol* 1988;159:604–607.

29. Taufield PA, Ales KL, Resnick LM, et al: Hypocalcuria in preeclampsia. *N Engl J Med* 1987;316:715–718.

30. Sibai BM, Villar MA, Mabie BC: Acute renal failure in hypertensive disorders of pregnancy. Pregnancy outcome and remote prognosis in thirty-one consecutive cases. *Am J Obstet Gynecol* 1990;162:777–783.

31. Alexopoulos E, Tambakoudis P, Bili H, et al: Acute renal failure in pregnancy. *Renal Fail* 1993;15:609–613.

32. Grünfeld JP, Pertuiset N: Acute renal failure in pregnancy: 1987. *Am J Kidney Dis* 1987; 9:359–362.

33. Frangieh SA, Friedman SA, Audibert F: Maternal outcome in women with eclampsia. *Am J Obstet Gynecol* 1996;174:453.

34. Audibert F, Friedman SA, Frangieh AY, Sibai BM: Diagnostic criteria for HELLP syndrome: Tedious or "HELLPful"? *Am J Obstet Gynecol* 1996;174:454.

35. Cunningham FG: Liver disease complicating pregnancy. In: *Williams Obstetrics*, ed 19 (suppl 1). Norwalk, CT: Appleton & Lange; 1993.

36. Knox TA, Olans LB: Liver disease in pregnancy. *N Engl J Med* 1996;335:569–576.

37. Barton JR, Riely CA, Adamec TA, et al: Hepatic histopathologic condition does not correlate with laboratory abnormalities in HELLP syndrome (hemolysis, elevated liver enzymes, and low platelet count). *Am J Obstet Gynecol* 1992;167:1538–1543.

38. Manas KJ, Welsh JD, Rankin RA, Miller DD: Hepatic hemorrhage without rupture in preeclampsia. *N Engl J Med* 1985;312:424–426.

38a. Isler CM, Rinehart BK, Terrone RW, et al: Maternal mortality associated with HELLP syndrome. *Am J Obstet Gynecol* 1999 (in press).

39. Smith LG Jr, Moise KJ Jr, Dildy GA III, Carpenter RJ Jr: Spontaneous rupture of liver during pregnancy: Current therapy. *Obstet Gynecol* 1991;77:171–175.

40. Stain SC, Woodburn DA, Stephens AL, et al: Spontaneous hepatic hemorrhage associated with pregnancy. Treatment by hepatic arterial interruption. *Ann Surg* 1996;224:72–78.

41. Rinehart BK, Terrone DA, Magann EF, et al: Preeclampsia-associated hepatic hemorrhage and rupture: Mode of management versus maternal–perinatal outcome. *Am J Obstet Gynecol* 1998;178:S119.

42. Hunter SK, Martin M, Benda JA, Zlatnik FJ: Liver transplant after massive spontaneous hepatic rupture in pregnancy complicated by preeclampsia. *Obstet Gynecol* 1995;85:819–822.

43. Oosterhof H, Voorhoeve PG, Aarnoudse JG: Enhancement of hepatic artery resistance to blood flow in preeclampsia in presence or absence of HELLP syndrome (hemolysis, elevated liver enzymes, and low platelets). *Am J Obstet Gynecol* 1994;171:526–530.

44. De Boer K, Büller HR, Ten Cate JW, Treffers PE: Coagulation studies in the syndrome of haemolysis, elevated liver enzymes and low platelets. *Br J Obstet Gynaecol* 1991;98:42–47.

45. Pritchard JA, Weisman R Jr, Ratnoff OD, Vosburgh G: Intravascular hemolysis, thrombocytopenia and other hematologic abnormalities associated with severe toxemia of pregnancy. *N Engl J Med* 1954;250:89–98.

46. Weinstein L: Preeclampsia–eclampsia with hemolysis, elevated liver enzymes, and thrombocytopenia. *Obstet Gynecol* 1985;66:657–660.

47. Sibai BM, Ramadan MK, Usta I, et al: Maternal morbidity and mortality in 442 pregnancies with hemolysis, elevated liver enzymes, and low platelets (HELLP syndrome). *Am J Obstet Gynecol* 1993;169:1000–1006.

48. Briggs R, Chari RS, Mercer B, Sibai B: Postoperative incision complications after cesarean section in patients with antepartum syndrome of hemolysis, elevated liver enzymes, and low platelets (HELLP): Does delayed primary closure make a difference? *Am J Obstet Gynecol* 1996;175:893–896.

49. Sibai BM, Ramadan MK, Chari RS, Friedman S: Pregnancies complicated by HELLP syndrome (hemolysis, elevated liver enzymes, and low platelets): Subsequent pregnancy outcome and long-term prognosis. *Am J Obstet Gynecol* 1995;172:125–129.

50. Sullivan CA, Magann EF, Perry KG Jr, et al: The recurrence risk of the syndrome of hemolysis, elevated liver enzymes, and low platelets (HELLP) in subsequent gestations. *Am J Obstet Gynecol* 1994;171:940–943.

51. Brown CEL, Cunningham FG, Pritchard JA: Convulsions in hypertensive, proteinuric primiparas more than 24 hours after delivery: Eclampsia or some other cause? *J Reprod Med* 1987;32:499–503.

52. Lubarsky SL, Barton JR, Friedman SA, et al: Late postpartum eclampsia revisited. *Obstet Gynecol* 1994;83:502–505.

53. Belfort M, Wihman I, Grunewald C, et al: Preeclamptic women with headache are much more likely to have abnormal cerebral perfusion than those without. *Am J Obstet Gynecol* 1998;178:S3.

53a. Williams K, Wilson S: Cerebral hyperperfusion change in eclampsia persists for up to 24 hours. *Am J Obstet Gynecol* 1999 (in press).

54. Morriss MC, Twickler DM, Hatab MR, et al: Cerebral blood flow and cranial magnetic resonance imaging in eclampsia and severe preeclampsia. *Obstet Gynecol* 1997;89:561–568.

55. Belfort MA, Saade GR, Moise KJ Jr: The effect of magnesium sulfate on maternal retinal blood flow in preeclampsia: A randomized placebo-controlled study. *Am J Obstet Gynecol* 1992;167:1548–1553.

56. Sibai BM, Spinnato JA, Watson DL, et al: Eclampsia. IV. Neurological findings and future outcome. *Am J Obstet Gynecol* 1985;152:184–192.

57. Rosenbaum M, Maltby G: Cerebral dysrhythmia in relation to eclampsia. *Arch Neurol Psychiatr* 1943;49:204–213.

58. Sheehan HL: Pathological lesions in the hypertensive toxaemias of pregnancy. In: Hammond J, Browne FJ, Wolstenholme GEW, eds. *Toxaemias of Pregnancy, Human and Veterinary*. Philadelphia: Blakiston; 1950.

59. Sheehan HL, Lynch JB, eds: Cerebral lesions. In: *Pathology of Toxaemia of Pregnancy*. Baltimore: Williams & Wilkins; 1973, chap 32.

60. Strandgaard S, Paulson OB: Cerebrovascular consequences of hypertension. *Lancet* 1994; 344:519–521.

61. Govan ADT: The pathogenesis of eclamptic lesions. *Pathol Microbiol* 1961;24:561–575.

62. Brown CEL, Purdy PD, Cunningham FG: Head computed tomographic scans in women with eclampsia. *Am J Obstet Gynecol* 1988a;159:915–920.

63. Witlin AG, Friedman SA, Egerman RS, et al: Cerebrovascular disorders complicating pregnancy—beyond eclampsia. *Am J Obstet Gynecol* 1997;176:1139–1148.

64. Giannina G, Belfort MA, Abadejos P, Dorman K: Comparison of intraocular pressure between normotensive and preeclamptic women in the peripartum period. *Am J Obstet Gynecol* 1997;176:1052–1055.

65. Herzog TJ, Angel OH, Karram MM, Evertson LR: Use of magnetic resonance imaging in the diagnosis of cortical blindness in pregnancy. *Obstet Gynecol* 1990;76:980–982.

66. Cunningham FG, Fernandez CO, Hernandez C: Blindness associated with preeclampsia and eclampsia. *Am J Obstet Gynecol* 1995;172:1291–1298.

67. Lövestam-Adrian M, Agardh CD, Agardh AE: Pre-eclampsia is a potential risk factor for deterioration of retinopathy during pregnancy in type 1 diabetic patients. *Diabet Med* 1997;14:1059–1065.

68. Hinchey J, Chaves C, Appignani B, et al: A reversible posterior leukoencephalopathy syndrome. *N Engl J Med* 1996;334:494.

69. Pritchard JA, Cunningham FG, Mason RA: Coagulation changes in eclampsia: Their frequency and pathogenesis. *Am J Obstet Gynecol* 1976;124:855–864.

70. Nolan TE, Smith RP, DeVoe LD: Maternal plasma D-dimer levels in normal and complicated pregnancies. *Obstet Gynecol* 1993;81:235–238.

71. Katz VL, Thorp JM Jr, Rozas L, Bowes WA Jr: The natural history of thrombocytopenia associated with preeclampsia. *Am J Obstet Gynecol* 1990;163:1142–1143.

72. Romero R, Mazor M, Lockwood CJ, et al: Clinical significance, prevalence, and natural history of thrombocytopenia in pregnancy-induced hypertension. *Am J Perinatol* 1989;6:32–38.

73. Leduc L, Wheeler JM, Kirshon B, et al: Coagulation profile in severe preeclampsia. *Obstet Gynecol* 1992;79:14–18.

73a. Terrone DA, Isler CM, May WL, et al: Cardiopulmonary morbidity as a complication of severe preeclampsia HELLP syndrome. *Am J Obstet Gynecol* 1999 (in press).

74. Torres PJ, Escolar G, Palacio M, et al: Platelet sensitivity to prostaglandin E_1 inhibition is reduced in preeclampsia but not in nonproteinuric gestational hypertension. *Br J Obstet Gynaecol* 1996;103:19–24.

75. Samuels P, Main EK, Tomaski A, et al: Abnormalities in platelet antiglobulin tests in preeclamptic mothers and their neonates. *Am J Obstet Gynecol* 1987;157:109–113.

76. Burrows RF, Hunter DJS, Andrew M, Kelton JG: A prospective study investigating the mechanism of thrombocytopenia in preeclampsia. *Obstet Gynecol* 1987;70:334–338.

77. Kelton JG, Hunter DJS, Naeme PB: A platelet function defect in preeclampsia. *Obstet Gynecol* 1995;65:107–109.

78. Thiagarajah S, Bourgeois FJ, Harbert GM, Caudle MR: Thrombocytopenia in preeclampsia: Associated abnormalities and management principles. *Am J Obstet Gynecol* 1984;150:1–7.

79. Pritchard JA, Cunningham FG, Pritchard SA, Mason RA: How often does maternal preeclampsia–eclampsia incite thrombocytopenia in the fetus? *Obstet Gynecol* 1987;69:292–295.

80. Cunningham FG, Lowe T, Guss S, Mason R: Erythrocyte morphology in women with severe preeclampsia and eclampsia. *Am J Obstet Gynecol* 1985;153:358–363.

81. Sanchez-Ramos L, Adair CD, Todd JC, et al: Erythrocyte membrane fluidity in patients with preeclampsia and the HELLP syndrome: A preliminary study. *J Matern Fetal Invest* 1994;4:237–239.

82. Grisaru D, Zwang E, Peyser R, et al: The procoagulant activity of red blood cells from patients with severe preeclampsia. *Am J Obstet Gynecol* 1997;177:1513–1516.

83. Hastings S, Knowlton J, Nelson L, et al: Obstetrical and medical complications in women with the Factor V Leiden mutation. *Am J Obstet Gynecol* 1998;178:S104.

84. Dizon-Townson DS, Nelson LM, Jang H, et al: The incidence of the factor V Leiden mutation in an obstetric population and its relationship to deep vein thrombosis. *Am J Obstet Gynecol* 1997;176:883–886.

85. Dizon-Townson DS, Nelson LM, Easton K, Ward K: The factor V Leiden mutation may predispose women to severe preeclampsia. *Am J Obstet Gynecol* 1996;175:902–905.

86. Assali NS, Douglas RA, Baird WW: Measurement of uterine blood flow and uterine metabolism. *Am J Obstet Gynecol* 1953;66:248–256.

87. Metcalfe J, Romney SL, Ramsey LH, et al: Estimation of uterine blood flow in normal human pregnancy at term. *J Clin Invest* 1955;34:1632–1638.

88. Browne JCM, Veall N: The maternal placental blood flow in normotensive and hypertensive women. *J Obstet Gynaecol Br Emp* 1953;60:141–147.

89. Weis EB Jr, Bruns PD, Taylor ES: A comparative study of the disappearance of radioactive sodium from human uterine muscle in normal and abnormal pregnancy. *Am J Obstet Gynecol* 1958;76:340–346.

90. Brosens IA, Robertson WB, Dixon HG: The role of the spiral arteries in the pathogenesis of preeclampsia. *Obstet Gynecol Ann* 1972;1:177–191.

91. Everett RB, Porter JC, MacDonald PC, Gant NF: Relationship of maternal placental blood flow to the placental clearance of maternal plasma dehydroisoandrosterone sulfate through placental estriol formation. *Am J Obstet Gynecol* 1980;136:435–439.

92. Fritz MA, Stanczyk FZ, Novy MJ: Relationship of uteroplacental blood flow to the placental clearance of maternal dehydroepiandrosterone through estradiol formation in the pregnant baboon. *J Clin Endocrinol Metab* 1985;61:1023–1030.

93. Worley RJ, Everett RB, MacDonald PC, Gant NF: Placental clearance of dehydroisoandrosterone sulfate and pregnancy outcome in three categories of hospitalized patients with pregnancy-induced hypertension. *Gynecol Obstet Invest* 1975;6:28–29.

94. Gant NF, Madden JD, Siiteri PK, MacDonald PC: The metabolic clearance rate of dehydroisoandrosterone sulfate. IV. Acute effect of induced hypertension, hypotension, and natriuresis in normal and hypertensive pregnancies. *Am J Obstet Gynecol* 1976;124:143–148.

95. Fleischer A, Schulman H, Farmakides G, et al: Uterine artery Doppler velocimetry in pregnant women with hypertension. *Am J Obstet Gynecol* 1986;154:806–813.

96. Trudinger BJ, Cook CM: Doppler umbilical and uterine flow waveforms in severe pregnancy hypertension. *Br J Obstet Gynaecol* 1990;97:142–148.

96a. Irion O, Massé J, Forest J-C, Montaquin J-M: Prediction of preeclampsia, low birthweight for gestation, and prematurity by uterine artery flow velocity waveform analysis in low risk nulliparous women. *Br J Obstet Gynaecol* 1998;105:422–429.

97. Hanretty KP, Whittle MJ, Rubin PC: Doppler uteroplacental waveforms in pregnancy-induced hypertension: A re-appraisal. *Lancet* 1988;1:850–852.

98. Fairlie FM, Moretti M, Walker JJ, Sibai BM: Determinants of perinatal outcome in pregnancy-induced hypertension with absence of umbilical artery end-diastolic frequencies. *Am J Obstet Gynecol* 1991;164:1084–1089.

99. Kofinas AD, Penry M, Nelson LH, et al: Uterine and umbilical artery flow velocity waveform analysis in pregnancies complicated by chronic hypertension or preeclampsia. *South Med J* 1990;83:150–155.

100. Thaler I, Weiner Z, Itskovitz J: Systolic or diastolic notch in uterine artery blood flow velocity waveforms in hypertensive pregnant patients: Relationship to outcome. *Obstet Gynecol* 1992;80:277–282.

101. Pirhonen JP, Erkkola RU, Ekblad UU: Uterine and fetal flow velocity waveforms in hypertensive pregnancy: The effect of a single dose of nifedipine. *Obstet Gynecol* 1990;76:37–41.

102. Puzey MS, Ackovic KL, Lindow SW, Gonin R: The effect of nifedipine on fetal umbilical artery Doppler waveforms in pregnancies complicated by hypertension. *S Afr Med J* 1991;79:192–194.

103. Ramos-Santos E, Devoe LD, Wakefield ML, et al: The effects of epidural anesthesia on the Doppler velocimetry of umbilical and uterine arteries in normal and hypertensive patients during active term labor. *Obstet Gynecol* 1991;77:20.

104. Ducey J, Schulman H, Farmakides G, et al: A classification of hypertension in pregnancy based on Doppler velocimetry. *Am J Obstet Gynecol* 1987;157:680–685.

105. Atkinson MW, Maher JE, Owen J, et al: The predictive value of umbilical artery Doppler studies for preeclampsia or fetal growth retardation in a preeclampsia prevention trial. *Obstet Gynecol* 1994;83:609–612.

106. Zimmerman P, Eirio V, Koskinen J, et al: Doppler assessment of the uterine and uteroplacental circulation in the second trimester in pregnancies at high risk for pre-eclampsia and/or intrauterine growth retardation: Comparison and correlation between different Doppler parameters. *Ultrasound Obstet Gynecol* 1997;9:330–338.

107. Cameron AD, Nicholson SF, Nimrod CA, et al: Doppler waveforms in the fetal aorta and umbilical artery in patients with hypertension in pregnancy. *Am J Obstet Gynecol* 1988;158:339–345.

108. Lowery CL Jr, Henson BV, Wan J, Brumfield CG: A comparison between umbilical artery velocimetry and standard antepartum surveillance in hospitalized high-risk patients. *Am J Obstet Gynecol* 1990;162:710–714.

109. Villar MA, Sibai BM, González AR, et al: Plasma volume, umbilical artery Doppler flow, and antepartum fetal heart testing in high-risk pregnancies. *Am J Perinatol* 1989;6:341–346.

110. Francis ST, Duncan KR, Moore RJ, et al: Non-invasive mapping of placental perfusion. *Lancet* 1998;351:1397–1399.

6

Prediction and Differential Diagnosis

Steven A. Friedman and Marshall D. Lindheimer

In the first edition of this text, Chesley devoted but two pages to predictive tests, reflecting the paucity of data regarding changes in circulating substances and identification of risk factors associated with preeclampsia that had been researched prior to the mid 1970s. In fact, of the three possible predictors he highlighted, indices of exchangeable sodium, the flicker fusion test (the point at which a rapidly flickering light is perceived as steady), and a variety of pressor responses ranging from angiotensin infusion to the roll-over test, none are in widespread use as we start the 21st century. Throughout Chesley's text, however, more space was devoted to distinguishing between preeclampsia and less ominous forms of the hypertensive disorders complicating pregnancy, primarily transient hypertension in late pregnancy. This differential remains a challenge today.

Predictive tests are those performed on asymptomatic patients to determine which members of that population will later develop a particular disease. The classic example of a successful predictive (or screening) test is the Pap smear. Similarly, diagnostic tests are performed on patients with similar symptoms, such as hypertension, to determine which members of the population have the disease of interest, in this case preeclampsia.

For such tests to become reality, detailed knowledge of the pathogenesis of preeclampsia is required, and such knowledge is presently lacking. To be sure, preeclampsia remains a syndrome, defined by its complex and varied clinical manifestations, and efforts to study this disease have been impaired by the lack of a diagnostic "gold standard," a pathognomonic biochemical, biophysical, histologic, or radiologic probe. As a result, much of the published literature on preeclampsia is inadequate primarily because the authors failed to use sufficiently specific criteria to define the disease. In addressing this problem, Chesley[1] noted that only half of all women diagnosed clinically with mild preeclampsia actually have the disease. He correctly argued that this overdiagnosis in the clinical setting is appropriate, since "so-called mild preeclampsia or even barely recognizable preeclampsia is potentially lethal." In the research setting, however, such diagnostic errors lead to erroneous and contradictory conclusions. "What have we been studying," he asked, "thinking that the disorders were preeclampsia?" Chesley therefore proposed the following strict diagnostic criteria for the purposes of including hypertensive women in research studies of preeclampsia: (1) nulliparity; (2) abundant proteinuria; (3) reliable history of cardiovascular and renal normality or, better, follow-up studies proving it; (4) age less than 25 years; and (5) hyperuricemia. Such strict criteria would incorrectly exclude a small number of women with true preeclampsia, but they would no doubt correctly exclude a larger number of women with other diseases such as transient hypertension, chronic hypertension, and chronic renal disease.

Since Chesley's guidelines were enunciated more than 20 years ago, subsequent investigations should have incorporated some or all of these criteria into the study design. Sadly, however, such is not the case, and even at the present time a disturbingly large proportion of reports must be discarded because the disease actually observed may not have been preeclampsia. On the other hand, reality dictates that the requirement to meet all of these criteria may render certain protocols prohibitive so at a minimum, hypertension, proteinuria, and nulliparity would seem to be reasonable basic requirements for most studies.

With the above considerations in mind, we shall review some aspects of the pathogenesis of preeclampsia and then describe the major efforts that have been made to develop accurate tests for the prediction of and for the diagnosis of preeclampsia.

PREDICTION

Pathogenesis of Preeclampsia

Several chapters in this text (Chaps. 11–14) address the pathophysiology and pathogenesis of preeclampsia. In this chapter we briefly underscore the area of pathogenesis which impacts on prediction and diagnosis. Although new mechanisms and insights are continually unfolding,[2-8] the etiology of preeclampsia remains unknown. Because there is no "gold standard" for identifying the disorder, this pregnancy-specific syndrome continues to be defined by its clinical manifestations, namely hypertension, proteinuria, and edema occurring in the latter stages of pregnancy. Predisposing factors include nulliparity, maternal vascular disease, and decreased maternal exposure to paternal or foreign antigens.[9] Research over the past several decades has implicated decreased placental perfusion (absolute or relative), widespread endothelial cell dysfunction, and systemic manifestations resulting from vasospasm, capillary leak, and activation of the coagulation system in the pathophysiology of preeclampsia (Fig. 6–1). Note that hypertension is but one manifestation of disease that occurs relatively late in the pathophysiologic cascade.

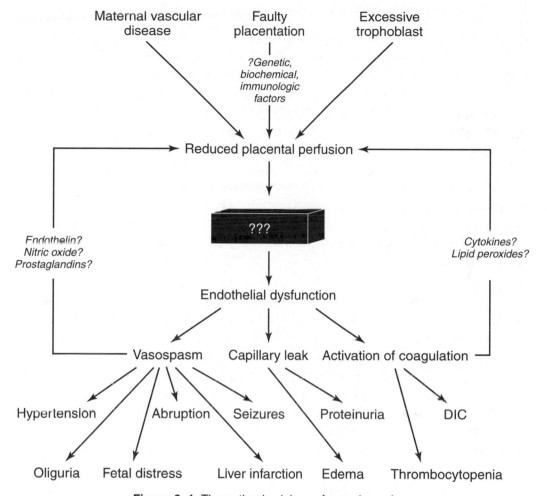

Figure 6–1. The pathophysiology of preeclampsia.

The view that hypertension is not the only important component of preeclampsia, and that there are other serious systemic manifestations of the disorder, are described elsewhere in the text. Of interest are several series of women with eclampsia, in which approximately 20% of women did not meet the diagnostic criteria for hypertension (at least 140 mm Hg systolic or 90 mm Hg diastolic).[10,11] Thus, identifying women with preeclampsia involves more than simply diagnosing late-pregnancy hypertension.[12]

Prediction of Preeclampsia

In the past, efforts to develop screening tests to predict the subsequent development of preeclampsia centered on attempts to detect the known manifestations of disease (hypertension, proteinuria, hyperuricemia, increased vascular resistance, excessive weight gain) at an earlier period of the pregnancy. More recent efforts have focused on detection of more proximal events in the pathogenesis of preeclampsia depicted in Figure 6–1. Thus, investigators have sought to detect early markers of faulty placentation, reduced placental perfusion, endothelial dysfunction, and activation of coagulation. After a brief discussion of screening tests in general, a number of selected tests that have been used with varying degrees of success to predict the subsequent development of preeclampsia will be described.

Using the Pap smear as a prototype, Grimes[13] described ten attributes of an ideal screening test (Table 6–1). The first four attributes pertain to the disease for which the screening test has been developed, and the last six pertain to characteristics of the test itself.

Preeclampsia appears to be an appropriate disease for which to develop a screening test. It is certainly an important disease, since it increases maternal mortality threefold and perinatal mortality fivefold. Although the only definitive therapy available is delivery, intensified maternal and fetal surveillance could be offered to women at high risk of developing the disease. There is ample evidence that a preclinical phase of disease exists, during which women destined to develop preeclampsia exhibit biochemical and biophysical signs of impending disease.[4] And finally, preeclampsia is relatively common, complicating 6 to 7% of pregnancies in healthy nulliparas[14,15] and up to 20% or more of pregnancies in high-risk populations especially in women with underlying thrombophilias.[16a,16b]

For several decades, investigators have attempted to develop screening tests that will predict the onset of preeclampsia several weeks or months before clinically apparent disease. The major problem with the preponderance of literature on predictive tests lies in the definition of the outcome of interest, preeclampsia. Until recently, the outcome reported in virtually all large studies was merely hypertension that occurred in the second half of pregnancy, what would be called gestational hypertension today. In most cases, no mention was made of proteinuria, so that the major causes of gestational hypertension—transient hypertension, chronic hypertension, and preeclampsia—cannot be distinguished, even retrospectively. Such a distinction is extremely important, since proteinuric hypertension is associated with increased maternal and fetal morbidity and mortality, whereas mild isolated

---

TABLE 6–1. CRITERIA FOR AN IDEAL SCREENING TEST

1. Important disease
2. Acceptable and available diagnosis and treatment
3. Recognizable latent or early symptomatic stage of disease
4. Prevalent disease
5. Safe test
6. Test acceptable to the population
7. Reliable results (reproducible among different practitioners)
8. Valid test (sensitive and specific)
9. Appropriate test for the population being screened
10. Economical cost

From Grimes DA: Screening tests: What they are and what they aren't. *Contemp Obstet Gynecol* 1982;20:69–80.

hypertension (transient hypertension) is not.[17] Thus, the bulk of the past literature on predictive tests reflects the ability of those tests to predict gestational hypertension, which is of little consequence in the majority of patients.

It is well beyond the scope of this chapter to review each study individually. Instead, the surprisingly small number of studies that attempt to predict the development of true preeclampsia, rather than merely gestational hypertension, will be highlighted. At a minimum, the studies reviewed will have proteinuric hypertension as an outcome variable. Ideally, the study subjects are nulliparous, and when the reviewed reports contain subjects of mixed parity, data on the nulliparous patients are extracted, when possible. In addition, these studies had to be cohort studies reporting sufficient information to construct a 2 × 2 table, permitting calculation of sensitivity, specificity, positive and negative predictive values, and likelihood ratios. The likelihood ratio is "the likelihood that a person with a disease would have a particular test divided by the likelihood that a person without the disease would have that result."[18] Table 6–2 provides an interpretation of the magnitude of likelihood ratios.[19] Since likelihood ratios convey the relative probability of disease given a positive test, a test must have high sensitivity for the likelihood ratio to be clinically useful.

Table 6–3 lists the major predictive tests reported in the English-language medical literature. Most studies used hypertension as their primary outcome; consequently, they do little to elucidate useful approaches to predicting preeclampsia.

Table 6–4 contains data from those studies that use new-onset proteinuric hypertension as their primary outcome. Results of several of them have been pooled when the reports contained the same tests applied to similar populations.

The major components of antepartum obstetric visits are measurement of blood pressure, urine protein, and weight. As screening tests, these measurements are safe, acceptable to the population, reliable, appropriate for the population, and economical. Several studies have assessed the ability of these measurements, taken in the second trimester, to predict the later development of preeclampsia.

Blood Pressure

Several approaches have been taken to assess the value of second-trimester blood pressure measurements for the prediction of preeclampsia. Friedman and Neff[23] determined the maximum mean arterial pressure recorded in the midtrimester and

TABLE 6–2. MAGNITUDE OF LIKELIHOOD RATIOS

Likelihood Ratio	Change Between Pretest and Posttest Probability
> 10 or < 0.1	Large and often conclusive
5–10 or 0.1–0.2	Moderate
2–5 or 0.2–0.5	Small (but sometimes important)
1–2 or 0.5–1	Small (and rarely important)

From Jaeschke R, Guyatt GH, Sackett DL (for the Evidence-Based Medicine Working Group): User's guide to the medical literature. III. How to use an article about a diagnostic test. B. What are the results and will they help me in caring for my patients? *JAMA* 1994;271:703–707.

TABLE 6–3. SCREENING TESTS FOR GESTATIONAL HYPERTENSION

I. Routine components of antepartum care performed in the second trimester
   Measurement of blood pressure[20-33]
   Detection of proteinuria (microalbuminuria)[34-37]
   Measurement of weight[38,39]
   Measurement of serum β-hCG[40-43]

II. Early detection of vasoconstriction
   Intravenous infusion of angiotensin II[44-50]
   Roll-over test[48,51-66]
   Hand-grip (isometric exercise) test[25,63,67,68]
   Platelet angiotensin II receptors[49,69,70]
   Platelet calcium response to arginine vasopressin[71,72]

III. Early detection of altered renal function
   Serum (plasma) uric acid[28,73-76]
   Urinary excretion of calcium[35,75,77,78]
   Urinary kallikrein[79-81]

IV. Early detection of altered hemodynamics
   Cardiac output[82]

V. Detection of placental hypoperfusion/ischemia
   Doppler waveforms of uterine arteries[74,83-88]
   Fetal fibronectin in plasma[89] or amniotic fluid[90]

VI. Detection of endothelial activation, disruption, or injury
   Plasma fibronectin (soluble, cellular)[91-98]
   Urinary excretion of prostacyclin metabolites[99]
   Plasma endothelial cell adhesion molecules[100]

VII. Detection of an activated coagulation/fibrinolytic system
   Plasma antithrombin III[28,98,101-104]
   Platelet count[28,75,102,105]
   Platelet volume[28,106]
   Platelet activation (CD63 expression)[107]
   Factor VIII-related antigen/coagulant[103,108]
   Plasminogen activator inhibitor-1[98,102,103]

chose 90 mm Hg as a cutoff. Massé et al.,[28] Ales et al.,[27] and Conde-Agudelo et al.[29] used mean arterial pressure measurements at single visits during the second trimester and chose the cutoff based on receiver–operator characteristics curves. Overall, midtrimester mean arterial pressure measurements have sensitivities ranging from 43 to 67%, low positive predictive values ranging from 3 to 23%, and likelihood ratios of approximately 2 and 3. Thus, elevations of mean arterial pressure in the second trimester are poor predictors of preeclampsia.

As part of two large multicenter trials in the United States involving healthy nulliparous women, second-trimester systolic blood pressures in the upper end of the normal range were evaluated for their abilities to predict preeclampsia.[31,33] A positive test was defined as a systolic blood pressure of ≥ 120 mm Hg, with the upper limit of normal being slightly different between the two studies. Overall, systolic blood pressure had a low sensitivity (18%), a low positive predictive value (13%), and a low likelihood ratio (1.9). In the 1995 study,[31] the authors noted that the predictive ability of systolic blood pressure was superior to that of mean blood pressure or diastolic blood pressure. Of note, systolic blood pressure has been given short shrift in the hypertension literature in general, and in the obstetric literature in particular. Clearly, this is an area for further research.

In an excellent study, Higgins et al.[32] examined the ability of 24-hour ambulatory blood pressure measurement in the second trimester to predict preeclampsia. The predictor variables studied were systolic, diastolic, and mean blood pressures averaged during daytime, nighttime, and overall during the 24 hours. The cut-off points chosen were the 95th percentile values in the group of women with normal pregnancy outcomes. The authors found the 24-hour mean diastolic blood pressure to be the most effective predictor of preeclampsia. Nevertheless, the sensitivity and positive predictive value are low (22% and 15%, respectively). The high likelihood ratio (8.0) is mitigated by the low sensitivity, since less than one preeclamptic woman in four will be identified by a positive test.

Proteinuria

None of the studies of proteinuria or microalbuminuria provided suitable evidence to determine their value as predictors of preeclampsia, either because the outcome did not explicitly require proteinuria or because predictive data were not reported.

Weight Gain

Studies by Nelson[38] and Thomson and Billewicz[39] examined the predictive ability of weight gain from 20 to 30 weeks. With few exceptions, these studies included only low-risk, nulliparous women with singleton gestations. From the data, it is immediately apparent that sensitivity or specificity may be maximized by careful selection of the cut-off values. In any case, positive predictive values and likelihood ratios remain very low, rendering weight determination of little value in predicting preeclampsia.

Serum β-Human Chorionic Gonadotrophin

Determination of serum beta-human chorionic gonadotrophin (β-hCG) has become a frequent component of routine prenatal care as part of the so-called triple screen for prediction of Down syndrome. After initial associations were reported between elevated serum levels of β-hCG in the second trimester and subsequent preeclampsia, several studies[41-43] were performed to determine the predictive ability of β-hCG levels in larger populations. Sorensen et al.[41] studied women of mixed parity. Ashour et al.[43] also studied women of mixed parity but reported results separately for nulliparas and multiparas; consequently, only data on nulliparous women have been included in Table 6-4. Vaillant et al.[42] included only nulliparous women. From the combined data, it is apparent that choosing a cutoff of ≥ 2 MoM (multiples of the mean) maximizes sensitivity (which is still quite low), whereas a cutoff of ≥ 3 MoM maximizes specificity. In either case, the positive predictive values and likelihood ratios render this test a poor predictor of preeclampsia.

Angiotensin II Infusion

When first reported,[44] the angiotensin infusion test held great promise as an effective predictor of preeclampsia. Subsequent studies in larger numbers of women have failed to confirm the initially stunning results. Only four studies specified pro-

TABLE 6–4. SCREENING TESTS FOR TRUE PREECLAMPSIA (PROTEINURIC HYPERTENSION), INCLUDING SENSITIVITY, SPECIFICITY, POSITIVE AND NEGATIVE PREDICTIVE VALUES, AND LIKELIHOOD RATIOS

Test	Cutoff	1st Author	Patients (No.)	Sensitivity	Specificity	PPV	NPV	LR
MAP 2nd trimester	≥ 90 mm Hg	Friedman[23]	22,582	64	62	6	98	1.7
	≥ 87 mm Hg	Massé[28]	504	47	80	23	92	2.4
	≥ 85 mm Hg	Ales[27]	730	67	81	3	99.7	3.6
	≥ 85 mm Hg	Conde-Agudelo[29]	580	43	78	8	97	2.0
	Combined MAP ≥ 85		**1310**	**48**	**80**	**5**	**99**	**2.4**
Systolic BP	120–134 mm Hg	Sibai[31]	1500	36	82	12	95	2.0
	120–136 mm Hg	Sibai[33]	4314	13	94	14	93	2.0
	Combined		**5814**	**18**	**91**	**13**	**93**	**1.9**
Ambulatory BP	mean diastolic ≥ 71 mm Hg	Higgins[32]	1048	22	97	15	98	8.0
Weight gain	≥ 10 lbs from 20–30 wks	Nelson[38]	1492	73	43	10	94	1.3
	≥ 8 lbs from 20–30 wks	Thomson[39]	4214	85	25	7	96	1.1
	≥ 12 lbs from 20–30 wks		4214	53	66	10	95	1.6
Serum β-hCG	≥ 2 MoM	Sorensen[41]	426	69	70	7	99	2.3
	≥ 3 MoM		426	15	94	7	97	2.5
	≥ 2 MoM	Vaillant[42]	434	69	85	15	99	4.6
	≥ 2 MoM	Ashour[43]	2737	12	89	5	96	1.1
	≥ 3 MoM		2737	5	97	8	96	2.0
	Combined ≥ 2 MoM		**3597**	**23**	**86**	**7**	**96**	**1.7**
	Combined ≥ 3 MoM		**3163**	**6**	**97**	**8**	**96**	**2.0**
Angiotensin II infusion	≤ 8 ng/kg/min	Morris[45]	26	33	39	7	82	0.6
	≤ 10 ng/kg/min		26	67	30	11	88	1.0
	≤ 10 ng/kg/min	Öney[46]	231	85	82	38	98	4.8

Test	Criterion	Reference	n	Sens	Spec	PPV	NPV	LR
Roll-over	≤ 8 ng/kg/min	Dekker[48]	90	78	96	70	98	21
	≤ 10 ng/kg/min		90	89	83	36	99	5.1
	≤ 10 ng/kg/min	Kyle[50]	495	25	84	6	96	1.6
	≤ 8 ng/kg/min	**Combined**	**116**	**67**	**84**	**32**	**96**	**4.1**
	≤ 10 ng/kg/min	**Combined**	**842**	**64**	**82**	**21**	**97**	**3.6**
Roll-over	↑ diastolic ≥ 20 mm Hg	Dekker[48]	90	33	93	33	93	4.5
Hand-grip	↑ diastolic ≥ 20 mm Hg	Baker[67]	200	80	92	20	99	10.0
Uric acid (plasma)	≥ 350 μmol/L (≥ 5.9 mg/dL)	Jacobson[74]	135	54	89	33	95	4.7
(serum)	not specified	Conde-Agudelo[75]	387	53	65	6	97	1.5
Urinary calcium	≤ 195 mg/dL	Sanchez-Ramos[77]	103	88	84	32	99	5.5
	not specified	Conde-Agudelo[75]	387	33	77	5	96	1.4
Urinary kallikrein	IUK:creatinine ratio ≤ 170	Millar[79]	307	83	99.7	91	99	246
	IUK:creatinine ratio ≤ 170	Kyle[81]	458	80	71	11	99	2.8
Uterine artery doppler	RI ≥ 0.58	Jacobson[74]	136	64	64	17	94	1.8
	RI ≥ 0.58	Steel[86]	1014	63	89	10	99	5.9
	early diastolic notch	Bower[87]	2026	78	96	28	99.5	17.3
	placental-side RI > 0.57	North[88]	446	27	89	8	97	2.4
	placental-side AC > 90th %ile	North[88]	446	53	88	14	98	4.6
Fibronectin (plasma)	≥ 230 mg/L	Paarlberg[97]	376	69	59	12	96	1.7
Platelet count	?	Conde-Agudelo[75]	387	47	59	5	96	1.1
Platelet activation	platelet CD63 ≥ 2%	Konijnenberg[107]	244	47	76	13	95	1.9

PPV = positive predictive value; NPV = negative predictive value; LR = likelihood ratio; MAF = mean arterial pressure; BP = blood pressure; IUK = inactive urinary kallikrein; RI = resistance index; AC = systolic to early diastolic ratio.

teinuria as a mandatory part of the diagnosis of preeclampsia. The test was performed in essentially the same way in all studies. After a baseline blood pressure is established, angiotensin II is infused in a stepwise fashion until an effective pressor dose is reached. The effective pressor dose is the dose of angiotensin II that causes a rise of 20 mm Hg in the diastolic blood pressure. In all four studies, this test was performed at the beginning of the third trimester. Two of the studies[45,48] contained results using two different cut-off values to define an effective pressor dose; the other studies[46,50] chose the higher cut-off value. From the combined data, it would seem that the cut-off value 8 ng/kg/min maximizes positive predictive value without sacrificing sensitivity. Compared to the other tests already discussed, the angiotensin infusion test has a much higher positive predictive value. Nevertheless, because it is cumbersome, time-consuming, invasive, and expensive, it is not a useful test for mass screening purposes. It may, however, have a role in research studies in which the investigator wishes to identify a population of women at relatively high risk for preeclampsia.

Roll-over Test

In contrast, the roll over test, or supine pressor test, is a safe, acceptable, and economical test that may easily be applied to large numbers of women. With the woman in the recumbent position, blood pressure is taken in the upper arm until a stable value is observed. She is then turned onto her back, and blood pressure is again measured. A rise in the diastolic blood pressure of at least 20 mm Hg is a positive test. Surprisingly, only one study required proteinuria for the diagnosis of preeclampsia. Dekker et al.[48] performed the roll-over test in 90 healthy nulliparous women. Although the predictive value of a positive test (33%) was similar to that of the angiotensin infusion test, the low sensitivity (33%) precludes its use as a predictive test for preeclampsia.

Hand-Grip (Isometric Exercise) Test

Several authors have described their experience with the hand-grip (isometric exercise) test.[25,63,67,68] The test is considered positive when the diastolic blood pressure rises by at least 20 mm Hg after a brief hand-grip exercise. This test, which takes approximately 30 minutes to perform, is safe, acceptable, appropriate, and economical. Only the study by Baker and Johnson[67] required proteinuria for the diagnosis of preeclampsia. The test was performed on 200 healthy nulliparous women between 28 and 32 weeks' gestation. Although the sensitivity and specificity were high (80% and 92%, respectively), the positive predictive value was only 20%. It should be noted that only five women in this study developed preeclampsia. Clearly, a definitive assessment of the value of the hand-grip test awaits larger trials.

Uric Acid

Because of its association with established preeclampsia, plasma or serum uric acid levels have been investigated for their ability to predict preeclampsia. Jacobson et al.[74] studied 135 women of mixed parity who were at "high risk" for preeclampsia (incidence 10%). Plasma uric acid levels were determined at 24 weeks, with values above 350 μmol/L (5.9 mg/dL) considered abnormal. In contrast, Conde-Agudelo et al.[75] studied 387 women at 27 weeks. The definition of an abnormal value was not given. Both studies found a sensitivity around 50%, with a considerably higher positive predictive value in the high-risk population. The low sensitivity renders this test unhelpful for widespread use.

Urinary Calcium

Since the report by Taufield et al.[109] describing hypocalciuria in association with preeclampsia, several studies have been performed to determine whether urinary calcium excretion in the second trimester might predict the subsequent development of preeclampsia. In only two of these studies was proteinuria required for the diagnosis of preeclampsia as well as providing sufficient data to calculate predictive statistics. Sanchez-Ramos et al.[77] measured 24-hour urinary calcium excretion in 103 nulliparous women between 10 and 24 weeks (mean 17.3 weeks). The sensitivity was 88%, the positive predictive value was 32%, and the likelihood ratio was 5.5. Although a 24-hour urine collection is cumbersome, it is safe and relatively inexpensive. Of the tests described thus far, the 24-hour urinary excretion seems to have the greatest potential for practical use, but its validity awaits confirmation by other investigators. Conde-Agudelo et al.[75] measured the calcium/creatinine ratio in single urine samples collected from 387 nulliparous women at 27 weeks. While sample collection is much simpler than in the 24-hour urinary calcium excretion test, the low sensitivity and positive predictive values preclude the use of the calcium/creatinine ratio as a predictive test.

Inactive Urinary Kallikrein

Renal kallikrein is believed to be an important paracrine regulator of blood pressure. Kallikrein excreted in the urine is believed to reflect renal production. Millar et al.[79] hypothesized that reduced urinary kallikrein excretion might precede the clinical signs and symptoms of preeclampsia and might therefore be a reliable predictor. Accordingly, they measured the inactive urinary kallikrein:creatinine ratio in spot urine samples from 307 healthy gravidas of mixed parity. Using a receiver–operator characteristics curve, they defined a positive test as an inactive urinary kallikrein:creatinine ratio of 170 or less, and reported an astonishing 83% sensitivity, 91% positive predictive value, and a likelihood ratio of 246 for true preeclampsia. But as with so many tests before it, the promising results of this study could not be confirmed by others. Kyle et al.[80] measured inactive urinary kallikrein:creatinine ratios in spot urine samples from 458 healthy nulliparous women. They likewise used a receiver–operator characteristics curve and chose 170 as the cut-off value for a positive test. The specificity, positive predictive value, and likelihood ratio were substantially lower than those reported by Millar et al. (see Table 6–4). In addition, despite the large number of women tested, only 32 women from the two studies combined actually developed preeclampsia. Clearly, then, this test would need to be repeated on many more women who actually developed preeclampsia before its true value can be assessed.

Uterine Artery Doppler Velocimetry

Presumably as a result of impaired trophoblastic invasion of the spiral arteries during the second trimester,[110] uteroplacental blood flow is reduced in pregnancies destined to develop preeclampsia.[4] Consequently, numerous investigators have used Doppler ultrasound to detect reduced uterine blood flow as a screening test for preeclampsia. There is no consensus regarding which feature(s) of the flow velocity waveform (resistance index, systolic to end-diastolic ratio, systolic to early diastolic ratio, pulsatility index, presence of an early diastolic notch) best expresses the degree of abnormality. Jacobson et al.[74] measured the resistance index in both uterine arteries of 136 "high-risk" women of mixed parity at 20 to 24 weeks' gestation. They chose a resistance index ≥ 0.58 (two standard deviations above the mean for a normal pregnant population) to define a positive test. With a sensitivity of 64% and a positive predictive value of 17%, they concluded that measurement of the resistance index was not a clinically useful screening test. Steel et al.[86] performed the same test at 16 to 22 weeks and then, if abnormal, again at 24 weeks in 1014 nulliparous women. Again, a resistance index equaling or exceeding 0.58 defined an abnormal test. Sensitivity (63%) was similar to that of the previous study; positive predictive value (10%) was lower. Bower et al.[87] screened 2026 unselected women using a two-stage approach. They first screened women at 18 to 22 weeks, and re-screened those with abnormal tests at 24 weeks. They defined a positive test as the presence of an early diastolic notch in either artery at the 24-week screen. Compared to the two previous studies, Bower et al. achieved a higher sensitivity (78%), a higher positive predictive value (28%), and a higher likelihood ratio (17.3). Finally, North et al.[88] screened 446 healthy nulliparas between 19 and 24 weeks. They defined a positive test as a placental-side resistance index greater than 0.57 or a placental side systolic to early diastolic (AC) ratio above the 90th percentile for gestational age. Compared to the two previous studies that employed resistance index, the North study reported a lower sensitivity (27%) and a lower positive predictive value (8%). The ability to predict preeclampsia improved somewhat using the systolic to early diastolic ratio, but did not approach that of the diastolic notch reported by Bower et al.[87] Irion et al.[87a] found that Doppler was not a reliable screening test in 1311 low-risk women. Thus, Doppler does not appear to be useful in screening low-risk patients but may have a role in research protocols seeking to define a high-risk population. Currently, the presence of an early diastolic notch seems most promising.

Fibronectin

The fibronectins are a group of ubiquitous, high-molecular-weight glycoproteins that are involved in a number of fundamental cellular interactions, such as adhesion, migration, opsonization, hemostasis, and fibrinolysis. Most of the circulating fibronectin, termed plasma fibronectin, is secreted primarily by hepatocytes.[111] Cellular fibronectin is less soluble, is synthesized by endothelial cells and fibroblasts, and is released from endothelial cells and extracellular matrix after endothelial injury.[94,112] Fetal fibronectin, a third isoform, can be secreted by trophoblast into the extracellular matrix and detected in the maternal circulation or cervical secretions.[89,113] Of the many reports of plasma, cellular, and fetal fibronectin in women with impending or manifest preeclampsia, only one provides data from which predictive statistics can be inferred. Paarlberg et al.[97] measured plasma fibronectin during the second trimester in 347 healthy nulliparous women. Using receiver–operator characteristics curves, they chose plasma fibronectin concentrations above 230 mg/L as the definition of a positive test. They did not report predictive statistics for the group's preeclamptic (proteinuric hypertension) vs. nonpreeclamptic (normal plus nonproteinuric hypertension) subjects, but these statistics can be inferred from the data provided. Sensitivity and specificity were somewhat low at 69% and 59%, respectively. The positive predictive value was 12% and the likelihood ratio 1.7, rendering this an ineffective screening test for low-risk populations. Plasma levels of the cellular isoform of fibronectin are known to rise, on average, weeks or months before the onset of clinically apparent disease,[93,94] but the predictive statistics reflecting its value as a screening test have not been reported. Sakura et al.[90] have reported elevated levels of fetal fibronectin in second-trimester amniotic fluid from women who later became preeclamptic. Because their study was a nested case-control study, predictive values cannot be calculated. Nevertheless, even if this test were highly predictive, it is unlikely that it would be used to a large degree in women who were not otherwise having amniocentesis.

Platelet Count

Although thrombocytopenia is frequently observed in preeclampsia, there is no evidence that platelet count is a useful screening test for the disorder. Conde-Agudelo et al.[75] measured platelet count at 27 weeks in 387 healthy nulliparous women. The cut-off value for defining an abnormal test was not specified. Reporting a sensitivity of 47% and a positive predictive value of 5%, the authors correctly concluded that second-trimester platelet counts were of little value in predicting preeclampsia.

Platelet Activation

Konijnenberg et al.[107] investigated the ability of platelet activation, as evidenced by surface CD63 expression, to predict the subsequent development of preeclampsia. They collected blood during the first and second trimesters from 244 women of mixed parity who had "risk factors for preeclampsia." Using receiver–operator characteristics curve analysis, they defined a cut-off value as 2% of platelets with expression of CD63 on their surface. When the test was performed in the first trimester, the sensitivity was 47%, the positive predictive value 13%, and the likelihood ratio 1.9. Of interest, these researchers reported that the test was even less efficacious when performed in the second trimester. When first-trimester platelet activation was combined with first-visit diastolic blood pressure (cut-off value 75 mm

Hg), the sensitivity remained low (41%), but the positive predictive value and like-lihood ratio improved (41% and 9.4, respectively). While this combined test may be somewhat useful in research protocols, it is unlikely to be worthwhile for mass screening since it fails to identify more than half of the women who will become preeclamptic.

Summary

It is evident at the present time that there is no screening test for preeclampsia that is safe, acceptable to the population, reliable, valid, appropriate for the population, and economical. Perhaps advances in our understanding of the underlying patho-physiology of preeclampsia will lead to the development of effective screening tests.

DIFFERENTIAL DIAGNOSIS

Because there is no gold standard diagnostic test, the differential diagnosis of preeclampsia remains a challenge to the practicing obstetrician. The cardinal clini-cal signs of preeclampsia—hypertension plus proteinuria—may be shared, in part or in whole, by a variety of other conditions. Additional laboratory testing may clarify or obfuscate the diagnosis. The distinction between preeclampsia and other diseases that present similarly is particularly important in midpregnancy (weeks 20–30), when the choice of management scheme may have enormous consequences for mother and fetus. Because preeclampsia is a multisystem disorder, a complete differential diagnosis can be virtually endless. The discussion that follows encom-passes the most frequent and the most important diagnostic dilemmas that the practicing obstetrician is likely to face.

Preeclampsia vs. Chronic Hypertension, Transient Hypertension, and Intrinsic Renal Disease (see also Chap. 19)

The inherent inaccuracy in diagnosing the clinical syndrome preeclampsia has been demonstrated by investigators at the University of Chicago–Pritzker School of Medicine. In their original report of 1959[114] and their follow-up report 22 years later,[115] these researchers described postpartum renal biopsy findings in primi-parous and multiparous women with the clinical diagnosis of preeclampsia. Eighty-seven of the 104 primigravidas (84%) had biopsy-proven glomerular capil-lary endotheliosis, the characteristic renal lesion of preeclampsia. In eight of these women, there was additional evidence of nephrosclerosis, intrinsic renal disease, or both. The remaining 17 women all had nephrosclerosis, renal disease, or both; none had normal histology. In contrast, 27 of 72 multiparas (38%) had glomerular capil-lary endotheliosis, either alone (17) or in combination with nephrosclerosis and/or intrinsic renal disease (10). Thirty-seven multiparas (51%) had nephrosclerosis, renal disease, or both, and eight (11%) had normal histology. Thus, the clinical diagnosis of preeclampsia was usually correct (84%) in primigravid women, although a surprising 24% had unsuspected nephrosclerosis or renal disease. Conversely, the diagnosis of preeclampsia was usually incorrect (62%) in multiparous women, with underlying nephrosclerosis or renal disease present in the majority (65%). Since renal biopsy is rarely warranted in clinical practice today, numerous attempts have been made to distinguish these conditions based on clinical or laboratory evidence.

Chronic Hypertension

Ideally, the diagnosis of chronic hypertension should be based on blood pressure readings of at least 140 mm Hg systolic or 90 mm Hg diastolic prior to pregnancy. If prepregnancy blood pressures are unknown, then these blood pressure elevations prior to 20 weeks' gestation are usually considered sufficient to make the diagnosis. During pregnancy, in both normal and chronically hypertensive women, midtrimester nadirs in blood pressure are observed. Often, it is during this time that women first present for prenatal care. Later, when blood pressure returns toward its prepregnancy values, women with chronic hypertension may be erroneously diagnosed with preeclampsia.

Women with chronic hypertension are at increased risk of developing preeclampsia.[16] In women with known chronic hypertension, changes in blood pressure and proteinuria, rather than absolute measurements, must be used for diagnosis. Because proteinuria can occur in women with chronic hypertension, a baseline 24-hour urine collection, along with baseline serum creatinine and uric acid, should be obtained early in pregnancy as a basis for later comparison. In women suspected of having chronic hypertension, physical signs of longstanding hypertension such as arteriovenous nicking of the retinal vasculature or left ventricular hypertrophy may be sought.

A number of laboratory tests may help to distinguish preeclampsia from chronic hypertension. For quantifying proteinuria, 24-hour urine collection is the method of choice, since semiquantitative dipstick measurements can often be misleading.[116-118] The likelihood of preeclampsia is increased by the presence of certain specific laboratory abnormalities, such as thrombocytopenia, elevated serum transaminases, and elevated lactate dehydrogenase. Hyperuricemia has been correlated with the presence and severity of preeclampsia when the diagnosis was determined by renal biopsy.[119] It may be helpful, therefore, in diagnosing superimposed preeclampsia in women with chronic hypertension (likelihood ratio 2.5 using a cut-off value of 5.5 mg/dL).[120] Antithrombin III concentrations[121] and activity[122] remain normal in women with chronic hypertension in pregnancy but are reduced in women with preeclampsia. Antithrombin III may fall in conjunction with other conditions such as viral illness and pyelonephritis.[14] Taufield et al.[109] found that hypocalciuria was helpful in distinguishing chronic hypertension, on the one hand, from isolated preeclampsia or, on the other, from preeclampsia superimposed on chronic hypertension. The number of patients studied was small, a cut-off value for defining hypocalciuria was not defined, and therefore predictive statistics were not calculated. Quantifying urinary calcium is relatively inexpensive, widely available, and probably underutilized.

Transient Hypertension

Transient hypertension is generally a benign condition characterized by late-pregnancy hypertension in the absence of signs or symptoms suggesting preeclampsia or preexisting hypertension. It has little effect on maternal or perinatal morbidity or mortality. Transient hypertension may be the preproteinuric phase of preeclampsia, the return to baseline chronic hypertension after a midpregnancy nadir, or the unmasking by pregnancy of incipient essential hypertension.[17] Redman and Jeffries[123] reported that adopting a stricter definition of hypertension increases the likelihood that a woman with hypertension in pregnancy would have preeclampsia. The criteria that they advocated were an initial diastolic blood pressure less than 90 mm Hg, a rise of at least 25 mm Hg, and a maximum reading of at least 90 mm Hg.

Hypocalciuria may be effective in distinguishing transient hypertension from preeclampsia. Taufield et al.[109] noted that there was "little or no overlap" in urinary calcium excretion rates between women with preeclampsia and women with transient hypertension. Sanchez-Ramos et al.[124] measured urinary calcium excretion in healthy women suspected of having preeclampsia. After pregnancy, women were classified as having had preeclampsia (hypertension and proteinuria), gestational hypertension (hypertension alone), or normal pregnancy. Hypocalciuria was defined as a urinary calcium concentration below 12 mg/dL in a 24-hour collection. They reported a sensitivity of 85% and a specificity of 91% for detecting preeclampsia.

Hyperuricemia, on the other hand, does not appear helpful in one study, where its abilities to diagnose preeclampsia in the setting of new-onset hypertension late in pregnancy was weak (likelihood ratio 1.4).[120] Likewise, Weenink et al.[121] did not find a difference in antithrombin III levels in newly hypertensive pregnant women with and without proteinuria. Although circulating concentrations of both plasma[97] and cellular[94] fibronectin are higher in women with preeclampsia than in women with transient hypertension, predictive statistics are not provided to assess their clinical utility. These tests are not widely available in hospital-based clinical laboratories and are unlikely to prove useful. Activin A, advocated as a highly specific marker of preeclampsia,[125,126] has been reported in one study[125] to be significantly higher in preeclampsia than in chronic hypertension, transient hypertension, and normal pregnancy. This finding awaits confirmation by other investigators. In the meantime, this test is not available for widespread use.

Intrinsic Renal Disease

As pointed out by Spargo et al.[114] and Fisher et al.[115] chronic renal disease and nephrosclerosis are important components of the differential diagnosis of late-pregnancy hypertension and proteinuria. The pathologic diagnoses reported in the

31 women who had isolated intrinsic renal disease were chronic glomerulonephritis (16), tubulointerstitial lesions (6), membranous nephropathy (4), sickle-cell nephropathy (2), acute poststreptococcal glomerulonephritis (1), lipoid nephrosis (1), and diabetic nephropathy (1). Women with chronic renal disease are at high risk for the development of preeclampsia, although the best way to diagnose preeclampsia in such patients is controversial. Cunningham et al.[127] reported on a group of 37 women with moderate (serum creatinine 1.4–2.5 mg/dL) or severe (serum creatinine > 2.5 mg/dL) renal insufficiency. Eighty percent of the women with chronic hypertension and one-third of the women without chronic hypertension developed preeclampsia.

Few studies have been performed to distinguish preeclampsia clinically from intrinsic renal disease. The definitive diagnostic test is renal biopsy, which is rarely indicated in pregnancy.[128] Chronic renal disease may be suggested by an abnormal serum creatinine, creatinine clearance, or 24-hour urinary protein excretion obtained early in pregnancy as a baseline study. Acute nephritis presents clinically as hypertension, proteinuria, edema, and hematuria. Red blood cell casts on a urinalysis are strongly suggestive, but they can occur with preeclampsia (albeit more rarely). Specific causes of glomerulonephritis can sometimes be identified with blood tests, such as antistreptolysin O, streptozyme panel and the complement profile in poststreptococcal glomerulonephritis, or screening tests for collagen vascular disease, but a renal biopsy is often required for definitive diagnosis.

Weiner and Bonsib[129] performed renal biopsies in 12 women diagnosed with severe early-onset preeclampsia (gestational age 30 ± 3 weeks). They correlated the biopsy findings with plasma antithrombin III activity. They noted that antithrombin III was reduced in women with pure preeclampsia or preeclampsia superimposed on underlying renal disease, and was normal in women with underlying renal disease alone. This study, however, is too limited for firm conclusions.

Severe Preeclampsia vs. Lupus Nephritis Flare

Distinguishing a flare of lupus nephritis from severe preeclampsia can be one of the most challenging problems in clinical obstetrics. Although both conditions are characterized by hypertension and proteinuria, occasionally the distinction may be made on clinical grounds alone. If a patient with a history of lupus nephritis develops hypertension and proteinuria along with other evidence of flare, such as arthralgias, myalgias, skin rash, and pleuritis, then the diagnosis of lupus flare can be made with some confidence. Conversely, if hypertension and proteinuria are accompanied by hyperuricemia, thrombocytopenia, hemoconcentration, and elevated serum transaminases in the absence of the usual manifestations of lupus flare in that particular patient, then severe preeclampsia may be inferred. Rarely, however, is the distinction so clear.

Laboratory evaluation may be helpful in differentiating these two disorders. Serum concentrations of C3, C4, and CH50 are usually normal or mildly elevated during both uncomplicated and preeclamptic pregnancies. Serum C3, C4, and

TABLE 6–5. COMPARISON OF COMMON LABORATORY TESTS IN PREECLAMPSIA AND LUPUS NEPHRITIS

Clinical Measure	Preeclampsia	Lupus Nephritis
C3, C4, CH50	Decrease unusual	Commonly low
Urinalysis	Red blood cell (RBC) casts rare	RBC casts frequent
Onset of proteinuria	Usually abrupt	Gradual or abrupt
Serum aminotransferases	May be increased	Rarely abnormal
Quantitative proteinuria	Does not differentiate	
Thrombocytopenia	Does not differentiate	
Hyperuricemia	Does not differentiate	
Level of hypertension	Does not differentiate	

Adapted from Lockshin MD, Druzin ML: Rheumatic disease. In: Barron WM, Lindheimer MD, eds. *Medical Disorders during Pregnancy*, ed. 2. St. Louis: Mosby; 1995:307–337.

CH50 concentrations are low, however, in women with lupus, especially when measured in association with a flare.[130,131] In addition, antibodies to double-stranded (native) DNA, which may or may not be present during clinical quiescence, increase markedly prior to lupus flare.[132,133] Coincident with the appearance of clinical manifestations, anti-dsDNA antibodies begin to fall but remain significantly elevated for at least 1 to 2 weeks. Thus, the occurrence of low levels of complement (C3, C4, CH50) in association with high anti-dsDNA titers is highly suggestive of lupus flare. Moreover, results from a recent study[130] suggest that a decreased ratio of CH50 to Ba (a product of the alternative complement pathway) is highly sensitive and specific in distinguishing lupus flare from preeclampsia. Table 6–5 compares the results of common laboratory tests in preeclampsia and lupus nephritis.[134]

HELLP Syndrome vs. Thrombotic Thrombocytopenic Purpura, Hemolytic Uremic Syndrome, and Acute Fatty Liver of Pregnancy

HELLP Syndrome

In 1982, Weinstein[135] proposed the term *HELLP syndrome* (*H* for hemolysis, *EL* for elevated liver enzymes, *LP* for low platelets) to describe a severe variant of preeclampsia. Unfortunately, there has been no consensus regarding the exact laboratory criteria required to make this diagnosis. The strictest, and, hence, the most specific criteria have been proposed by Sibai et al.[136] (Table 6–6), although other criteria have been reported.[137,138] Of importance, any abnormality in the tests associated with the acronym (↑LDH, AST, hemolysis; e.g., schistocytes, liver abnormalities alone, or just thrombocytopenia), is enough to treat the patient as a severe preeclamptic.

In a large series of women with HELLP syndrome, Sibai et al.[136] reported a high rate of serious maternal complications. In 442 women with HELLP, they noted disseminated intravascular coagulopathy in 21% (16% secondary to placental abruption, peripartum hemorrhage, or liver hematoma, 5% de novo), placental abruption

TABLE 6–6. CRITERIA FOR THE DIAGNOSIS OF HELLP SYNDROME[a]

Hemolysis

Abnormal peripheral smear (schistocytes, burr cells)

Lactate dehydrogenase (LDH) > 600 U/L or bilirubin > 1.2 mg/dL

Elevated liver enzymes

Aspartate aminotransferase (AST) > 70 U/L

Low platelets

Platelet count < 100,000/μL

[a]These values are those suggested by Sibai et al.[136] and represent an average twice the upper limits of normal at the University of Tennessee, Memphis Medical Center for LDH and AST. These suggested values will differ, therefore, from center to center.
From Sibai BM, Ramadan MK, Usta I, et al: Maternal morbidity and mortality in 442 pregnancies with hemolysis, elevated liver enzymes, and low platelets (HELLP syndrome). *Am J Obstet Gynecol* 1993; 169:1000–1006.

in 16%, acute renal failure in 8%, severe ascites in 8%, pulmonary edema in 6%, and cerebral edema, or adult respiratory distress syndrome in 1%. In 49 maternal deaths associated with HELLP syndrome, 45% were due to cerebral hemorrhage.[138a]

Thrombotic thrombocytopenic purpura (TTP) and hemolytic uremic syndrome (HUS) may simply denote slightly different manifestations of the same disease.[137–140a] Both disorders may occur as a single episode or as a chronic relapsing condition.[141] In TTP, the classic clinical pentad consists of microangiopathic hemolysis, thrombocytopenia, central nervous system abnormality, renal dysfunction, and fever. During the course of disease, 40% of patients exhibit all five manifestations, and 74% exhibit the first three.[142] In HUS, renal dysfunction is predominant and is associated with hemolysis and thrombocytopenia. Both disorders have a female preponderance, TTP typically occurring in adults, HUS occurring primarily in children or puerperal women. Plasmapheresis is the cornerstone of therapy in TTP, but its efficacy in HUS is less well established.[142]

Acute fatty liver of pregnancy (AFLP) is a rare complication of third-trimester pregnancies. It is characterized by manifestations of hepatic insufficiency or failure: hyperbilirubinemia, coagulopathy, cerebral disturbance, and hypoglycemia. Presenting complaints, usually nonspecific, include nausea or vomiting (76%), abdominal pain (43%), anorexia (21%), and jaundice (16%).[145] About one-half of patients have hypertension, proteinuria, or edema,[145] and in a recent series, 9 of 14 patients had an admitting diagnosis of preeclampsia.[144] Whether AFLP resembles preeclampsia or merely coexists with it is unclear, since some authors consider the two conditions part of a spectrum of disease.[145] Although ultrasound and computed tomography of the liver may be helpful, definitive diagnosis is based on liver biopsy which, of course, is rarely indicated.[143,145] Maternal mortality, once above 90%, is now probably less than 10%,[144] due possibly to improved management, but more likely to recognition of milder forms of the disease. Supportive care and prompt delivery remain the only cure for AFLP.

TABLE 6–7. DIFFERENTIAL DIAGNOSIS OF HELLP SYNDROME, TTP, HUS, AND AFLP

Clinical/Laboratory Finding	HELLP	TTP	HUS	AFLP
Hypertension	77%	rare	present	25–50%
Proteinuria	90%	variable	present	variable
Thrombocytopenia	100%	100%	50% (onset)	variable
LDH	↑	↑	↑↑	↑
PT and PTT	↔	↔	↔	↑
Fibrinogen	↔	↔	↔	↓
Fibrin degradation products	↔	↔	↑	↑
Antithrombin III	↓	↔	↔	↓
Bilirubin	↑	↑	↑	↑↑
Ammonia	↔	↔	↔	↑↑
Hyperglycemia	↔	↔	↔	↓↓
Renal abnormalities	↑	↔	↑↑	↑
Neurologic abnormalities	↑	↑↑	↔	↑
Fever	↔	↑	↑	↔

TTP = thrombotic thrombocytopenic purpura; HUS = hemolytic uremic syndrome; AFLP = acute fatty liver of pregnancy; LDH = lactate dehydrogenase; PT = prothrombin time; PTT = partial thromboplastin time. From Sibai BM, Kustermann L, Velasco J: Current understanding of severe preeclampsia, pregnancy-associated hemolytic uremic syndrome, thrombotic thrombocytopenic purpura, hemolysis, elevated liver enzymes, and low platelet syndrome, and postpartum acute renal failure: Different clinical syndromes or just different names? *Curr Opin Nephrol Hypertens* 1994;3:436–445.

Because these disorders share clinical and laboratory features and may coexist, differential diagnosis may be problematic. Yet, differential diagnosis is vitally important, since the preferred treatment—delivery for HELLP and AFLP, plasmapheresis for TTP, dialysis and plasmapheresis for HUS—depends on an accurate diagnosis. Shown in Table 6–7 is the differential diagnosis of Sibai et al.[146] In the last analysis one should remember that HELLP occurs much more frequently than the other disorders, and patience is required if we are to avoid undue invasive therapy.

CONCLUSION

The literature is replete with studies of screening tests that predict the development of hypertension at the end of pregnancy. These investigations have little value, since isolated late-pregnancy hypertension has no appreciable effect on maternal or perinatal morbidity or mortality. Studies of tests that predict the development of new-onset hypertension and proteinuria in nulliparous women are much more important steps in the quest to identify women at high risk for developing true preeclampsia. Unfortunately, at the present time there is no predictive test for preeclampsia that meets all of the criteria defined by Grimes[13] for an ideal screening test. Similarly, there is no ideal diagnostic test for preeclampsia in women who are symptomatic. It is hoped that future progress in elucidating the pathophysiology of preeclampsia will lead to the development of clinically useful predictive and diagnostic tests.

REFERENCES

1. Chesley LC: Diagnosis of preeclampsia. *Obstet Gynecol* 1985;65:423–425.
2. Friedman SA: Preeclampsia: A review of the role of prostaglandins. *Obstet Gynecol* 1988; 71:122–137.
3. Roberts JM, Taylor RN, Musci TJ, et al: Preeclampsia: An endothelial disorder. *Am J Obstet Gynecol* 1989;161:1200–1204.
4. Friedman SA, Taylor RN, Roberts JM: Pathophysiology of preeclampsia. *Clin Perinatol* 1991;18:661–682.
5. Friedman SA, Lubarsky SL, Ahokas RA, et al: Preeclampsia and related disorders. Clinical aspects and relevance of endothelin and nitric oxide. *Clin Perinatol* 1995;22:343–355.
6. Poranen AK, Ekblad U, Uotila P, Ahotupa M: Lipid peroxidation and antioxidants in normal and pre-eclamptic pregnancies. *Placenta* 1996;17:401–405.
7. Rajkovic A, Catalano PM, Malinow MR: Elevated homocyst(e)ine levels with preeclampsia. *Obstet Gynecol* 1997;90;168–171
8. Conrad KP, Benyo DF: Placental cytokines and the pathogenesis of preeclampsia. *Am J Reprod Immunol* 1997;37:240–249.
9. Taylor RN: Review: Immunobiology of preeclampsia. *Am J Reprod Immunol* 1997;37:79–86.
10. Chesley LC: *Hypertensive Disorders in Pregnancy.* New York: Appleton-Century-Crofts; 1978.
11. Sibai BM: Eclampsia. VI. Maternal-perinatal outcome in 254 consecutive cases. *Am J Obstet Gynecol* 1990;163:1049–1054.
12. Roberts JM, Redman CWG: Pre-eclampsia: More than pregnancy-induced hypertension. *Lancet* 1993;341:1447–1451.
13. Grimes DA: Screening tests: What they are and what they aren't. *Contemp Obstet Gynecol* 1982;20:69–80.
14. Sibai BM, Caritis SN, Thom E, et al: Prevention of preeclampsia with low-dose aspirin in healthy, nulliparous pregnant women. *N Engl J Med* 1993;329:1213–1218.
15. Levine RJ, Hauth JC, Curet LB, et al: Trial of calcium to prevent preeclampsia. *N Engl J Med* 1997;337:69–76.
16. Caritis SN, Sibai BM, Hauth J, et al: Low-dose aspirin to prevent preeclampsia in women at high risk. *N Engl J Med* 1998;338:701–705.
16a. Kupferminc MJ, Eldor A, Steinman N, et al: Increased frequency of genetic thrombophilias in women with complications of pregnancy. *N Engl J Med,* in press, Jan. 1999.
16b. van Pampus MG, Dekker GA, Wolf H: High prevalence of hemostatic abnormalities in women with a history of preeclampsia. *Am J Obstet Gynecol,* in press, 1999.
17. National High Blood Pressure Education Program Working Group Report on High Blood Pressure in Pregnancy. *Am J Obstet Gynecol* 1990;163.1691–1712.
18. Browner WS, Newman TB, Cummings SR: Designing a new study: III. Diagnostic tests. In: Hulley SB, Cummings SR, eds. *Designing Clinical Research.* Baltimore: Williams & Wilkins; 1988:87–97.
19. Jacschke R, Guyatt GH, Sackett DL (for the Evidence-Based Medicine Working Group): Users' guide to the medical literature. III. How to use an article about a diagnostic test. B. What are the results and will they help me in caring for my patients? *JAMA* 1994; 271:703–707.
20. Fallis NE, Langford HG: Relation of second trimester blood pressure to toxemia of pregnancy in the primigravid patient. *Am J Obstet Gynecol* 1963;87:123–125.
21. Page EW, Christianson R: The impact of mean arterial pressure in the middle trimester upon the outcome of pregnancy. *Am J Obstet Gynecol* 1976;125:740–746.
22. Phelan JP: Enhanced prediction of pregnancy-induced hypertension by combining supine pressor test with mean arterial pressure of middle trimester. *Am J Obstet Gynecol* 1977; 129:397–400.
23. Friedman EA, Neff RK: *Pregnancy Hypertension: A Systematic Evaluation of Clinical Diagnostic Criteria.* Littleton, MA: PSG; 1977:212–219.
24. Moutquin JM, Rainville C, Giroux L, et al: A prospective study of blood pressure in pregnancy: Prediction of preeclampsia. *Am J Obstet Gynecol* 1985;151:191–196.

25. Marya RK, Rathee S, Mittal R: Evaluation of three clinical tests for predicting pregnancy-induced hypertension (letter). *Am J Obstet Gynecol* 1988;158:683–684.

26. Villar MA, Sibai BM: Clinical significance of elevated mean arterial blood pressure in second trimester and threshold increase in systolic or diastolic blood pressure during third trimester. *Am J Obstet Gynecol* 1989;160:419–423.

27. Ales KL, Norton ME, Druzin ML: Early prediction of antepartum hypertension. *Obstet Gynecol* 1989;73:928–933.

28. Massé J, Forest J-C, Moutquin J-M, et al: A prospective study of several potential biologic markers for early prediction of the development of preeclampsia. *Am J Obstet Gynecol* 1993;169:501–508.

29. Conde-Agudelo A, Belizán JM, Lede R, Bergel EF: What does an elevated mean arterial pressure in the second half of pregnancy predict—gestational hypertension or preeclampsia? *Am J Obstet Gynecol* 1993;169:509–514.

30. Kyle PM, Clark SJ, Buckley D, et al: Second trimester ambulatory blood pressure in nulliparous pregnancy: A useful screening test for preeclampsia? *Br J Obstet Gynaecol* 1993;100:914–919.

31. Sibai BM, Gordon T, Thom E, et al: Risk factors for preeclampsia in healthy nulliparous women: A prospective multicenter study. *Am J Obstet Gynecol* 1995;172:642–648.

32. Higgins JR, Walshe JJ, Halligan A, O'Brien E, et al: Can 24-hour ambulatory blood pressure measurement predict the development of hypertension in primigravidae? *Br J Obstet Gynaecol* 1997;104:356–362.

33. Sibai BM, Ewell M, Levine RJ, et al: Risk factors associated with preeclampsia in healthy nulliparous women. *Am J Obstet Gynecol* 1997;177:1003–1010.

34. Lopez-Espinoza I, Dhar H, Humphreys S, Redman CWG: Urinary albumin excretion in pregnancy. *Br J Obstet Gynaecol* 1986;93:176–181.

35. Rodriguez MH, Masaki DI, Mestman J, et al: Calcium/creatinine ratio and microalbuminuria in the prediction of preeclampsia. *Am J Obstet Gynecol* 1988;159:1452–1455.

36. Konstantin-Hansen KF, Hesseldahl H, Pedersen SM: Microalbuminuria as a predictor of preeclampsia. *Acta Obstet Gynecol Scand* 1992;71:343–346.

37. Das V, Bhargava T, Das SK, Pandey S: Microalbuminuria: A predictor of pregnancy-induced hypertension. *Br J Obstet Gynaecol* 1996;103:928–930.

38. Nelson TR: A clinical study of pre-eclampsia. *J Obstet Gynaecol Br Emp* 1955;62:48–57.

39. Thomson AM, Billewicz WZ: Clinical significance of weight trends during pregnancy. *Br Med J* 1957;1:243–247.

40. Gonen R, Perez R, David M, et al: The association between unexplained second-trimester maternal serum hCG elevation and pregnancy complications. *Obstet Gynecol* 1992;80:83–86.

41. Sorensen TK, Williams MA, Zingheim RW, et al: Elevated second-trimester human chorionic gonadotropin and subsequent pregnancy-induced hypertension. *Am J Obstet Gynecol* 1993;169:834–838.

42. Vaillant P, David E, Constant I, et al: Validity in nulliparas of increased β-human chorionic gonadotrophin at mid-term for predicting pregnancy-induced hypertension complicated with proteinuria and intrauterine growth retardation. *Nephron* 1996;72:557–563.

43. Ashour AMN, Lieberman ES, Wilkins Haug LE, Repke JT: The value of elevated second-trimester β-human chorionic gonadotropin in predicting development of preeclampsia. *Am J Obstet Gynecol* 1997;176:438–442.

44. Gant NF, Daley GL, Chand S, et al: A study of angiotensin II pressor response throughout primigravid pregnancy. *J Clin Invest* 1973;52:2682–2689.

45. Morris JA, O'Grady JP, Hamilton CJ, Davidson EC: Vascular reactivity to angiotensin II infusion during gestation. *Am J Obstet Gynecol* 1978;130:379–384.

46. Öney T, Kaulhausen H: The value of the angiotensin sensitivity test in the early diagnosis of hypertensive disorders in pregnancy. *Am J Obstet Gynecol* 1982;142:17–20.

47. Nakamura T, Ito M, Matsui K, et al: Significance of angiotensin sensitivity test for prediction of pregnancy-induced hypertension. *Obstet Gynecol* 1986;67:388–394.

48. Dekker GA, Makovitz JW, Wallenburg HCS: Prediction of pregnancy-induced hyperten-

sive disorders by angiotensin II sensitivity and supine pressor test. *Br J Obstet Gynaecol* 1990;97:817–821.

49. Baker PN, Broughton Pipkin F, Symonds EM: Comparative study of platelet angiotensin II binding and the angiotensin II sensitivity test as predictors of pregnancy-induced hypertension. *Clin Sci* 1992;83:89–95.

50. Kyle PM, Buckley D, Kissane J, et al: The angiotensin sensitivity test and low-dose aspirin are ineffective methods to predict and prevent hypertensive disorders in nulliparous pregnancy. *Am J Obstet Gynecol* 1995;173:865–872.

51. Gant NF, Chand S, Worley RJ, et al: A clinical test useful for predicting the development of acute hypertension in pregnancy. *Am J Obstet Gynecol* 1974;120:1–7.

52. Gusdon JP Jr, Anderson SG, May WJ: A clinical evaluation of the "roll-over test" for pregnancy-induced hypertension. *Am J Obstet Gynecol* 1977;127:1–3.

53. Karbhari D, Harrigan JT, Lamagra R: The supine hypertensive test as a predictor of incipient pre-eclampsia. *Am J Obstet Gynecol* 1977;127:620–622.

54. Marshall GW, Newman RL: Roll-over test. *Am J Obstet Gynecol* 1977;127:623–625.

55. Phelan JP, Everidge GJ, Wilder TL, Newman C: Is the supine pressor test an adequate means of predicting acute hypertension in pregnancy? *Am J Obstet Gynecol* 1977;128:173–176.

56. Didolkar SM, Sampson MB, Johnson WL, Petersen LP: Predictability of gestational hypertension. *Obstet Gynecol* 1979;54:224–225.

57. Marx GF, Husain FJ, Shiau HF: Brachial and femoral blood pressures during the prenatal period. *Am J Obstet Gynecol* 1980;136:11–31.

58. Kassar NS, Aldridge J, Quirk B: Roll over test. *Obstet Gynecol* 1980;55:411–413.

59. Kuntz WD: Supine pressor (roll-over) test: An evaluation. *Am J Obstet Gynecol* 1980;137:764–768.

60. Andersen GJ: The roll-over test as a screening procedure for gestational hypertension. *Aust NZ J Obstet Gynaecol* 1980;20:144–150.

61. Verma UL, Tejani NA, Chatterjee S, Weiss RR: Screening for SGA by the roll-over test. *Obstet Gynecol* 1980;56:591–594.

62. Tunbridge RD, Donnai P: Pregnancy-associated hypertension, a comparison of its prediction by 'roll-over test' and plasma noradrenaline measurement in 100 primigravidae. *Br J Obstet Gynaecol* 1983;90:1027–1032.

63. Degani S, Abinader E, Eibschitz I, et al: Isometric exercise test for predicting gestational hypertension. *Obstet Gynecol* 1985;65:652–654.

64. Okonofua FE, Onwudiegwu U, Odunsi AO, et al: Does standing up improve the predictive value of the supine pressor test for gestational hypertension? *Obstet Gynecol* 1990;76:332–335.

65. Louden KA, Broughton Pipkin F: Prediction of pregnancy-induced hypertensive disorders by angiotensin II sensitivity and supine pressor test (letter; comment). *Br J Obstet Gynaecol* 1991;98:231–232.

66. Conde-Agudelo A, Lede R, Belizán J: Evaluation of methods used in the prediction of hypertensive disorders of pregnancy. *Obstet Gynecol Surv* 1994;49:210–222.

67. Baker PN, Johnson IR: The use of the hand-grip test for predicting pregnancy-induced hypertension. *Eur J Obstet Gynecol Reprod Biol* 1994;56:169–172.

68. Tomoda S, Kitanaka T, Ogita S, Hidaka A: Prediction of pregnancy-induced hypertension by isometric exercise. *Asia Oceania J Obstet Gynaecol* 1994;20:249–255.

69. Yang Y, Jones DM, Pawlak MA, et al: Accuracy of single concentration estimations of platelet angiotensin II receptor number. Its usefulness in screening for pregnancy-induced hypertension. *Am J Hypertens* 1994;7:989–995.

70. Pouliot L, Forest J-C, Moutquin J-M, et al: Platelet angiotensin II binding sites and early detection of preeclampsia. *Obstet Gynecol* 1998;91:591–595.

71. Zemel MB, Zemel PC, Berry S, et al: Altered platelet calcium metabolism as an early predictor of increased peripheral vascular resistance and preeclampsia in urban black women (published erratum appears in *N Engl J Med* 1992;326:647). *N Engl J Med* 1990;323:434–438.

72. Kyle PM, Jackson MC, Buckley DC, et al: Platelet intracellular free calcium response to argi-

nine vasopressin is similar in preeclampsia and normal pregnancy. *Am J Obstet Gynecol* 1995;172:654–660.

73. Redman CWG, Williams GF, Jones DD, Wilkinson RH: Plasma urate and serum deoxy-cytidylate deaminase measurements for the early diagnosis of pre-eclampsia. *Br J Obstet Gynaecol* 1977;84:904–908.

74. Jacobson S-L, Imhof R, Manning N, et al: The value of Doppler assessment of the utero-placental circulation in predicting preeclampsia or intrauterine growth retardation. *Am J Obstet Gynecol* 1990;162:110–114.

75. Conde-Agudelo A, Belizán JM, Lede R, Bergel E: Prediction of hypertensive disorders of pregnancy by calcium/creatinine ratio and other laboratory tests (letter). *Int J Gynecol Obstet* 1994;47:285–286.

76. Calvert SM, Tuffnell DJ, Haley J: Poor predictive value of platelet count, mean platelet volume and serum urate in hypertension in pregnancy. *Eur J Obstet Gynecol Reprod Biol* 1996;64:179–184.

77. Sanchez-Ramos L, Jones DC, Cullen MT: Urinary calcium as an early marker for preeclampsia. *Obstet Gynecol* 1991;77:685–688.

78. Raniolo E, Phillipou G: Prediction of pregnancy-induced hypertension by means of the urinary calcium:creatinine ratio. *Med J Aust* 1993;158:98–100.

79. Millar JGB, Campbell SK, Albano JDM, et al: Early prediction of pre-eclampsia by measurement of kallikrein and creatinine on a random urine sample. *Br J Obstet Gynaecol* 1996;103:421–426.

80. Kyle PM, Campbell S, Buckley D, et al: A comparison of the inactive urinary kallikrein:creatinine ratio and the angiotensin sensitivity test for the prediction of pre-eclampsia. *Br J Obstet Gynaecol* 1996;103:981–987.

81. Kyle P, Redman C, de Swiet M, Millar G: A comparison of the inactive urinary kallikrein:creatinine ratio and the angiotensin sensitivity test for the prediction of pre-eclampsia (letter reply). *Br J Obstet Gynaecol* 1997;104:969–974.

82. Easterling TR, Benedetti TJ, Schmucker BC, Millard SP: Maternal hemodynamics in normal and preeclamptic pregnancies: A longitudinal study. *Obstet Gynecol* 1990;76:1061–1069.

83. Campbell S, Pearce JMF, Hackett G, et al: Qualitative assessment of uteroplacental blood flow: Early screening test for high-risk pregnancies. *Obstet Gynecol* 1986;68:649–653.

84. Arduini D, Rizzo G, Romanini C, Mancuso S: Utero-placental blood flow velocity waveforms as predictors of pregnancy-induced hypertension. *Eur J Obstet Gynecol Reprod Biol* 1987;26:335–341.

85. Steel SA, Pearce JM, Chamberlain GV: Doppler ultrasound of the uteroplacental circulation as a screening test for severe pre-eclampsia with intra-uterine growth retardation. *Eur J Obstet Gynecol Reprod Biol* 1988;28:279–287.

86. Steel SA, Pearce JM, McParland P, Chamberlain GVP: Early doppler ultrasound screening in prediction of hypertensive disorders of pregnancy. *Lancet* 1990;335:1548–1551.

87. Bower S, Bewley S, Campbell S: Improved prediction of preeclampsia by two-stage screening of uterine arteries using the early diastolic notch and color Doppler imaging. *Obstet Gynecol* 1994;82:78–83.

87a. Irion O, Massé J, Forest J-C, Montquin J-M: Prediction of pre-eclampsia, low birthweight for gestation and prematurity by uterine blood flow velocity waveform analysis in low risk nulliparous women. *Br J Obstet Gynaecol* 1998;105:422–429.

88. North RA, Ferrier C, Long D, et al: Uterine artery Doppler flow velocity waveforms in the second trimester for the prediction of preeclampsia and fetal growth retardation. *Obstet Gynecol* 1994;83:378–386.

89. Friedman SA, de Groot CJ, Taylor RN, Roberts JM: Circulating concentrations of fetal fibronectin do not reflect reduced trophoblastic invasion in preeclamptic pregnancies. *Am J Obstet Gynecol* 1992;167:496–497.

90. Sakura M, Nakabayashi M, Takeda Y, Sato K: Elevated fetal fibronectin in midtrimester amniotic fluid is involved with the onset of preeclampsia. *J Obstet Gynaecol Res* 1998;24:73–76.

91. Lazarchick J, Stubbs TM, Romein L, et al: Predictive value of fibronectin levels in nor-

motensive gravid women destined to become preeclamptic. *Am J Obstet Gynecol* 1986; 154:1050–1052.

92. Ballegeer V, Spitz B, Kieckens L, et al: Predictive value of increased plasma levels of fibronectin in gestational hypertension. *Am J Obstet Gynecol* 1989;161:432–436.

93. Lockwood CJ, Peters JH. Increased plasma levels of ED1+ cellular fibronectin precede the clinical signs of preeclampsia. *Am J Obstet Gynecol* 1990;162:358–362.

94. Taylor RN, Crombleholme WR, Friedman SA, et al: High plasma cellular fibronectin levels correlate with biochemical and clinical features of preeclampsia but cannot be attributed to hypertension alone. *Am J Obstet Gynecol* 1991;165:895–901.

95. Jones I, Cowley D, Andersen M, et al: Fibronectin as a predictor of preeclampsia: A pilot study. *Aust NZ J Obstet Gynaecol* 1996;36:1–3.

96. Arnaud C, Chau C, Dizier B, et al: Plasma fibronectin: Predictive factor in gestational hypertension? *Pathol Biol* (Paris) 1997;45:487–490.

97. Paarlberg KM, De Jong CLD, Van Geijn HP, et al: Total plasma fibronectin as a marker of pregnancy-induced hypertensive disorders: A longitudinal study. *Obstet Gynecol* 1998;91: 383–388.

98. Halligan A, Donnar J, Sheppard B, et al: Haemostatic, fibrinolytic and endothelial variables in normal pregnancies and preeclampsia. *Br J Obstet Gynaecol* 1994;101:488–492.

99. Fitzgerald DJ, Entman SS, Mulloy K, FitzGerald GA: Decreased prostacyclin biosynthesis preceding the clinical manifestation of pregnancy-induced hypertension. *Circulation* 1987; 75:956–963.

100. Krauss T, Kuhn W, Lakoma C, Augustin HG: Circulating endothelial cell adhesion molecules as diagnostic markers for the early identification of pregnant women at risk for development of preeclampsia. *Am J Obstet Gynecol* 1997;177:443–449.

101. Weiner CP, Brandt J: Plasma antithrombin III activity: An aid in the diagnosis of preeclampsia–eclampsia. *Am J Obstet Gynecol* 1982;142:275–281.

102. Caron C, Goudemand J, Marey A, et al: Are haemostatic and fibrinolytic parameters predictors of preeclampsia in pregnancy-associated hypertension? *Thromb Haemost* 1991;66: 410–414.

103. Ho C-H, Yang Z-L: The predictive value of the hemostasis parameters in the development of preeclampsia. *Thromb Haemost* 1992;67:214–218.

104. Savelieva GM, Efimov VS, Grishin VL, et al: Blood coagulation changes in pregnant women at risk of developing preeclampsia. *Int J Gynaecol Obstet* 1995;48:3–8.

105. Redman CWG, Bonnar J, Beilin L: Early platelet consumption in preeclampsia. *Br Med J* 1978;1:467–469.

106. Walker JJ, Cameron AD, Bjornsson S, et al: Can platelet volume predict progressive hypertensive disease in pregnancy? *Am J Obstet Gynecol* 1989;161:676–679.

107. Konijnenberg A, van der Post JAM, Mol BW, et al: Can flow cytometric detection of platelet activation early in pregnancy predict the occurrence of preeclampsia? A prospective study. *Am J Obstet Gynecol* 1997;177:434–442.

108. Redman CWG, Denson KWE, Beilin LJ, et al: Factor-VIII consumption in pre-eclampsia. *Lancet* 1977;2:1249–1252.

109. Taufield PA, Ales KL, Resnick LM, et al: Hypocalciuria in preeclampsia. *N Engl J Med* 1987;316:715–718.

110. Brosens IA, Robertson WB, Dixon HG: The role of the spiral arteries in the pathogenesis of pre-eclampsia. *Obstet Gynecol Annu* 1972;1:177–191.

111. Hynes RO: *Cell Biology of Extracellular Matrix.* New York: Plenum Press; 1981:295–334.

112. Peters JH, Maunder RJ, Woolf AD, et al: Elevated plasma levels of ED1+ ("cellular") fibronectin in patients with vascular injury. *J Lab Clin Med* 1989;113:586–597.

113. Lockwood CJ, Senyei AE, Dische MR, et al: Fetal fibronectin in cervical and vaginal secretions as a predictor of preterm delivery. *N Engl J Med* 1991;325:669–674.

114. Spargo B, McCartney CP, Winemiller R: Glomerular capillary endotheliosis in toxemia of pregnancy. *Arch Pathol* 1959;68:593–599.

115. Fisher KA, Luger A, Spargo BH, Lindheimer MD: Hypertension in pregnancy: Clinical–pathological correlations and remote prognosis. *Medicine* 1981;60:267–276.

116. Kuo VS, Koumantakis G, Gallery EDM: Proteinuria and its assessment in normal and hypertensive pregnancy. *Am J Obstet Gynecol* 1992;167:723–728.
117. Meyer NL, Mercer BM, Friedman SA, Sibai BM: Urinary dipstick protein: A poor predictor of absent or severe proteinuria. *Am J Obstet Gynecol* 1994;170:137–141.
118. Brown MA, Buddle ML: Inadequacy of dipstick proteinuria in hypertensive pregnancy. *Aust N Z J Obstet Gynaecol* 1995;35:366–369.
119. Pollak VE, Nettles JB: The kidney in toxemia of pregnancy: A clinical and pathologic study based on renal biopsies. *Medicine* 1960;39:469–526.
120. Lim K-H, Friedman SA, Ecker JL, et al: The clinical utility of serum uric acid measurements in hypertensive diseases of pregnancy. *Am J Obstet Gynecol* 1998;178:1067–1071.
121. Weenink GH, Borm JJJ, Ten Cate JW, Treffers PE: Antithrombin III levels in normotensive and hypertensive pregnancy. *Gynecol Obstet Invest* 1983;16:230–242.
122. Weiner CP, Kwaan HC, Xu C, et al: Antithrombin III activity in women with hypertension during pregnancy. *Obstet Gynecol* 1985;65:301–306.
123. Redman CWG, Jeffries M: Revised definition of pre-eclampsia. *Lancet* 1988;1:809–812.
124. Sanchez-Ramos L, Sandroni S, Andres FJ, Kaunitz AM: Calcium excretion in preeclampsia. *Obstet Gynecol* 1991;77:510–513.
125. Petraglia F, Aguzzoli L, Gallinelli A, et al: Hypertension in pregnancy: Changes in activin A maternal serum concentration. *Placenta* 1995;16:447–454.
126. Muttukrishna S, Knight PG, Redman CWG, Ledger WL: Activin A and inhibin A as possible endocrine markers for pre-eclampsia. *Lancet* 1997;349:1285–1288.
127. Cunningham FG, Cox SM, Harstad TW, et al: Chronic renal disease and pregnancy outcome. *Am J Obstet Gynecol* 1990;163:453–459.
128. Davison JM, Lindheimer MD: Chronic renal disease. In: Gleicher N, ed. *Principles and Practice of Medical Therapy in Pregnancy.* Norwalk, CT: Appleton & Lange; 1992:928–938.
129. Weiner CP, Bonsib SM: Relationship between renal histology and plasma antithrombin III activity in women with early onset preeclampsia. *Am J Perinatol* 1990;7:139–143.
130. Buyon JP, Tamerius J, Ordorica S, et al: Activation of the alternative complement pathway accompanies disease flares in systemic lupus erythematosus during pregnancy. *Arthritis Rheum* 1992;35:55–61.
131. Abramson SB, Buyon JP: Activation of the complement pathway: Comparison of normal pregnancy, preeclampsia, and systemic lupus erythematosus during pregnancy. *Am J Reprod Immunol* 1992;28:183–187.
132. Weinstein A, Bordwell B, Stone B, et al: Antibodies to native DNA and serum complement (C3) levels. Application to diagnosis and classification of systemic lupus erythematosus. *Am J Med* 1983;74:206–216.
133. Swaak AJG, Groenwold J, Bronsveld W: Predictive value of complement profiles and anti-dsDNA in systemic lupus erythematosus. *Ann Rheum Dis* 1986;45:359–366.
134. Lockshin MD, Druzin ML: Rheumatic disease. In: Barron WM, Lindheimer MD, eds. *Medical Disorders during Pregnancy,* ed 2. St. Louis: Mosby; 1995:307–337.
135. Weinstein L: Syndrome of hemolysis, elevated liver enzymes, and low platelet count: A severe consequence of hypertension in pregnancy. *Am J Obstet Gynecol* 1982;142:159–167.
136. Sibai BM, Ramadan MK, Usta I, et al: Maternal morbidity and mortality in 442 pregnancies with hemolysis, elevated liver enzymes, and low platelets (HELLP syndrome). *Am J Obstet Gynecol* 1993;169:1000–1006.
137. Martin JN Jr, Blake PG, Lowry SL, et al: Pregnancy complicated by preeclampsia–eclampsia with the syndrome of hemolysis, elevated liver enzymes, and low platelet count: How rapid is postpartum recovery? *Obstet Gynecol* 1990;76:737–741.
138. Visser W, Wallenburg HCS: Temporising management of severe preeclampsia with and without the HELLP syndrome. *Br J Obstet Gynaecol* 1995;102:111–117.
138a. Isler CM, Rinehart BK, Terrone RW, et al: Maternal mortality associated with HELLP syndrome. *Am J Obstet Gynecol* 1999 (in press).
139. Remuzzi G: HUS and TTP: Variable expression of a single entity (clinical conference). *Kidney Int* 1987;32:292–308.

140. Egerman RS, Witlin AG, Friedman SA, Sibai BM: Thrombotic thrombocytopenic purpura and hemolytic uremic syndrome in pregnancy: Review of 11 cases. *Am J Obstet Gynecol* 1996;175:950–956.

140a. Dashe JS, Ramin SM, Cunningham FG: The long-term consequences of thrombotic microangiopathy (thrombocytopenic purpura and hemolytic uremic syndrome) in pregnancy. *Obstet Gynecol* 1998;91:662–668.

141. Ridolfi RL, Bell WR: Thrombotic thrombocytopenic purpura. Report of 25 cases and review of the literature. *Medicine* 1981;60:413–428.

142. Badr KF, Brenner BM: Vascular injury to the kidney. In: Fauci AS, Braunwald E, Isselbacher KJ, et al, eds. *Harrison's Principles of Internal Medicine*, ed 14. New York: McGraw-Hill; 1998:1558–1562.

143. Bacq Y: Acute fatty liver of pregnancy. *Semin Perinatol* 1998;22:134–140.

144. Usta IM, Barton JR, Amon EA, et al: Acute fatty liver of pregnancy: An experience in the diagnosis and management of fourteen cases. *Am J Obstet Gynecol* 1994;171:1342–1347.

145. Riely CA, Latham PS, Romero R, Duffy TP: Acute fatty liver of pregnancy. A reassessment based on observations in nine patients. *Ann Int Med* 1987;106:703–706.

146. Sibai BM, Kustermann L, Velasco J: Current understanding of severe preeclampsia, pregnancy-associated hemolytic uremic syndrome, thrombotic thrombocytopenic purpura, hemolysis, elevated liver enzymes, and low platelet syndrome, and postpartum acute renal failure: Different clinical syndromes or just different names? *Curr Opin Nephrol Hypertens* 1994;3:436–445.

IV

Pathology and Pathophysiology of Preeclampsia

7

Pathology of the Kidney, Liver, and Brain

Lillian W. Gaber and Marshall D. Lindheimer

Chapter 4 in Chesley's first edition of this text was entitled "Structural Lesions." It focused on gross and microscopic descriptions emanating from autopsy reports dating from epochs when mortality rates for both preeclampsia and eclampsia were considerably higher than today. In line with the style and scholarship throughout Chesley's text, there was an extensive historical review which bears rereading, but in this specific chapter he relied primarily on the observations described by the celebrated pathologist Harold Sheehan. The latter had overseen 677 autopsies on obstetric patients dying from all causes, mainly performed at the Glasgow Royal Maternal Hospital during the period of 1935 through 1946. The uniqueness of this series was that the majority of these autopsies were performed within 2 hours after death, thus avoiding postpartum artifacts, and that specimens from 377 of these cases were reexamined using a variety of special staining techniques. The data included 112 cases classified as normal and at least 200 where a diagnosis of preeclampsia–eclampsia seems secure. The findings are discussed in detail in a book by Sheehan and Lynch, *Pathology of Toxaemia of Pregnancy* (published jointly by Williams & Wilkins, Baltimore, and the Longman Group, Ltd., Churchill Livingstone, Edinburgh in 1973).[1] This monograph, too, bears rereading, for like Chesley, Sheehan was compulsive and scholarly, the historical reviews in his book ranking with those in the first edition of this text. Also, there are extensive autopsy descriptions and excellent photomicrographs for the reader to review.

Another focus in Chesley's "Structural Lesions" chapter was renal pathology, as this area had "exploded" once renal biopsies started to be performed on preeclamptic women in the 1950s. Here, the concern of postmortem changes was eliminated, but as Sheehan pointed out, other artifacts, such as limited sampling may have taken its place.

The majority of this chapter will focus on renal pathology, including biopsy material reviewed by the first author. The reason for this is that the pathophysiology of preeclampsia, generalized arteriolar spasm, and functional derangement of endothelial cells, which may be associated with coagulation abnormalities, are usually associated with the development of a nephropathy quite characteristic of the disorder. In fact, proteinuria has traditionally been considered a cardinal sign and requisite for the diagnosis (often the reason for biopsy), making a renal lesion almost universal to all cases. Indeed, the kidney manifests an array of reversible structural and functional lesions which may be responsible for a variety of alterations in kidney function described in Chapter 8. Another reason for focusing on the kidney (as Chesley did) is that the use of renal biopsies have demonstrated to us our clinical frailties, that is, how difficult it can be to distinguish by clinical criteria alone between preeclampsia, essential or secondary hypertension, renal disease, or combinations of these entities. For example, in 1960, Pollak and Nettles[2] showed the rate of concordance between clinical impression and biopsy diagnosis in patients presenting with hypertension complicating pregnancy to be but 58%. Fisher et al.,[3] in 1981, evaluated the clinical and histologic features of 176 women biopsied because of hypertension complicating pregnancy. The etiology of hypertension was correctly established by clinical parameters in 75% of the nulliparas, while in multiparas the agreement was only 50%. Despite the recent advances in laboratory testing, a firm diagnosis of preeclampsia (pure or superimposed) can still be difficult, as shown by Weiner and Bonsib,[4] who were able to demonstrate preeclamptic nephropathy in only 4 of 12 patients who presented with early onset "preeclampsia."

Still another area where renal biopsy has proved revealing are those variants of preeclampsia where the microangiopathy is particularly evident in other organs resulting in a complex clinical picture that combines the nephropathy with a variety of extrarenal and hematologic lesions. The diagnosis of the multisystemic variant of preeclampsia is often challenging, as the symptoms overlap with other pregnancy-associated disorders such as acute fatty liver of pregnancy, thrombotic thrombocytopenic puerpera, hemolytic uremia-like syndromes, and certain types of rapidly progressive or acute postpartum forms of renal failure. These disorders, however, may be a spectrum of one disease, sharing the same pathogenetic vascular–endothelial injury with varied end-organ effect. Some of these problems, too, will be emphasized below.

THE KIDNEY

Gross Description

In the series described by Sheehan and Lynch[1] kidneys from women dying after eclampsia usually had a pale and broad cortex, which they ascribed to tubular dilation. The kidneys were also enlarged compared to those from "normal" cases but variance was such that the changes were not statistical. Few, if any other gross changes were observed.

Renal Histopathology in Preeclampsia

Insight into the pathology of preeclampsia evolved from several landmark studies performed after the adoption of new technologies in the histopathologic examination and assessment of renal biopsies. In 1918, the initial descriptions of glomerular morphology in preeclampsia by Lohlein[5] claimed that the renal lesion was characterized by increased glomerular cellularity, and these findings led to speculation that preeclampsia was an inflammatory hypercellular response, i.e., a form of glomerulonephritis. (Note that this hypothesis has recently been revised by investigators of animal models where the disease is evoked by endotoxin [see Chapter 15].) This view was disputed a few years later when renal specimens were studied with the aid of special histochemical stains, namely the periodic-acid Schiff (PAS) stain. The latter, which permitted better visualization of the glomerular tuft elements and the glomerular basement membrane demonstrated an impressive increase in glomerular basement membrane width, which contributed to the fullness of the glomerular tuft, but with a modest increase in glomerular cellularity. Thus, the renal lesions of preeclampsia were next categorized as a membranous glomerulonephritis.[6,7] This, too, was to be proven incorrect, especially when electron microscopic technology was applied to renal biopsies. Sheehan, whose unique and outstanding autopsy series was described above, provided elaborate descriptions of the renal histopathology of preeclampsia as early as 1950.[1,8] Because, as noted, his autopsies were performed so quickly after death, and autolysis was minimal, most of his findings have been proven correct in the renal biopsy–electron microscopy studies which appeared in the late 1950s and are considered milestones in relation to our understanding of renal pathology in preeclampsia. Still, one should recognize that the lesions described by Sheehan pertained to a subset of patients who suffered a fatal form of the disease.

In the late 1950s through the early part of the 1970s, the increasing application of percutaneous needle biopsy in the diagnosis of renal disorders made it possible to examine the renal pathology of preeclampsia during different stages in its development, offering a better understanding of the natural history of the disease during pregnancy and after delivery. It was also possible to observe the histologic changes that develop in the atypical cases and in cases with varying clinical manifestations and severity. In addition, the application of immunofluorescence and electron microscopy in the diagnosis of renal disorders helped to define the lesions beyond just their morphologic appearance and suggested pathogenetic mechanisms that inspired many investigators. Dieckmann et al.[9] and other investigators at the University of Chicago interested in gestational hypertension, focused on the histologic and clinical aspects that distinguish "pure preeclampsia" from other conditions that lead to a secondary form of preeclampsia. They were able to distinguish the natural history of reversible "pure preeclampsia" from that of patients with preexisting hypertension or renal disease.[9,10] In addition, Spargo et al.[10] elaborated on ultrastructural glomerular lesions and proposed "endotheliosis," a term which became synonymous with preeclampsia, to describe the alterations in the glomerular endothelial cells. Their findings had significant implications, as it became evident that the glomerular endothelium was the primary target for injury in preeclampsia.* Studies by Chesley et al.[11] suggested the benign nature of preeclamptic nephropathy, for not only do signs and symptoms reverse completely after delivery but there is no remote evidence of cardiovascular or renal disease when nulliparous eclamptics are reexamined decades after the putative illness. Kincaid-Smith et al. studied the pathogenetic mechanism of the disease and its natural history.[12,13]

More recently, there has been a marked decline in published studies which address the renal pathology in preeclampsia, probably due to the appropriately stringent criteria that now limit the indications for a renal biopsy in women whose pregnancies are complicated by hypertension. The few that have appeared have concentrated on two issues. One is the expression of different vasoactive mediators and products of endothelial cells in the kidney and placenta during preeclampsia, in the hope to clarify the yet undetermined pathway of endothelial cell damage. The second is the application of morphometric techniques to enhance understanding of the relationship between the hemodynamic and the structural changes in preeclampsia and to address the issue of the development of focal segmental glomerulosclerosis-like lesions in a subset of patients.

Light Microscopy

Glomerular Alterations. The light microscopy of preeclamptic nephropathy is typically characterized by moderate glomerular hypertrophy and decreased glomerular capillary space area, resulting from swelling of the glomerular endothelium and increased capillary wall thickness without significant change in glomerular cellularity. This pattern of glomerular injury is both diffuse and global in distribution, i.e., involves most of the glomerular tuft surface area in greater than 50% of the glomeruli in a sample.

Since the early descriptions of the renal histopathology in patients with preeclampsia, most investigators report a moderate increase in glomerular size. These observations are based on subjective examination of renal biopsy or autopsy material from patients with preeclampsia. To our knowledge, Sheehan was the first to attempt measuring the glomerular diameter in pregnant women who died from true preeclampsia or other hypertensive gestational disorders.[1,14] In his analysis, Sheehan found that gravidas with severe eclampsia had a glomerular diameter of 216 μm, while women who died from other incidental obstetric complications and with presumably normal glomeruli had a lower mean glomerular diameter of

---

* Actually, glomerular endothelial swelling had been noted as early as 1924 by Mayer (see Mayer A: Changes in the endothelium during eclampsia and their significance. (translated from Germ.) *Klin Wochenzetschrift* 1924;H27).

193 μm (statistical significance was not determined) (Fig. 7–1). Three decades later, new quantitative data are beginning to emerge by using the current imaging-computed techniques to measure the different glomerular parameters in biopsies from gravid women with gestational hypertension. Nochy et al.[15] demonstrated a statistically significant increase in the glomerular surface area (21,540 μm^2) in pregnant women with preeclampsia compared to nonpregnant women with sporadic benign hematuria (17,950 μm^2), while glomerular size in non-preeclamptic gestational hypertension was generally less than normal. Unfortunately, most of our information regarding glomerular size change in preeclampsia is derived from comparisons to gravid women with other renal diseases or to normal, nondiseased glomeruli from nongravid females. Little is known, however, about glomerular size change in preeclampsia in comparison to the physiologic pregnancy-induced glomerular hypertrophy.

Hypertrophy, rather than proliferation of the mesangial and endothelial cells, dominates the cellular alterations associated with preeclampsia.[14-16] Most investigators agree that glomerular cellularity is within normal limits or at least the increase in cellularity is very mild. For example, Seymour et al.[17] reported a twofold increase in the number of endothelial and mesangial cells by counting cells in standard tissue sections. These findings, however, may be atypical, since the biopsy material analyzed displayed characteristics of very severe preeclamptic lesions, the

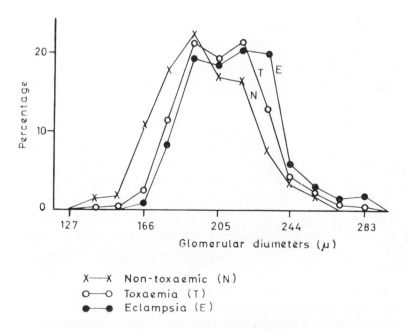

Figure 7–1. Distribution of mean glomerular diameters in relation to preeclampsia. Percentage of patients whose glomerular diameter exceeds 205 μm is much higher in the groups of patients with preeclampsia and eclampsia than in the control groups. (*Reprinted, with permission, from Sheehan HL, Lynch JB:* Pathology of Toxaemia of Pregnancy. *Baltimore: Williams & Wilkins; 1973:807.*)

prevalence of mesangial and capillary loop abnormalities being much greater than that generally reported in the literature. Although there are other reports of increased glomerular cellularity in preeclampsia, most are subjective in nature, based on the general impressions made during the evaluation.[18]

One of the characteristic features of preeclampsia is the obstructed hypovascular appearance of the glomerular tufts, often referred to as "bloodless glomeruli" (Fig. 7–2). Narrowing of the glomerular capillary loops is a multifactorial process, resulting from a combination of apparent structural alterations in the glomerular endothelium, biochemical and structural changes in the capillary wall and possibly in the mesangium, and finally the effects of hemodynamic and vasoactive mediators on the vascular tone. Endothelial hypertrophy, a characteristic feature of the microvascular pathology of preeclampsia, is partly responsible for the compromise of the vascular spaces in the glomeruli.[8,14,16] The variability in the reported incidence of endothelial hypertrophy in renal biopsies is the result of the different methods used to evaluate the intravascular pathology. For instance, light microscopy is sufficient when the cellular changes are pronounced; the hypertrophied

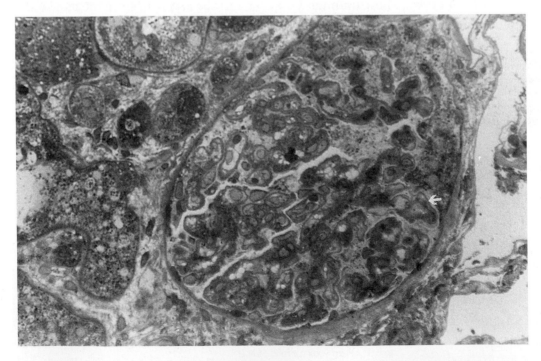

Figure 7–2. Light microscopy of a glomerulus depicting a conglomerate of lesions characteristic of preeclampsia. The capillary loops are completely or partially obliterated by swollen endothelial cells. Lipid deposits and clear vacuoles expand the cytoplasm of the endothelial cells. The glomerular podocytes are granulated and moderately enlarged. Occasional segments of the glomerular basement membrane depict a "double-contour" pattern (*arrow*). Also note the presence of numerous protein droplets in the tubular epithelial cells. (Toluidine blue-stained, spur-embedded, 1 μm thick sections; ×350)

endothelial cells become readily detectable by virtue of their voluminous, densely eosinophilic and vacuolated cytoplasm. However, mild degrees of cellular hypertrophy may not be appreciated by routine light microscopy, and a better method to depict the cellular pathology is through use of the electron microscope. Spargo et al.[10] determined from the ultrastructural findings that endothelial enlargement and cytoplasm alterations are almost universal to all biopsies of preeclampsia. Characteristic of the alterations in the cytoplasm is the presence of clear vacuoles and lipid droplets. When the cytoplasm is displaced by massive intracellular lipid deposits, the cells acquire a foamy appearance, hence described as "foam cells."

Whether all intracapillary foam cells are of endothelial cell origin or are derived from mononuclear cells or even mesangial cells is still questionable. The use of special stains such as Sudan stain or Oil red O increases the sensitivity of light microscopy in the detection of intraglomerular fat deposits; however, these stains are only applied to frozen tissue to bypass lipid solvents used during processing for routine light microscopy.[14] In general, electron microscopy is the most sensitive in the detection of intracellular lipid deposits, even when present in small quantities. Intraglomerular foam cells have been detected with a much higher frequency in postpartum biopsies as opposed to biopsies during pregnancy, suggesting that they represent an involutional stage of the disease process. It is not surprising that the reported frequency of intraglomerular foam cells is quite variable, generally between 4 and 35%, depending on the timing of the biopsy, method of tissue processing and staining, and the sensitivity of the technique used to detect the intraglomerular fat.[10,14] Other changes that can be appreciated by light microscopic assessment of the glomerular endothelial cells include cytoplasmic edema and accumulation of PAS-positive intracytoplasmic fibrillary deposits.[14,16]

As noted, Bell,[6] and later Allen,[7] impressed by the capillary wall thickening, identified the dominant pattern of glomerular injury in preeclampsia as a "membranous glomerulonephritis," a misleading term that generally implies an immune-complex mediated glomerular disease, which is not the case in preeclampsia. Substantial amounts of plasma-derived proteins and/or IgM deposited along the inner surface of the basement membrane are the primary causes of basement membrane alterations, when present. These deposits, which can be visualized in PAS-stained sections by their fibrillary or amphophilic appearance, are major contributors to capillary wall thickening, as they expand the lamina interna and the subendothelial zone. Capillary loop thickening has also been considered a consequence of mesangial matrix expansion and interposition, which first affect the segments of the basement membrane close to the mesangial aspect of the capillary loop, then eventually progress to involve most or the entire circumference of the loop creating a "double-contour" pattern. Mesangial interposition in preeclampsia was first described in 1961, and for several years became a controversial issue because of the great variation in its frequency. Seymour et al.[17] reported widespread mesangial interposition and basement membrane splitting in 14 renal biopsies performed within 2 weeks postpartum. Tribe et al.[18] also reported mesangial interposition in 7 of 11 biopsies (64%), showing moderate or severe lesions of preeclampsia. The extent of mesangial interposition in different reports seemed to correspond to the severity of the disease, with no mesangial interposition observed in biopsies with mild disease in contrast to severe mesangial expansion leading to complete obliteration of the capillary lumen "strangulated loop" in the most severe case. Other large biopsy series, such as those reported by Spargo, Kincaid-Smith, Pirani, and their respective colleagues,[10,13,16,19,20] did not identify mesangial interposition to be either a dominant or a widespread histologic finding, although they studied both pre- and postpartum biopsies, a wide range of histologic disease severity, and varied clinical presentations with both typical and atypical manifestations. In essence, in the majority of preeclamptic women biopsied there is little or no basement membrane pathology, and when present may represent severe disease. Ironically, however, restrictions of indications to biopsy to patients with severe and/or atypical disease may be one reason why, in the more recent literature, descriptions of basement membrane changes in biopsies from preeclamptic women seem to be discussed more often.

The empty, bloodless glomerular tufts with obstructed capillary loops dominate the glomerular pathology of preeclampsia. In addition, there are other less common lesions that affect but a small number of glomeruli, and although they are not unique or specific to preeclampsia, they most likely are the result of exaggerated, yet localized alterations in the capillary loops. One of these patterns is the "cigar-shaped" loops which describe a localized cluster of simplified, elongated loops, often obliterated by mildly enlarged endothelial cells and connected to poorly defined mesangial stalks.[19] The second pattern is almost the reverse of the above, with the glomerular capillaries showing enormous expansion and dilation by markedly swollen endothelial cells and foam cells, hence termed "ballooned loops." Adhesions may be present connecting the ballooned loops to the capsule. The ballooned capillary loops are usually located near the tubular pole of the glomerulus and often herniate through the initial segment of the proximal connecting tubule, a process known as "pouting" (Fig. 7–3).[1,14] Of note, however, "pouting" is a nonspecific occurrence which is present in a variety of renal diseases, particularly when the glomeruli are enlarged.

In addition to capillary loop pathology, there may be changes in the mesangial areas as well as in the glomerular epithelium. However, the alterations in the glomerular mesangium are difficult to appreciate by light microscopy, unless there is pronounced interposition of the mesangium in the glomerular capillary loops. Also, Sheehan[14] has described a peculiar change in the mesangium, commonly associated with the healing stages of the disease, characterized by vacuolization of the mesangial stalks and resembling a "string of beads." The mesangial regions are expanded by swollen mesangial cells and by a complex fibrillary network which extend from the axial mesangium at the glomerular vascular pole down to the peripheral mesangial stalks that connect directly to the loops. However, comprehensive analysis of glomerular pathology by methods other than light microscopy indicate a quantitative as well as a qualitative change in the mesangium. Expansion of the mesangial matrix is better shown by ultrastructural evidence of encroachment of the capillary

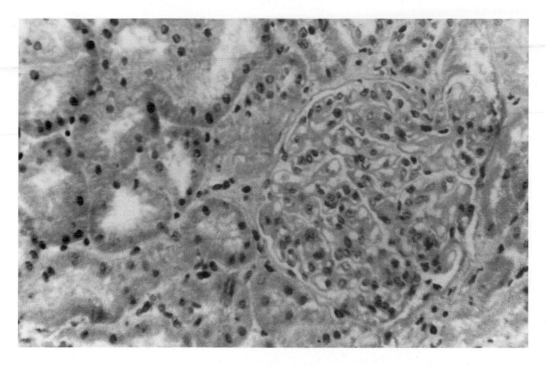

Figure 7–3. Example of a glomerulus with mild lesions of preeclampsia and with apparent pouting. The glomerular tuft is mildly enlarged, and the capillary loops are constricted. A portion of glomerular tuft herniates into the proximal segment of the proximal convoluted tubules. (H&E; ×350)

loops by mesangial matrix and cells and also by morphometric estimates of mesangial volume. The lesions in the mesangial regions are usually focal in nature. However, approximately 8% of the cases associated with severe disease manifest a generalized dilation of the mesangium and distortion of the capillary loops.[14]

Hypertrophy of the visceral glomerular epithelial cells (podocytes) is more appreciated in biopsies performed during pregnancy and also in clinically severe preeclampsia. The epithelial cells are often distended by clear vacuoles or large hyaline, eosinophilic droplets, which are also present but to a lesser extent in the peripolar glomerular cells, in some mesangial cells, and in the epithelial cells lining the proximal renal tubules (Fig. 7–4). As will be detailed later in the electron microscopy section of this chapter, the major components of the intracellular droplets are IgM, fibrin, and albumin.[21] Speculation regarding the nature of the intracellular droplets has vacillated between a secretory process vs. clearing of immunoglobulins and other proteins that leak into damaged glomeruli. Overall, more clinical and histologic evidence support the latter view. These reactive vacuolated epithelial cells are concentrated around segments of the glomerular tufts with ample subendothelial deposits of plasma proteins. Similar hyperplastic and reactive changes occur in the visceral epithelium in a variety of renal diseases, e.g., focal segmental glomerulosclerosis, HIV-associated glomerulosclerosis, collapsing glomerulopathy,

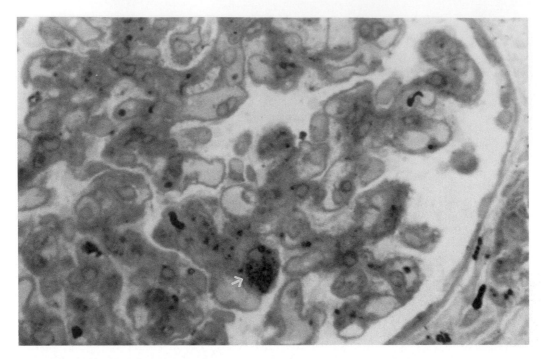

Figure 7–4. Portion of a glomerulus from a patient with preeclampsia, showing large hyaline droplets in the podocytes. (Toluidine blue; ×600)

and lupus glomerulonephritis, all of which have proteinuria and structural evidence of glomerular damage as common denominators. On the other hand, when proteinuria is present without apparent structural damage, as in minimal change disease, the visceral epithelium does not exhibit the large intracytoplasmic hyaline droplets, despite showing features of hypertrophy and cytoplasmic vacuolization. Thus, hypertrophy of the glomerular podocytes and accumulation of protein transport droplets should not be viewed as unique to preeclamptic nephropathy but a manifestation of the heavy proteinuria combined with glomerular basement membrane injury.

A second, but far more rare change in the glomerular epithelium is the development of epithelial crescents. We identified epithelial crescents in 15% of the biopsies from patients with atypical, severe preeclampsia.[8,19] The etiology of crescent formation in this disorder remains largely unknown, but is presumably caused by localized ischemia and necrosis of the capillary loops. Infarcted or preinfarcted glomeruli are extremely rare in biopsies with classic preeclampsia lesions. Likewise, glomerular thrombi are not common, but if found, one should exclude the presence of lupus anticoagulant or coagulopathy associated with the "HELLP" syndrome (see Chap. 10).

Focal Segmental Glomerulosclerosis and Preeclampsia. Sheehan and Lynch[1] were the first to observe focal fibrosis of one or two lobules of the glomerular tuft

in occasional glomeruli in postmortem samples. In a later report, Sheehan[14] reiterated the finding of focal glomerular fibrosis in a series of renal biopsies; however, he cautioned against interpreting this process as evidence for a progressive disease secondary to preeclampsia, mainly because he recognized similar lesions with the same incidence in the normal control population of gravid patients who died due to conditions other than preeclampsia. Shortly after, other investigators reported the presence of a lesion similar to that of focal and segmental glomerulosclerosis in a subset of their biopsies and referred to this finding as "de novo focal segmental glomerulosclerosis."[21-23] The incidence of focal segmental glomerulosclerosis in biopsies with otherwise typical changes of preeclampsia varied between 6 and 25% in several ethnic populations, while the number of glomeruli that displayed segmental sclerosis ranged from 10 to 60% in the different series. The affected segments of the glomerular tuft commonly displayed localized occlusion or near complete occlusion of the capillary loops by voluminous intracapillary mesangial–endothelial cells and usually foam cells. The podocyte covering this segment became enlarged and often packed with large protein resorption droplets. Localized hyaline deposits (hyalinosis), splitting of the glomerular basement membrane (double-contour), and synechia are occasionally found. It has to be taken into account that the described lesions of focal segmental glomerulosclerosis are almost identical to the generalized changes of preeclampsia nephropathy except for the segmental localization and accentuation of the morphologic alterations. Such a histopathologic picture is analogous to the "early cellular lesion" or the "glomerular tip lesion" variants of focal segmental glomerulosclerosis (FSGS).[24]

Perhaps the most unsettled issue during the late 1990s, is how to interpret the histologic pattern that resembles FSGS when it is observed for the first time in the setting of rather typical preeclamptic nephropathy, and, accordingly, whether to consider patients who develop this combination of lesions as a unique clinicopathologic group that should be distinguished from classic preeclampsia patients. There are two possible explanations for the mechanisms leading to the development of FSGS in these biopsies. One theory recognizes focal sclerosis in biopsies with preeclampsia as a true pathologic change induced by the hemodynamic stress of pregnancy in a manner similar to hyperfiltration-induced focal segmental glomerulosclerosis, while the second considers the lesion of focal sclerosis a mere histologic aberration caused by localized accentuation of the capillary loop lesions and endothelial damage. The distinction between these two mechanisms is essential because of the possible grave clinical implications on the long-term outcome of the disease. Unlike preeclampsia, FSGS is a progressive renal disease that carries a relatively high risk for renal failure. Thus far, there is no evidence to indicate that women with the histologic lesions of FSGS and preeclampsia appear any different from those without glomerulosclerosis. The rate of resolution of proteinuria and hypertension in patients with FSGS preeclampsia appears similar to that in patients without glomerulosclerosis; albeit, it takes the former group of patients

a longer time to achieve clinical remission. Moreover, recurrence of gestational hypertension, characteristic of primary renal diseases including FSGS, is not a feature of preeclampsia. Evidence for the benign course of patients who develop histologic lesions of FSGS in the background of preeclampsia was presented in separate studies by Nochy et al.[25] and Nagai et al.[26] Both studies demonstrated that complete remission of the proteinuria and hypertension following delivery was the rule for the preeclamptic patients with histologic FSGS, without recurrence of proteinuria or gestational hypertension in any of the subsequent pregnancies. In contrast, patients with FSGS, although they may present at the time of pregnancy with a clinical picture that can be confused with preeclampsia, have the postpartum course of their primary renal disease which is characterized by persistent or recurrent proteinuria and hypertension, frequent relapses with subsequent pregnancies, and eventually progression to chronic renal insufficiency in the majority of the patients.[27]

Hemodynamic factors known to be associated with the appearance of FSGS in nongravid patients, including glomerular morphologic and functional hypertrophy, and glomerular capillary hypertension, have been suggested as perhaps causal in the evolution of FSGS during preeclampsia (i.e., peripheral blood pressure is elevated, and glomerular filtration rate, though reduced, is still usually above nonpregnant values). In normal pregnancy, the increments in the glomerular filtration are largely a direct result of increased renal plasma blood flow. Physiologic glomerular adaptation and hyperfiltration during pregnancy do not appear to be accompanied by intraglomerular hypertension and is nondamaging to the kidneys, even in repetitive pregnancies, at least in animal models. Studies measuring renal permselectivity to neutral dextrans, combined with mathematical modeling suggest the glomerular capillary pressure is not increased in human gestation (see Chap. 8 for both human and animal studies). In preeclampsia, the renal blood flow and subsequently the glomerular filtration rate (GFR) are often reduced compared to the normal gestational levels, probably due, in part, to the systemic vasoconstriction, reduced plasma volume, and decreased caliber of the glomerular capillaries. Lafayette et al.,[28] using morphometric techniques, have recently demonstrated that the decrements in the GFR in preeclampsia may parallel the density of subendothelial deposits and the mesangial interposition, establishing a correlation between the functional and the histologic alterations. Using modeling techniques, these researchers also estimate the ultrafiltration coefficient is decreased 37% compared to normal nonpregnant controls. Such data would suggest that glomerular capillary pressure will be increased, which could dispose the patient's kidneys to the development of FSGS. In general, preliminary data from morphometric studies indicate the absence of significant differences in either glomerular size or glomerular filtration surface area between biopsies with preeclampsia alone and those with preeclampsia lesions of FSGS. Nochy et al.[25] demonstrated a trend toward increased glomerular volume when FSGS was present in combination with preeclampsia rather than in preeclampsia alone, but the difference was not statisti-

cally significant. On the other hand, compared to gravid patients with primary FSGS, the glomerular filtration surface area in preeclampsia is significantly decreased.[27]

We identified FSGS in 35% of 20 consecutive postpartum biopsies, demonstrating the histopathologic lesions of preeclampsia.[29] Patients with combined lesions of FSGS and preeclampsia were predominantly African Americans (80%), averaging 23 years of age, who had a higher incidence of hypertension and nephrotic range proteinuria compared to patients with pure preeclampsia lesions on biopsy. The histologic lesions of FSGS were apparent in 2 to 10% of the glomeruli (Fig. 7–5) in the affected biopsies, which showed localized glomerular scarring, capillary collapse and capsular adhesions. Of interest, evidence of arteriosclerosis and interstitial fibrosis were identified in 100% and 86% of the biopsies with FSGS, respectively. While only one-third of biopsies with classic preeclampsia alone had mild interstitial or vascular-sclerosing lesions (Table 7–1), all biopsies with FSGS and preeclampsia had evidence of chronic-sclerosing lesions in the interstitium and/or the arteries. The dominance of focal glomerular scarring in black patients who inherently are at risk for nephrosclerosis even at a young age, together with the

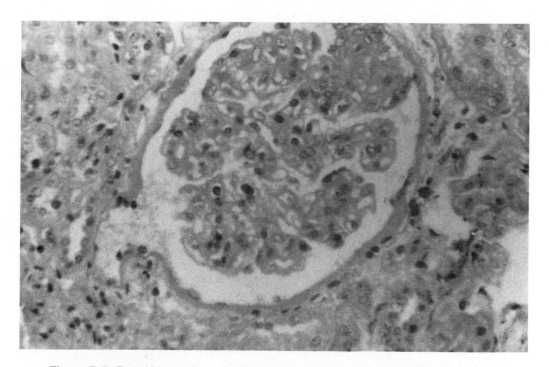

Figure 7–5. Renal biopsy from a patient with early onset preeclampsia, showing focal segmental glomerulosclerosis (FSGS). There is segmental effacement of the tuft architecture with increased extracellular matrix, loss of capillary loops, and adhesion to Bowman's capsule. This pattern of segmental glomerulosclerosis was frequently recognized in our series in association with interstitial fibrosis or arterial sclerosis. Note that it shows more mesangial sclerosis than the cellular variant of FSGS, commonly described in the other studies of preeclampsia and FSGS. (H&E; ×350)

TABLE 7-1. CLINICAL AND HISTOLOGIC CHARACTERISTICS OF 20 WOMEN WTH ATYPICAL PREECLAMPSIA

Patient	Age	Race	Parity	Onset of Hypertension (gestational wk)	Indication for Renal Biopsy	Biopsy Performed (postpartum day)	Total No. of Glomeruli	PIN	FSGS (%)	Global Sclerosis (%)	Cellular Crescents (%)	Tubulo-interstitial Changes	Vascular Lesions
1	28	B	M	32	Severe preeclampsia (HELLP syndrome)—persistent postpartum hypertension	15	3	+	—	—	—	—	—
2	27	W	M	25	Early onset of severe preeclampsia with HELLP syndrome	11	17	++	—	6	—	+	++
3	26	B	M	32	Hypertension with marked nephrotic proteinuria	10	26	++	8	8	—	+	++
4	32	B	M	28	Early onset of severe preeclampsia	7	29	++	—	—	—	+	—
5	19	B	N	34	Persistent postpartum hypertension	11	33	++	7	—	9	+	++
6	19	W	M	34	Eclampsia and persistent postpartum hypertension	7	20	++	4	—	4	+	+
7	20	B	N	29	Early onset of preeclampsia	6	37	++	—	—	—	—	—
8	30	W	N	33	Persistent postpartum hypertension	21	4	++	—	—	—	—	—
9[a]	18	B	N	19	Early onset of preeclampsia and eclampsia	5	66	+++	2	3	—	+	NA

10[a]	19	B	M	24	Early onset of severe preeclampsia	8	113	++	—	—	—	+	+
11	22	B	M	22	Early onset of severe preeclampsia	10	17	+	—	—	—	—	—
12	21	B	N	33	Persistent postpartum hypertension	6	19	—	—	—	—	—	—
13	18	B	N	32	Severe preeclampsia	5	5	++	10	—	20	+	NA
14	25	B	N	28	Early onset of nephrotic syndrome and hypertension	7	50	+++	—	—	—	—	—
15	18	B	N	37	Postpartum hypertension and seizures in a diabetic patient	9	30	+	—	—	—	—	—
16	15	B	M	28	Early onset preeclampsia	6	13	++	—	8	—	—	+
17	18	B	M	32	Severe hypertension and nephrotic proteinuria	5	20	++	—	—	—	+	+
18	23	B	M	27	Early onset of severe preeclampsia	6	20	+++	10	—	—	+	+
19	36	W	N	34	Persistent postpartum hypertension and nephrotic range proteinuria	4	36	++	10	—	10	+	+
20	17	B	N	39	Persistent postpartum hypertension	7	20	+	—	—	—	—	+

[a] Patients 9 and 10 are the same women biopsied after successive hypertensive gestations.

B = black; W = white; N = nullipara; M = multipara; HELLP syndrome = hemolysis, elevated liver enzymes and low platelet counts; PIN = pregnancy-induced nephropathy (i.e., preeclampsia changes only; glomerular capillary swelling +, ++, +++ = mild, moderate and severe respectively); FSGS = focal segmental glomerulosclerosis; NA = inadequate material for diagnosis.

Reprinted, with permission, from Gaber LW, Spargo BH: Pregnancy-induced nephropathy: The significance of focal segmental glomerulosclerosis. Am J Kidney Dis 1987;9:317–323.

prevalence of vascular and interstitial lesions in biopsies exhibiting FSGS, led us to conclude that the presence of FSGS in the preeclampsia biopsies in this series of patients was precipitated by underlying nephrosclerosis and is not a feature or a complication of preeclampsia.

Coexistence of arteriolar sclerosis and preeclampsia lesions in young primigravidas has also been identified in earlier studies with an incidence close to that seen in our patients. In 1960, Pollak and Nettles[2] biopsied 50 patients with gestational hypertension to find isolated nephrosclerosis in 20% of the cases, while 70% of the biopsies showed lesions of preeclampsia alone or in combination with arteriolar sclerosis (23%). The mean age of the patients with the combined lesions was 23 years, but unlike the patients in our study, the majority of the patients in the study by Pollak and Nettles were white. Another study by Smythe et al.[30] identified preeclampsia superimposed on arteriolar vascular disease in 17% of the patients, averaging 18 years of age, and biopsied for gestational hypertension. The authors, however, did not elaborate on the glomerular findings other than to indicate whether endotheliosis was present or absent. Therefore, the incidence of focal glomerulosclerosis or interstitial fibrosis in this cohort is unknown. Clinicopathologic studies, including those reporting FSGS in the biopsies, confirm the reversibility of the histologic and the clinical manifestations of preeclampsia and resolution of proteinuria, asserting the general consensus that preeclampsia is a reversible disease process. A large study conducted at the University of Chicago analyzed the clinical and the pathologic characteristics of a cohort of 176 gravidas biopsied because of suspected preeclampsia. The researchers were also able to follow the remote prognosis of about half of these subjects. Women who had preeclampsia as nulliparas had a remote prevalence of hypertension which was similar to that expected from age and race matched population surveys. Only six patients with clinically atypical preeclampsia developed latent hypertension. Similar findings were reported by Chesley et al. in their follow-up of 267 patients.[11] In the studies of Fisher et al.[3] and Chesley et al.,[11] as well as another large study by Bryans,[31] the incidence of remote hypertension in nulliparous gravidas presenting with typical preeclampsia or eclampsia was similar to that in the general population.

In summary, localized lesions resembling those of FSGS are identified in approximately 20% of patients with the clinical diagnosis of preeclampsia. To date, there is no evidence that this subset of patients will have any long-term renal dysfunction, albeit, they may present with atypical or severe preeclampsia. There are two existing interpretations of this change; one considers this lesion as "de novo FSGS" and the second recognizes the association of FSGS with preexisting subclinical nephrosclerosis. The implication that a secondary form of FSGS develops in patients with preeclampsia carries serious health and social consequences for the patients because of the adverse course of FSGS. Therefore, it is vital that terms such as "de novo focal segmental glomerulosclerosis" should not be used until enough follow-up data on this subset of patients are available. Future studies should distinguish biopsies with lesions that resemble the early cellular type of FSGS, which may be a localized accentuation of the rather classic diffuse lesions of preeclampsia from biopsies that show segmental sclerosis and scarring of the glomerular tuft. Furthermore, interstitial and vascular lesions indicative of premature nephrosclerosis should be looked for and quantified.

Tubules and Interstitium. Tubulo-interstitial lesions in preeclampsia are infrequent and nonspecific.[1,8] Intracytoplasmic hyaline droplets similar to those forming in the glomerular epithelial cells can also be found in the epithelial cells of the proximal convoluted tubules.[13,14] The protein transport droplets in the tubular epithelial cells are predominantly composed of fibrin and albumin. Lipid droplets are also found in the tubular epithelial cells, particularly in biopsies from patients with nephrotic syndrome. Simplification of the tubular epithelium and mild tubular dilation can be seen in the most severe forms of the disease. Rarely, acute tubular necrosis may develop secondary to localized ischemia of the renal cortex; some of these cases may also have evidence of glomerular ischemia in the form of massive ectasia and congestion of the capillary loops (preinfarcted glomeruli), epithelial crescents, or infarcted glomeruli. A second cause of acute tubular necrosis is hemolysis and hemoglobinuria, leading to pigmentary acute tubular necrosis. Interstitial fibrosis, atrophy of the renal tubules, or tubular drop out are not features of preeclampsia; if found in the biopsy, preexisting renal disease or nephrosclerosis should be considered.

Arteries and Juxtaglomerular Apparatus. Vascular changes in preeclampsia are more functional than structural. In vitro studies of resistance-sized arteries removed from patients with preeclampsia at the time of caesarean section demonstrate abnormalities in both contraction and relaxation when tested with pharmacologic probes.[32] Radiologic evidence has also been presented demonstrating the abnormal intrarenal vasculature in preeclampsia.[33,34] The finding of hyaline arteriolosclerosis should imply the prior existence of a minor degree of nephrosclerosis regardless of the patient's age. Minor degrees of incipient nephrosclerosis in young individuals have been shown to correlate with seemingly trivial blood pressure elevations.[35] Nephrosclerosis is not only a manifestation of hypertension, but is also a process of microvascular aging that progresses over time. The evolution of arterionephrosclerosis was the focus of several epidemiologic studies that assessed the structure of the intrarenal arteries by quantitative measures in different groups of victims of violent or unexpected death. Surprisingly, measurable intimal fibrosis in the intrarenal arteries can occur in young individuals, even between the ages of 10 and 19 years, with no or trivial elevation of the arterial blood pressure. The rate of growth of the fibrous intima and hyalinosis seem to follow an exponential pattern with advancement in age, but the fastest rate of growth appears between the ages of 35 to 60 years. Gender, race, and environmental factors also influence the incidence and the rate of progression of intimal fibroplasia. Therefore, one should be alarmed to the finding of intimal fibrosis and hyalinosis in these young gravidas and should not attribute them to preeclampsia, as these changes may possibly be precursors of a hypertensive state. In this context, the focal scarring of the glomeruli in these young gravidas is theoretically part of this premature vascular aging.

Evaluation of the juxtaglomerular apparatus in these hypertensive patients has been limited by the need for special histochemical or immunohistologic techniques to properly evaluate the J–G cells and their intracellular granular products. Altchek et al.[20] reported hyperplasia and degranulation of the epithelioid J–G cells on PAS-stained sections of biopsies with lesions of preeclampsia. More recent studies using specific antirenin antisera and ultrastructural evaluation show a diminished number of renin-containing cells and irregular intracellular distribution of the renin granules.[36,37]

Morphometric Studies

Morphometric studies of biopsies with preeclampsia concentrated on quantifying glomerular and mesangial volume. Quantitative objective measurements of glomerular size and glomerular components are particularly useful in studying the hemodynamics of preeclampsia, and the structural correlates to the functional changes. Furthermore, investigators applied morphometric techniques to explore the current controversy regarding the relationship between focal segmental glomerulosclerosis and preeclampsia. It is very apparent that more data are needed in this area, since the current morphometric studies are sparse and hard to generalize because they are limited to small groups of patients, and each is uniquely compared to pregnant or nonpregnant patients with preexisting diseases such as hypertension or FSGS.

As noted earlier, Nochy et al.[15] compared glomerular parameters in biopsy specimens showing the classic lesions of preeclampsia alone or in combination with the early lesions of FSGS, biopsies from gravid women with gestational hypertension, or biopsies from nonpregnant women presenting with isolated hematuria as normal controls. Measurements of digitized images of representative glomeruli from these biopsies disclosed the glomerular surface area in pregnancies with isolated preeclamptic nephropathy to be 21,540 μm^2 and 23,665 μm^2 if FSGS was present; both measurements were significantly higher than the control mean glomerular surface area of 17,950 μm^2 (P < 0.05). Women with essential hypertension or those manifesting de novo hypertension of late pregnancy alone, had significantly smaller glomeruli (16,800 μm^2), particularly those patients whose increased blood pressure was apparent early in pregnancy. These results confirm the glomerular hypertrophy that develops in preeclampsia but do not provide comparisons to glomerular size in uncomplicated normal pregnancy. Morphometric data also indicate an increase in mesangial matrix volume, which is more apparent in biopsies with combined FSGS and preeclampsia lesions.

Morphometric analysis of the biopsies comparing the severity of structural alterations to determinants of glomerular function disclose a strong correlation between the degree of endothelial swelling and the density of subendothelial fibrin to decrements in glomerular permeability, while the interposition of the mesangial matrix into the peripheral capillaries further curtailed the effective filtration surface.[28,38,39] These results suggest that the structural changes that develop in preeclampsia influence the intrinsic glomerular ultrafiltration capacity.

Immunohistology

Vassalli et al.[40] and Morris et al.[41] were probably the first to note the dominant fibrin deposition in glomeruli from preeclamptic patients. In both studies fibrin/fibrin-related products were detected in 80 and 100% of the biopsies, respectively, within 2 to 300 days after delivery. The most intense staining for intraglomerular fibrin was observed during the first 2 weeks following delivery. Most investigators who studied glomerular immunofluorescence in preeclampsia conclude that immunoglobulins play little or no role in the pathogenesis of the renal lesions of preeclampsia. In most reports IgM and fibrin within the glomerular capillary loops are the most commonly detected immune reactants. However, there have been some discrepancies in the reported frequency of intraglomerular fibrin in preeclampsia, and occasional reports describing immunoglobulin deposits other than IgM. Petrucco et al.[42] observed deposits of IgG and IgM and complement in 67 and 77% of the biopsies from women with preeclampsia, respectively, noting a correlation between the intensity of immunostaining and the severity of the histologic lesions. Although these researchers identified fibrin in all biopsies, they speculated such deposition was a secondary phenomenon that followed initial immune complex-mediated glomerular damage. Fisher et al.,[3] however, found intraglomerular fibrin deposition less often, as it was present in only 44% of the patients whose biopsies were subjected to immunofluorescent testing. Moreover, in over half of the cases reactive to fibrin antisera, the intensity of staining was low grade (1+ on a scale of 1 to 4).[2,3] They also noted low intensity staining of IgG and IgM in 23 and 51% of the biopsies, respectively (Table 7–2). Meanwhile, Nochy et al.[43] identified

TABLE 7–2. IMMUNOFLUORESCENCE FINDINGS IN BIOPSIES DEPICTING GLOMERULAR ENDOTHELIOSIS

	Frequency of Glomerular Deposition	
	All Cases	**Greater than 1+**
Fibrin	20 of 45	8 of 45 (18)[a]
AHG[b]	5 of 10	1 of 10 (10)
IgC	10 of 43	3 of 43 (7)
IgM	23 of 45	16 of 45 (36)
IgA	6 of 43	2 of 43 (5)
IgE	9 of 36	2 of 36 (6)
C3	8 of 40	1 of 40 (3)
C4	15 of 36	10 of 36 (28)

[a] Values in parentheses are percentages.
[b] AHG = Antihemophilic globulin.
Reprinted, with permission, from Fisher KA, Luger A, Spargo BH, Lindheimer MD: Hypertension in pregnancy: Clinical–pathological correlations and late prognosis. *Medicine* 1981;60:267–276.

codeposition of fibrin-related products and IgM in 50% of the biopsies with preeclampsia. These results do not necessarily undermine the importance of fibrin in preeclampsia or favor an immune complex-induced glomerular injury either. The discrepancies can be explained in several ways. First, the patient population in some of these studies may be heterogenous. Second, quantitative data of the ultra-structural changes support early resolution of glomerular fibrin during the first 2 weeks after delivery; therefore, timing of the biopsy may influence the results. Both fibrin and IgM glomerular deposition are secondary to glomerular injury and leakage of plasma proteins across the injured capillary wall.

Quantitative and qualitative alterations in the protein composition of the ex-tracellular matrix occur in the glomeruli, affecting the glomerular basement mem-brane and to a lesser extent, the mesangium. Alteration in the biochemical structure of the glomerular basement membrane augments the negative effect of the glomerular morphologic lesions on the glomerular filtration capacity. The bio-chemical structure of the glomerular basement membrane and the mesangium in preeclamptic nephropathy has been studied by antibodies directed against the dif-ferent matrix proteins and their integrins, using either immunofluorescence or im-munoperoxidase techniques. In 1983, Foidart et al.[44] were among the first of a hand-ful of investigators to explore the question of distribution of the extracellular matrix in hypertensive pregnancies. They demonstrated the focal accumulation of type IV collagen, laminin, and proteoglycan in the thickened segments of the glomerular basement membrane, as well as fibronectin, a protein that is exclusively localized to the mesangium in normal glomeruli. The pattern of immunostaining was also in-teresting, in that the basement membrane segments with the highest staining den-sity were not only thickened, but also disclosed a single or a bilaminar pattern of immunostaining. Fibronectin and fibrin were also localized in these severely al-tered segments. It should be noted that a comparable distribution of basement membrane patterns and fibronectin was also detected in glomeruli of patients with other types of gestational hypertension, including chronic hypertension or recur-rent gestational hypertension. Confirmation of these results came in a recent study by Shiiki et al.,[45] who detected focal accumulation of the fibrin and intrinsic base-ment membrane proteins, tenascin, and fibronectin receptors along the suben-dothelial layer of the glomerular basement membrane. Segments of the glomerular tuft with localized sclerosis exhibited increased staining for type IV collagen, laminin, fibronectin, vitronectin, and tenacin, whereas the fibronectin receptors and vitronectin receptors were greatly decreased. The patients in this study presented with nephrotic range proteinuria.

Mediators suspected of inducing glomerular injury in preeclampsia have been looked for in kidney samples by immunohistochemistry as well. Among these me-diators is endothelin$_1$ (ET$_1$), a product of the endothelial cells with a strong vaso-constricting effect and multiple hemoregulatory functions including augmentation of the sensitivity to angiotensin II. Serum levels of ET$_1$ vary in preeclamptic patients (see Chap. 6), with some reports describing elevated levels that are presumably re-lated to endothelial damage, while others fail to detect similar elevations. The expression of ET_1 in kidney samples from pregnant women with preeclamptic nephropathy or preexisting renal disease and samples from nonpregnant women with nephrotic syndrome or normal renal tissue were tested by the avidin–biotin peroxidase method.[46] Identification of ET_1 in the glomeruli of pregnant women, whether they have preeclampsia or underlying renal disease, appeared equally diminished from that in nonpregnant groups. The role of ET_1 and endothelium receptors and how they may influence vascular tone are discussed further in Chapter 8. Another vasoactive mediator evaluated in biopsy studies is renin. Intensity of its antibody staining has been reported to be decreased in the juxtaglomerular region in pregnancies with either preeclampsia or hypertensive nephrosclerosis.[47]

In summary, immunohistologic analysis of renal biopsies from gravid patients with preeclampsia disclosed the nature of the subendothelial deposits, being formed of extracellular glomerular matrix proteins and plasma-derived proteins, and affirming the localized interposition of the mesangium. The expression of vasoactive mediators in the kidneys with preeclamptic nephropathy is inconsistent, and its significance is still unclear. Diminished glomerular expression of substances such as ET_1 or renin may be the consequence of endothelial injury and exhaustion of the renin–angiotensin system, respectively, or may be a pregnancy-induced adaptation that is not unique to preeclampsia.

Electron Microscopy

The characteristic ultrastructural alterations in preeclampsia are those of endothelial hypertrophy, segmental basement membrane expansion, and accumulation of subendothelial electron-dense deposits. The endothelial cells exhibit both nonspecific features of hypertrophy as well as intracytoplasmic alterations more typical of preeclampsia. Enlargement of the endothelial cells can be extremely variable from one glomerulus to the other and among the capillary loops within the same glomerulus. Pronounced hypertrophy of the endothelium leads to complete or near complete occlusion of the capillary lumen, obliteration of the endothelial fenestrae, and extensive folding of the cell surface, producing a complex arcade network on the surface and pseudovesicles (Fig. 7–6). The cytoplasm is rich in mitochondria, enlarged vacuolated lysosymes, and vacuoles of different morphologic appearance.[48] Clear, membrane-bound, lipid vacuoles are one type that is particularly abundant in the glomerular endothelial cells but can also be detected in the mesangial cells. On occasion myelin figures are present, which are caused by intracellular accumulation of saturated proteins. Excessive intracellular fat deposition leads to displacement of the cytoplasmic organelles, as the entire cell appears to be filled with fat droplets (foam cells) (Fig. 7–7). Other nonspecific clear vacuoles are created by massive enlargement and vacuolization of the cellular organelles, mainly the lysosomes and mitochondria as well as pseudovacuoles formed by the exaggerated cytofols. Farqhuar[49] and Spargo et al.[10] separately reported the dominance of the endothelial cell swelling and vacuolization and their obstructive effect on the capillary endothelium. Spargo and associates proposed the term "glomerular capillary

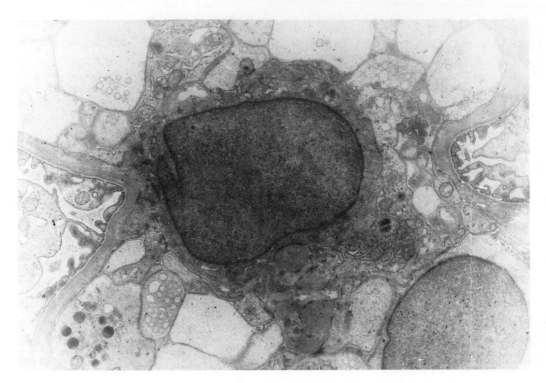

Figure 7–6. Electron micrograph of a segment of the glomerular tuft depicting enlarged obstructing endothelial cells with excessive folding of the cell membrane and formation of pseudocysts. (*Courtesy of Ben Spargo, MD, University of Chicago.*)

endotheliosis" to describe this pronounced form of endothelial hypertrophy which represents an extreme degree of cellular reactive changes. These endothelial reactive changes are characteristic of, but not unique to, preeclampsia and have been described in a variety of other related hypertensive disorders in pregnancy. Similar reactive endothelial cell changes have been found in renal biopsies from gravid women with severe abdominal bleeding secondary to abruptio placentae, hydatidiform mole, and ectopic pregnancy.[50]

The second most significant ultrastructural finding is the expansion of the subendothelial zone by acellular deposits which are composed of plasma-derived proteins, as proven by immunofluorescent studies (Fig. 7–8). These deposits are usually homogeneous and electron-dense and may contain fibrils that are most likely the product of organization of the fibrin. Rarely, typical fibrin tactoids with periodicity characteristic of fibrin are found within these subendothelial deposits, in addition to their presence in the urinary space and inside of the epithelial cytoplasmic vacuoles. The lamina densa is never altered in preeclampsia, but the lamina interna rara may be expanded by flocculent material similar to the ultrastructural lesions characterized by thrombotic microangiopathy present in hemolytic uremic syndrome, thrombotic thrombocytopenic purpura (TTP), and postpartum acute renal failure. Endothelial cell injury, central to preeclampsia and thrombotic

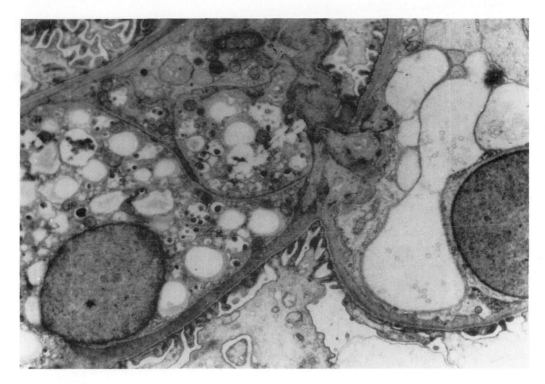

Figure 7–7. Electron micrograph of a segment of the glomerular capillary loop, showing exuberant swelling of the endothelial cell cytoplasm and intracytoplasmic membrane-bound lipid droplets, a few with myelin figures. (*Courtesy of Ben Spargo, MD, University of Chicago.*)

microangiopathy, allows the escape of plasma proteins into the subendothelial zone and the lamina interna, appearing as flocculent deposits accumulating under the endothelium. This process is much more profound in biopsies with microangiopathies rather than preeclampsia to the point where the endothelium becomes detached and widely separated from the basement membrane. Differentiation between severe preeclampsia and thrombotic microangiopathy in gravidas with HELLP syndrome by ultrastructural features may be difficult, but the presence of thrombosis, arteriolopathy, and a massive expansion of the subendothelial layer are more in favor of a pregnancy-associated thrombotic microangiopathy (TTP or postpartum acute renal failure), depending on the clinical circumstances.

Expansion of the mesangial areas and migration of mesangial matrix and cells toward the capillary loops, separating the endothelium from the underlying basement membrane, is best illustrated by ultrastructural examination. Interposition of the mesangium exaggerates the widening of the glomerular capillary wall and the narrowing of the vascular spaces. The combination of endothelial swelling and mesangial interposition occasionally results in occlusion and stretching of the capillary loops which acquire a "cigar-shaped" appearance (Fig. 7–9). Some cases demonstrate mesangial deposits of fat droplets in the mesangial cells and matrix similar to those detected in the loop endothelium.

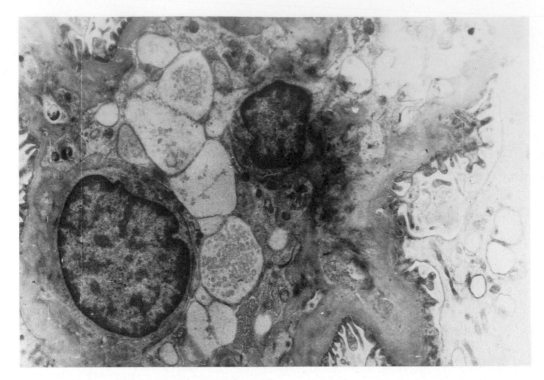

Figure 7–8. Electron micrograph of a glomerular capillary loop, showing inconspicuous dense deposits along the subendothelial lamina of the basement membrane. Note that the endothelial cell lining this capillary possesses exuberant cytofolds and pseudovacuoles. (*Courtesy of Ben Spargo, MD, University of Chicago.*)

The epithelial cells show hypertrophy of the cytoplasmic organelles, vacuolation, and accumulation of hyaline droplets. Immunogold-labeling technique reveals that protein droplets in the epithelium are composed of an inner, dense core of fibrinogen enclosed within a less intensely stained peripheral rim rich in IgM.[21] Albumin was randomly identified within the droplets without any particular zonal distribution. Effacement of the epithelial podocytes is described as focal, regardless of the level of proteinuria.

Involution and Reversibility of Lesions of Preeclamptic Nephropathy

The general consensus is that the lesions of preeclampsia disappear gradually after delivery, without inducing any permanent damage to the kidney. Regression of some of the glomerular lesions can be seen as early as the first week postpartum.[1,13,51-53] Repeat biopsies performed within months and up to 2 years after the initial diagnosis of preeclampsia show complete resolution of the glomerular lesions, except for a few reports of persistent glomerular adhesions or vascular pathology in the repeat biopsies. These latter findings are suspect as they do not rule out preexisting renal pathology. The restrictive indications for renal biopsy in

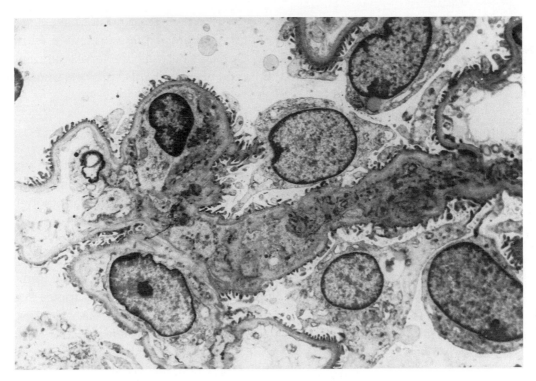

Figure 7–9. Electon micrograph of a streched mesangial area leading into partially obstructed capillary loops. The podocytes are enlarged, but there is an effacement of the foot processes. (*Courtesy of Ben Spargo, MD, University of Chicago.*)

gravid patients, selects patients with clinically atypical disease for biopsy, who usually have a high incidence of underlying kidney disease.

The time table for regression of preeclampsia lesions is not clearly defined, but it appears from comparing biopsies before and after labor that the lesion most likely to disappear in the first week postpartum is the subendothelial fibrin. Substantial amounts of subendothelial electron-dense deposits accumulate in the capillary loops during pregnancy, strongly correlating with the degree of impairment of glomerular permeability, while the deposits are rare in the postpartum biopsies.[38] In contrast, foam cells are more commonly identified in the postpartum biopsies, linking these cells to the healing stage. The volume of the glomerular endothelial cells, the frequency of cellular swelling, and mesangial interposition are similar for biopsies before or after delivery. The longest reported time for persistence of cellular swelling was 2 years. Studies of remote cardiovascular prognosis of women who developed preeclampsia are in accord with the reversibility of the renal lesions.[3,11,31] The controversial FSGS-like lesion that appears during preeclampsia resolves after delivery, as discussed earlier. Reports of persistent renal damage following preeclampsia should be carefully evaluated. The possibility that the glomerulosclerosis, adhesions, and tubulo-interstitial lesions had antedated the pregnancy should be considered. In fact, some reports describe an extremely high percentage of globally scarred glomeruli which could not have developed over a period of a few months without the patients having presented with a rapidly progressive renal failure.[54,55] The discrepancy between the level of chronicity in these biopsies and the clinical presentation of the patients supports preexisting renal damage.

Indications for Renal Biopsy in Pregnancy

Evaluation of renal biopsies performed during pregnancy or the immediate puerperium have enhanced our understanding of the pathology and pathophysiology immensely. Most were performed at a time when clinician–investigators thought that biopsy interpretation would influence their management of the gestation and/or produce information of prognostic value to the patient in regard to future pregnancies. This has not proven to be the case and currently there are very few indications for the performance of a renal biopsy during pregnancy or in the immediate puerperium. While risks of renal biopsy of pregnant women now appear similar to those of nonpregnant subjects, patients with preeclampsia may have additional risks due to their labile, and at times, hectic hypertension, and to the coagulation abnormalities. In fact, pregnancy was once considered a relative contraindication to biopsy owing to earlier, albeit anecdotal, reports of excessive bleeding and other complications, at a time when the majority of biopsies were performed in relation to the hypertensive complications of gestation.

Our own recommendations are as follows: Biopsy should be considered when there is sudden deterioration of renal function and no obvious cause is present. This is due to the belief that certain forms of rapidly progressive glomerulonephritis, when diagnosed early, may respond to aggressive therapeutic regimens including pulse steroids, chemotherapy, and perhaps plasma exchange. Another indication is symptomatic nephrotic syndrome presenting prior to gestational week 32. Even at this point some might consider a therapeutic trial of steroids, but we prefer to determine first whether the lesion is likely to respond to steroids before subjecting the gravida to high-dose prednisone. On the other hand, proteinuria alone, even in the nephrotic range, in a normotensive woman with well-preserved renal function who has neither marked hypoalbuminemia nor intolerable edema, would lead us to examine the patient at more frequent intervals and defer the biopsy until the postpartum period. This is because prognosis is determined primarily by the level of renal function and the presence or absence of hypertension rather than the nature of the renal lesion. A similar view is taken in the management of pregnancies with symptomatic hematuria alone, when neither stone nor tumor is suggested on ultrasonographic examination. The reason why renal biopsies are not performed after gestational week 32 is that at this stage the pregnancy will end successfully in any case, the decision to terminate the gestation is often made quickly and independent of biopsy results.

With the above limitations on renal biopsy, it should be obvious why so few procedures are performed or indicated when gestation is complicated by preeclampsia. Decisions to end the pregnancy are not based on the biopsy, there being a host of biochemical and other tests to monitor maternal well being. The remote prognosis of preeclampsia is relatively benign, and in most nulliparas the disorder does not repeat. Under such circumstances, the risks outweigh benefits and preclude the procedure. Thus as we approach the year 2000, most reports of renal biopsy associated with preeclampsia seem to be focused on women with severe or atypical disease, as it is no longer ethical to suggest biopsies for patients with more routine forms of the disorder.

THE LIVER

Clinically evident liver disease in preeclampsia is detected in only a minority of patients, usually those with severe disease, but evidence of subclinical hepatic involvement is present in over 70% of patients diagnosed with the disorder.[56] Patients with severe preeclampsia and liver abnormalities are at risk for developing hepatic rupture and fatal intraabdominal bleeding. However, the prevalence of microscopic liver disease in preeclampsia may not be as infrequent as previously thought. Laparoscopic examination of the liver surface at the time of caesarean section in a random sample of women with preeclampsia disclosed varying degrees of subcapsular hemorrhage from punctate hemorrhage to subcapsular hematoma in almost all of the patients (Fig. 7–10).[36]

Gross Description

Visually the liver appeared normal in 40% of the preeclamptic–eclamptic women autopsied by Sheehan and Lynch or their associates.[1] Still, as described below, microscopic pathology was to be found in one-third of these cases. Also noted were occasional petechiae either on the surface or in sections (20%), but in a large number of instances (40%), the petechiae were confluent or obvious infarcts were present. Sheehan and Lynch[1] also described subcapsular hematomas which on occasion had ruptured into the peritoneal cavity and were given as the proximal cause of death. Their series, however, differed from that of the laparoscopic experience of Dani et al.,[57] who noted that hematomas were unusual. More surprising, such hemorrhages were more apt to occur in multiparas.

Microscopic Findings

Sheehan and Lynch[1] describe two characteristic microscopic lesions in their autopsy material. One is hemorrhage into the hepatic cellular columns at their periportal bases, the hepatocytes pushed up in their stromal sleeves but not necrotic. They noted that the hemorrhage was replaced with fibrin, beginning 3 hours after the convulsion and completed at 18 hours, unless the lesion was "frozen" within the infarct. These periportal hemorrhages were present in 70% of women dying after eclampsia, but only 30% of autopsies on preeclamptics who had not convulsed

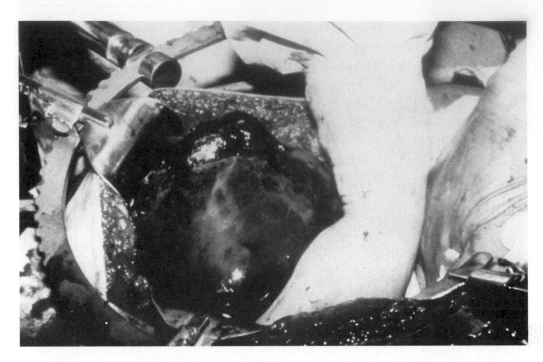

Figure 7–10. Gross appearance of the liver of a patient with preeclampsia and hepatic complications. At exploratory laparotomy the liver surface shows numerous petechiae and a subcapsular hematoma. (*Courtesy of Baha M. Sibai, MD, University of Tennessee, Memphis.*)

revealed such findings. The second lesion highlighted by Sheehan and Lynch was infarction. These were said to present later than the periportal hemorrhages, were variable in extent, and were attributed to severe vasospasm.

Liver biopsy studies concur with the autopsy findings described above, and extend them by noting considerable pathology in women deemed to have less severe forms of preeclampsia. In the study of Dani et al.,[57] performed during laparoscopy at caesarean section, there were intracellular fatty changes in all patients, irrespective of the clinical severity of preeclampsia. The hemorrhage was not related to either the amount of microvesicular fatty change or to the presence of hepatocellular necrosis. Other biopsy findings when preeclampsia was associated with abnormal liver enzymes were hemorrhagic and necrotizing lesions in the liver that seemed to begin at the periportal zone and expanded with increasing severity of the disease, very similar to changes described earlier by Sheehan and Lynch. The histopathology of the liver in preeclampsia includes focal, periportal hemorrhage and sinusoidal fibrin deposition, with varying degrees of hepatocellular fatty change and necrosis. Intraparenchymal hemorrhage and subcapsular hematomas usually develop in the right lobe of the liver in severe cases. Focal areas of ischemic hepatic necrosis can also be seen in severe disease, while confluent multilobular necrosis leading to hepatic infarction and rupture are fortunately rare.

The macro- and microvesicular fatty changes resemble the histopathology of acute fatty liver of pregnancy; this histologic similarity, in addition to the similarities in the clinical features and the etiology of both diseases, supports the possibility that preeclampsia and acute fatty liver of pregnancy are different manifestations or stages of the same disease.

THE BRAIN

The pathophysiology of the central nervous system in preeclampsia–eclampsia is highlighted in Chapter 5. They range from visual disturbances (scotoma), hyperreflexia, severe headache, the convulsions of eclampsia, transient cortical blindness, and cerebral hemorrhage. Lateralizing neurologic signs or symptoms unrelated to hemorrhage are rare, anecdotal, and point to causes other than preeclampsia. The pathogeneses of the cerebral pathology are disputed. They include vasospasm, leading to ischemia, and increased cerebral perfusion pressure and/or perfusion, secondary to the severity of hypertension, especially when it exceeds the autoregulatory threshold. The latter would be akin to what occurs in nonpregnant patients with hypertensive encephalopathy. Still another theory ascribes pathogenesis to the coagulopathy of preeclampsia, i.e., infiltration of the vascular wall with fibrinoid material leading to focal edema, thrombosis, and rupture. These topics are beyond the scope of this chapter. Of interest, is a growing literature which is utilizing noninvasive technology including computed tomographic scanning, magnetic resonance imaging, and Doppler ultrasound to gain insight into the cerebral pathophysiology and pathology of preeclampsia–eclampsia. These subjects are discussed further in Chapters 5 and 17.

Gross and Microscopic Descriptions

In the autopsy series of Sheehan and Lynch[1] the brain was usually firm, and its weight was not increased. There was little or no evidence of edema, which led the authors to conclude that edema was a late and even postseizure event, i.e., not a cause of the eclamptic convulsion. The major findings were those of cerebral hemorrhages, not surprisingly present more often if the subject expired within 48 hours of an eclamptic fit (60%). Cerebral softening was another feature in their descriptions. The authors classified the hemorrhages into eight types (pia-arachnoid, cortical petechia, multiple focal softenings or petechia in the white matter or midbrain, subcortical hemorrhages, medium-sized hemorrhages in the outer white matter, large hemorrhage in the white matter, hemorrhage into basal ganglia, and hemorrhage into the pons). All this seems to underscore the protean manifestations of the preeclampsia syndrome, and gives little insight to pathogenesis.

Histologic features suggest that the naked eye observation of petechia relates to vascular disturbances producing local ischemia. Numerous microscopic hemorrhages are present, some diffusely into brain substance, without forming ring hemorrhages. Others are confined to the Virchow–Robin spaces. In some instances the precapillaries and capillaries are distended apparently in stasis, while in other instances precapillaries are thrombosed, many consisting of solid fibrin which occludes the lumen. These thrombi are always in close proximity to the hemorrhages. Sheehan and Lynch have produced a series of outstanding microphotographs and their monograph bears review.[1] Finally, pituitary necrosis was observed in 8% of the brain necropsies. This compares with the presence of such pathology in 40% of women dying as a result of placental abruption.

CONCLUSION

This chapter reviewed the pathologic changes associated with preeclampsia–eclampsia in the kidney, liver, and brain, organs vital to maternal well being. Lesions have also been described in other organs including the adrenal glands, intestines, and heart; they tend to be minor, appear nonspecific, and their relationships to preeclampsia–eclampsia, or other preterminal complications, are often obscure. The pathology of the placenta, the "fetus's vital organ" is described in Chapter 11. Most of this chapter was devoted to the kidney, the organ most frequently associated with the signs and pathologic changes of the disease including proteinuria, as well as decreased glomerular filtration and urate clearance. It is also the organ where light and electron microscopy have been used to dissect the glomerular pathology of preeclampsia, where Spargo, in 1958, coined the term glomerular "endotheliosis," a lesion used by others to characterize the clinical–pathologic correlations of the disease, and later cited as one piece of evidence by those who ascribe the pathogenesis of preeclampsia to a disordered vascular endothelium.

REFERENCES

1. Sheehan HL, Lynch JB: *Pathology of Toxaemia of Pregnancy*. Baltimore: Williams & Wilkins Co; 1973; 807.*
2. Pollak VE, Nettles JB: The kidney in toxemia of pregnancy: A clinical and pathological study based on renal biopsies. *Medicine* 1960;39:469–526.
3. Fisher KA, Luger A, Spargo BH, Lindheimer MD: Hypertension in pregnancy: Clinical–pathological correlations and late prognosis. *Medicine* 1981;60:267–276.
4. Weiner CP, Bonsib SM: Relationship between renal histology and plasma antithrombin III activity in women with early onset preeclampsia. *Am J Perinatol* 1990;7:139–143.
5. Lohlein M: Zur pathogenese der nierenkrankheiten: Nephritis und nephrose mit besonderer berucksichtigung der nephropathia gravidarum. *Dtsch Med Wochenschr* 1918;44:1187–1189.
6. Bell ET: Renal lesions in the toxemias of pregnancy. *Am J Pathol* 1932;8:1–41.
7. Allen AC: *The Kidney: Medical and Surgical Diseases*. New York: Grune & Stratton; 1962.

---

* This monograph, by Sheehan and Lynch, contains over 1500 references, some of considerable historical interest.

8. Sheehan HL: Pathological lesions in the hypertensive toxaemias of pregnancy. In: CIBA *Foundation Symposium on Toxemias of Pregnancy,* London: Churchill; 1950.

9. Dieckmann WM, Potter EL, McCartney CP: Renal biopsies from patients with toxemia of pregnancy. *Am J Obstet Gynecol* 1957;73:1–16.

10. Spargo BH, McCartney C, Winemiller R: Glomerular capillary endotheliosis in toxemia of pregnancy. *Arch Pathol* 1959;13:593–599.

11. Chesley LC, Annitto JE, Cosgrove RA: Long-term follow-up study of eclamptic women, sixth periodic report. *Am J Obstet Gynecol* 1976;124:446–459.

12. Kincaid-Smith P: The similarity of lesions and underlying mechanisms in preeclampsia toxemia and postpartum renal failure. In: Kincaid-Smith P, Mathew TH, Becker EL, eds: *Glomerulonephritis: Morphology, Natural History and Treatment.* New York: John Wiley & Sons; 1973:1013.

13. Kincaid-Smith P: The renal lesion of preeclampsia revisited. *Am J Kidney Dis* 1991;17:144–148.

14. Sheehan HL: Renal morphology in preeclampsia. *Kidney Int* 1980;18:241–252.

15. Nochy D, Heudes D, Glotz D, et al: Preeclampsia associated focal and segmental glomerulosclerosis and glomerular hypertrophy with a morphometric analysis. *Clin Nephrol* 1994;42:9–17.

16. Pirani CL, Pollak VE, Lannigan R, Folli G: The renal glomerular lesions of pre-eclampsia: Electron microscopic studies. *Am J Obstet Gynecol* 1963;87:1047–1070.

17. Seymour AE, Petrucco OM, Clarkson AR, et al: Morphological evidence of coagulopathy in renal complications of pregnancy. In: Lindheimer MD, Katz AI, Zuspan FP, eds. *Hypertension in Pregnancy,* New York: John Wiley & Sons; 1976:139–153.

18. Tribe CR, Smart GE, Davies DR, Mackenzie JC: A renal biopsy study in toxemia of pregnancy. *J Clin Pathol* 1979;32:681–692.

19. Gaber LW, Spargo BH, Lindheimer MD: The nephrology of preeclampsia–eclampsia. In: Tisher CC, Brenner BM, eds. *Renal Pathology,* ed 2. Philadelphia: Lippincott; 1994;419–441.

20. Altchek A, Albright NL, Sommers SC: The renal pathology of toxemia of pregnancy. *Obstet Gynecol* 1968;31:595–607.

21. Nakajima M, Mathews D, Hewitson T, Kincaid-Smith P: Modified immunogold labelling applied to the study of protein droplets in glomerular diseases. *Virchows Arch* 1989;415:429–499.

22. Kida H, Takeda S, Yokoyama H, et al: Focal segmental glomerulosclerosis in preeclampsia. *Clin Nephrol* 1985;24:221–227.

23. Nochy D, Gaudry C, Hinglais N, et al: Can focal segmental glomerulosclerosis appear in preeclampsia? *Adv Nephrol* 1985;24:221–227.

24. Schwartz MM, Korbet SM: Primary focal segmental glomerulosclerosis: Pathology, histological variants, and pathogenesis. *Am J Kidney Dis* 1993;22:874–883.

25. Nochy D, Hinglais N, Jacquot C, et al: De novo focal segmental glomerulosclerosis in preeclampsia. *Clin Nephrol* 1986;25:116–121.

26. Nagai Y, Washizawa Y, Hirata K, et al: A renal biopsy study in preeclampsia: Clinical–pathological correlations in 20 cases. *Nippon Jinzo Gakkai* 1989;13:1179–1186.

27. Lee HS, Kim TS: A morphometric study of preeclamptic nephropathy with focal segmental glomerulosclerosis. *Clin Nephrol* 1995;44:14–21.

28. Lafayette RA, Druzin M, Sibley R, et al: Nature of glomerular dysfunction in preeclampsia. *Kidney Int* 1998;54:1240–1249 (see also Chapman A: accompanying editorial).

29. Gaber LW, Spargo BH: Pregnancy-induced nephropathy: The significance of focal segmental glomerulosclerosis. *Am J Kidney Dis* 1987;9:317–323.

30. Smythe CM, Bradham WS, Dennis EJ, et al: Renal arteriolar disease in young primiparas. *J Lab Clin Invest* 1964;63:562–573.

31. Bryans CI Jr: The remote prognosis of toxemia of pregnancy. *Clin Obstet Gynecol* 1966;9:973–990.

32. Pascoal IF, Lindheimer MD, Nalbantian-Brandt C, Umans JG: Preeclampsia selectively impairs endothelium-dependent relaxation and leads to oscillatory activity in small omental arteries. *J Clin Invest* 1998;101:464–470.

33. Aber GM: Intrarenal vascular lesions associated with preeclampsia. *Nephron* 1978; 21:297–309.

34. Richard RB, Boyd WM, Aber GM: Structural and functional changes in the renal circulation after complicated pregnancy. *Nephron* 1979;24:183–192.
35. Tracy RE, Berenson G, Wattigrey W, Barrett TJ: The evolution of benign arterionephrosclerosis from age 6 to 70 years. *Am J Pathol* 1990;136:429–439.
36. Hill PA, Fairley KF, Kincaid-Smith P, et al: Morphologic changes in the renal glomerulus and the juxtaglomerular apparatus in human preeclampsia. *J Pathol* 1988;156:291–303.
37. Nochy D, Bariety J, Camilbieri JR, et al: Diminished number of renin-containing cells in kidney biopsy samples from hypertensive women immediately postpartum: An immunomorphologic study. *Kidney Int* 1984;26:85–87.
38. Packham DK, Mathews DC, Fairley KF, et al: Morphometric analysis of pre-eclampsia in women biopsied in pregnancy and post partum. *Kidney Int* 1988;34:704–711.
39. Ishitobi F, Sagiya A, Ueda Y, et al: Morphometric analysis of the glomerular capillary area—A comparison of minimal change nephrotic syndrome, focal glomerular sclerosis, and preeclampsia. *J Pathol* 1991;165:329–336.
40. Vassalli PO, Morris RH, McCluskey RT: The pathogenic role of fibrin deposition in the glomerular lesions of toxemia of pregnancy. *J Exp Med* 1963;118:467–479.
41. Morris RH, Vassalli P, Beller FK, McCluskey RT: Immunofluorescent studies of renal biopsies in the diagnosis of toxemia of pregnancy. *Obstet Gynecol* 1964;24:32–46.
42. Petrucco OM, Thomson NM, Laurence JR, Weldon MV: Immunofluorescent studies in renal biopsies in preeclampsia. *Br Med J* 1974;1:473–476.
43. Nochy D, Birembaut P, Hinglais N, et al: Renal lesions in the hypertensive syndrome of pregnancy: Immunomorphological and ultrastructural studies in 114 cases. *Clinic Nephrol* 1980;13:155–162.
44. Foidart JM, Nochy D, Nusgens B, et al: Accumulation of several basement membrane proteins in glomeruli of patients with preeclampsia and other hypertensive syndromes of pregnancy: Possible role of renal prostaglandins and fibronectin. *Lab Invest* 1983;49:250–259.
45. Shiiki H, Nishino T, Uyama H, et al: Alterations in extracellular matrix components and integrins in patients with preeclamptic nephropathy. *Virchows Arch* 1996;427:567–573.
46. Nagai Y, Hara N, Yamaguchi S, et al: Immunohistochemical study of endothelin-1 in preeclamptic nephropathy. *Am J Kidney Dis* 1997;29:345–354.
47. Nochy D, Bariety J, Camilleri JP, et al: Diminished number of renin-containing cells in kidney biopsy samples from hypertensive women immediately postpartum: An immunomorphologic study. *Kidney Int* 1984;26:85–87.
48. Faith GC, Trump BF: The glomerular capillary wall in human kidney disease, acute glomerulonephritis: Systemic lupus erythematosus, preeclampsia–eclampsia. *Lab Invest* 1966;15:1682–1719.
49. Farquhar M: Review of normal and pathologic glomerular ultrastructures. In: *Proceedings of the 10th Annual Conference on the Nephrotic Syndrome*. New York: National Kidney Disease Foundation; 1959:2–29.
50. Gaber LW, Spargo BH, Lindheimer MD: Renal pathology in pre-eclampsia. *Clin Obstet Gynaecol* (Baillière) 1994;8:443–468.
51. Fadel H, Sabour MS, Mahran M, et al: Reversibility of the renal lesion and functional impairment in preeclampsia diagnosed by renal biopsy. *Obstet Gynecol* 1969;4:528–534.
52. Oe PL, Ooms ECM, Uttendorfsky OT, et al: Postpartum resolution of glomerular changes in edema–proteinuria–hypertensive gestosis. *Renal Physiol* 1980;3:375–379.
53. Pollak VE, Pirani CL, Kark RM, et al: Reversible glomerular lesions in toxemia of pregnancy. *Lancet* 1956;ii:59–62.
54. Heaton JM, Turner DR: Persistent renal damage following pre-eclampsia: A renal biopsy study of 13 patients. *J Pathol* 1985;147:121–126.
55. Grcevska L, Polenakovic M: Focal glomerular sclerosis (FGS)-like lesions are not rare in preeclampsia. *Clin Nephrol* 1992;38:233–235.
56. Byrd DE, Riely CA: Liver disease in preeclampsia. *Gastroenterologist* 1996;4:65–69.
57. Dani R, Mendes GS, Medeiros J deL, et al: Study of the liver changes occurring in preeclampsia and their possible pathogenetic connection with acute fatty liver of pregnancy. *Am J Gastroenterol* 1996; 91, 2:292–294.

8

Renal and Cardiovascular Alterations

Kirk P. Conrad and Marshall D. Lindheimer

Leon Chesley was among a select group of investigators who, between 1930 and 1960, pioneered the modern era of renal physiology. One of his earliest contributions, in fact, included a formula for calculating urea clearances at low urine flow rates. Thus, it was only natural that his interests in normal and pathological pregnancies focused on the kidney. Indeed, the description of renal physiology and pathophysiology in the first edition of this book was encyclopedic in scope. The authors of this chapter wish to honor Dr. Chesley by attempting to be as comprehensive as he was when we discuss the kidney, but the text will be more "traditional" when reviewing other cardiovascular changes in pregnancy.

An appreciation for the alterations in maternal renal and cardiovascular physiology, as well as volume homeostasis during normal pregnancy is a prerequisite to complete understanding, proper diagnosis, and medical management of preeclampsia. General cardiovascular and volume homeostatic adaptations to normal pregnancy are reviewed elsewhere in this book. In this chapter, the specific alterations in renal hemodynamics and glomerular filtration during normal pregnancy will be considered first. Then, the disturbances in renal hemodynamics and glomerular filtration which transpire during preeclampsia will be addressed. Although the filtration, reabsorption, and excretion of many solutes change in pregnancy, only the renal handling of uric acid and of proteins will be discussed because of their clinical significance to preeclampsia. Last, we will highlight some of the other perturbations of cardiovascular function during preeclampsia with emphasis on newer findings and concepts.

RENAL HEMODYNAMICS AND GLOMERULAR FILTRATION RATE DURING NORMAL PREGNANCY

Decreased vascular resistance of *nonreproductive* organs is one of the earliest physiologic adaptations to occur in normal pregnancy leading to a profound decrease in total peripheral vascular resistance. The kidneys make a major contribution to this reduction in total peripheral vascular resistance; a nadir in renal vascular resistance and peak in renal blood flow and glomerular filtration rate are reached by the end of the first trimester. Thus, the kidneys and presumably other nonreproductive organs of high vascular conductance vasodilate even further during early gestation, effectively serving as large "arteriovenous shunts." In turn, the reduction in total peripheral vascular resistance initiates a chain of events which ultimately results in the gestational rise of cardiac output. This early gestational rise in cardiac output *anticipates* the tremendous increase in uteroplacental blood flow, as well as the oxygen and nutrient demands of the nascent fetoplacental unit(s). Indeed, the oxygen content difference between arterial and mixed-venous blood narrows during early pregnancy in both humans and rats.[1] In summary, the reduction in vascular resistance of nonreproductive organs such as the kidney is a fundamental adaptation to pregnancy, and insight into the hormonal signals and molecular mechanisms may be particularly critical because in preeclampsia, both renal and systemic vasodilation are compromised.*

Renal Clearances of para-Aminohippurate and Inulin

The most comprehensive investigations of renal hemodynamics and glomerular filtration rate (GFR) were reported by Sims and Krantz,[2] de Alvarez,[3] Assali et al.,[4] Dunlop,[5] Roberts et al.,[6] and Chapman et al.[7] These studies are noteworthy because of their superior experimental design and methodologies, i.e., (1) the same women were serially studied during gestation and either preconception[7] or in the postpartum period;[2-6] (2) the renal clearances of para-aminohippurate (C_{PAH}) and inulin (C_{IN}), which provide measures of effective renal plasma flow (ERPF) and GFR, respectively, were determined by constant infusion technique; and (3) the potential problem of urinary tract dead space, which can lead to inadequate collection of urine, and thereby introduce error into the determination of C_{PAH} and C_{IN}, was circumvented by instigating a water diuresis and/or by irrigating the bladder after each clearance period.** Taking care to avoid dead space error is particularly important in pregnancy when the urinary tract is dilated and when the bladder may fail to drain completely.[8,9]

To facilitate comparison of the studies, data of GFR and ERPF (or RPF; RPF = ERPF/0.9) from each investigation are illustrated in Figure 8–1 with the exception of Chapman et al.[7] Because the work of Chapman et al. was particularly comprehensive, including the evaluation of renal function in women during the midfollicular phase of the menstrual cycle before conception, and then on six occa-

---

* An agriculture analogy can be used to illustrate the significance of the early increase in cardiac output during pregnancy. That is, it is more beneficial to construct canals for irrigation of new crops which stem from the Mississippi rather than the Rio Grande River.

** Although irrigation of the bladder with water and then air helps to improve urine collection, largely because of the increased risk of urinary tract infection, this procedure is currently considered to be inappropriate for research purposes. On the other hand, increasing urine flow rate by instigating a water diuresis is an acceptable and effective means to minimize urinary tract dead space error.

A

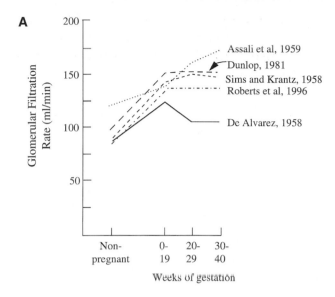

B

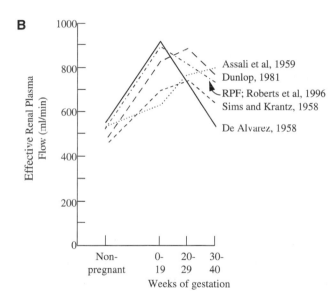

Figure 8–1. **A.** Serial studies of glomerular filtration rate (C_{IN}) during pregnancy and in the postpartum period (nonpregnant values). **B.** Serial studies of effective renal plasma flow (C_{PAH}) or renal plasma flow (RPF = ERPF/0.9) during pregnancy and in the postpartum period (nonpregnant values). See text for details. (*Modified, with permission, from Conrad KP: Renal changes in pregnancy.* Urol Ann *1992;6:313–340 and Davison JM, Dunlop W: Changes in renal hemodynamics and tubular function induced by normal human pregnancy.* Semin Nephrol *1984;4:198–207.*)

sions throughout pregnancy, these data are presented separately in Figure 8–2. Upon consideration of all of these studies, both GFR and ERPF (or RPF) markedly increased during the first half of pregnancy. Peak values were approximately 40 to 65% and 50 to 85% above nonpregnant levels for GFR and ERPF (or RPF), respectively. In general, the filtration fraction fell during the first half of gestation. The pattern of change for GFR was similar in all the studies except that of de Alvarez. In the latter, GFR declined during the last half of pregnancy toward nonpregnant levels, whereas in the other investigations, GFR remained at elevated values throughout gestation. The reason for this discrepancy is uncertain, but ERPF also fell sooner and more precipitously in the study by de Alvarez. The ERPF declined during the final stages of pregnancy in all studies except that of Assali et al. Thus,

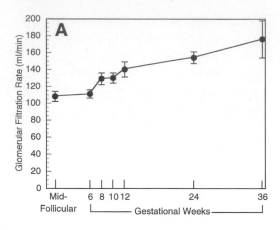

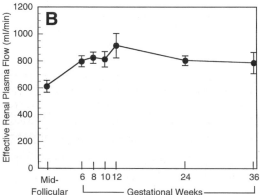

Figure 8–2. A. Serial study of glomerular filtration rate (C_{IN}) before pregnancy in the midfollicular phase of the menstrual cycle and then throughout pregnancy in 10 women. **B.** Serial study of effective renal plasma flow (ERPF) in the same women. All values during pregnancy are significantly different from those obtained during the midfollicular phase of the menstrual cycle before pregnancy. (*Adapted, with permission, from Chapman AB, Abraham WT, Zamudio S, et al: Temporal relationships between hormonal and hemodynamic changes in early human pregnancy. Kidney Int* 1998;54:2056–2063.)

with the exception of the investigation by Assali et al., filtration fraction (FF) generally rose during the final stages of pregnancy, mainly because ERPF fell while GFR was relatively well maintained. Since position (e.g., supine, sitting, etc.) may compromise renal hemodynamics and GFR during the clearance experiments by mechanical effects of the enlarged gravid uterus, particularly in late gestation (see below), Ezimokhai et al.[10] measured C_{IN} and C_{PAH} while the subjects were in the left lateral position. This posture helps prevent compression of major vessels by the gravid uterus, thus preserving perfusion of the kidneys as well as other organs. In their study, Ezimokhai and coworkers found that ERPF but not GFR significantly declined during the final stages of pregnancy (748 ± 20 to 677 ± 20 mL/min), suggesting the decline in ERPF is not solely an artifact of posture.

Elevated GFR during pregnancy is reflected by reciprocal changes in plasma concentration of creatinine,[2,6,11] which is decreased throughout gestation. The reason for this is as follows: plasma levels are determined by the clearance of creatinine from the body by glomerular filtration and there appears to be little change in the production of creatinine by skeletal muscle during gestation. Therefore, when GFR increases during pregnancy, plasma levels of creatinine are accordingly reduced. Although renal handling of urea is more complicated, it is also freely filtered by the kidney; consequently, plasma levels are lower during pregnancy, again primarily because renal clearance of urea is increased.[2,12] Average values for plasma creatinine and urea nitrogen during gestation are 0.5 and 9.0 mg/dL, respectively, compared to nonpregnant values of 0.8 and 13.0 mg/dL, respectively.[2,6,11,12] Of interest, GFR was noted to rise during pregnancy in renal allograft recipients and in women with a single kidney (albeit to a lesser degree), demonstrating a pattern of change similar to that observed in normal gravid women.[13,14] Thus, despite compensatory functional and anatomic hypertrophy, the renal allograft and single kidney can adapt even further during pregnancy and undergo gestational hyperfiltration. (Because the renal allograft is a denervated kidney, renal nerves are probably not crucial for gestational increases in GFR.) In the same vein, the kidneys of both gravid women and rats demonstrate further increases in GFR and ERPF in response to intravenous infusion of amino acids, and the percentage increases are comparable to those observed in the nonpregnant condition.[15,16]

Creatinine Clearance

The 24-hour renal clearance of endogenous creatinine (C_{CR}) is routinely used as an estimate of GFR. However, this is due to a fortuitous chain of events. Creatinine undergoes proximal tubular secretion as well as glomerular filtration, but circulating levels are overestimated because of the presence of a chromagen in plasma which is measured along with true creatinine. When GFR is normal, the two events cancel. However, when GFR falls, tubular secretion may represent a greater proportion of urinary creatinine, and the influence of the chromagen on plasma levels decreases. Under such circumstances, creatinine clearance may overestimate GFR, sometimes by 25 to 50%.[17]

Using the 24-hour C_{CR}, Davison and Noble provided evidence that GFR rises 25% by the second week postconception.[18] This investigation supports the concept that the physiologic adaptations in the renal circulation during human pregnancy are among the earliest to occur. A recent report by Chapman et al. both corroborates and extends the findings of Davison and Noble, insofar as both C_{IN} and C_{PAH} were found to be significantly increased by 4 weeks postconception (or 6 weeks after the last menstrual period), the earliest timepoint investigated (Fig. 8–2).[7]

Several investigators concurrently measured the renal clearance of inulin throughout pregnancy and in the postpartum period using the constant infusion technique, and compared these values to the 24-hour endogenous C_{CR}.[2,3,19] On balance, the 24-hour C_{CR} was not consistently greater or less than the C_{IN}. The changes in GFR during pregnancy as measured by C_{IN} and the 24-hour C_{CR} were comparable, except possibly in the last few weeks before delivery. Although 24-hour C_{CR} declined at 35 to 38 weeks' gestation in the study by Davison and Hytten, the short-term C_{CR}, as assessed by constant infusion of creatinine in the same study, did not decrease and was similar to C_{IN}.[19] This last finding suggested that the renal handling of creatinine did not change at this stage of pregnancy, and substantiated the C_{CR} as a valid measure of GFR in this setting.

In the only comprehensive study of the last few weeks of pregnancy immediately before delivery, Davison et al. performed weekly, serial 24-hour C_{CR} measurements in 10 subjects.[20] These authors demonstrated that 24-hour C_{CR} decreased and plasma creatinine increased over this time period to levels not significantly different from nonpregnant values (Figure 8–3). Because creatinine is not only filtered but also secreted, the authors did not conclude definitely that this decline in 24-hour C_{CR} in fact reflected a fall in GFR.[20] On the other hand, taken together with the study of Davison and Hytten,[19] it is likely that the fall in 24-hour C_{CR} which occurred prior to delivery did indicate a true decline in GFR. Because the 24-hour C_{CR} is performed while the subject goes about her normal daily activities, it may be a more realistic and physiologic measure of GFR. Possibly during late pregnancy, extended periods of standing during the day or lying supine at night may compro-

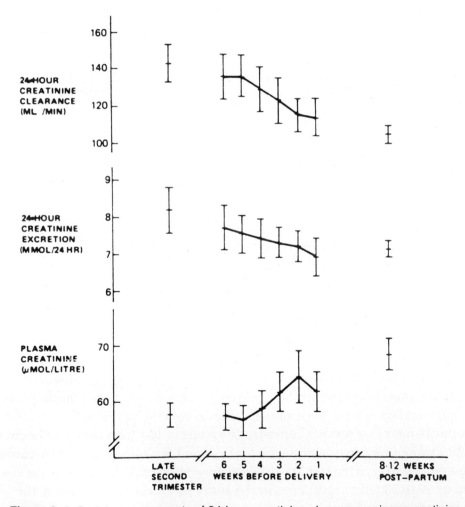

Figure 8–3. Serial measurements of 24-hour creatinine clearance, urinary creatinine excretion, and plasma creatinine in 10 healthy women during the late second trimester, last 6 weeks before delivery, and 8 to 12 weeks postpartum. (*Reprinted, with permission, from Davison JM, Dunlop W, Ezimokhai M: 24-hour creatinine clearance during the third trimester of normal pregnancy.* Br J Obstet Gynaecol *1980;87:106–109.*)

mise renal perfusion and GFR, which is then reflected by a reduced 24-hour C_{CR} (see next section). Such potentially protracted periods of reduced GFR would be missed by short-term measurements of C_{IN} or C_{CR} performed under the artificial conditions in a laboratory setting.

Possible Influence of Posture on Renal Hemodynamics and GFR during Late Pregnancy

Pritchard et al.[21] and Sims and Krantz[2] observed no compromise of C_{PAH} and C_{IN} when gravid subjects turned from the lateral recumbent to the supine position. In contrast, Chesley and Sloan studied 10 women between 34 to 43 weeks' gestation demonstrating decreases of $19 \pm 3\%$ and $21 \pm 5\%$ in C_{PAH} and C_{IN}, respectively, when the subjects assumed the supine position.[22] These decreases were accompanied by comparable percent increases in serum para-aminohippurate and inulin, indicating a true compromise of renal function, rather than an artifact of inadequate urine collection. The authors concluded that when in late gestation a subject assumes a supine position, the enlarged uterus compresses the great veins which, in turn, impairs venous return, decreasing both cardiac output and renal perfusion. Similar findings and conclusions were made by Pippig.[23]

Dunlop studied 18 healthy women at approximately 36 weeks' gestation and again 8 weeks postpartum.[24] He measured C_{PAH} and C_{IN} in three positions: supine, sitting, and lateral recumbency. Although the subjects demonstrated the expected gestational increases in ERPF and GFR, there was no significant influence of posture. Specifically, these variables were not reduced by the supine position. Finally, Lindheimer and Weston, in a study designed to determine mechanisms of renal salt handling, noted decrements in GFR in 11 of 13 volume expanded third-trimester women when these subjects changed from a lateral recumbent to a supine position.[25] In summary, whether change of position from lateral recumbency to supine can compromise renal hemodynamics and GFR during late pregnancy remains controversial. Indeed, Assali et al. demonstrated that renal hemodynamics and GFR decreased markedly in response to quiet standing, especially in the third trimester.[4] This decrease of renal function persisted even after postural hypotension had subsided.

Possible Mechanisms for Alterations of Renal Hemodynamic and GFR

Our understanding of the mechanism(s) responsible for the increase of ERPF, and consequently, of GFR in pregnancy is improving. Reduction in renal vascular resistance underlies the phenomenon. An attractive and plausible theory is that the altered hormonal environment plays an important causal role. Unfortunately, so many hormones undergo change during pregnancy that it has been difficult to know which ones first deserve investigative attention. Because of obvious ethical considerations as well as feasibility issues, many of the investigations dealing with mechanisms of gestational changes in renal hemodynamics and GFR have employed animal models.

Renal Hyperfiltration during Pregnancy

The Munich–Wistar rat has been extensively studied by renal physiologists because this breed manifests glomeruli belonging to superficial cortical nephrons at the kidney surface that are accessible by micropuncture.[26] Thus, much of our current understanding of glomerular hemodynamics is based on investigations using this rat strain. The single nephron GFR (SNGFR) is determined by the Starling forces, both hydrostatic and oncotic pressures within the glomerular capillary and Bowman's space, as well as the ultrafiltration coefficient, K_f, which is the product of the glomerular capillary hydraulic permeability and surface area. Applying the renal micropuncture technique to Munich–Wistar rats during midgestation when whole kidney RPF and GFR are increased, Baylis showed that the gestational rise in SNGFR can be attributed to an increase in glomerular plasma flow and that the transglomerular hydrostatic pressure difference remains unchanged.[27] Thus, the higher glomerular plasma flow effectively decreases the rate of rise of oncotic pressure along the glomerular capillary leading to increased net pressure of ultrafiltration and SNGFR. In essence, a comparable reduction in both afferent and efferent arteriolar resistances accounts for both the unchanged glomerular hydrostatic pressure and increase in glomerular plasma flow during gestation. In this study, plasma oncotic pressure was not significantly different between nonpregnant and pregnant rats, and because the animals were in filtration equilibrium, only a minimum value for the ultrafiltration coefficient K_f could be derived; nevertheless, these determinants of glomerular ultrafiltration most likely contributed little to the gestational rise in SNGFR in the pregnant rat model. Thus, SNGFR rises because glomerular plasma flow increases during pregnancy.[27]

Whether similar mechanisms occur in human gestation is ultimately a matter of conjecture, because glomerular dynamics cannot be directly evaluated. Nevertheless, the parallel rise in RPF and GFR suggests a similar mechanism governing the gestational rise in GFR. Indeed, recent mathematical modeling by Roberts et al.[6] based on renal clearances and other measurements obtained from pregnant women suggested that the renal hyperfiltration of human gestation is almost completely due to a rise in RPF. Although small decrements in plasma oncotic pressure may contribute slightly, there was no evidence for alterations in the transglomerular hydrostatic pressure difference or in the K_f.

Conrad adapted the technique developed by Gellai and Valtin for chronic instrumentation of rats to the investigation of renal function in pregnancy.[28,29] Because renal, cardiovascular, and endocrine parameters are markedly perturbed by anesthesia and acute surgical stress, physiologic studies in chronically instrumented, conscious animals are critical for the investigation of underlying mechanisms. Thus, the same chronically instrumented, conscious rats were serially examined before, during, and after gestation.[29] Comparable to human pregnancy, the conscious rat demonstrates both renal vasodilation and hyperfiltration throughout most of gestation. Thus, the gravid rat has been extensively investigated to determine the mechanisms underlying these changes in the renal circulation during pregnancy.

Plasma Volume Expansion

Pregnancy is associated with tremendous expansion of extracellular and plasma volume (see Chap. 4). Nevertheless, *acute* expansion of plasma volume by 10 to 15% failed to increase the GFR, SNGFR, or glomerular plasma flow in virgin female Munich–Wistar rats.[30] Furthermore, volume expansion had been shown to suppress tubuloglomerular feedback activity, which could conceivably permit the gestational increases in both glomerular plasma flow and SNGFR.[31] However, tubuloglomerular feedback activity was not suppressed in gravid Munich–Wistar rats, rather the mechanism was reset to the higher level of SNGFR manifested by the pregnant animals. Thus, the authors concluded that the volume expansion of pregnancy may actually be perceived as "normal." This contention logically follows from the concept that reductions in total peripheral vascular resistance (the "arteriolar underfilling" stimulus theory of normal pregnancy) and the consequent vascular filling are tightly linked and temporally inseparable, although a dissociation has been discerned by some investigators.[32,33]

Whether *chronic* volume expansion can elicit changes in the renal circulation comparable to those observed in pregnancy needs to be investigated further. Most instances of chronic volume expansion that occur in nature, other than pregnancy of course, are the result of pathology such as congestive heart failure or cirrhosis in which renal function is frequently reduced rather than elevated. However, in the rare instances of primary mineralocorticoid excess, which is associated with volume expansion, the GFR rises but not to the same extent as observed in pregnancy. Also, prolonged administration of either arginine vasopressin or oxytocin to chronically instrumented rats allowed free access to water results in considerable expansion of total body water, reduction in plasma osmolality, as well as increases in both ERPF and GFR comparable in magnitude to that observed in gestation.[34] Thus, the possibility exists that chronic volume expansion may contribute either to the initiation or maintenance of elevated ERPF and GFR during pregnancy.

Pseudopregnancy

The study of the renal circulation in rats that become pseudopregnant may shed light on mechanisms contributing to renal vasodilation and hyperfiltration during pregnancy. By mating a female rat with a vasectomized male, pseudopregnancy—a condition which physiologically mimics the first half of gestation in rats, but lacks fetoplacental development—is produced. This condition mimics the increases in ERPF and GFR that are observed during early pregnancy in rats.[35,36] Thus, maternal factors alone may be sufficient to initiate the changes in the renal circulation during pregnancy (see below).

Menstrual Cycle

Of interest, Davison and Noble[18] showed that the 24-hour endogenous C_{CR} increased by 20% in the luteal phase of the menstrual cycle. This finding has been corroborated by other investigators using the renal C_{CR},[37,38] Cr 51-EDTA,[37,39] or inulin.[40,41] Furthermore, ERPF measured either by the renal clearance of PAH or iodine 125-hippuran was also reported to be increased in two studies,[39,41] but not significantly so in another.[40] Thus, the gestational increases in ERPF and GFR are most likely observed, albeit on a smaller scale, in the luteal phase of the menstrual cycle. This finding may provide insights into underlying mechanisms, because several hormones which rise during early pregnancy also increase during the luteal phase of the menstrual cycle (e.g., the corpus luteal hormones, progesterone and relaxin, see below).

Hormonal Regulation: Sex Steroids

Based on both acute and chronic administration of *estrogens* to humans and laboratory animals, this hormone has little or no influence on RPF or GFR, although it can clearly increase blood flow to other nonreproductive and reproductive organs.[42-46] On the other hand, *progesterone* is a potential candidate. Chesley and Tepper administered 300 mg/d IM progesterone to 10 nonpregnant women for 3.5 days.[43] They found that the hormone produced a 15% increase in C_{IN} and C_{PAH}. The authors speculated that more prolonged administration of progesterone might produce the magnitude of increase in GFR and ERPF seen in normal pregnancy. Similar findings were published by Atallah et al.[47] In the 4-hour period following the IM administration of 200 mg of progesterone to 9 nonpregnant women, plasma levels of the steroid rose on average from 7 to 30 ng/mL, and endogenous C_{CR} increased from 103 to 118 mL/min—a significant rise of about 15%. By extrapolation, the investigators suggested that the level of progesterone observed in pregnancy, which is considerably higher than that attained in their study, might fully account for the 40 to 65% gestational increase of GFR. Three hours after IM administration of 310 μmol progesterone to male subjects, ERPF rose significantly by 15% irrespective of the sodium content in the diet, although GFR was unaffected.[48] In the same report, IM administration of 155 μmol progesterone twice daily for 3 days produced comparable changes in ERPF, but again, no change in the GFR. Finally, subcutaneous injection of 2 mg/kg/d progesterone for 3 days to intact female rats produced a 26% increase in GFR; however, ERPF was not measured in this study.[49] Based on the results from these reports, further study of progesterone seems warranted as a factor contributing to the alterations in renal hemodynamics and GFR during pregnancy.

Hormonal Regulation: Peptide Hormones

Peptide hormones of maternal origin may contribute to the early gestational increases in ERPF and GFR. In this regard, *prolactin* has been considered. Indeed, the hormone surges in both pseudopregnant and pregnant rats coincident with the increases in ERPF and GFR as discussed above. Unfortunately, whether prolactin can raise renal hemodynamics and GFR remains controversial[50] and, as such, requires further investigation.

Relaxin may contribute to the changes in renal and possibly other organ circulations during pregnancy. In gravid rats and women, circulating relaxin originates from the corpus luteum of the ovary.[51] In the latter, human chorionic gonadotrophin (hCG) is a major stimulus for relaxin secretion.[51] There are several compelling, albeit circumstantial, reasons to consider relaxin as a potential mediator of renal vasodilation and hyperfiltration during pregnancy.

First, plasma relaxin rapidly increases after conception in women[51] corresponding with the large increase in GFR and ERPF during the first trimester.[18,19] Second, plasma relaxin also increases during the luteal phase of the menstrual cycle[51-54] correlating with the transient 10 to 20% increase in GFR and ERPF.[18,37-41] Third, the early gestational rise in relaxin corresponds with another early physiologic adaptation in human pregnancy; namely, osmoregulatory changes[55] (see Chap. 4). Indeed, these changes were mimicked by administering hCG to women in the luteal phase of the menstrual cycle and intact female rats, but not to men or ovariectomized rats, suggesting the intermediary role of an ovarian hormone.[56-58] Associated with the osmoregulatory changes observed in women after administration of hCG was a 15 to 20% rise in GFR, which again was not observed in males administered the hormone (J.M. Davison, personal communication). Furthermore, administration of synthetic human relaxin to ovariectomized rats for 7 days produced a significant fall in plasma osmolality without a change in plasma arginine vasopressin comparable to the osmoregulatory changes observed in normal pregnancy.[59] Fourth, chronic administration of relaxin was shown to reduce blood pressure and vasoconstrictor responses in the mesenteric circulation of spontaneously hypertensive rats,[60,61] while acute treatment increased coronary blood flow and reduced platelet aggregation via nitric oxide and guanosine 3',5'-cyclic monophosphate.[62,63]

Although renal vasodilation and hyperfiltration are apparent in gravid rats as early as gestational day 5, before measurable increases in ovarian and plasma relaxin, there is a marked jump in renal function between gestational days 8 and 12, when ovarian and circulating relaxin levels surge.[29,51] Indeed, it was recently reported in a preliminary communication that chronic, but not acute, administration of porcine relaxin or of recombinant human relaxin to chronically instrumented, conscious female rats increases both ERPF and GFR to levels observed during pregnancy.[64] Furthermore, this response was not dependent on the presence of ovaries and may be mediated by nitric oxide (L.A. Danielson and K.P. Conrad, unpublished observations).

Endothelium-Derived Relaxing Factors

Other possible mechanisms for gestational increases of renal hemodynamics and GFR during pregnancy include endothelial factors, e.g., vasodilatory *prostaglandins* (PGs) and *endothelium-derived relaxing factor*. The potential role of PGs has been tested in gravid animal models. Gestational increases in ERPF and/or GFR were unaffected by administration of inhibitors of PG synthesis to chronically instrumented, conscious pregnant rabbits and rats.[65-67] Furthermore, measurements of vasodilatory PG production by relevant renal tissues in vitro failed to show increased synthesis by the tissues from pregnant animals.[68,69] Although intravenous infusion may not necessarily be expected to exert the same physiologic actions as locally produced PGs, intravenous infusion of prostacyclin to male volunteers did not significantly affect either ERPF or GFR.[70] Finally, indomethacin increased total peripheral vascular resistance by only 5% in pregnant women without significantly affecting either mean arterial pressure or cardiac output, and this increase was slight compared to the overall decrease in total peripheral resistance observed in pregnancy.[71] Similarly, meclofenamate failed to significantly augment total peripheral vascular resistance in conscious, pregnant guinea pigs.[72] On balance, therefore, a role for vasodilatory prostaglandins in the gestational elevation of ERPF, GFR, and cardiac output, as well as the reduction in both renal and total peripheral vascular resistances seems doubtful.

Guanosine 3',5'-cyclic monophosphate (cGMP), a second messenger of endothelium-derived relaxing factor/nitric oxide (NO) may contribute to gestational renal vasodilation and hyperfiltration during pregnancy.[50,73] Because extracellular levels of cGMP most likely reflect intracellular production, plasma concentration, urinary excretion, and "metabolic production rate" of cGMP were investigated in conscious rats. Increases in all of these parameters were observed throughout pregnancy and pseudopregnancy.[50,73,74] Similar increases in urinary excretion or plasma concentration of cGMP were reported for human gestation.[75-77] The urinary excretion of nitrate and nitrite (NO_x), the stable metabolites of nitric oxide, also increased during pregnancy and pseudopregnancy in rats consuming a low-NO_x diet, paralleling the rise in urinary cGMP excretion.[74] The gestational rise in urinary NO_x was inhibited by chronic administration of nitro-L-arginine methyl ester (L-NAME), an inhibitor of nitric oxide synthase, suggesting that it derived from nitric oxide. Plasma levels of NO_x were also increased during pregnancy, and NO-hemoglobin was detected in the red blood cells of pregnant rats by electron paramagnetic resonance spectroscopy, but was not detected in the red blood cells of nonpregnant rats.[74] These results demonstrated that endogenous NO production is increased in gravid rats, and although the sources of gestational increases in NO production were not identified, the possibility that NO may contribute to maternal vasodilation was raised. Similar increases in plasma levels and urinary excretion of NO_x were recently reported for gravid ewes.[78] The status of NO biosynthesis during normal pregnancy in women (and in women with preeclampsia) is presently controversial.[79,80]

The renal circulation participates in the maternal vasodilatory response to pregnancy. Peak renal vasodilation and hyperfiltration are observed in rats at midgestation.[29] In chronically instrumented conscious rats acutely administered analogs of L-arginine which inhibit nitric oxide synthase, GFR, ERPF, and effective renal vascular resistance converged in the midpregnant and virgin control animals[80,81] (Figs. 8–4A and 8–4B). Compared with virgin rats, the gravid animals were more responsive to acute NO synthase inhibition, showing a greater decline in GFR and ERPF, and a greater rise in effective renal vascular resistance. Consistent with these in vivo observations was the finding that myogenic reactivity of small renal arteries isolated from midpregnant rats was reduced relative to virgin control animals, and inhibitors of nitric oxide synthase restored this reduced myogenic reactivity to virgin levels.[82] (Fig. 8–4C). Thus, nitric oxide appears to play an important

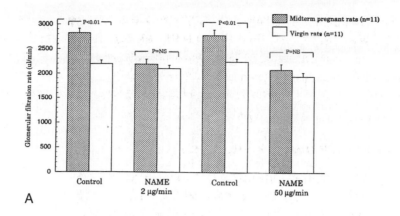

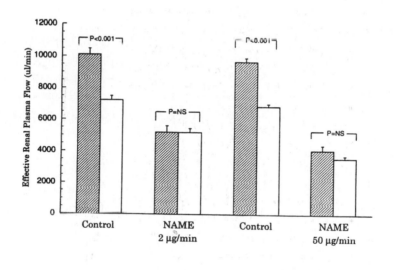

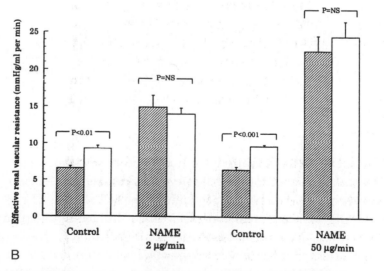

Figure 8–4. Effect of N$^\omega$-nitro-L-arginine methyl ester (NAME) on glomerular filtration rate (**A**) and effective renal plasma flow and renal vascular resistance (**B**) in midterm pregnant (hatched bar; N = 11) and virgin control (open bar; N = 11) rats. (*Continued*)

Figure 8–4. (*Continued*) (**C**) Percent increase in diameter over baseline of small renal arteries in response to a 20 mm Hg increase of lumenal pressure. Hatched bar, NAME; open bar, control. Midterm pregnant rats show reduced myogenic reactivity, which is restored to nonpregnant levels by nitric oxide synthase inhibition with NAME. N = 8 virgin and 8 midterm pregnant rats. *P < 0.05 midterm pregnant vs. nonpregnant; [†]P < 0.05 midterm pregnant NAME vs. midterm pregnant control.[82] (*Modified, with permission, from Sladek SM, Magness RR, Conrad KP: Nitric oxide and pregnancy.* Am J Physiol 1997;272:R441–R463.)

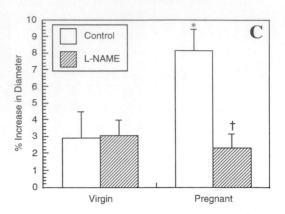

role in the renal circulatory adjustments during pregnancy in conscious rats. Of interest, a compensatory vasodilatory mechanism was recruited to maintain renal hyperfiltration and vasodilation in gravid rats relative to virgin controls during *chronic* blockade of nitric oxide synthase. In this setting, however, renal function was equalized in the two groups of rats during acute inhibition of prostaglandin synthesis by meclofenamate.[83] Prostaglandin inhibition alone, however, did not affect renal function in conscious virgin or pregnant rats.[66,67,83]

The renal regulation of nitric oxide during pregnancy can occur at several levels including: (1) regulation of nitric oxide synthase mass; (2) modulation of nitric oxide synthase activity by availability of cofactors or substrates; (3) intracellular targeting of the enzyme; and (4) alteration in nitric oxide catabolism. All of these possibilities require systematic investigation as they pertain to the three isoforms of nitric oxide synthase. So far, the possibility that the activity of endothelial nitric oxide synthase may be enhanced in the kidneys during pregnancy by calcium-dependent means has been entertained.

In this regard, the *endothelins* (ET) are a recently discovered family of peptides of 21 amino acids each. They are produced by many cell types including endothelium. Although ET is commonly known as a potent vasoconstrictor by interacting with ET_A and ET_B receptor subtypes on vascular smooth muscle,[84] ET has also been shown to increase intracellular calcium in endothelial cells, thereby stimulating prostacyclin, nitric oxide, and possibly other relaxing factors by an ET_B receptor subtype.[85-88] In view of the reputation of ET as a potent vasoconstrictor, it was surprising to find that disruption of the ET-1 gene in heterozygous mice produced elevated blood pressure,[89] and specific blockade of the endothelial ET_B receptor subtype in chronically instrumented conscious male rats with the pharmacologic antagonist, RES-701-1, *produced marked renal vasoconstriction*.[90] These unexpected findings are consistent with a *major role for endogenous ET in maintaining low renal vascular tone* via the RES-701-1-sensitive, endothelial ET_B receptor subtype either by tonic stimulation of endothelial-derived relaxing factors and/or restraint of ET production.[85-88,91] Similar conclusions were reached by using mixed $ET_{A/B}$ antago-

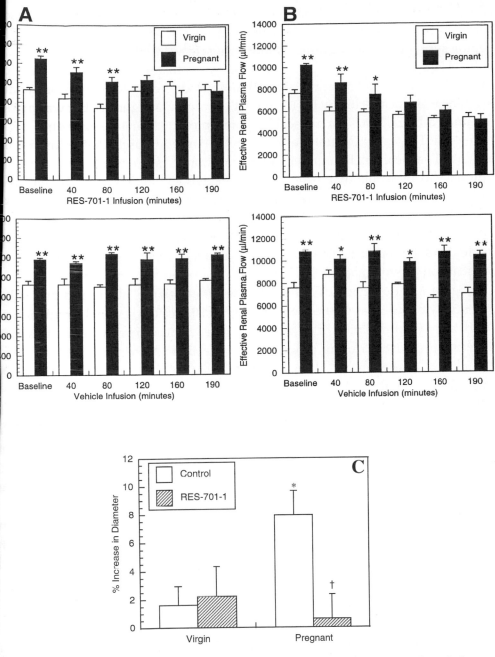

Figure 8–5. Effect of RES-701-1 on glomerular filtration rate (**A.** upper panel), and effective renal plasma flow (**B.** upper panel) in midterm pregnant (solid bar; N = 6) and virgin control (open bar; N = 7) rats. In the lower panels, the time-control experiments with infusion of vehicle rather than RES-701-1 are depicted (N = 4 midterm pregnant and 5 virgin rats). **P < 0.001, *P < 0.05 midterm pregnant vs. virgin rats.[95] **C.** Percent increase in diameter over baseline of small renal arteries in response to a 20 mm Hg increase of lumenal pressure. Hatched bar, RES-701-1; open bar, control. Midterm pregnant rats show reduced myogenic reactivity, which is restored to nonpregnant levels by inhibition of the endothelium ET_B receptor by RES-701-1. N = 5 virgin and 5 midterm pregnant rats. *P < 0.05 midterm pregnant vs. nonpregnant rats; †P < 0.05 midterm pregnant RES-701-1 vs. midterm pregnant control.[82]

nists,[92,93] although the renal vasoconstriction was moderat
tor" ET_B receptor subtype on the endothelium and the "
ceptor subtype on the vascular smooth muscle were blo
is, RES-701-1 is relatively selective for the "vasodilator" E
the endothelium. The renal vasoconstriction produced by I
arginine was not affected by BQ123 (an ET_A receptor antago
attenuated by SB209670 (a mixed $ET_{A/B}$ receptor antagoni
ence of an ET_B receptor subtype on vascular smooth musc
ates renal vasoconstriction under these conditions.[94] Moreo
tion elicited by sarafatoxin 6C (S6C), a selective ET_B agoni
RES-701-1 and nitro-L-arginine[94] (M. Gellai, personal comr
RES-701-1-sensitive, ET_B receptor subtype, located on the er
low renal vascular tone in conscious rats most likely by ton
oxide. Under pharmacologic or pathophysiologic condition
constriction predominates.[94]

Because endogenous ET acting through the endothelial
potentially contributes to the low vascular resistance of the r
likely by tonic stimulation of nitric oxide, it was logical to tes
nism is unregulated during pregnancy.[95] Indeed, acute adm
dothelial ET_B receptor antagonist RES-701-1 led to a conver
and effective renal vascular resistance in conscious gravid ar
8–5A and 8–5B), as well as restoration of reduced myogenic r
nal arteries from gravid rats in vitro[82] (Fig. 8–5C), analogous
inhibitors of nitric oxide synthase (see above). More recent
shown that the crucial role of endogenous endothelin in renal
perfiltration during pregnancy is indeed mediated by the nitri
way (K.P. Conrad, unpublished data).

Finally, autoregulation was found to be preserved during
thetized rats and rabbits.[96,97] The threshold blood pressure for a
nal blood flow was reduced in late-pregnant rats commensurate
resting blood pressure.

Summary

Recent studies using the gravid rat as a model have greatly en
standing of mechanisms underlying the remarkable changes in t
during pregnancy. Hyperfiltration appears to be almost comple
crease in renal plasma flow, the latter attributable to profound r
vascular resistance. Several mechanisms which may cause ren
pregnancy have been reviewed. Those that hold promise include a
nancy of several hormones and autocoids including progesterone
ide, and endothelin. In addition, whether the chronic volume exp
istic of pregnancy is involved in the initiation and/or maintena
renal changes warrants further investigation. Studies are needec

grate these above discussed mechanisms further, and to investigate whether they apply to other animal models, especially nonhuman primates, as well as to women.

RENAL HEMODYNAMICS AND GLOMERULAR FILTRATION RATE IN PREECLAMPSIA

Chesley was the first to measure ERPF and GFR in normal pregnant women and in women with preeclampsia,[98,99] and his pioneering work was followed by numerous reports on the subject. Table 8–1 is a summary of those investigations that, in addition to women with preeclampsia, included an appropriate control group of late-pregnant women. Twenty-three publications met this criterion, though on many occasions the data from these two subject groups were published separately by the investigators; however, they came from the same laboratory. Furthermore, in 9 of these 23 publications, nonpregnant women were also studied.

An additional qualification for inclusion in Table 8–1 was a reasonably clear presentation of the criteria used to make the diagnosis of preeclampsia. These criteria included onset of hypertension in late gestation and proteinuria, and in many instances, there was also evidence for the absence of hypertension before or during early pregnancy, or that the blood pressure normalized in the postpartum period. Several investigators remarked that most of their preeclamptic subjects were primiparous, which in retrospect, is believed to improve the likelihood of correctly diagnosing the disease based on the clinical evidence alone.[126] Whenever possible, subjects not fulfilling the above discussed diagnostic criteria for preeclampsia were excluded from the mean values calculated for Table 8–1.

A word about the methodologies used. In the majority of cases, the subjects were hydrated by oral intake of water, in order to increase urine flow rate, thereby decreasing dead space error and improving the accuracy of the urine collection and renal clearance measurements. As well, an indwelling bladder catheter was routinely used in most of the studies (a practice deemed unacceptable today), which also enabled more complete and accurate urine collections. In many instances, the renal clearances of inulin and para-aminohippurate, respectively, were used to measure GFR and ERPF. However, occasionally the renal clearance of thiosulfate, mannitol, or creatinine was employed, and at best, these provided an "estimate" of GFR. As well, the renal clearance of diodrast was frequently used to "estimate" ERPF. Few investigators commented on the position of their subjects during the study. Out of convenience, most women were probably studied while in the supine position. However, this position may depress renal function, particularly in late gestation (see "Possible Influence of Posture on Renal Hemodynamics and GFR during Late Pregnancy," above). Finally, most investigators normalized GFR and ERPF for 1.73 m^2 body surface area as assessed during pregnancy, a practice which has been abandoned in recent times because the gestational changes in renal hemodynamics and GFR are believed to be functional in nature, and not related to renal hypertrophy.[127]

TABLE 8–1. RENAL HEMODYNAMICS AND GLOMERULAR FILTRATION RATE IN PREECLAMPSIA[a]

1st Author & Reference No.	Nonpregnant Women				Normal Pregnancy–Last Trimester				Preeclampsia–Eclampsia			
	N	GFR	ERPF	FF (%)	N	GFR	ERPF	FF (%)	N	GFR	ERPF	FF (%)
Chesley[98,99]	8–9	57 ± 1	518 ± 15	11.4 ± 0.4	8	79 ± 6[b]	610 ± 38	12.2 ± 0.5	17	77 ± 4[b]	560 ± 39	14.8 ± 1.3
Wellen,[100] Welsh[101]	—	—	—	—	7–17[c]	121 ± 6	588 ± 40	19.9 ± 1.0	4–6[d]	94 ± 15	636 ± 70	14.7 ± 1.6
Dill[102]	—	—	—	—	7	113 ± 7	614 ± 45	18.6 ± 0.9	6–7[e]	83 ± 15	432 ± 58	17.7 ± 2.5
Kariher[103]	—	—	—	—	8[f]	150	754	20.9	17[f]	102	512	19.8
Schaffer[104]	—	—	—	—	9	117 ± 9	—	—	7[g]	86 ± 14	—	—
Chesley[105]	—	—	—	—	10	125 ± 9	—	—	8[h]	93 ± 7	—	—
Bucht[106,107]	23	122 ± 5	557 ± 30	22.7 ± 1.0	10	156 ± 10	571 ± 25	28.9 ± 1.2	8 (< 33 wks)	102 ± 18	495 ± 72	22.0 ± 3.6
									18 (> 33 wks)	98 ± 8	423 ± 36	24.6 ± 3.1
Assali[108]	—	—	—	—	7	109[i]	699	15.7	9	77 ± 6[i]	557 ± 47	14.7 ± 1.4
Brandstetter[109,110]	10	117 ± 4	584 ± 30	20.1 ± 0.7	11	128 ± 4	661 ± 27	19.4 ± 0.6	5 (preeclampsia)	77 ± 5	466 ± 27	16.5 ± 0.8
									3 (eclampsia)	59 ± 8	399 ± 36	14.5 ± 0.8
Friedberg[111]	—	—	—	—	6	112 ± 7	635 ± 58	18 ± 1	10	93 ± 5	571 ± 36	17 ± 1
Lanz[112]	12	115 ± 4[k]	585 ± 25	20 ± 1	5[j]	125[k]	700	18	8	91 ± 5[k]	529 ± 27	17 ± 1
Page[113]	—	—	—	—	12	181 ± 10	—	—	9	75 ± 6	—	—
Lovotti[114]	5	121 ± 7[k]	551 ± 54	22.3 ± 1.4	5	151 ± 9[k]	641 ± 34	23.6 ± 1.5	10	101 ± 5[k]	452 ± 40	23.6 ± 3.0
Hayashi[115]	—	—	—	—	14 (< 32 wks)	129 ± 1	—	—	5 (< 32 wks)	63 ± 9	—	—
					23 (> 32 wks)	108 ± 6	—	—	21 (> 32 wks)	99 ± 6	—	—
Chesley[116]	17	124 ± 6	—	—	11	145 ± 7	—	—	13	103 ± 8	—	—

Reference	N	GFR	ERPF	FF	N	GFR	ERPF	FF	N	GFR	ERPF	FF
Buttermann[117]	11	122 ± 5	624 ± 29	19.3 ± 0.9	26	132 ± 5	647 ± 28	20.9 ± 0.8	33	59 ± 5	341 ± 21	17.0 ± 0.6
Schlegel[118]	10	133 ± 8	659 ± 21	21 ± 1	12	132 ± 6	593 ± 28	23 ± 1	11	93 ± 11	454 ± 59	21.6 ± 1.7
Friedberg[119]	—	—	—	—	10	132 ± 5	586 ± 15	22.5 ± 0.8	14	105 ± 3	480 ± 16	22.2 ± 0.8
McCartney[120]	—	—	—	—	7	133 ± 8	—	—	6	90 ± 12	—	—
Bocci[121]	16	—	573 ± 36	—	14	—	560 ± 24	—	5	—	391 ± 43	—
Sarles[122]	—	—	—	—	5	175[l]	825[l]	21.2	9	115[l]	550[l]	20.9
Sismondi[123]	—	—	—	—	24	—	601 ± 6	22.5	12	—	406 ± 15	—
Chesley[124]	—	—	—	—	14	170 ± 9	755 ± 45	22.5	13	114 ± 9	606 ± 42	19.6 ± 1.3
Grand mean		**114**	**581**	**19.5**		**133**	**649**	**20.4**		**90**	**487**	**18.7**

[a] Mean ± SEM. All renal clearances are expressed as mL/min or mL/min × 1.73 m². N = number of subjects. Glomerular filtration rate (GFR) was measured by the renal clearance of inulin, or estimated by the renal clearances of creatinine, mannitol, or thiosulfate. Effective renal plasma flow (ERPF) was measured by the renal clearances of para-aminohippurate or diodrast. Women with preeclampsia and eclampsia were evaluated separately or together. FF, filtration fraction (GFR/ERPF).

[b] GFR was estimated by the renal clearance of creatinine.

[c] Four subjects who were in the first or second trimester were excluded from the analyses.

[d] Patients without proteinuria during pregnancy or persistent hypertension after pregnancy at a follow-up clinic were excluded from the analyses.

[e] Two patients without proteinuria were excluded from the analyses; also, one subject with an average C_D of 1189 mL/min/1.73 m² was deleted as an outlier. Despite bladder catheterization and oral hydration, the authors suggested that low urine flow rate shown by some of the subjects may have compromised measurements of GFR and ERPF. Therefore, subjects with a urine flow of < 1.0 cc/min were also excluded.

[f] Only mean values were provided. For preeclampsia, mild (N = 7), severe (N = 7), and eclamptic (N = 3) women were combined. However, the mean values for eclampsia provided by the authors were considerably lower than either mild or severe preeclampsia which were comparable.

[g] One subject without proteinuria was excluded from the analysis.

[h] Two subjects were excluded from analysis due to oliguria.

[i] The renal clearance of mannitol was used as an estimate of GFR. Only mean values were provided for normal pregnancy.

[j] Only 5 subjects were apparently studied after 24 weeks of gestation, and the data points were plotted on a graph. Because mean values were not provided, they were estimated from the graph.

[k] GFR was estimated by the renal clearance of thiosulfate.

[l] Mean values were not provided, rather they were estimated from bar graphs.

In Table 8–1, the means ± SEM have been recalculated from the measurements provided for all subjects, when they were presented in the original publications. In some instances, the measurements for each subject were not provided, rather mean values and/or standard deviations were reported, and these were incorporated directly into Table 8–1. (The standard deviation was converted to standard error by dividing the former by the square root of N.) Perhaps the most convenient way to assimilate all of the data from the 23 studies presented in Table 8–1 is to examine the percentage change in GFR, ERPF, and filtration fraction (FF) between preeclamptic and late-pregnant women, and between preeclamptic and nonpregnant women as depicted in Table 8–2. In all 23 reports, there was a reduction in GFR of preeclamptic subjects compared to late-pregnant women, on average by 32%. In all but one publication, there was also a depression of ERPF, on average by 24%. In all but one of the nine studies which also included data for nonpregnant women, GFR and ERPF were reduced by comparison in the preeclamptic subjects both by 22%. Thus, GFR and ERPF are compromised in preeclampsia compared to late-pregnant and nonpregnant women, a conclusion that Chesley reached based on his survey of the literature in 1971.[124] To our knowledge, more recent studies reporting measurements of GFR and ERPF in women with preeclampsia using renal clearance techniques have not been reported except in abstract form.[*,128]

The study of Assali et al.[108] is noteworthy because of their succinct statement about the diagnosis of preeclampsia which was frequently lacking in other reports: ". . . the presence of hypertension, edema, and proteinuria after the 24th week of gestation, together with the absence of a history of hypertension prior to pregnancy, and the return of the blood pressure to normal levels following delivery." In this study, GFR and ERPF were significantly reduced by 29.4 and 20.3%, respectively, compared to normal women in the late pregnancy. Also deserving of emphasis are the reports by McCartney et al.[120] and Sarles et al.[122] who based the diagnosis of preeclampsia not only on clinical grounds, but also according to the finding of glomerular endotheliosis on renal biopsy obtained in the postpartum or intrapartum period, respectively. McCartney et al. also studied their subjects in the lateral recumbent position which circumvented any potential, artifactual decrease in renal function due to compression of the great vessels by the gravid uterus.[120] Thus, using the renal clearance of inulin, McCartney et al. identified a 32.3% reduction of GFR in women with preeclampsia (diagnosis validated by renal biopsy) com-

---

* In other recent work, Irons et al. measured ERPF and GFR by the renal clearances of para-aminohippurate and inulin, respectively, in women with normal pregnancy (N = 10) and women with preeclampsia (N = 10). The normotensive gravidae demonstrated an ERPF and GFR of 766 ± 52 and 153 ± 13 mL/min at 32 weeks' gestation, respectively, which decreased to 486 ± 17 and 87 ± 3 mL/min 4 months postpartum. The preeclamptic women who were primiparous, as well as normotensive during gestational weeks 12–18, showed > 2 g protein/24 h and blood pressure > 140/90 at 33.5 weeks' gestation. ERPF and GFR were 609 ± 24 and 97 ± 7 mL/min, respectively, which changed to 514 ± 22 and 109 ± 7 mL/min 4 months postpartum. Thus, consistent with previous investigations, both GFR and ERPF were compromised during preeclampsia, the former to a greater degree. (Irons DW, Baylis PH, Davison JM: Atrial natriuretic peptide in pre-eclampsia: Metabolic clearance, renal hemodynamics and sodium excretion. *Hypertens Pregnancy* 1997;16:66.)

TABLE 8–2. PERCENTAGE CHANGE IN GFR, ERPF, AND FILTRATION FRACTION BETWEEN PREECLAMPSIA/ECLAMPSIA AND LATE PREGNANT OR NONPREGNANT LEVELS[a]

1st Author & Reference No.	% Change from Late Pregnant			% Change from Nonpregnant		
	GFR	ERPF	FF	GFR	ERPF	FF
Chesley[98,99]	−2.5	−8.2	+21.3	+35.1	+8.1	+29.8
Wellen,[100] Welsh[101]	−22.3	+8.2	−26.1	—	—	—
Dill[102]	−26.6	−29.6	−4.8	—	—	—
Kariher[103]	−32	−32.1	−5.3	—	—	—
Schaffer[104]	−26.5	—	—	—	—	—
Chesley[105]	−25.6	—	—	—	—	—
Bucht[106,107]						
< 33 wks	−34.6	−13.3	−23.9	−16.4	−11.1	−3.1
> 33 wks	−37.2	−25.9	−14.9	−19.7	−24.1	+8.4
Assali[108]	−29.4	−20.3	−6.4	—	—	—
Brandstetter[109,110]						
preeclampsia	−39.8	29.5	−15.0	−34.2	−20.2	−17.9
eclampsia	−53.9	−39.6	−25.3	−49.6	−31.7	−27.9
Friedberg[111]	−17.0	−10.1	−5.6	—	—	—
Lanz[112]	−27.2	−24.4	−5.6	−20.9	−9.6	−15.0
Page[113]	−58.6	—	—	—	—	—
Lovotti[114]	−33.1	−29.5	0.0	−16.5	−18.0	+5.8
Hayashi[115]						
< 32 wks	−51.2	—	—	—	—	—
> 32 wks	−8.3	—	—	—	—	—
Chesley[116]	−29.0	—	—	−16.9	—	—
Buttermann[117]	−55.3	−47.3	−18.7	−51.6	−45.4	−11.9
Schlegel[118]	−29.6	−23.4	−6.1	−30.1	−31.1	+2.9
Friedberg[119]	−20.5	−18.1	−1.3	—	—	—
McCartney[120]	−32.3	—	—	—	—	—
Bocci[121]	—	−30.2	—	—	−31.8	—
Sarles[122]	−34.3	−33.3	−1.4	—	—	—
Sismondi[123]	—	−32.5	—	—	—	—
Chesley[124]	−32.9	−19.7	−12.9	—	—	—
Grand mean	**−32%**	**−24%**	**−9%**	**−22%**	**−22%**	**−3%**

[a] The percentage changes were calculated based on the mean values for GFR, ERPF, and filtration fraction shown in Table 8–1. See footnotes to Table 8–1 for an explanation of the abbreviations.

pared to normal women in late pregnancy (Fig. 8–6A). Similarly, Sarles et al.[122] observed a 34.3% and 33.3% reduction in the renal clearances of inulin and para-aminohippurate, respectively, in women with preeclampsia (diagnosis again validated by renal biopsy) compared to normal women in late pregnancy. Last, but not least, is the well-controlled study by Chesley and Duffus in which the women were studied in the lateral recumbent position, and the GFR and ERPF were corrected for 1.73 m^2 based on *prepregnancy* body surface area. The investigators noted a 32.9%

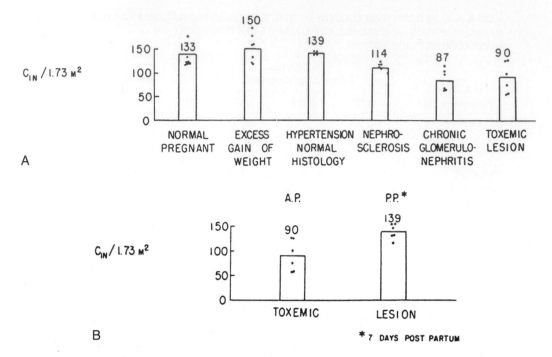

Figure 8–6. A. Individual inulin clearance data and the mean values for six different patient groups. In particular, note the 32% reduction of glomerular filtration rate in pregnant women with preeclampsia (as documented by postpartum renal biopsy) compared to healthy pregnant women. **B.** Individual inulin clearance data and the mean values for pregnant women with preeclampsia documented by postpartum renal biopsy. AP, antepartum; PP, postpartum day 7. See text for further details. (*Reprinted, with permission, from McCartney CP, Spargo B, Lorincz AB, et al: Renal structure and function in pregnant patients with acute hypertension. Am J Obstet Gynecol 1964;90:579–590.*)

and 19.7% decline in GFR and ERPF, respectively, for the women with preeclampsia compared to normal women in late pregnancy.[124]

The mechanism(s) ultimately responsible for the compromise of the renal circulation in preeclampsia is, of course, unknown. It may stem, however, from vascular endothelial damage as first proposed by Stubbs et al.,[129] and as reflected by the finding of glomerular endothelial swelling first reported by Mayer in 1924.[130] Thus, "endothelial dysfunction" is widely believed to be a fundamental mechanism in the pathogenesis of the disease leading to widespread vasospasm and organ hypoprofusion.[131] Interestingly, the endothelium-derived relaxing factor, nitric oxide, is implicated in the renal vasodilation and hyperfiltration of *normal* pregnancy as previously described (see "Renal Hemodynamics and Glomerular Filtration Rate during Normal Pregnancy," above), and possibly this mechanism is compromised by the "endothelial dysfunction" which is believed to affect women with preeclampsia, thereby contributing to the reduction in GFR and ERPF. Irrespective of the inciting agent(s), renal vascular resistance is inappropriately high which accounts for reduced renal blood flow. Based on indirect calculations of the renal afferent and efferent arteriolar, as well as venular resistances,[125] the increase in total renal vascular resistance is mainly, if not solely, due to an increase in the afferent arteriolar resistance (Table 8–3). On the one hand, this finding is not wholly unexpected because the FF, which is actually used in the calculation of the renal segmental arteriolar resistances shows only a 9% decline in preeclampsia (see Table 8–2). That is, if GFR and ERPF are reduced in proportion such that the ratio or FF is unchanged, then a reduction only in the afferent arteriolar resistance is inferred.[132] On the other hand, although the decline in FF is small, it is a consistent finding in preeclampsia, indicating that the compromise of GFR may slightly exceed that of ERPF (see Table 8–2). Although a *simultaneous reduction* in renal efferent arteriolar or venular resistance could theoretically account for this finding, the calculated segmental resistances do not support this argument (see Table 8–3). Rather, a reduction in the glomerular ultrafiltration coefficient is a more likely explanation, perhaps stemming from perturbations in the glomerular basement membrane or in the glomerular capillary surface area available for filtration.

A final consideration relates to the recovery of renal function during the puerperium in women who suffered preeclampsia during pregnancy. Table 8–4 lists those investigations that included postpartum as well as antepartum measurements of GFR and/or ERPF in women with preeclampsia. Also listed is the average number of days or weeks after delivery when the measurements of renal function were made. From the studies of Schaffer et al.,[104] Chesley and Williams,[105] as well as McCartney et al.[120] (Fig. 8–6B), there was notable improvement of the GFR dur-

TABLE 8–3. ESTIMATED SEGMENTAL RENAL VASCULAR RESISTANCES IN PREECLAMPSIA[a]

1st Author & Reference No.	Diagnosis	N	Renal Vascular Resistance (dynes × sec × cm^{-5})[b]			
			Total	Afferent Arteriolar	Efferent Arteriolar	Venular
Assali[108]	Normal pregnancy	7	5,178	1,883	1,531	1,751
	Preeclampsia	9	10,229	6,666	1,405	2,228
Friedberg[111]	Normal pregnancy	6	6,144	2,085	1,781	2,333
	Preeclampsia	10	11,321	6,887	2,057	2,470
Brandstetter[110]	Normal pregnancy	44	6,640	2,430	2,080	2,130
	Preeclampsia	5	17,643	12,896	1,864	2,884
	Eclampsia	3	21,522	16,611	1,694	3,417
Buttermann[117]	Normal pregnancy	26	7,410	3,055	2,125	1,960
	Preeclampsia	33	18,740	13,270	1,788	3,682
Bocci[121]	Normal pregnancy	14	7,300	3,167	1,870	2,275
	Preeclampsia	5	16,500	11,440	1,867	3,174
Grand mean	**Normal pregnancy**		**6,534**	**2,524**	**1,877**	**2,090**
	Preeclampsia/ Eclampsia		**15,994**	**11,296**	**1,779**	**2,976**

[a] Segmental renal vascular resistances were estimated according to the calculations of Gómez.[125]
[b] Mean values are shown.

TABLE 8–4. ANTEPARTUM AND POSTPARTUM RENAL FUNCTION IN WOMEN WITH PREECLAMPSIA[a]

1st Author & Reference No.	Antepartum				Postpartum				Average Time
	N	GFR	ERPF	FF (%)	GFR	ERPF	FF (%)		
Corcoran[133]	3–13	99 ± 7	659 ± 6	13.5 ± 1.2	109 ± 5	478 ± 11	22.3 ± 0.4		13 wks
Dill[102]	6–7	83 ± 15	432 ± 58	17.7 ± 2.5	129 ± 8	429 ± 38	28.5 ± 2.4		Not cited
Welsh[101]	4–6	94 ± 5	636 ± 70	14.7 ± 1.6	107 ± 5	540 ± 28	20.2 ± 0.9		5 wks
Kariher[103]	17	102	512	19.8	124	568	21.3		≥ 12 days
Schaffer[104]	3	93 ± 28	—	—	121 ± 15	—	—		8 days
Chesley[105]	8	93 ± 7	—	—	106 ± 6	—	—		6–9 days
Odell[134]	4	93 ± 17	—	—	182 ± 27	—	—		Not cited
Bucht[107]	18–26	98	423	24.6	119	426	27.9		2–7 wks
Lanz[112]	3	78 ± 1	598 ± 10	13 ± 0	108 ± 6	559 ± 50	19 ± 1		10 wks
Page[113]	9	75 ± 6	—	—	109 ± 6	—	—		Several weeks
Butterman[117]	33	59 ± 5	341 ± 21	17.0 ± 0.6	98 ± 6	418 ± 17	24.0 ± 1.3		Immediately after delivery
Schlegel[118]	4	92 ± 24	504 ± 143	20.3 ± 2.9	121 ± 19	532 ± 56	23.3 ± 3.9		14–22 days
McCartney[120]	6	90 ± 12	—	—	139 ± 13	—	—		7 days
Grand mean		88	513	17.6	121	494	22.7		

[a] Mean ± SEM. All renal clearances are expressed as mL/min or mL/min × 1.73 m^2 body surface area. See footnotes to Table 8–1 for an explanation of the abbreviations.

ing the first 7 to 8 days postpartum. This rapid progress toward recovery apparently occurred despite the persisting abnormalities in glomerular structure observed on renal biopsy which suggested that the compromise of GFR during preeclampsia is mainly functional in origin. Unfortunately, these investigators did not measure ERPF, but it appears from the other studies listed in Table 8–4 that ERPF may have remained depressed during the same postpartum period. On the other hand, Buttermann[117] studied the women immediately after delivery, and found GFR markedly, and ERPF somewhat improved (see Table 8–4).

Summary

A review of 23 reports on renal function in preeclampsia shows that GFR and ERPF are decreased, on average by 32% and 24%, respectively, from normal, late-pregnant values. The GFR and ERPF are also decreased in preeclampsia compared to nonpregnant levels, but to a lesser degree. Although the criteria used for the diagnosis of preeclampsia in these studies were often not presented or failed to meet modern standards, the work of Assali et al.[108] is exceptional because of the rigorous diagnostic criteria used. In this study, GFR and ERPF were reduced by 29% and 20%, respectively. So too, in the studies by McCartney et al.[120] and Sarles et al.,[122] the clinical diagnosis of preeclampsia was corroborated by renal histology. In these reports, GFR and/or ERPF were also observed to be modestly reduced in women with preeclampsia compared to normal pregnant women. Several investigators calculated the renal segmental vascular resistances, and only the preglomerular arteriolar resistance was increased in the disease; no alterations in postglomerular arteriolar resistances were noted. Because the reduction in GFR generally exceeded that of ERPF, yet only preglomerular arteriolar resistance was increased, these findings when taken together, suggest a reduction in the glomerular ultrafiltration coefficient during preeclampsia. Interestingly, GFR appears to rapidly recover during the first week after delivery, despite persisting structural abnormalities on renal histology. On the other hand, ERPF may recover more slowly. The mechanism(s) for compromised GFR and ERPF is unknown, but may relate to the generalized "endothelial dysfunction" believed to account for widespread vasospasm and organ hypoperfusion in preeclampsia (see Chap. 12). Conceivably, the endothelium-derived relaxing factors, most notably nitric oxide, which promote renal vasodilation and hyperfiltration in normal pregnancy, at least in the gravid rat model, are compromised in the disease.

RENAL HANDLING OF URIC ACID

Normal Pregnancy

Uric acid is the end product of purine metabolism in humans.[135] Purines are both dietary in origin and endogenously produced, the latter being the major source of uric acid production. Most circulating uric acid is produced in the liver, and in humans approximately two-thirds of this solute is excreted by the kidney. The remaining one-third is excreted by the gastrointestinal tract. Five percent of circulating uric acid is bound to plasma proteins, thus almost all of this circulating solute is freely filtered by the glomeruli. Once filtered, it undergoes both reabsorption and secretion, mainly in the proximal tubule. In humans, however, net reabsorption occurs, and the bulk of filtered uric acid—88 to 93%—is reabsorbed by the renal tubules back into the blood, and only 7 to 12% of the filtered load reaches the urine.[135]

Serum levels of uric acid are significantly decreased from nonpregnant values by approximately 25 to 35% throughout most of normal human pregnancy.[136-139] During late gestation, they rise toward nonpregnant values. Theoretically, serum concentrations of uric acid are determined by several factors during pregnancy including dietary intake of purines and metabolic production of uric acid by mother and fetus, as well as renal and gastrointestinal excretion.[135,140,141] Alterations in any one or in several of these factors could underlie the changes of serum uric acid that occur in normal pregnancy.

Of the parameters that determine serum uric acid concentration in pregnancy, renal handling of uric acid has received the most investigative attention. Dunlop and Davison serially investigated 24 normal women at approximately 16, 26, and 36 weeks' gestation as well as 8 weeks postpartum.[137] The patients were not fasted, and they were studied in the sitting position. Following instigation of a water diuresis to minimize urinary tract dead space error, GFR was determined by the renal clearance of inulin using the constant infusion technique. Plasma and urine uric acid were measured by an enzymatic technique. In another investigation, Semple et al. serially studied 13 healthy women at approximately 14, 26, and 35 weeks' gestation as well as 10 weeks postpartum.[139] Methodologies were similar to those used by Dunlop and Davison except that the patients were given a purine restricted diet for 3 days before each experiment, and they were fasted overnight prior to each study.

The results are summarized in Table 8–5. Briefly, the pattern of change in blood concentration of uric acid in both investigations was as described above; namely, a decline of about 25 to 35% was observed throughout most of pregnancy, followed by a return toward nonpregnant levels during late gestation. The renal handling of uric acid, however, was somewhat different in the two studies. Dunlop and Davison reported increased renal clearance and urinary excretion of uric acid throughout gestation.[137] These variables were elevated, because filtered load of uric acid was increased, and fractional reabsorption was decreased. A lower fractional reabsorption signified that the tubular transport of uric acid was compromised by normal pregnancy. Since urate undergoes bidirectional transport mainly in the proximal tubule (see above), either the absorptive component was decreased by pregnancy and/or the secretory component increased. In contrast, Semple et al. did not observe a significant rise in urinary excretion of uric acid, although an enhanced renal clearance of the compound throughout pregnancy was reported.[139] The augmented renal clearance of uric acid was a consequence of reduced serum levels ($C_{urate} = U_{urate} \times V/P_{urate}$). The filtered load of uric acid was not increased by pregnancy in this study except at 30 to 40 weeks, and fractional reabsorption

TABLE 8–5. RENAL HANDLING OF URIC ACID DURING NORMAL HUMAN PREGNANCY[a]

Variable	Calculation	Study	Weeks of Gestation			6–15 Weeks Postpartum
			10–19	20–29	30–40	
Plasma or serum uric acid (μmol/L)[b]		Dunlop & Davison	168[c]	178[c]	202	219
		Semple et al.	180[c]	190[c]	230[c]	280
Urinary excretion rate of uric acid (μmol/min)	$U_{urate} \times V$	Dunlop & Davison	3.5[c]	3.6[c]	3.5[c]	2.5
		Semple et al.	2.6	2.8	3.4	2.7
Renal clearance of uric acid (mL/min)	(2)/(1)	Dunlop & Davison	22.0[c]	20.5[c]	17.6[c]	11.8
		Semple et al.	14.2[c]	15.3[c]	15.8[c]	9.8
Renal clearance of inulin, GFR (mL/min)	$U_{IN} \times V/P_{IN}$	Dunlop & Davison	149[c]	153[c]	156[c]	98
		Semple et al.	135[c]	145[c]	145[c]	96
Filtered load of uric acid (μmol/min)	(4) × (1)	Dunlop & Davison	24.9[c]	27.6[c]	31.0[c]	21.4
		Semple et al.[d]	24.3	27.6	33.4	26.9
Fractional excretion of uric acid × 100(%)	(2)/(5) or (3)/(4)	Dunlop & Davison	14.8[c]	13.3[c]	11.5	12.0
		Semple et al.	10.5	10.6	10.9	10.2
Fractional reabsorption of uric acid × 100(%)	100−(6)	Dunlop & Davison	85.3[c]	86.8[c]	88.5	88.0
		Semple et al.[d]	89.5	89.4	89.1	89.8

[a] Mean values are depicted. Dunlop and Davison[137] serially studied 24 healthy women, and Semple et al.[139] investigated 13 healthy women throughout pregnancy and in the postpartum period. See text for details. Data obtained from Dunlop and Davison[137] Semple et al.[139]

[b] To convert μmol/L to mg/100 mL multiply by 1.68×10^{-2}.

[c] Significantly different from postpartum values.

[d] Filtered load and fractional reabsorption of uric acid were not provided by Semple et al., but they were calculated from the data provided.

289

was not changed at any gestational period. These findings may be analogous to the situation of plasma creatinine in pregnancy: circulating levels decline secondary to increased glomerular filtration and a transient increase in urinary excretion. Then, a new steady state is reached whereby circulating levels remain low because now the filtered load results in urinary creatinine excretion in amounts that virtually balance production. Because the reports of Dunlop and Davison[137] and Semple et al.[139] are not in complete agreement, it is difficult to determine whether the handling of urate by the renal tubules changes during pregnancy. Nevertheless, pregnancy increased the renal clearance of uric acid in both studies by virtue of increased GFR and filtered load, reduced tubular reabsorption, or both, which likely accounts for the reduced circulating levels. The return of plasma uric acid concentrations toward nonpregnant values in late gestation can be explained by progressively increasing tubular reabsorption (and consequently, falling renal clearance), at least in the report by Dunlop and Davison.[137]

Preeclampsia

In 1917, Slemons and Bogert first reported that maternal concentrations of circulating uric acid in preeclampsia and eclampsia are elevated.[142] In primiparous women, four of whom had preeclampsia and two with eclampsia, they observed a mean ± SEM of 7.6 ± 0.5 mg% compared to uncomplicated pregnancies in which the values ranged from 2 to 5 mg%. In 1925, and again, in 1934, Stander et al.[143,144] confirmed this observation of Slemons and Bogert, and concluded that "The blood uric acid is increased in eclampsia and preeclampsia . . . [and] . . . may be regarded as a fairly safe criterion of the severity of the disease." Subsequently, numerous investigators have substantiated hyperuricemia in preeclampsia and eclampsia.[140,141,145-171]

Indeed, with one exception,[154] the majority of investigators found a relationship between the degree of hyperuricemia and disease severity.[144,153,157,159-162,168] Of particular note is the study by Pollak and Nettles.[157] They measured the serum uric acid concentration in 30 healthy pregnant women in the third trimester, 10 pregnant women with hypertensive vascular disease, and 33 women with preeclampsia (Fig. 8–7). The diagnosis in the last two groups was established by histologic findings of "glomerular endotheliosis" on antepartum percutaneous renal biopsy. The mean values ± SEM of serum uric acid for the three groups were 3.6 ± 0.1, 3.7 ± 0.3, and 6.3 ± 0.3 mg/%, respectively (P < 0.001 preeclampsia vs. other groups). Moreover, there was a significant correlation between the renal histologic severity of the preeclamptic lesion (degree of "glomerular swelling and ischemia") and the serum uric acid (P < 0.014 by rank correlation test). Although several investigators have suggested that elevated circulating uric acid concentrations be included among the diagnostic criteria for preeclampsia,[153,159] one can see in Figure 8–7, that several women with the renal histologic diagnosis of mild preeclampsia had serum uric acid concentrations in the normal range. As well, a few of the patients with hypertensive vascular disease without evidence for the renal histologic changes of preeclampsia had elevated serum uric acid. Thus, there is

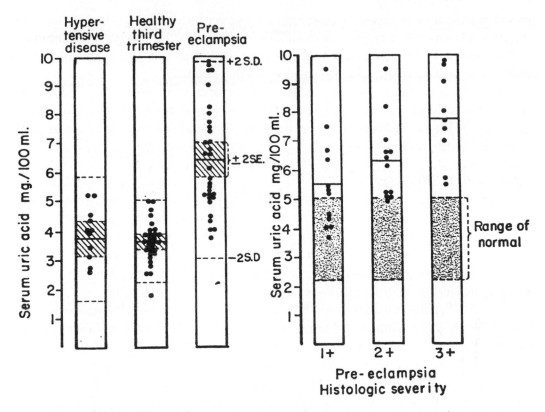

Figure 8–7. Left Panel: Serum uric acid in normal pregnant women and pregnant women with hypertension or preeclampsia. The latter diagnosis was corroborated by the renal histologic findings on antepartum percutaneous renal biopsy. Right Panel: Serum uric acid according to the severity of the renal histologic findings in women with preeclampsia. See text for details. (*Reprinted, with permission, from Pollak VE, Nettles JB: The kidney in toxemia of pregnancy: A clinical and pathologic study based on renal biopsies.* Medicine *1960;39:469–526.*)

considerable overlap of the patient groups when the circulating uric acid levels are only modestly increased. Nevertheless, based mainly on the work of Pollak and Nettles, inclusion of elevated circulating uric acid as an additional criterion for the diagnosis of preeclampsia is reasonable in addition to hypertension and protein-uria, particularly if one demands that the value should be one or two standard deviations above the mean for normal pregnant subjects adjusted for gestational age.[138] It is important to take into account the gestational age due to the changes in circulating uric acid observed in normal pregnancy (see "Renal Handling of Uric Acid—Normal Pregnancy," above).

Redman et al. reported that hyperuricemia is a relatively early change in preeclampsia.[166] Specifically, they observed at 25 ± 4 ($\pm$ 1 SD) weeks' gestation, a 2.0 mg/% rise in plasma uric acid above the first measurement made at 17 ± 3 weeks. In contrast, a 5.0 mg/% rise in urea or the appearance of proteinuria did not occur until 28 ± 3 and 29 ± 3 weeks' gestation, respectively. In 1976, Redman et al.[165] further noted that "perinatal mortality was markedly increased when mater-nal plasma urate concentrations were raised, generally in association with severe preeclampsia of early onset . . . [being] . . . a better indicator than blood pressure of prognosis for the fetus." Sagen et al.[169] later confirmed this association between higher circulating levels of uric acid and poor fetal outcome, i.e., perinatal death, distress, or intrauterine growth restriction < 5th percentile.

Theoretically, the potential mechanisms for increased circulating concentrations of uric acid in preeclampsia may relate to increases in urate production or dietary purine intake, reductions in the metabolic or renal clearance of uric acid, or a combination thereof.

Production of Uric Acid

Both Slemons and Bogert[142] and Crawford[146] observed that the severity and length of labor were associated with increased circulating concentrations of uric acid in normal pregnancy and preeclampsia. Furthermore, the seizure activity of eclampsia was also reported to raise uric acid levels.[145,171] However, uric acid levels clearly are increased during preeclampsia in the absence of convulsions and remote from labor, which suggests other etiologies.

In 1956, Seitchik evaluated the fate of injected nitrogen 15-urate stable isotope in healthy pregnant women and women with preeclampsia and concluded that the rate of production was increased in the latter.[140] However, in 1958,[141] Seitchik retracted this conclusion (citing inadequate control of protein intake and miscalculation of results in the 1956 study), and reported that ". . . the rate of production of urate was not increased as previously reported . . . [and] . . . faulty renal function is the sole causative factor in urate accumulation in acute toxemia." In 1969, Fadel et al.[162] revisited the issue of increased uric acid production in preeclampsia, and postulated that production by the placenta may be increased in the disease due to cellular destruction caused by "multiple infarcts" leading to increased purines, the substrate for xanthine dehydrogenase/oxidase, and uric acid formation. However, the same investigators later showed that the uterine venous concentration of uric acid was actually somewhat less than (not greater than) that measured in simultaneously obtained peripheral venous plasma providing no evidence for either increased release of uric acid by the placenta in preeclampsia or a placental contribution to the raised systemic levels observed in the disease.[163] Similar negative data were reported by Hayashi et al. who found no significant difference in oxypurine levels in the peripheral blood and "intervillous space" blood of preeclamptic women.[155]

As a matter of fact, the human placenta was thought to be devoid of xanthine dehydrogenase/oxidase activity until recently,[172] and the concept that placental activity is increased in preeclampsia was again considered.[173] However, in light of the studies cited above, it seems unlikely that the placental activity is sufficiently increased to affect circulating levels of uric acid in the disease.

Dietary Intake

Although dietary intake of purines can affect circulating levels of uric acid,[135] this mechanism seems unlikely to account for elevated levels in preeclampsia. A multitude of investigators from around the world have reported increased circulating uric acid in preeclampsia over the years despite the failure to control dietary intake, suggesting that the latter is not a critical factor. Even when preeclamptic and normal pregnant control women were studied on a metabolic ward and received rigidly controlled diets with respect to calories, protein, and purine intake, hyperuricemia in preeclampsia was still observed.[141]

Disposal of Uric Acid

Another possible mechanism for increased circulating uric acid in preeclampsia is reduced metabolic clearance. Stander and Cadden[144,145] suggested that impairment in liver catabolism of uric acid occurred in preeclampsia. Later work, however, showed that this mechanism is untenable as the enzyme uricase, which degrades uric acid to allantoin in the liver, is absent in humans.[174]

Renal Excretion of Uric Acid in Preeclampsia

Virtually all instances of hyperuricemia of preeclampsia can be accounted for by reduced renal clearance.[148-152,156,158,164,168,174] Table 8–6A and 8–6B present a tabulation of the results from ten investigations in which the renal handling of uric acid was measured in the last trimester of normal pregnancy, as well as in women with preeclampsia and pregnant subjects with chronic hypertension. First, hyperuricemia was a characteristic feature of preeclampsia, and the degree of elevation generally correlated with disease severity ("mild" vs. "severe"), or as in the study by Hayashi[152] with the early onset of disease (before 32 weeks' gestation). Second, in all of the investigations, the renal clearance of uric acid was reduced in preeclamptic compared to healthy pregnant women or pregnant women with chronic hypertension. Roughly speaking, the reduction in the renal clearance of uric acid by one-half observed in preeclampsia would be expected to produce the twofold elevation in circulating levels (see the grand means listed in Table 8–6A and 8–6B). Third, the decrease in uric acid clearance can be accounted for by two factors: increased net reabsorption of uric acid by the renal tubules and reduced glomerular filtration. The former is the more universal mechanism, because in several of the studies depicted in Table 8–6A and 8–6B, and upon close inspection of the data for individual subjects which were reported by some of the investigators, there was often little, if any, apparent reduction in GFR, yet the circulating levels and net renal reabsorption of uric acid were both elevated.

Studies by Hayashi[152] and Czaczkes et al.[156] using Probenecid to inhibit tubular reabsorption of uric acid support the conclusion that abnormal renal handling of uric acid in preeclampsia contributes significantly to elevated circulating levels in the disease. The report by Czaczkes et al. is particularly thorough. Fifteen preeclamptic women with edema, proteinuria, and hypertension, as well as three healthy pregnant women were studied. The 24-hour renal creatinine and uric acid clearances were first assessed during a 3- to 4-day control period. Then, these variables were again measured over the subsequent 5 to 6 days while the subjects received 0.5 g of Probenecid t.i.d., as well as over several days after cessation of Probenecid administration. The renal clearance of creatinine in this study was not

TABLE 8-6A. RENAL HANDLING OF URIC ACID IN PREECLAMPSIA[a]

1st Author & Reference No.	Normal Pregnancy—Last Trimester					Preeclampsia–Eclampsia				
	N	P_{UA} (mg %)	C_{UA} (mL/min)	GFR (mL/min)	FR_{UA} (%)	N	P_{UA} (mg %)	C_{UA} (mL/min)	GFR (mL/min)	FR_{UA} (%)
Schaffer[148,b]	8	3.7 ± 0.3	33.6 ± 2.7	117 ± 10	70.2 ± 3.0	6	6.0 ± 0.3	18.9 ± 4.0	85 ± 16	77.5 ± 2.0
Chesley[149]	10	3.8 ± 0.2	15.2 ± 1.1	125 ± 9	87.5 ± 0.8	8[c]	6.6 ± 0.5	7.5 ± 0.6	93 ± 7	91.8 ± 0.6
Bonsnes[150]	7[d]	—	12.2 ± 2.4	—	—	32[e]	—	6.4 ± 2.0	—	—
Chesley[174]	29[f]	—	16.7 ± 1.3	—	—	30	—	7.8 ± 0.5	—	—
Seitchik[151]	8	3.7 ± 0.3	16.3 ± 1.1	153 ± 8[g]	89.5 ± 0.5	12, mild	5.1 ± 0.4	8.6 ± 0.8	130 ± 9[g]	93.2 ± 0.4
						2, severe	9.0	7.2	102	93.3
Hayashi[152]	16 < 32 wks	3.2 ± 0.2	18.4 ± 1.2	129 ± 11	85.7[h]	8 < 32 wks	7.5 ± 1.1	4.8 ± 0.6	63 ± 9	92.4[h]
	27 > 32 wks	3.0 ± 0.3	13.0 ± 0.8	108 ± 6	88.0[h]	25 > 32 wks	6.0 ± 0.3	6.5 ± 0.5	99 ± 6	93.4[h]
Czaczkes[156,i]	3	3.7 ± 0.2	8.6 ± 0.2	101 ± 4	91.8 ± 0.6	15	6.9 ± 0.4	3.7 ± 0.2	101 ± 1	96.3 ± 0.2
Handler[158]	10	4.3 ± 0.4	8.8 ± 1.1	109 ± 7	92.1 ± 0.8	11, preeclampsia	5.6 ± 0.6	8.1 ± 1.8	105 ± 13	92.9 ± 1.1
						3, eclampsia	9.0 ± 1.2	2.0 ± 0.7	66 ± 6	96.9 ± 1.0
Fadel[164,j]	13	4.2	14.0	160	91.1	17	6.7	7.2	122	94.2
Dunlop[168]	13	258 ± 16[k]	10.5 ± 1.1	110 ± 7	89.4 ± 0.9	18, mild	329 ± 24[k]	7.7 ± 0.7	95 ± 7	91.9 ± 0.4
						10, severe	365 ± 25[k]	7.1 ± 1.0	90 ± 7	92.3 ± 0.7
Grand mean[l]		3.8	13.4	124	89.4		6.7	6.5	96	93.5

TABLE 8-6B. RENAL HANDLING OF URIC ACID IN CHRONIC HYPERTENSION

1st Author & Reference No.	N	Chronic Hypertension			
		P_{UA} (mg %)	C_{UA} (mL/min)	GFR (mL/min)	FR_{UA} (%)
Hayashi[152]	22, < 32 wks	3.7 ± 0.3	14.5 ± 1.2	114 ± 10	87.3[h]
	26, > 32 wks	4.1 ± 0.2	14.2 ± 1.3	128 ± 12	88.9[h]
Handler[158]	4	4.2 ± 0.3	9.0 ± 1.1	123 ± 5	92.7 ± 1.1
Fadel[164,j]	22	5.5	9.9	135	92.4
Dunlop[168]	5	261 ± 25[k]	13.1 ± 2.6	132 ± 22	90.2 ± 0.9
Grand mean		**4.4**	**12.6**	**126**	**90.3**

[a] Mean ± SEM. All renal clearances are expressed as mL/min or mL/min × 1.73 m² body surface area. N = number of subjects; P_{UA} = plasma or serum uric acid; C_{UA} = renal clearance of uric acid; GFR = glomerular filtration rate. Unless otherwise indicated, GFR was assessed by the renal clearance of inulin or creatinine. FR_{UA} = fractional reabsorption of uric acid $(1.0 - C_{UA}/C_{IN}) \times 100(\%)$.

[b] Fractional reabsorption of uric acid was not provided by Schaffer. It was calculated from the C_{UA} and C_{IN} presented for each subject. Only those subjects with simultaneous renal clearances for uric acid and inulin were tabulated, and one subject without proteinuria was omitted from the preeclamptic group. In this study, the generally high values for the renal clearance of uric acid may be attributable to infused diodrast (for measurement of ERPF) which interferes with renal uric acid reabsorption.[135]

[c] Two subjects were omitted from the analysis due to oliguria which diminishes the accuracy of renal clearance measurements. One subject had antepartum eclampsia.

[d] An unspecified number of these 7 subjects were pregnant. However, the authors stated that there was no difference in the renal clearances of uric acid between nonpregnant and pregnant women.

[e] Included are 3 subjects who had antepartum eclampsia and another 2 with postpartum eclampsia.

[f] Normal pregnant subjects ranged from 8–40 weeks' gestation.

[g] The renal clearance of mannitol was used as an estimate of GFR.

[h] FR_{UA} was not given. It was, therefore, calculated based on the average values for C_{UA} and GFR.

[i] Renal clearance data were based on 24-h urine collections.

[j] Only mean values were reported.

[k] Expressed as μmol/L. To convert μmol/L to mg/100mL, multiply by 1.68×10^{-2}.

[l] The C_{UA} is high and the FR_{UA} is low in the work by Schaffer et al.[148] because, in addition to inulin, diodrast was also infused to measure effective renal plasma flow. However, diodrast, a radiocontrast agent, interferes with the tubular reabsorption of uric acid.[135] Therefore, these results of Schaffer et al. were omitted from the grand means.

reduced in preeclampsia compared to normal pregnancy, nor was it affected by Probenecid in either group of subjects. The plasma uric acid was modestly reduced by the drug from 3.7 to 3.3 mg/% in normal pregnancy due to augmented renal clearance (8.6–12.5 mL/min) and reduced net renal reabsorption of uric acid (91.8–87.0%). Probenecid had a more dramatic effect in preeclampsia; the renal clearance of uric acid was greatly augmented (3.7–18.8 mL/min) while net tubular reabsorption was reduced (96.3–81%). Most important, the plasma uric acid was completely restored to normal pregnancy levels by the drug, *6.9 to 3.2 mg/%*. Thus, by correcting the augmented renal reabsorption of uric acid in preeclampsia, the elevated circulating levels of the organic anion can be completely restored to normal pregnancy levels. Because Probenecid inhibits tubular reabsorption of uric acid, these results indicate that abnormal renal retention of uric acid in preeclampsia is secondary to enhanced tubular reabsorption and not to reduced secretion. Finally, it is noteworthy to point out that Hayashi reported "no clinical change was observed [in the women with preeclampsia receiving Probenecid suggesting that] hyperuricemia alone is not an important pathogenetic factor in pregnancy toxemia."[152]

There are three studies in which the renal handling of uric acid was evaluated in the same preeclamptic women during the antepartum and postpartum periods.[148-150] Similar to the reduction in GFR, the restoration to normal levels occurs rapidly in the postpartum period, generally within the first week. Of particular note is the work by Bonsnes and Stander who studied women daily in the immediate postpartum period.[150] A large recovery in the plasma level and renal clearance of uric acid was evident between the 5th and 7th postpartum days.

The factors capable of influencing renal tubular handling of uric acid include various hormones such as angiotensin II and norepinephrine which enhance net tubular reabsorption of uric acid.[135] In this regard, the circulating renin–angiotensin system is believed to be suppressed in preeclampsia.[175] On the other hand, sympathetic activity to the skeletal muscle has been reported to be increased in the disease.[176] However, whether renal sympathetic nerve activity or renal generation of angiotensin II is increased in preeclampsia is unknown. Estrogens are believed to augment the renal clearance of uric acid by reducing the net renal reabsorption,[135] thereby accounting for the lower circulating levels observed in female compared to male subjects. However, a considerable amount of investigation over the years has not produced compelling evidence that estrogen levels are different in preeclampsia compared to normal pregnancy. Even if estrogen levels are somewhat reduced as reported by some investigators,[177] the overall capacity of estrogens to affect the renal handling and plasma levels of uric acid seems relatively modest compared to the large reductions in renal clearance and elevations in circulating levels observed in preeclampsia.

Handler et al. suggested that increased plasma levels of lactate, presumably derived from the ischemic placenta, accounted for increased circulating uric acid in preeclampsia by enhancing net renal reabsorption of the organic anion.[158] Indeed, infusion of sodium lactate into normal pregnant women produced a marked decline in the renal clearance of uric acid secondary to increased net renal reabsorption.[158,164] However, whether circulating lactate is increased in preeclampsia is controversial.[158,164,178] Finally, lactate affects the renal handling of uric acid by inhibiting tubular secretion, not by enhancing reabsorption.[135] Thus, the lactate hypothesis conflicts with the reports by investigators who used Probenecid and established that the abnormality of renal uric acid handling in preeclampsia was enhanced tubular reabsorption and not reduced secretion.

The most likely mechanism for enhanced renal tubular reabsorption of uric acid in preeclampsia is the relative or absolute contraction of plasma volume. In general, volume contraction has been shown to be associated with increased renal tubular reabsorption of uric acid.[135] As preeclampsia is associated with reduced plasma volume,[179,180] this mechanism for augmented renal tubular reabsorption of uric acid seems most plausible. To our knowledge, the mechanism linking altered volume status and renal tubular handling of uric acid is unknown, although it is likely related to the coupling of sodium and urate transport in the proximal tubule.[135]

Summary

The serum levels of uric acid are decreased throughout much of human pregnancy by 25 to 35% from nonpregnant values. During late gestation, they rise toward non-pregnant values. Although several factors can theoretically contribute to the decline in circulating levels, altered renal handling likely makes a major contribution. That is, the renal clearance of uric acid is increased during gestation by virtue of raised GFR and filtered load, reduced tubular reabsorption, or both. In one study, the restoration of serum uric acid toward nonpregnant levels near term was explained by a progressively increasing renal tubular reabsorption.

Hyperuricemia accompanies preeclampsia. In fact, some investigators include it as a diagnostic criterion because of the strong correlation between hyperuricemia and the histologic finding of "glomerular endotheliosis" on antepartum percutaneous renal biopsy, which is believed to be characteristic of preeclampsia. Moreover, a significant correlation between the renal histologic severity of the preeclamptic lesion and the serum uric acid has been noted. Hyperuricemia is a relatively early change in preeclampsia and is correlated with poor fetal prognosis.

The hyperuricemia of preeclampsia is not due to increased metabolic production or reduced disposal, but altered renal handling is important. Specifically, the renal clearance of uric acid is decreased mainly because net tubular reabsorption is increased, although reduced GFR and filtered load may contribute. Probenecid, which inhibits renal tubular reabsorption of uric acid, restored the renal clearance and plasma levels of uric acid in preeclamptic women implicating enhanced tubular reabsorption rather than diminished secretion. The renal clearance and plasma levels of uric acid were restored rapidly to normal values by postpartum day 5 in women who suffered preeclampsia.

The precise etiology of exaggerated renal tubular reabsorption of uric acid in preeclampsia is uncertain, but most likely relates to plasma volume depletion which is also a typical feature of the disease. Presumably, the volume contraction leads to enhanced renal reabsorption of sodium, and therefore of uric acid by the proximal tubule, although the precise mechanism is unknown.

RENAL HANDLING OF PROTEINS

Normal Pregnancy

Circulating Proteins

Because the plasma concentrations of substances influence their filtered load, the circulating levels of various proteins in normal pregnancy must be considered. In this regard, there are many reports,[181-184] but perhaps the most comprehensive series of investigations were carried out by Studd and Wood.[183] They serially measured serum protein concentrations in the same women at several stages during pregnancy and 3 months postpartum. Significant decreases in albumin, thyroxine-binding prealbumin, IgG, and IgA were noted, whereas significant increases in α_1-

antitrypsin, transferrin, β-lipoprotein, complement fraction β_1-A–C, IgD, and α_2-macroglobulin were observed. Hemopexin, haptoglobin, and IgM were unchanged. Many of these findings were corroborated by other investigators.[182,184]

Using iodine 131-albumin, Honger showed that the intravascular mass of albumin was comparable between late-pregnant and nonpregnant women, and an increase in plasma volume accounted for the reduction in serum albumin concentration.[181] The extravascular mass of albumin tended to be lower in pregnancy suggesting that the capillary permeability was decreased or the lymphatic flow increased. Interestingly, the catabolic and synthetic rates were comparable indicating suppression of synthesis in normal pregnancy, because low serum albumin concentration is normally countered by an increase in synthesis. Honger suggested that estradiol or progesterone may mediate the reduced synthesis of albumin which was supported by later studies using derivatives of estradiol and progesterone.[183]

Urinary Excretion of Total Protein and Albumin

It is widely held that urinary protein excretion increases during normal pregnancy with an upper limit of approximately 300 mg/24 h. Although there are reports suggesting that urinary albumin excretion decreases[184] or remains unchanged during normal pregnancy,[185-189] the majority of publications support an increase.[190-203] In a cross-sectional study using spot urines, Cheung et al.[195] showed that the urinary excretion of albumin rose significantly from a nonpregnant median value of 1.19 to 1.76, 1.90, and 1.91 g/mol of creatinine during the first, second, and third trimesters, respectively. In this study, the urinary excretion of albumin was approximately 30% of total protein excretion.[195] In another carefully conducted study, Douma et al.[201] collected both 24-hour and separate 12-hour nighttime and daytime urines from nonpregnant women and women during the third trimester on an outpatient basis. Furthermore, they conducted a similar investigation on a metabolic ward with the subjects on strict bed rest. In both experimental settings, the 24-hour urinary excretion of albumin, as well as the nocturnal and diurnal urinary excretions of albumin were greater in pregnancy, and the difference between nonpregnant and pregnant subjects was greatest during the nighttime. In the outpatient setting, both the nonpregnant and pregnant women showed a significant day–night difference with lower excretion at night. Although this day–night difference was preserved for nonpregnant women on continuous bed rest in the metabolic ward, it was lost in pregnant subjects, which suggested a blunting of the intrinsic (i.e., independent of upright posture and normal daily activity) circadian variation in albumin excretion during pregnancy.[201] Perhaps the most meticulous study was conducted by Taylor and Davison.[203] Although the investigators have only studied 5 healthy women thus far, they first did so preconception, and then on 12 different occasions throughout gestation, and again 12 weeks postpartum. Urinary albumin excretion was significantly increased by 16 weeks' gestation, showing overall a 2- to 3-fold increase during pregnancy, and it returned to preconception levels by postpartum week 12. In contrast, the urinary excretion of total protein measured in the same samples was not significantly increased until the third trimester. Urinary albumin excretion was approximately 10% of the total protein excretion. This work generally corroborates an earlier study from the same laboratory, except that previously, the elevated urinary excretion of albumin persisted at least until 16 weeks postpartum; nonpregnant levels were observed by 12 months postpartum.[202] This interesting finding of persisting albuminuria in the postpartum period was also suggested in the investigations of McCance et al.,[196] Lopez-Espinoza et al.,[191] and Wright et al.[192] Thus, the alterations in renal function that affect urinary albumin excretion during normal pregnancy are not completely restored to nonpregnant levels until some time after delivery.

Urinary Excretion of Low Molecular Weight (LMW) Proteins

Because β2-microglobulin (β2-m), retinol-binding protein (RBP), and Clara cell protein are LMW proteins of 11.8, 21.4, and 15.8 kDa, respectively, they are considered to be freely filtered at the glomerulus. At the same time, they are virtually reabsorbed to completion by the proximal tubule. Thus, the concept has emerged that increased urinary excretion of these LMW proteins mainly reflects inadequate proximal tubular reabsorptive capacity.[204-206]

Most,[184,186,187,193,195,207] but not all,[208,209] investigators have observed increased urinary excretion of LMW proteins during normal pregnancy. Of particular note is the work of Bernard et al.[187] who observed a progressive increase in the urinary excretion of all three of these LMW proteins throughout pregnancy, which significantly exceeded nonpregnant values by the second and third trimesters. Because the plasma levels of these LMW proteins do not increase during normal pregnancy, and the pattern of increase in GFR does not correspond with that of the LMW protein excretion during normal pregnancy, Bernard et al. suggested a decrease in proximal tubular reabsorptive capacity which recovers after delivery. The urinary excretion of α_1-microglobulin (26–33 kDa)[187] and of immunoglobulin light chains (25 kDa)[186] were also increased in normal pregnancy, although these proteins are of more intermediate molecular weight and are not so freely filtered. Interestingly, the absolute urinary excretion or fractional excretion of other substances which are primarily reabsorbed by the proximal tubule such as glucose, amino acids, calcium, and uric acid is also increased during gestation[8,210] (see "Renal Handling of Uric Acid," above). Taken together, these data indicate a general, physiologic compromise of proximal tubular reabsorption during normal pregnancy.

Urinary Excretion of Enzymes

Most,[194,195,211-213] but not all,[208] investigators have also reported increased urinary excretion of several large molecular weight enzymes during normal human gestation. These enzymes are presumably of proximal tubular origin being located in the brush border (γ-glutamyl transferase, alanine aminopeptidase, and tissue nonspecific alkaline phosphatase) or in the lysosomes (β-glucoronidase, N-acetyl-β-D-glucosaminidase, α-galactosidase, β-galactosidase, and α-mannosidase). The urinary excretion of γ-glutamyl transferase was observed to be increased during pregnancy by Noble et al.,[211] Cheung et al.,[195] but not by Kelly et al.[208] Similar increases were reported for alanine aminopeptidase.[195,212] The urinary excretion of some of the lysomal enzymes such as N-acetyl-β-D-glucosamine and β-galactosidase were also reported to be increased.[194,195,212,213] A raised filtered load could contribute to the increased urinary excretion of these enzymes during gestation: the plasma concentration of N-acetyl-β-D-glucosamine and β-galactosidase are higher in pregnancy,[213] the GFR is also increased, and there may be subtle alterations in glomerular permeability or electrostatic charge allowing for greater filtration of these large molecular weight proteins. On the other hand, Jackson et al. observed that the molecular weights of the urinary lysosomal enzymes more closely matched those measured for the enzymes extracted from kidney homogenates than from the serum, suggesting a renal origin for the proteins.[213] On balance, these data further implicate physiologic alterations in the proximal tubule during normal gestation.

Glomerular Permselectivity

The cause of increased urinary albumin excretion observed by most investigators during normal gestation is probably multifactorial. On the one hand, the filtered load is increased by virtue of elevated GFR, although this is offset somewhat by a decline in circulating albumin concentration. On the other hand, studies to date have failed to detect any change in the permselectivity of larger molecular weight proteins in human gestation, at least on the basis of size or molecular weight alone. Indeed, Roberts et al.[202] actually demonstrated *reduced* fractional clearance of smaller neutral dextran particles (30–39 Å, ≈20 kDa) throughout normal human pregnancy, and no alteration in the fractional clearance of larger dextrans. Whether the anionic charge of the glomerular barrier is reduced allowing for greater passage of negatively charged plasma proteins has not been investigated. In this regard, however, Cheung et al.[195] showed that the rise in urinary excretion of transferrin greatly exceeded the rise in urinary excretion of albumin during normal pregnancy despite similar molecular weights, possibly indicating an alteration in the charge of the glomerular membrane as transferrin is considerably less anionic than albumin. Finally, based on the data dealing with urinary excretion of LMW proteins (see above), inadequate proximal tubular reabsorption may contribute to increased urinary albumin excretion in normal pregnancy.

PREECLAMPSIA

Circulating Proteins

With one exception,[214] both serum albumin[182,215-217] and IgG[182,215,216,218] concentrations were further decreased in preeclampsia relative to normal pregnancy. Serum α_2-macroglobulin levels were generally reported to be further increased in preeclampsia relative to normal pregnancy.[182,215,216,219] Again, with one exception,[182] serum transferrin concentration fell during the disease.[215,216,218] In fact, Studd et al. reported that the pattern of change in serum proteins in preeclampsia was remarkably similar to the nephrotic syndrome in general, i.e., reduced serum concentrations of albumin, total protein, thyroxine-binding prealbumin, IgG, and transferrin, as well as increased levels of α_2-macroglobulin, β-lipoprotein and β_1-A–C complement fraction. They concluded that these alterations in serum proteins in part reflected heavy urinary loss of intermediate molecular weight proteins with relative retention of the larger species.[215,216]

Using I 131-albumin, Honger analyzed the metabolic fate of albumin in preeclampsia relative to normal pregnancy.[217] He reported that the plasma volume and serum concentration of albumin, as well as the intravascular and total exchangeable mass of albumin were all reduced in the disease. The fractional rate of albumin disappearance was increased which he attributed approximately equally to urinary loss and hypercatabolism and/or increased gastrointestinal loss. Laakso and Paasio showed exaggerated loss of I 131-PVP (polyvinylpyrrolidone) into the feces of women who were preeclamptic 2 to 8 days postpartum most likely due to increased capillary permeability.[220] Although Honger showed that the rate of albumin synthesis was increased in preeclampsia relative to normal pregnancy, evidently it was insufficient as serum albumin concentrations were further reduced in the disease.[217] This finding is consistent with the generalized state of "systemic inflammation" and activation of the "acute phase response" which typifies the disease possibly compromising hepatic albumin synthesis.[221] Interestingly, the distribution of albumin between the intravascular and extravascular compartments was not different,[217] which is counterintuitive since generalized capillary leakiness is believed to be a disease manifestation of preeclampsia.[222]

Urinary Excretion of Total Protein and Albumin

In 1843, Lever first reported protein in the urine of a woman with eclampsia.[223] Today, in addition to fulfilling blood pressure criteria, proteinuria in excess of 300 mg/24 h is part of the clinical diagnosis of preeclampsia.[224] In fact, preeclampsia is the most common cause of nephrotic range proteinuria in pregnancy,[225] and the magnitude of the protein excretion correlates significantly with the histologic severity of the renal lesion.[126] The proteinuria consists of a number of different proteins as identified by many investigators over the years.[218,226-232] These urinary proteins mainly derived from the plasma include albumin, α_1 and α_2-globulin, β-globulin, γ-globulin (IgG, IgA, and occasionally IgM), ceruloplasmin, pseudocholinesterase, and α_2-macroglobulin.

Glomerular Permeability to Proteins

Normally, the glomerulus effectively retains proteins that are of the size of albumin or greater. The small amounts which do escape are reabsorbed in the proximal tubule, such that most urinary protein reflects tubular secretion, e.g., the Tamm–Horsfall protein which normally accounts for about one-half of urinary protein.[233] However, in glomerular disease when urinary protein exceeds 1 g/day, one can compare the renal clearances of plasma proteins relative to their molecular weights, thereby evaluating the integrity of the glomerular barrier. Several investigators have reported the renal clearances of plasma proteins and of dextran or the inert polymer polyvinylpyrrolidone (PVP) in women with preeclampsia. Dextran and PVP are exogenous compounds, and therefore must be administered intravenously. They come in a variety of molecular sizes, and are not reabsorbed or secreted by the renal tubules, making their renal clearance solely determined by glomerular filtration and the integrity of the glomerular filter. In general, the relationship between the log of the renal clearance of plasma proteins ranging in size from 69 kDa (albumin) to 1000 kDa (IgM), and the log of the molecular weight or particle size is inverse and linear. The same holds true for dextran or PVP. By convention, the renal clearances of selected plasma proteins are factored by the renal clearance of one of the smaller plasma proteins such as transferrin, and plotted against their respective molecular weights. Thus, a steeper or flatter slope, respectively, represents a more or less "selective" or "unselective" proteinuria, signifying the relative retention or loss of larger molecular weight proteins by the glomerular filter (Fig. 8–8A). Using this technique, MacLean et al.[234] as well as Robson[235] noted that the protein selectivity was in an "intermediate range" for preeclampsia. The measurement of dextran selectivity in five of the same subjects by MacLean et al. yielded similar results. These corroborative findings using dextran suggested that the protein selectivity data were indeed reflecting a glomerular abnormality, and not tubular changes in protein processing during preeclampsia. As well, because comparable results were obtained with both charged (plasma proteins) and uncharged (neutral dextran) molecules, significant alteration in the glomerular electrostatic barrier seemed unlikely. Robson commented that, when viewed in the context of primary glomerular diseases, the intermediate values for selectivity of protein in preeclampsia seemed out of proportion relative to the minor anatomic changes in the glomerulus (Fig. 8–8B). Clearly, there is a paucity of data on the simultaneous measurements of the renal clearances of plasma proteins and of dextran or PVP in women with preeclampsia; further investigation is needed to provide greater insight into the changes of the glomerular filter in the disease.

Using similar methodology, Simanowitz et al.[231] substantiated the finding of intermediate range protein selectivity in preeclampsia. By using an abbreviated technique of measuring the renal clearance of IgG relative to that of transferrin, Kelly and McEwan,[218] as well as Simanowitz and MacGregor[236] again observed intermediate range protein selectivity. Katz and Berlyne reported variable protein selectivity ranging from highly selective to unselective, but they did not actually calculate the renal clearances of the various plasma proteins.[232] It should be noted, however, that a "variable" pattern is not surprising given the microscopic picture of the disorder (see Chap. 7). That is, while neither basement membrane nor foot process changes are noted in many renal biopsies, such changes can be seen with very severe disease.

Finally, Wood et al.[237] evaluated the glomerular filter by testing the renal clearance of PVP (10,000–100,000 MW). They reported a "vasoactive pattern" for

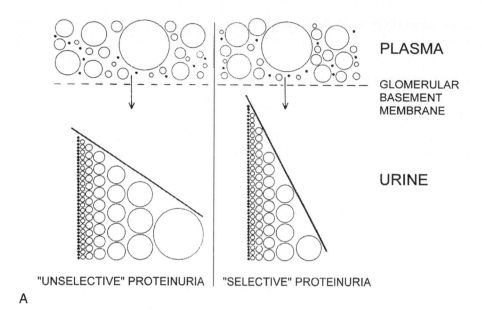

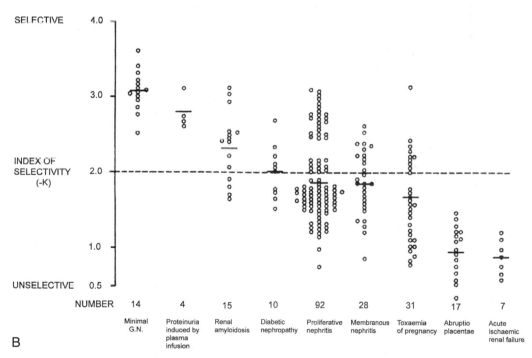

Figure 8–8. A. Illustration of the concept of glomerular selectivity for proteinuria. The slope, −k or the index of selectivity, is determined by the clearance of the proteins ranging in size from 60,000 to 2 million daltons ($U_{protein} \times V/P_{protein}$) expressed as a percentage of the clearance of the smaller plasma proteins such as albumin or transferrin. **B.** Indices of protein selectivity for a variety of glomerular diseases, preeclampsia, and abruptio placentae. Again, "−k" relates the molecular size of selected proteins to their renal clearance, the latter being normalized to the renal clearance of relatively small molecular weight proteins such as albumin or transferrin. (*Reprinted, with permission, from Robson JS: Proteinuria and the renal lesion in preeclampsia and abruptio placentae. In: Lindheimer MD, Katz Al, Zuspan FP:* Hypertension in Pregnancy. *New York: John Wiley & Sons; 1976.*

the PVP clearance–molecular radius relationship in gestational hypertension and mild preeclampsia comparable to that observed with the infusion of angiotensin II which increases intraglomerular pressure, thereby increasing the filtration of intermediate-sized molecules, and is fully reversible. This finding is consistent with the intermittent nature of proteinuria in preeclampsia as first reported by Chesley.[238] In moderate to severe disease, a "membranous pattern" was noted which Wood and colleagues postulated to be a consequence of intravascular coagulation and alterations in the glomerular basement membrane.[237]

An important component of the glomerular barrier is the negative charge associated with heparin sulfate-rich glycosaminoglycans mainly in the lamina rara interna and externa of the basement membrane, but also associated with the polyanionic glycoproteins on the endothelial surface.[239] Disruption of this electrostatic barrier is not detected by the clearance of neutral dextrans and PVP. The work of MacLean discussed above, showing comparable results for both the plasma protein and dextran clearance techniques, is not supportive of a major change in the electrostatic properties of the glomerular barrier in preeclampsia.[234] On the other hand, recent publications by Naicker et al.[240,241] provide experimental evidence for fewer polyethyleneimine-labeled anionic sites in the glomerular basement membrane on renal biopsies procured 2 weeks after delivery from women with early-onset preeclampsia, at least when compared to nonpregnant subjects who underwent partial nephrectomy due to trauma.

Urinary Excretion of Low Molecular Weight Proteins and Enzymes

Weise et al. reported urine excretory rates for β_2-m of 0.11 and 0.5 mg/24 h for normal pregnant and preeclamptic women, respectively.[242] Although Pedersen et al. did not find a significant difference in renal β_2-m excretion between preeclamptic and normal pregnant women in the third trimester (both were elevated relative to nonpregnant subjects, see "Normal Pregnancy," above), the increases persisted in the preeclamptic group 5 days postpartum with complete resolution not being observed until 3 months postpartum.[186] The same group of investigators, however, noted substantial increases in immunoglobulin light chain excretion in preeclampsia relative to third trimester control subjects which also persisted 5 days postpartum and resolved by 3 months.[186] In contrast, Øian et al. reported reduced renal β_2-m excretion in preeclampsia when compared to normal third trimester subjects.[207] Interestingly, Kreiger et al. observed elevated renal β_2-m excretion in subjects with pregnancy-induced hypertension, the majority of whom had proteinuria < 0.3 g/24 h and normal serum uric acid.[209] Because the LMW proteins are freely filtered at the glomerulus, the additional increase in urinary excretion observed by many investigators in preeclampsia relative to normal pregnancy probably indicates further impairment of proximal tubular function above and beyond that noted for normal pregnancy (see "Normal Pregnancy," above).

The renal excretion of enzymes in preeclampsia has been reported by several groups of investigators. Goren et al. found a significant increase in both the renal excretion of N-acetyl-β-D-glucosaminidase and alanine aminopeptidase in pre-eclamptic women compared to normal third trimester subjects.[212] Jackson et al. conducted an extensive investigation and observed that the urinary excretion and/or fractional excretion of five lysosomal enzymes were significantly increased in the disease.[243] Finally, Shaarawy et al. reported increased urinary excretion of nonspecific alkaline phosphatase, an enzyme localized to the proximal tubule, which correlated with the severity of preeclampsia.[244] The increase in renal excretion of enzymes relative to normal pregnancy reinforces the concept of some proximal tubular dysfunction in the disease.

Summary

The urinary excretion of total protein, albumin, LMW proteins, and of several renal tubular enzymes increases during normal human pregnancy. The increase in renal excretion of LMW proteins and of renal tubular enzymes is consistent with a physiologic impairment of proximal tubular function. (This concept is also supported by the finding of elevated urinary excretion or fractional excretion of glucose, amino acids, uric acid, and calcium during normal human gestation[8,210] [see "Renal Handling of Uric Acid," above.]) In addition to insufficient proximal tubular reabsorption, the elevated GFR of pregnancy and possibly an alteration in the electrostatic charge of the glomerular filter also contribute to gestational albuminuria. Available evidence does not indicate an increase in the glomerular permselectivity on the basis of size or molecular weight. As in the nonpregnant condition, much of the protein in normal pregnancy urine is probably Tamm Horsfall protein, and whether its secretion is increased during gestation has not been studied in detail.[245]

In preeclampsia, the urinary excretion of total protein, albumin, LMW proteins, and of several renal tubular enzymes is exaggerated compared to normal pregnancy. The further increase in renal excretion of LMW protein and renal tubular enzymes suggests additional compromise of proximal tubular function. The gross albuminuria and excretion of other plasma proteins is secondary to vasoconstriction, as well as alteration of both the molecular size constraints, possibly of the electrostatic properties of the glomerular filter, and perhaps compromised proximal tubular reabsorptive capacity. Further investigation of both the permselective and electrostatic properties of the glomerular filter in preeclampsia is needed. An unresolved paradox is the reduced reabsorptive capacity for proteins in preeclampsia implicating proximal tubular dysfunction, and the enhanced reabsorptive capacity for uric acid by the proximal tubule in the disease (see "Renal Handling of Uric Acid," above).

CARDIOVASCULAR ALTERATIONS IN PREECLAMPSIA

This final section is devoted to cardiovascular alterations in preeclampsia. In the first edition, Chesley combined hemodynamic alterations in normal gestation and preeclampsia into a single chapter, titled "Blood Pressure and Circulation." In this book, data relating to the physiologic alterations in cardiac performance and the control of blood pressure during normal gestation are detailed in Chapter 3. Here we summarize these changes briefly as background to the focus of this final section which deals with the heart (contractility and cardiac output) and vessels (systemic vascular resistance and pressor responses) in preeclampsia.

Normal Pregnancy

Blood pressure decreases rapidly after conception, such that by midpregnancy diastolic levels are approximately 10 mm Hg below nonpregnant values. Pressures then increase slowly and near term may return to nonpregnant levels, while in the immediate puerperium they may even rise transiently above the nongravid means. Cardiac output increases to levels 30 to 50% above nonpregnant values. Serial studies using noninvasive echocardiographic technology (see Chap. 3) have established that the rise starts very early in pregnancy and peaks about gestational week 16, after which levels are probably sustained until term (though some have noted small declines late in pregnancy which may relate to posture or other technical aspects of their studies).

Given the magnitude of the increments in cardiac output, the decrease in mean arterial pressure observed must be due to large decrements in peripheral vascular resistance, and indeed this is the case; *normal pregnancy is a markedly vasodilated state*. Factors responsible for these physiologic changes (including increased total arterial compliance, changed pressor or dilator autocoid production, and a variety of circulating substances) are further discussed in Chapter 3. Of importance is that knowledge of the cardiovascular changes in normal pregnancy enhances diagnostic skills. For instance, though technically classified as "normal," diastolic levels of 75 mm Hg in the second trimester and 85 mm Hg in the third trimester, or systolic values of 120 mm Hg at midpregnancy or 130 mm Hg in the last trimester are suspect. Indeed there is epidemiologic evidence that fetal death increases when diastolic pressure exceeds 85 mm Hg at any stage in gestation, as well as evidence of increased fetal growth retardation when mean arterial pressure exceeds 90 and 95 mm Hg during the second and third trimesters, respectively[246,247] (see Chap. 2).

Preeclampsia

Cardiac Performance and Systemic Vascular Resistance

Pulmonary edema is a complication of severe preeclampsia, yet the literature is unclear as to whether or not the disease directly affects the heart.[248] For example, myocardial necrosis compatible with coronary spasm has been noted in autopsy reports, and several investigators have highlighted decrements in the contractile state of the myocardium.[248] Also, as discussed below, there is no consensus on what happens to cardiac output and stroke volume in preeclampsia. A critical review of all these studies is beyond the scope of this chapter which will focus on a more recent approach to the evaluation of left ventricular function in preeclampsia, and will analyze in detail two seemingly divergent studies of cardiac output and peripheral vascular resistance in preeclamptic women.

Left Ventricular Mechanics.   Perusal of the literature devoted to ventricular function in preeclampsia reveals a host of problems with interpretation of data,[248] which are as follows. Most investigators use traditional ejection phase indices to describe left ventricular performance. These indices are unable to distinguish alterations in contractility from changes in ventricular load. Also, many reports contain patients who have preeclampsia superimposed on other disorders such as essential hypertension, diabetes, and kidney disease. Some investigators acquired their data during active labor, or when the women were receiving vasodilator therapy or volume-expanding infusates, including saline, albumin, or dextran.[248] Finally, the posture assumed during the study, which may affect cardiac output (especially in late pregnancy), was frequently not controlled.

One attempt to circumvent these problems is the study design used by Lang et al.[248] These authors evaluated ten nulliparous preeclamptics, defined by de novo hypertension and new-onset proteinuria, as well as hyperuricemia in late gestation. The women were studied on three occasions, first, just prior to induced labor or ceasarean section (when no antihypertensive medications had been administered, although magnesium sulfate therapy had usually been initiated), then one day postpartum when the subjects were still hypertensive, but magnesium therapy had been discontinued. The last test took place one month postpartum, when abnormal proteinuria was no longer present and blood pressures had normalized. The values of the ten preeclamptic women were similar to those of ten normotensive women studied at the same three time periods who served as controls. The investigators used noninvasive echocardiography to evaluate *load-independent left ventricular contractility* as well as cardiac output and total systemic resistance. The derivation of this index, and the experimental evidence to support its validity are discussed in the report, but a brief description is in order.

To assess *load-independent left ventricular contractility*, left end-systolic wall stress (in g/cm^2) is compared to the rate corrected velocity of fiber shortening (VCF$_c$) as depicted in Figure 8–9. Ventricular performance is evaluated by comparing the recorded observations in the patient to a mean contractility line and its confidence intervals in the graph which compares wall stress to VCF$_c$ (shaded area on Fig. 8–9). This "normal" area was derived from simultaneous echocardiographic and angiographic studies of volunteers tested under basal conditions, and during pharmacologic manipulation of afterload with vasoconstrictors and vasodilators. In essence, the mean contractility line and its confidence limits define normal contractility over the physiologic range. Furthermore, it is a sensitive index of contractility *independent of preload and heart rate, and incorporates afterload into its analysis.* A criticism in relation to this study, though, is that the healthy volunteers who underwent echocardiographic and angiographic studies, as well as pharmacologic manipulation, and whose data determine the normal contractility range were all nonpregnant. However, the data from the ten normotensive control studies pre- and

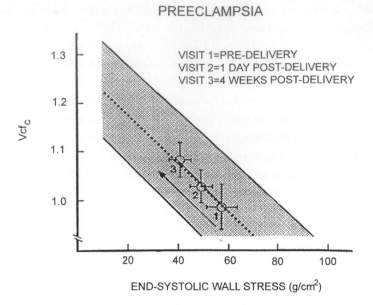

Figure 8–9. Average end-systolic wall stress (σ_{es})-rate-corrected velocity of fiber shortening (Vcf$_c$) data obtained in patients with preeclampsia before delivery, 1 day after delivery, and 4 weeks after delivery. From visit 1 to visit 3, data points shifted left-ward and upward (*arrow*) but still fell on the mean contractility line, indicating de-creased afterload without changes in contractility. (*Reprinted, with permission, from Lang RM, Pridjian G, Feldman T, et al: Left ventricular mechanics in preeclampsia. Am Heart J 1991;121:1768–1775.*)

postpartum in the study by Lang et al.,[248] all fell on the mean contractility line at each study period even though overall left ventricular performance was greater during, compared to studies performed one month after delivery.

As noted in Figure 8–9, values in the preeclamptic women were also on or near the normal contractility line at each test period. The data demonstrate decreased left ventricular performance when the disease was manifest, with normalization one month postpartum. However, contractility is normal. Stated otherwise, the de-creased performance represented a mechanically appropriate response to increased afterload and not a cardiomyopathic state. Of interest, using traditional approaches some would have interpreted the echocardiographic findings as showing decreased contractility.

Cardiac Output and Systemic Vascular Resistance During Preeclampsia.   A survey of the literature suggests that the systemic hemodynamic pattern in preeclampsia ranges from a high output–low resistance to a low output–high resis-tance state.[249,250] The main point of controversy is whether this wildly inconsistent view reflects experimental artifact, a wide spectrum of pathophysiology, or both.

Wallenburg made a strong case for the former. He suggested that older studies were confounded by a number of methodologic shortcomings, most notably, clini-cal intervention with magnesium sulfate, antihypertensive medications, and intravenous fluids, all of which can profoundly influence systemic hemodynamics.[249] (The Wallenburg work reviews studies from 1949–1988.)[249] In a 1991 investigation by Visser and Wallenburg,[251] the inclusion criteria consisted of: (1) gestational age less than 34 weeks; (2) singleton pregnancy with a live fetus; (3) no obstetric indication for immediate delivery; (4) unrestricted diet; (5) not in labor; (6) no signs of pulmonary edema; (7) no known preexisting hypertensive, cardiac, or renal disease; and (8) strict definition of severe preeclampsia including a diastolic pressure of 100 mm Hg or more on two occasions at least 4 hours apart and proteinuria of 0.5 g/L or more, both of which resolved after delivery, and development of symptoms after 20 weeks' gestation. In addition, they divided the patients into those who had not received any treatment whatsoever and those who had received treatment. There were 87 and 47 women in the untreated and treated groups, respectively. A control group of 10 normotensive parous women was also investigated. Using the Swan–Ganz pulmonary artery thermodilution technique, the investigators observed a remarkably consistent view of the hemodynamic status in the untreated severe preeclamptic patients irrespective of parity or position of the subject during the study, i.e., a low output–high resistance state associated with a normal pulmonary capillary wedge pressure. By contrast, in those subjects who had received treatment, the hemodynamic pattern was more varied; on average, the cardiac index was comparable to normal pregnancy, and the systemic vascular resistance was considerably improved (Table 8–7). These findings corroborate and extend those of a preliminary report by the same group of investigators.[252] (In the earlier publication,[252] the pulmonary capillary wedge pressure was very low in the preeclamptic patients presumably because they were on a "mildly sodium-restricted diet." The fact that these women were quite volume-contracted confounded this earlier work, but was not an issue in the later publication.[251]) Based on their results, Wallenburg and coworkers concluded that "the [previously] reported extremes of the hemodynamic profile appear to reflect clinical management rather than the pathophysiological state."[251] Of interest, similar findings were noted in noninvasive echocardiographic studies by Lang et al.,[248] which compared cardiac output and peripheral vascular resistance at term and one month postpartum in ten nulliparous, proteinuric preeclamptic women and ten normotensive matched controls. In this study, cardiac output and resistance were significantly lower and higher, respectively, at term in preeclamptic subjects compared to controls, while values were similar in both groups one month postpartum.

Another perspective championed by Easterling et al. is that a high output–low resistance state precedes the clinical onset of preeclampsia, and a "cross-over" to low output–high resistance may occur in the latter stages, particularly in severe preeclampsia.[253] This reasoning follows by analogy one view of the progression of essential hypertension.[254] Thus, as the argument goes, Wallenburg and coworkers captured the hemodynamic state in women with severe preeclampsia after the "cross-over."[251,252] Is it possible, therefore, that the disparate findings among many of the other publications (and even within a single publication) may be due to the timing of the measurements related to the progression of the disease, i.e., some

TABLE 8–7. HEMODYNAMIC PROFILE IN UNTREATED AND TREATED PREECLAMPTIC PATIENTS AND NORMOTENSIVE PREGNANT WOMEN

	Preeclamptics, Untreated (N = 87)	P^a	Normotensive Controls (N = 10)	P^b	Preeclamptics, Treated (N = 47)
Mean intraarterial pressure (mm Hg)	125 (92–156)	< 0.001	83 (81–29)	< 0.001	120 (80–154)^c
Cardiac index ($L \times min^{-1} \times m^{-2}$)	3.3 (2.0–5.3)	< 0.001	4.2 (3.5–4.6)	NS	4.3 (2.4–7.6)^c
Systemic vascular resistance index ($dyne \times sec \times cm^{-5} \times m^2$)	3003 (1,771–5,225)	< 0.001	1560 (1430–2019)	< 0.005	2212 (1057–3688)^c
Pulmonary capillary wedge pressure (mm Hg)	7 (−1–20)	NS	5 (1–8)	< 0.05	7 (0–25)

Values given are median (range).
[a] Differences between untreated preeclamptic patients and normotensive controls.
[b] Differences between pharmacologically treated preeclamptic patients and normotensive controls.
[c] P < 0.05 vs. untreated nulliparous patients.
NS, not significant.
Reprinted, with permission, from Visser W, Wallenburg HCS: Central hemodynamic observations in untreated preeclamptic patients. *Hypertension* 1991;17:1072–1077.

women were studied before and others after the "cross-over," manifesting high output–low resistance and low output–high resistance states, respectively. Clearly, the elegant work and conclusions of Wallenburg and colleagues stand,[251,252] but this alternative viewpoint may also have merit.

In brief, Easterling et al. prospectively studied throughout pregnancy the mean arterial pressure and cardiac output measured by noninvasive Doppler technique.[253] They obtained data for 179 nulliparous women, 9 of whom developed preeclampsia and 81 of whom developed gestational hypertension. The mean arterial pressure and cardiac output were significantly higher throughout gestation in the women destined to develop preeclampsia relative to the women who had normal pregnancy outcomes. The finding of increased mean arterial pressure early in gestation and remote from clinical disease is consistent with other reports.[255-260] However, the observation that the elevated systemic pressure before onset of disease is mediated by increased cardiac output rather than elevated systemic vascular resistance is provocative. There are several caveats which deserve mention. At best, the patients in the study by Easterling et al. fulfilled the diagnosis of mild preeclampsia, insofar as 7 of 9 had only 1+ proteinuria on dipstick, 7 of 9 failed to have plasma uric acid exceeding 1 SD above the normal for gestational age (see "Renal Handling of Uric Acid," above), the gestational age at delivery averaged 39.4 weeks, and the birth weight was within the normal range for gestational age and not significantly lower than the normal pregnancy group. Because the data for the women with gestational hypertension were not presented, one cannot assess whether the systemic hemodynamics are different between the two groups of hypertensive pregnant women. Of additional note is that the preeclamptic women were, on average, 12 kg heavier as reported at 23 weeks' gestation. (The BMIs calculated from the data on height and weight provided were 24.9 and 29.8 kg/m^2, respectively.) It is well known that "obese" women have higher cardiac outputs attributable mainly to peripheral vasodilation in organs such as the kidneys.[261] Therefore, the increase in cardiac output and decrease in systemic vascular resistance throughout gestation in the women with preeclampsia may have been related to an inherently higher BMI rather than to preeclampsia. The persistence of significantly elevated cardiac output and reduced systemic vascular resistance in the postpartum period in the women who suffered preeclampsia is consistent with this argument.

Clearly, further study is needed to resolve the provocative hypothesis raised by Easterling et al.[253] In this regard, using the same longitudinal approach which is necessary to address the status of systemic hemodynamics before clinical onset of preeclampsia, Boslo et al.[262] recently reported that women who developed the disease had significantly elevated cardiac outputs throughout the preclinical stage which is consistent with the findings of Easterling et al. In agreement with Wallenburg and colleagues,[251,252] they also found profoundly reduced cardiac output and increased systemic vascular resistance during the clinical phase. In contrast, women with gestational hypertension had significantly elevated cardiac output both before and after onset of clinical disease. The BMIs were not provided, but the investigators reported that cardiac output and peripheral resistance were not significantly different among the patient groups in the postpartum period. Although preliminary, this work corroborates both the findings of Easterling et al.,[253] as well as of Wallenburg et al.[251,252]

The recent work of Schobel et al.,[263] is both worthy of note and germane to the present topic regarding elevated systemic vascular resistance and blood pressure in preeclampsia. Except for the lack of a control hypertensive pregnant group (e.g., transient gestational hypertension), the patient selection and study design were virtually flawless. In particular, the diagnosis of preeclampsia was made based on rigorous criteria including hyperuricemia, and the interval between dihydralazine administration and study was at least 12 hours in those patients who received the medication. These researchers evaluated postganglionic sympathetic nerve activity in the blood vessels of skeletal muscle by using intraneural microelectrodes. Both baseline data and stimulated responses were recorded. Whether normalized to heart rate or not, the baseline sympathetic nerve firing was threefold higher in the preeclamptic women compared to normal nonpregnant and pregnant women, as well as to hypertensive nonpregnant women. Moreover, the sympathetic hyperactivity declined in parallel with the blood pressure in the same subjects 1 to 3 months after delivery. There was no difference among the groups in the sympathetic nerve activity in response to the Valsalva maneuver or cold pressor test. These data show a correlation between sympathetic hyperactivity as measured in the skeletal muscle of the leg and the elevated systemic vascular resistance and blood pressure of preeclampsia. Whether the finding of sympathetic overactivity can be generalized to other organ beds such as the kidney and liver is uncertain. In fact, the findings of Schobel et al.[263] are at variance with reports in the older literature, that autonomic blockade with tetraethylammonium chloride or imposition of spinal anesthesia (procaine) elicited substantial decreases in blood pressure in both normotensive gravidas or those with essential hypertension, but had minimal effects in preeclampsia.[264,265] Also, in view of the widely held belief that women with preeclampsia have contraction of plasma volume (see Chap. 9), it is possible that the increased sympathetic activity is compensatory rather than causal.

Summary

An emerging concept of the systemic hemodynamic status in preeclampsia is one of high output–low resistance before the clinical onset of the disease, and a "cross-over" to low output–high resistance after the appearance of clinical symptoms at least in severe disease. Clearly, further investigations are needed to substantiate this concept. Whether the initial hyperdynamic and vasodilated state exposes small arteries and capillaries to hemodynamic forces that damage the endothelium, thereby mediating disease manifestations as proposed by Easterling and Benedetti is unproven.[266] If so, it is difficult to reconcile this hypothesis with the conventional wisdom that substances originating from the placenta in response to local ischemia/hypoxia mediate endothelial damage in preeclampsia. Perhaps both mechanisms are at work.

Pressor Responses and Vascular Reactivity. The attenuation of pressor responsiveness to exogenous vasoconstrictors in normal pregnancy, and the loss of this attenuation in preeclampsia has been well documented over the years.[267,268] Perhaps the best illustration of this phenomenon was the classic study by Gant et al.[269] (Fig. 8–10). In particular, the group of women destined to develop preeclampsia lost the attenuated pressor responsiveness to infused angiotensin II prior to the onset of clinical disease relative to women with normal pregnancy outcome.[269]

There are several possible mechanisms for the altered pressor responsiveness to exogenous vasoconstrictors in normal pregnancy and preeclampsia which are unrelated to vascular reactivity. For example, different metabolic clearance rates of the vasoconstrictor can lead to different plasma concentrations reached during the

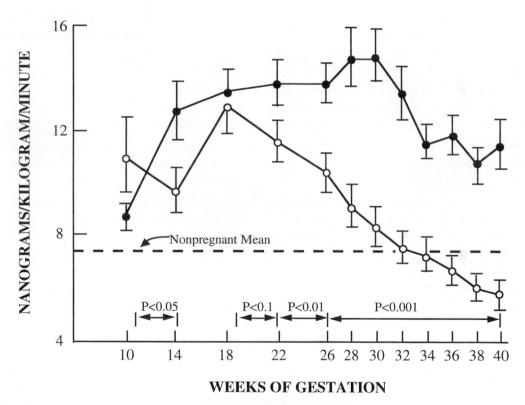

Figure 8–10. Comparison of the mean angiotensin II doses (ng/kg/min) required to evoke a pressor response in 120 primigravidas who remained normotensive and 72 primigravidas who ultimately developed pregnancy-induced hypertension. The nonpregnant mean is shown as a broken line. The horizontal bars represent the standard error of the mean. The black circles represent the results in 120 subjects who remained normal (769 infusions). The open circles represent the results obtained in 72 women who developed pregnancy-induced hypertension (421 infusions). The difference between the two groups became significant after week 23 (P < 0.01), and the two groups continued to widely diverge after the 26th week (P < 0.001). (*Reprinted from Gant NF, Daley GL, Chand S, et al: A study of angiotensin II pressor response throughout primigravid pregnancy.* J Clin Invest *1973;52:2682–2689, by copyright permission of the American Society for Clinical Investigation.*)

infusion in nonpregnant, normal pregnant, and preeclamptic women; pressure-dependent autoregulation contributes to pressor responses and may be different among the three groups of women; and baroreflex responses may also be dissimilar, thereby differentially affecting cardiac output and systemic vascular resistance during infusion of the vasoconstrictors. These confounding variables have not been comprehensively evaluated in normal human pregnancy and preeclampsia.

Nevertheless, there are indications that the enhanced pressor responsiveness of preeclampsia is at least partly related to augmented vascular reactivity. In an exemplary study, Nisell et al. measured cardiac output during infusion of norepinephrine (NE) in nonpregnant women, and in women with normal pregnancy as well as preeclampsia.[270] Physiologically relevant concentrations of NE were reached in the blood, and they were comparable among groups (9–10 nm). The nonpregnant women showed an increase in blood pressure caused by an increase in systemic vascular resistance partly offset by a small decline in cardiac output. In contrast, the comparable rise in blood pressure of normal pregnant women was solely due to a rise in cardiac output. Finally, the enhanced pressor response in preeclampsia was accounted for by an exaggerated rise in systemic vascular resistance. Thus, the vascular reactivity to NE is apparently reduced in normal pregnancy and augmented in preeclampsia.

Another way to evaluate vascular reactivity is by techniques such as venous occlusion plethysmography which provide data relevant to a particular limb. In normal pregnancy, hand blood flow was found to be increased, and the vascular response to NE reduced. Moreover, N^G-monomethyl-L-arginine (NMA), an inhibitor of NO synthase, produced a greater reduction in the hand blood flow of pregnant women compared to nonpregnant controls implying an important role for NO.[271] Using similar techniques, forearm blood flow was observed to be elevated in normal pregnancy, while the constrictor responses to angiotensin II and NMA were diminished and enhanced, respectively.[272] To our knowledge, such studies have not yet been reported for preeclampsia.

The assessment of vascular reactivity of blood vessels in vitro is another approach, which is further discussed in Chapter 3. By studying small arteries, it is apparent that vascular reactivity is altered in normal pregnancy and preeclampsia, although considerable vessel heterogenity exists. The mechanism(s), however, has not been clearly delineated and is likely to vary according to the vascular bed and vessel size. Possibilities include alterations in vasoconstrictor receptor density or affinity and receptor signal transduction, as well as changes in vascular smooth muscle and/or endothelial function. Recent data suggest that the density of platelet angiotensin II receptors is upregulated during preeclampsia, most likely reflecting the lower circulating levels of angiotensin II in the disease.[273,274] Given a similar change in the vascular smooth muscle, this finding could explain the alterations in pressor responsiveness to infused angiotensin II, although other mechanisms undoubtedly contribute.

Finally, in the first edition of this text, Chesley devoted a considerable portion of the chapter "Blood Pressure and Circulation" to discussions of regional blood

flows during both normal pregnancy and preeclampsia. The reader is referred to Tables 1 through 7 in the first edition for a scholarly review of older literature which attempts to define changes in flow to brain, liver, forearm, hand, and uterus. A critique of the methodologies used, the technical rigors of the study, and the validity of the diagnoses in this older literature, is beyond the scope of this chapter. Some more recent studies such as use of Doppler ultrasonography in the clinical assessment of uteroplacental circulation as well as the study of cerebral circulation in preeclampsia will be discussed in Chapters 3 and 5 of this text. Regional blood flow is another area that needs reassessment in preeclampsia. Given the advancements in noninvasive technology, this should now be much easier to evaluate.

Summary

Enhanced vascular reactivity most likely contributes to the well-described phenomenon of increased pressor responsiveness to infused vasoconstrictors in preeclampsia. To obtain an integrated picture, further investigations are needed in which cardiac output is measured as well as blood pressure so that changes in vascular reactivity to various vasoconstrictors can be determined. The application of techniques such as venous occlusion plethysmography to the study of vascular reactivity before and after the local infusion of pressor agents in preeclampsia would also be useful. Ultimately, the additional study of small resistance-sized blood vessels themselves is required to define the various molecular mechanisms which mediate the altered vascular reactivity in both normal pregnancy and preeclampsia relative to nonpregnant control subjects.

ACKNOWLEDGMENTS
The authors thank Sue Davis for expert secretarial support and the library staff of the Magee-Women's Hospital for their superb assistance. This work was supported by National Institutes of Health research grants RCDA K04 HD 01098, R01 HD30325, and 2 PO1 HD30367.

REFERENCES

1. Gilson GJ, Mosher MD, Conrad KP: Systemic hemodynamics and oxygen transport during pregnancy in chronically instrumented, conscious rats. *Am J Physiol* 1992;263:H1911–H1918.
2. Sims EAH, Krantz KE: Serial studies of renal function during pregnancy and the puerperium in normal women. *J Clin Invest* 1958;37:1764–1774.
3. de Alvarez RR: Renal glomerulotubular mechanisms during normal pregnancy. *Am J Obstet Gynecol* 1958;75:931–944.
4. Assali NS, Dignam WJ, Dasgupta K: Renal function in human pregnancy. *J Lab Clin Med* 1959;54:394–408.
5. Dunlop W: Serial changes in renal hemodynamics during normal human pregnancy. *Br J Obstet Gynaecol* 1981;88:1–9.
6. Roberts M, Lindheimer MD, Davison JM: Altered glomerular permselectivity to neutral dextrans and heteroporous membrane modeling in human pregnancy. *Am J Physiol* 1996; 270:F338–F343.

7. Chapman AB, Abraham WT, Zamudio S, et al: Temporal relationships between hormonal and hemodynamic changes in early human pregnancy. *Kidney Int* 1998;54:2056–2063.

8. Conrad KP: Renal changes in pregnancy. *Urol Ann* 1992;6:313–340.

9. Davison JM, Dunlop W: Changes in renal hemodynamics and tubular function induced by normal human pregnancy. *Semin Nephrol* 1984;4:198–207.

10. Ezinokhai M, Davison JM, Philips PR, Dunlop W: Non-postural serial changes in renal function during the third trimester of normal human pregnancy. *Br J Obstet Gynaecol* 1981; 88:465–471.

11. Kuhlbäck B, Widholm O: Plasma creatinine in normal pregnancy. *Scand J Clin Lab Invest* 1966;18:654–656.

12. Nice M: Kidney function during normal pregnancy. *J Clin Invest* 1935;14:575–578.

13. Davison JM: Changes in renal function in early pregnancy in women with one kidney. *Yale J Biol Med* 1978;51:347–349.

14. Davison JM: The effect of pregnancy on kidney function in renal allograft recipients. *Kidney Int* 1985;27:74–79.

15. Baylis C: Effect of amino acid infusion as an index of renal vasodilatory capacity in pregnant rats. *Am J Physiol* 1988;254:F650–F656.

16. Sturgiss SN, Wilkinson R, Davison JM: Renal reserve during human pregnancy. *Am J Physiol* 1996;271:F16–F20.

17. Smith HW: *The Kidney.* New York: Oxford University Press; 1951.

18. Davison JM, Noble MCB: Serial changes in 24 hour creatinine clearance during normal menstrual cycles and the first trimester of pregnancy. *Br J Obstet Gynaecol* 1981;88:10–17.

19. Davison JM, Hytten FE: Glomerular filtration during and after pregnancy. *Br J Obstet Gynaecol* 1974;81:588–595.

20. Davison JM, Dunlop W, Ezimokhai M: 24-hour creatinine clearance during the third trimester of normal pregnancy. *Br J Obstet Gynaecol* 1980;87:106–109.

21. Pritchard JA, Barnes AC, Bright RH: The effect of the supine position on renal function in the near-term pregnant woman. *J Clin Invest* 1955;34:777–781.

22. Chesley LC, Sloan DM: The effect of posture on renal function in late pregnancy. *Am J Obstet Gynecol* 1964;89:754–759.

23. Pippig L: Clinical aspects of renal disease during pregnancy. *Med Hygiene* 1969;27:181–216.

24. Dunlop W: Investigations into the influence of posture on renal plasma flow and glomerular filtration rate during late pregnancy. *Br J Obstet Gynaecol* 1976;83:17–23.

25. Lindheimer MD, Weston PV: Effect of hypotonic expansion on sodium, water, and urea excretion in late pregnancy: The influence of posture on these results. *J Clin Invest* 1969;48: 947–956.

26. Brenner BM, Troy JL, Daugharty TM: The dynamics of glomerular ultrafiltration in the rat. *J Clin Invest* 1971;50:1776–1780.

27. Baylis C: The mechanism of the increase in glomerular filtration rate in the twelve-day pregnant rat. *J Physiol* 1980;305:405–414.

28. Gellai M, Valtin H: Chronic vascular constrictions and measurements of renal function in conscious rats. *Kidney Int.* 1979;15:419–426.

29. Conrad KP: Renal hemodynamics during pregnancy in chronically catheterized, conscious rats. *Kidney Int* 1984;26:24–29.

30. Reckelhoff JF, Samsell L, Baylis C: Failure of an acute 10–15% plasma volume expansion in the virgin female rat to mimic the increased glomerular filtration rate (GFR) and altered glomerular hemodynamics seen at midterm pregnancy. *Clin Exper Hyper Pregnancy* 1989; B8:533–549.

31. Baylis C, Blantz RC: Tubuloglomerular feedback activity in virgin and 12-day-pregnant rats. *Am J Physiol* 1985;249:F169–F173.

32. Phippard AF, Horvath JS, Glynn EM, et al: Circulatory adaptation to pregnancy—serial studies of haemodynamics, blood volume, renin and aldosterone in the baboon (Papio hamadryas). *J Hypertension* 1986;4:773–779.

33. Robson SC, Hunter S, Boys RJ, Dunlop W: Serial study of factors influencing changes in cardiac output during human pregnancy. *Am J Physiol* 1989;256:H1060–H1065.

34. Conrad KP, Gellai M, North WG, Valtin H: Influence of oxytocin on renal hemodynamics and sodium excretion. *Ann NY Acad Sci* 1993;689:346–362.
35. Atherton JC, Bu'lock D, Pirie SC: The effect of pseudopregnancy on glomerular filtration rate and salt and water reabsorption in the rat. *J Physiol* 1982;324:11–20.
36. Baylis C: Glomerular ultrafiltration in the pseudopregnant rat. *Am J Physiol* 1982;234: F300–F305.
37. Paaby P, Brochner-Mortensen J, Fjeldborg P, et al: Endogenous overnight creatinine clearance compared with ^{51}Cr-EDTA clearance during the menstrual cycle. *Acta Med Scand* 1987;222:281–284.
38. Paaby P, Moller-Petersen J, Larsen CE, Raffn K: Endogenous overnight creatinine clearance, serum β_2-microglobulin and serum water during the menstrual cycle. *Acta Med Scand* 1987;221:191–197.
39. Brochner-Mortensen J, Paaby P, Fjeldborg P, et al: Renal haemodynamics and extracellular homeostasis during the menstrual cycle. *Scand J Clin Lab Invest* 1987;47:829–835.
40. Van Beek E, Houben AJI IM, Van Es PN, et al: Peripheral haemodynamics and renal function in relation to the menstrual cycle. *Clin Sci* 1996;91:163–168.
41. Chapman AB, Zamudio S, Woodmansee W, et al: Systemic and renal hemodynamic changes in the luteal phase of the menstrual cycle mimic early pregnancy. *Am J Physiol* 1997;273: F777–F782.
42. Christy NP, Shaver JC: Estrogens and the kidney. *Kidney Int* 1974;6:366–376.
43. Chesley LC, Tepper IH: Effects of progesterone and estrogen on the sensitivity to angiotensin II. *J Clin Endocr* 1967;27:576–581.
44. Nuwayhid B, Brinkman CR, Woods JR, et al: Effects of estrogen on systemic and regional circulations in normal and renal hypertensive sheep. *Am J Obstet Gynecol* 1975;123:495–504.
45. Rosenfeld CR, Morriss FH, Battaglia FC, et al: Effect of estradiol-17β on blood flow to reproductive and nonreproductive tissues in pregnant ewes. *Am J Obstet Gynecol* 1976; 124:618–629.
46. Magness RR, Phernetton TM, Zheng J: Systemic and uterine blood flow distribution during prolonged infusion of estradiol-17B. *Am J Physiol* 1998;44:731H–743H.
47. Atallah AN, Guimarães JAG, Gebara M, et al: Progesterone increases glomerular filtration rate, urinary kallikrein excretion and uric acid clearance in normal women. *Brazilian J Med Biol Res* 1988;21:71–74.
48. Oparil S, Ehrlich EN, Lindheimer MD: Effect of progesterone on renal sodium handling in man: Relation to aldosterone excretion and plasma renin activity. *Clin Sci Mol Med* 1975;49:139–147.
49. Omer S, Mulay S, Cernacek P, Varma DR: Attenuation of renal effects of atrial natriuretic factor during rat pregnancy. *Am J Physiol* 1995;268:F416–F422.
50. Conrad KP: Possible mechanisms for changes in renal hemodynamics during pregnancy: Studies from animal models. *Am J Kidney Dis* 1987;9:253–259.
51. Sherwood OD: Relaxin. In: Knobil E, et al, eds. *The Physiology of Reproduction.* New York: Raven Press; 1994:861–1009.
52. Stewart DR, Celniker AC, Taylor CA, et al: Relaxin in the peri-implantation period. *J Clin Endocrinol Metab* 1990;70:1771–1773.
53. Johnson MR, Carter G, Grint C, Lightman SL: Relationship between ovarian steroids, gonadotrophins and relaxin during the menstrual cycle. *Acta Endocrinol* 1993;129:121–125.
54. Wreje U, Kristiansson P, Aberg H, et al: Serum levels of relaxin during the menstrual cycle and oral contraceptive use. *Gynecol Obstet Invest* 1995;39:197–200.
55. Davison JM, Vallotton MB, Lindheimer MD: Plasma osmolality and urinary concentration and dilution during and after pregnancy: Evidence that lateral recumbency inhibits maximal urinary concentrating ability. *Br J Obstet Gynaecol* 1981;88:472–479.
56. Davison JM, Shiells EA, Philips PR, Lindheimer MD: Serial evaluation of vasopressin release and thirst in human pregnancy. *J Clin Invest* 1988;81:798–806.
57. Lindheimer MD, Barron WM, Davison JM: Osmoregulation of thirst and vasopressin release in pregnancy. *Am J Physiol* 1989;257:F159–F169.

58. Lindheimer MD, Davison JM: Osmoregulation, the secretion of arginine vasopressin and its metabolism during pregnancy. *Eur J Endocrinol* 1995;132:133–143.

59. Weisinger RS, Burns P, Eddie LW, Wintour EM: Relaxin alters the plasma osmolality–arginine vasopressin relationship in the rat. *J Endocrinol* 1993;137:505–510.

60. St-Louis J, Massicotte G: Chronic decrease of blood pressure by rat relaxin in spontaneously hypertensive rats. *Life Sci* 1985;37:1351–1357.

61. Massicotte G, Parent A, St-Louis J: Blunted responses to vasoconstrictors in mesenteric vasculature but not in portal vein of spontaneously hypertensive rats treated with relaxin. *Proc Soc Exp Biol Med* 1989;190:254–259.

62. Bani-Sacchi T, Bigazzi M, Bani D, et al: Relaxin-induced increased coronary flow through stimulation of nitric oxide production. *Br J Pharmacol* 1995;116:1589–1594.

63. Bani D, Bigazzi M, Masini E, et al: Relaxin depresses platelet aggregation: In vitro studies on isolated human and rabbit platelets. *Lab Invest* 1995;73:709–716.

64. Danielson LA, Conrad KP: Relaxin is a potent renal vasodilator in conscious rats. *J Soc Gynecol Invest* 1998;5:146A.

65. Venuto RC, Donker AJM: Prostaglandin E_2, plasma renin activity, and renal function throughout rabbit pregnancy. *J Lab Clin Med* 1982;99:239–246.

66. Conrad KP, Colpoys MC: Evidence against the hypothesis that prostaglandins are the vasodepressor agents of pregnancy. Serial studies in chronically instrumented, conscious rats. *J Clin Invest* 1986;77:236–245.

67. Baylis C: Renal effects of cyclooxygenase inhibition in the pregnant rat. *Am J Physiol.* 1987;253:F158–F163.

68. Conrad KP, Dunn MJ: Renal synthesis and urinary excretion of eicosanoids during pregnancy in rats. *Am J Physiol* 1987;253:F1197–F1205.

69. Brown GP, Venuto RC: Eicosanoid production in rabbit vascular tissues and placentas. *Am J Physiol* 1990;258:E418–E422.

70. Gallery EDM, Ross M, Grigg R, Bean C: Are the renal functional changes of human pregnancy caused by prostacyclin? *Prostaglandins* 1985;30:1019–1029.

71. Sorensen TK, Easterling TR, Carlson KL, et al: The maternal hemodynamic effect of indomethacin in normal pregnancy. *Obstet Gynecol* 1992;79:661–663.

72. Harrison GL, Moore LG: Blunted vasoreactivity in pregnant guinea pigs is not restored by meclofenamate. *Am J Obstet Gynecol* 1989;160:258–264.

73. Conrad KP, Vernier KA: Plasma level, urinary excretion, and metabolic production of cGMP during gestation in rats. *Am J Physiol* 1989;257:R847–R853.

74. Conrad KP, Joffe GM, Kruszyna H, et al: Identification of increased nitric oxide biosynthesis during pregnancy in rats. *FASEB J* 1993;7:566–571.

75. Conrad KP, Mosher MD: Nitric oxide biosynthesis in normal and preeclamptic pregnancy—a preliminary report. *J Am Soc Nephrol* 1995;6:657.

76. Kopp L, Paradiz G, Tucci JR: Urinary excretion of cyclic 3′,5′-adenosine monophosphate and cyclic 3′,5′-guanosine monophosphate during and after pregnancy. *J Clin Endocrinol Metab* 1977;44:590–594.

77. Sala C, Campise M, Ambroso G, et al: Atrial natriuretic peptide and hemodynamic changes during normal human pregnancy. *Hypertension Dallas* 1995;25:631–636.

78. Yang D, Lang U, Greenberg SG, et al: Elevation of nitrate levels in pregnant ewes and their fetuses. *Am J Obstet Gynecol* 1996;174:573–577.

79. Baylis C, Suto T, Conrad K: Importance of nitric oxide in control of systemic and renal hemodynamics during normal pregnancy: Studies in the rat and implications for preeclampsia. *Hypertension Pregnancy* 1996;15:147–169.

80. Sladek SM, Magness RR, Conrad KP: Nitric oxide and pregnancy. *Am J Physiol* 1997;272: R441–R463.

81. Danielson LA, Conrad KP: Acute blockade of nitric oxide synthase inhibits renal vasodilation and hyperfiltration during pregnancy in chronically instrumented conscious rats. *J Clin Invest* 1995;96:482–490.

82. Gandley RE, KP Conrad, McLaughlin MK: Endothelin and nitric oxide regulate myogenic behavior in the renal resistance vasculature at mid-pregnancy in the rat. *J Am Soc Nephrol* 1997;8:328A.

83. Danielson LA, Conrad KP: Prostaglandins maintain renal vasodilation and hyperfiltration during chronic nitric oxide synthase blockade in conscious, pregnant rats. *Circ Res* 1996;79: 1161–1166.

84. Haynes WG: Endothelins as regulators of vascular tone in man. *Clin Sci* 1995;88:509–517.

85. Yokokawa K, Johnson J, Kohno M, et al: Phosphoinositide turnover signaling stimulated by ET-3 in endothelial cells from spontaneously hypertensive rats. *Am J Physiol* 1994;267: R635–R644.

86. Hirata Y, Hayakawa H, Suzuki E, et al: Direct measurements of endothelium-derived nitric oxide release by stimulation of endothelin receptors in rat kidney and its alteration in salt-induced hypertension. *Circulation* 1995;91:1229–1235.

87. Tsukahara H, Ende H, Magazine HI, et al: Molecular and functional characterization of the non-isopeptide-selective ET$_B$ receptor in endothelial cells. *J Biol Chem* 1994;269:21778–21785.

88. Hirata Y, Emori T, Eguchi S, et al: Endothelin receptor subtype B mediates synthesis of nitric oxide by cultured bovine endothelial cells. *J Clin Invest* 1993;91:1367–1373.

89. Kurihara Y, Kurihara H, Suzuki H, et al: Elevated blood pressure and craniofacial abnormalities in mice deficient in endothelin-1. *Nature* 1994;368:703–710.

90. Gellai M, Fletcher T, Pullen M, Nambi P: Evidence for the existence of endothelin-B receptor subtypes and their physiological roles in the rat. *Am J Physiol* 1996;271:R254–R261.

91. Kourembanas S, McQuillan LP, Leung GK, Faller DV: Nitric oxide regulates the expression of vasoconstrictors and growth factors by vascular endothelium under both normoxia and hypoxia. *J Clin Invest* 1993;92:99–104.

92. Qui C, Samsell L, Baylis C: Actions of endogenous endothelin on glomerular hemodynamics in the rat. *Am J Physiol* 1995;269:R469–R473.

93. Dobrowolski L, Endlich K, Sadowski J, Steinhausen M: Cardiovascular and renal effects of endothelin receptor blockade with PD145065 and interaction with urodilatin. *Acta Physiol Scand* 1997;159:7–13.

94. Gellai M. Physiological role of endothelin in cardiovascular and renal hemodynamics: Studies in animals. *Curr Opin Nephrol Hypertension* 1997;6:64–68.

95. Conrad KP, Gandley RE, Ogawa T, et al: Endothelin mediates renal vasodilation and hyperfiltration during pregnancy in conscious rats. *J Am Soc Nephrol* 1997;8:327A.

96. Woods LL, Mizelle HL, Hall JE: Autoregulation of renal blood flow and glomerular filtration rate in the pregnant rabbit. *Am J Physiol* 1987;252:R69–R72.

97. Reckelhoff JF, Yokota SD, Baylis C: Renal autoregulation in midterm and late-pregnant rats. *Am J Obstet Gynecol* 1992;166:1546–1550.

98. Chesley LC, Chesley ER: The diodrast clearance and renal blood flow in normal pregnant and nonpregnant women. *Am J Physiol* 1939;127:731–739.

99. Chesley LC, Connell EJ, Chesley ER, et al: The diodrast clearance and renal blood flow in toxemias of pregnancy. *J Clin Invest* 1940;19:219–224.

100. Wellen I, Welsh CA, Taylor HC: The filtration rate, effective renal blood flow, tubular excretory mass and phenol red clearance in specific toxemia of pregnancy. *J Clin Invest* 1942;21: 63–70.

101. Welsh CA, Wellen I, Taylor HC: The filtration rate, effective renal blood flow, tubular excretory mass and phenol red clearance in normal pregnancy. *J Clin Invest* 1942;21:57–61.

102. Dill LV, Isenhour CE, Cadden JF, Schaffer NK: Glomerular filtration and renal blood flow in the toxemias of pregnancy. *Am J Obstet Gynecol* 1942;43:32–42.

103. Kariher DH, George RH: Toxemias of pregnancy and the inulin-diodrast clearance tests. *Proc Soc Exp Biol Med* 1943;52:245–247.

104. Schaffer NK, Dill LV, Cadden JF: Uric acid clearance in normal pregnancy and pre-eclampsia. *J Clin Invest* 1943;22:201–206.

105. Chesley LC, Williams LO: Renal glomerular and tubular function in relation to the hyperuricemia of pre-eclampsia and eclampsia. *Am J Obstet Gynecol* 1945;50:367–375.

106. Bucht H: Studies on renal function in man. *Scand J Clin Lab Invest* 1951;3:5–64.

107. Bucht H, Werkö: Glomerular filtration rate and renal blood flow in hypertensive toxaemia of pregnancy. *J Obstet Gynaec Bri Emp* 1953;60:157–164.

108. Assali NS, Kaplan SA, Fomon SJ, Douglass RA: Renal function studies in toxemia of pregnancy. *J Clin Invest* 1953;32:44–51.

109. Brandstetter F, Schüller E: Nierenclearance in der normalen schwangerschaft. *Zentralblatt für Gynakologie* 1954;76:181–190.
110. Brandstetter VF, Schüller E: Die clearanceuntersuchung in der gravidität. *Fortschritte der geburtshilfe und gynäkologie. Bibliotheca Gynaecol* 1956;4:1–99.
111. Friedberg V: Über die clearancemethode als nierenfunktionsprüfung in der schwangerschaft. *Zentralblatt für Gynakologie* 1954;76:2135–2147.
112. Lanz VR, Hochuli E. Über die nierenclearance in der normalen schwangerschaft und bei hypertensiven spättoxikosen, ihre beeinflussung durch hypotensive medikamente. *Schweizerische Med Wochenschrift* 1955;85:395–400.
113. Page EW, Glendening MB, Dignam W, Harper HA: The reasons for decreased histidine excretion in pre-eclampsia. *Am J Obstet Gynecol* 1955;70:766–773.
114. Lovotti A: La filtrazione glomerulare ed il flusso plasmatico renale nella tossicosi gravidica. *Revista d Obstetricia e Ginecologia Pratica* 1956;38:323–332.
115. Hayashi T: Uric acid and endogenous creatinine clearance studies in normal pregnancy and toxemias of pregnancy. *Am J Obstet Gynecol* 1956;71:859–870.
116. Chesley LC, Valenti C, Rein H: Excretion of sodium loads by nonpregnant and pregnant normal, hypertensive and pre-eclamptic women. *Metabolism* 1958;7:575–588.
117. Buttermann K: Clearance-untersuchungen in der normalen und pathologischen schwangerschaft. *Archiv für Gynäkologie* 1958;190:448–492.
118. Schlegel VC: Ergebnisse und prognostische bedeutung der nierenclearance bei spätschwangerschaftstoxikosen. *Zentralblatt für Gynäkologie* 1959;81:869–893.
119. Friedberg VV. Die veränderungen des wasser-und elektrolythaushaltes in der schwangerschaft. *Anaesthetist* 1961;10:334–339.
120. McCartney CP, Spargo B, Lorincz AB, et al: Renal structure and function in pregnant patients with acute hypertension. *Am J Obstet Gynecol* 1964;90:579–590.
121. Bocci A, Bartoli E, Revelli E, et al: L'emodinamica renale nella gravidanza normale e nella sindrome gestosica. *Minerva Ginecol* 1966;18:203–207.
122. Sarles HE, Hill SS, LeBlanc AL, et al: Sodium excretion patterns during and following intravenous sodium chloride loads in normal and hypertensive pregnancies. *Am J Obstet Gynecol* 1968;102:1–7.
123. Sismondi P, Massobrio M, Coppo F: Studio delle correlazioni intercorrenti tra flusso plasmatico renale e flusso ematico miometriale nella gravidanza normale e nella sindrome gestosica. *Minerva Ginecol* 1969;21:96–99.
124. Chesley LC, Duffus GM: Preeclampsia, posture and renal function. *Obstet Gynecol* 1971; 38:1–5.
125. Gómez DM. Evaluation of renal resistances, with special reference to changes in essential hypertension. *J Clin Invest* 1951;30:1143–1155.
126. Fisher KA, Luger A, Spargo BH, Lindheimer MD: Hypertension in pregnancy: Clinical–pathological correlations and remote prognosis. *Medicine* 1981;60:267–276.
127. Hytten FE, Leitch I: *The Physiology of Human Pregnancy.* London: Blackwell Scientific; 1971:139.
128. Roberts M, Milne J, Lindheimer M, Davison J: Glomerular dynamics and membrane porosity in gravidas with renal disease and preeclampsia. *Am J Obstet Gynecol* 1998;178:S109.
129. Stubbs TM, Lazarchick J, Horger EO: Plasma fibronectin levels in preeclampsia: A possible biochemical marker for vascular endothelial damage. *Am J Obstet Gynecol* 1984;150: 885–887.
130. Mayer A: Changes of the endothelium during eclampsia and their significance. *Klinische Wochenzeitschrift* 1924:H27.
131. Roberts JM, Taylor RN, Musci TJ, et al: Preeclampsia: An endothelial cell disorder. *Am J Obstet Gynecol* 1989;161:1200–1204.
132. Valtin H, Schafer JA: *Renal Function,* ed 3. Boston: Little, Brown and Co.; Boston 1995;98–101.
133. Corcoran AC, Page IH: Renal function in late toxemia of pregnancy. *Am J Med Sci* 1941; 201:385–396.
134. Odell LD: Renal filtration rates in pregnancy toxemia. *Am J Med Sci* 1947;213:709–714.
135. Sica DA, Schoolwerth AC: Renal handling of organic anions and cations and renal excretion

of uric acid. In: Brenner BM, ed. *The Kidney,* ed 5. Philadelphia: W.B. Saunders Co.; 1996; 607–626.

136. Boyle JA, Campbell S, Duncan AM, et al: Serum uric acid levels in normal pregnancy with observations on the renal excretion of urate in pregnancy. *J Clin Path* 1966;19: 501–503.

137. Dunlop W, Davison JM: The effect of normal pregnancy upon the renal handling of uric acid. *Br J Obstet Gynaecol* 1977;84:13–21.

138. Lind T, Godfrey KA, Otun H: Changes in serum uric acid concentrations during normal pregnancy. *Br J Obstet Gynaecol* 1984;91:128–132.

139. Semple PF, Carswell W, Boyle JA: Serial studies of the renal clearance of urate and inulin during pregnancy and after the puerperium in normal women. *Clin Sci Mol Med* 1974; 47:559–565.

140. Seitchik J: The metabolism of urate in pre-eclampsia. *Am J Obstet Gynecol* 1956;72:40–47.

141. Seitchik J, Szutka A, Alper C: Further studies on the metabolism of N^{15}-labeled uric acid in normal and toxemic pregnant women. *Am J Obstet Gynecol* 1958;76:1151–1155.

142. Slemons JM, Bogert LJ: The uric acid content of maternal and fetal blood. *J Biol Chem* 1917; 32:63–69.

143. Stander HJ, Duncan EE, Sisson WE: Chemical studies on the toxemias of pregnancy. *Bull Johns Hopkins Hosp* 1925;36:411–427.

144. Stander HJ, Cadden JF: Blood chemistry in preeclampsia and eclampsia. *Am J Obstet Gynecol* 1934;28:856–871.

145. Cadden JF, Stander HJ: Uric acid metabolism in eclampsia. *Am J Obstet Gynecol* 1939; 37:37–47.

146. Crawford MD: The effect of labour on plasma uric acid and urea. *J Obstet Gynaecol Br Emp* 1939;46:540–553.

147. Nayar ASM: Eclampsia. A clinical and biochemical study. *J Obstet Gynaecol Br Emp* 1940; 47:404–436.

148. Schaffer NK, Dill LV, Cadden JF: Uric acid clearance in normal pregnancy and pre-eclampsia. *J Clin Invest* 1943;22:201–206.

149. Chesley LC, Williams LO: Renal glomerular and tubular function in relation to the hyper-uricemia of pre-eclampsia and eclampsia. *Am J Obstet Gynecol* 1945;50:367–375.

150. Bonsnes RW, Stander HJ: A survey of the twenty-four-hour uric acid and urea clearances in eclampsia and severe preeclampsia. *J Clin Invest* 1946;25:378–385.

151. Seitchik J: Observations on the renal tubular reabsorption of uric acid. *Am J Obstet Gynecol* 1953;65:981–985.

152. Hayashi T: Uric acid and endogenous creatinine clearance studies in normal pregnancy and toxemias of pregnancy. *Am J Obstet Gynecol* 1956;71:859–870.

153. Lancet M, Fisher IL: The value of blood uric acid levels in toxaemia of pregnancy. *J Obstet Gynecol Br Emp* 1956;63:116–119.

154. Hayashi TT: The effect of Benemid on uric acid excretion in normal pregnancy and in pre-eclampsia. *Am J Obstet Gynecol* 1957;73:17–22.

155. Hayashi TT, Gillo D, Robbins H, Sabbagha RE: Simultaneous measurement of plasma and erythrocyte oxypurines. *Gynecol Invest* 1972;3:221–236.

156. Czaczkes WJ, Ullmann TD, Sadowsky E: Plasma uric acid levels, uric acid excretion, and response to probenecid in toxemia of pregnancy. *J Lab Clin Med* 1958;51:224–229.

157. Pollak VE, Nettles JB: The kidney in toxemia of pregnancy: A clinical and pathologic study based on renal biopsies. *Medicine* 1960;39:469–526.

158. Handler JS: The role of lactic acid in the reduced excretion of uric acid in toxemia of pregnancy. *J Clin Invest* 1960;39:1526–1532.

159. McFarlane CN: An evaluation of the serum uric acid level in pregnancy. *J Obstet Gynaecol Br Emp* 1963;70:63–68.

160. Widholm O, Kuhlbäck B: The prognosis of the fetus in relation to the serum uric acid in toxaemia of pregnancy. *Acta Obstet Gynecol Scandinav* 1964;43:137–139.

161. Connon AF, Wadsworth RJ: An evaluation of serum uric acid estimations in toxaemia of pregnancy. *Aust NZ J Obstet Gynaecol* 1968;8:197–201.

162. Fadel HE, Sabour MS, Mahran M, et al: Serum uric acid in pre-eclampsia and eclampsia. *J Egyptian Med Assoc* 1969;52:12–23.

163. Fadel HE, Osman L: Urterine-vein uric acid in EPH-gestosis and normal pregnancy. *Schweiz Z Gynäk Geburtsh* 1970;1:395–398.

164. Fadel HE: Northrop G, Misenhimer HR. Hyperuricemia in pre-eclampsia. *Am J Obstet Gynecol* 1976;125:640–647.

165. Redman CWG, Beilin LJ, Bonnar J, Wilkinson RH: Plasma–urate measurements in predicting fetal death in hypertensive pregnancy. *Lancet* 1976;1:1370–1373.

166. Redman CWG, Beilin LJ, Bonnar J: Renal function in preeclampsia. *J Clin Path* 1976; 29:91–94.

167. Redman CWG, Bonnar J, Beilin L: Early platelet consumption in pre-eclampsia. *Br Med J* 1978;1:467–469.

168. Dunlop W, Hill LM, Landon MJ, et al: Clinical relevance of coagulation and renal changes in pre-eclampsia. *Lancet* 1978;2:346–349.

169. Sagen N, Haram K, Nilsen ST: Serum urate as a predictor of fetal outcome in severe pre-eclampsia. *Acta Obstet Gynecol Scand* 1984;63:71–75.

170. Fischer RL, Bianculli KW, Hediger ML, Scholl TO: Maternal serum uric acid levels in twin gestations. *Obstet Gynecol* 1995;85:60–64.

171. Crawford MD: Plasma uric acid and urea findings in eclampsia. *J Obstet Gynaecol Br Emp* 1941;48:60–72.

172. Many A, Westerhausen-Larson A, Kanbour-Shakir A, Roberts JM: Xanthine oxidase/dehydrogenase is present in human placenta. *Placenta* 1996;17:361–365.

173. Many A, Hubel CA, Roberts JM: Hyperuricemia and xanthine oxidase in preeclampsia, revisited. *Am J Obstet Gynecol* 1996;174:288–291.

174. Chesley LC: Simultaneous renal clearances of urea and uric acid in the differential diagnosis of the late toxemias. *Am J Obstet Gynecol* 1950;59:960–969.

175. Brown MA, Wang J, Whitworth JA: The renin-angiotensin-aldosterone system in pre-eclampsia. *Clin Exper Hypertension* 1997;19:713–726.

176. Schobel HP, Fischer T, Heuszer K, et al: Preeclampsia—a state of sympathetic overactivity. *N Engl J Med* 1996;335:1480–1485.

177. Zamudio S, Leslie KK, White M, et al: Low serum estradiol and high serum progesterone concentrations characterize hypertensive pregnancies at high altitude. *J Soc Gynecol Invest* 1994;1:197–205.

178. Schaffer NK, Barker SB, Summerson WH, Stander HJ: Relation of blood, lactic acid and acetone bodies to uric acid in pre-eclampsia and eclampsia. *Proc Soc Exp Biol Med* 1941; 8:237–240.

179. Redman CWG. Maternal plasma volume and disorders of pregnancy. *Br. Med J* 1984;288: 955–956.

180. Brown MA, Zammit VC, Mitar DM: Extracellular fluid volumes in pregnancy-induced hypertension. *J Hypertens* 1992;10:61–68.

181. Honger PE: Albumin metabolism in normal pregnancy. *Scand J Clin Lab Invest* 1968;21: 3–9.

182. Horne CHW, Howie PW, Goudie RB: Serum alpha$_2$-macroglobulin, transferrin, albumin, and IgG levels in preeclampsia. *J Clin Path* 1970;23:514–516.

183. Studd JW, Wood S: Serum and urinary proteins in pregnancy. In: Wynn RM, ed. *Obstetrics and Gynecology Annual* 1976;5:103–123.

184. Beetham R, Dawnay A, Menabawy M, Silver A: Urinary excretion of albumin and retinol-binding protein during normal pregnancy. *J Clin Pathol* 1988;41:1089–1092.

185. Misiani R, Marchesi D, Tiraboschi G, et al: Urinary albumin excretion in normal pregnancy and pregnancy-induced hypertension. *Nephron* 1991;59:416–422.

186. Pederson EB, Rasmussen AB, Johannesen P, et al: Urinary excretion of albumin, beta-2-microglobulin and light chains in pre-eclampsia, essential hypertension in pregnancy and normotensive pregnant and non-pregnant control subjects. *Scand J Clin Lab Invest* 1981;41: 777–784.

187. Bernard A, Thielemans N, Lauwerys R, Van Lierde M: Selective increase in the urinary ex-

cretion of protein 1 (Clara cell protein) and other low molecular weight proteins during normal pregnancy. *Scand J Clin Lab Invest* 1992;52:871–878.

188. Brown MA, Wang M-X, Buddle ML, et al: Albumin excretory rate in normal and hypertensive pregnancy. *Clin Sci* 1994;86:251–255.
189. MacRury SM, Pinion S, Quin JD, et al: Blood rheology and albumin excretion in diabetic pregnancy. *Diabetic Med* 1995;12:51–55.
190. Irgens-Moller L, Hemmingsen L, Holm J: Diagnostic value of microalbuminuria in preeclampsia. *Clinica Chimica Acta* 1986;157:295–298.
191. Lopez-Espinoza I, Dhar H, Humphreys S, Redman CWG: Urinary albumin excretion in pregnancy. *Br J Obstet Gynaecol* 1986;93:176–181.
192. Wright A, Steele P, Bennet JR, et al: The urinary excretion of albumin in normal pregnancy. *Br J Obstet Gynaecol* 1987;94:408–412.
193. Gerö G, Anthony F, Davis M, et al: Retinol-binding protein, albumin and total protein excretion patterns during normal pregnancy. *J Obstet Gynaecol* 1987;8:104–108.
194. Skrha J, Perusicova J, Sperl M, et al: N-acetyl-β-glucosaminidase and albuminuria in normal and diabetic pregnancies. *Clinica Chimica Acta* 1989;182:281–288.
195. Cheung CK, Lao T, Swaminathan R: Urinary excretion of some proteins and enzymes during normal pregnancy. *Clin Chem* 1989;35:1978–1980.
196. McCance DR, Traub AI, Harley JMG, et al: Urinary albumin excretion in diabetic pregnancy. *Diabetologia* 1989;32:236–239.
197. Helkjaer PE, Holm J, Hemmingsen L: Intra-individual changes in concentrations of urinary albumin, serum albumin, creatinine, and uric acid during normal pregnancy. *Clin Chem* 1992;38:2143–2144.
198. Erman A, Neri A, Sharoni R, et al: Enhanced urinary albumin excretion after 35 weeks of gestation and during labour in normal pregnancy. *Scand J Clin Lab Invest* 1992;52:409–413.
199. Konstantin-Hansen KF, Hesseldahl H, Pedersen SM: Microalbuminuria as a predictor of preeclampsia. *Acta Obstet Gynecol Scand* 1992;71:343–346.
200. Higby K, Suiter CR, Phelps JY, et al: Normal values of urinary albumin and total protein excretion during pregnancy. *Am J Obstet Gynecol* 1994;171:984–989.
201. Douma CE, Van Der Post JAM, Van Acker BAC, et al: Circadian variation of urinary albumin excretion in pregnancy. *Br J Obstet Gynaecol* 1995;102:107–110.
202. Roberts M, Lindheimer MD, Davison JM: Altered glomerular permselectivity to neutral dextrans and heteroporous membrane modeling in human pregnancy. *Am J Physiol* 1996;270:F338–F343.
203. Taylor AA, Davison JM: Albumin excretion in normal pregnancy. *Am J Obstet Gynecol* 1997;177:1559–1560.
204. Peterson PA, Evrin P-E, Berggard I: Differentiation of glomerular, tubular, and normal proteinuria: Determinations of urinary excretion of β2-microglobulin, albumin, and total protein. *J Clin Invest* 1969;48:1189–1198.
205. Strober W, Waldmann TA: The role of the kidney in the metabolism of plasma proteins. *Nephron* 1974;13:35–66.
206. Maack T, Johnson V, Kau ST, et al: Renal filtration, transport, and metabolism of low-molecular-weight proteins: A review. *Kidney Int* 1979;16:251–270.
207. Øian P, Monrad-Hansen I I-P, Maltau JM: Serum uric acid correlates with β2-microglobulin in pre-eclampsia. *Acta Obstet Gynecol Scand* 1986;65:103–106.
208. Kelly AM, McNay MB, McEwan HP: Renal tubular function in normal pregnancy. *Br J Obstet Gynaecol* 1978;85:190–196.
209. Krieger MS, Moodley J, Norman RJ, Jialal I: Reversible tubular lesion in pregnancy-induced hypertension detected by urinary β2-microglobulin. *Obstet Gynecol* 1984;63:533–536.
210. Lindheimer MD, Katz AI: The normal and diseased kidney in pregnancy. In: Schrier RW, Gottshalk CW, eds. *Diseases of the Kidney*, ed 6. Boston: Little Brown Co.; 1997;2063–2097.
211. Noble MCB, Landon MJ, Davison JM: The excretion of γ-glutamyl transferase in pregnancy. *Br J Obstet Gynaecol* 1977;84:522–527.
212. Goren MP, Sibai BM, El-Nazar A: Increased tubular enzyme excretion in preeclampsia. *Am J Obstet Gynecol* 1987;157:906–908.

213. Jackson DW, Carder EA, Voss CM, et al: Altered urinary excretion of lysosomal hydrolases in pregnancy. *Am J Kidney Dis* 1993;22:649–655.
214. McCartney CP, Schumacher GFB, Spargo BH: Serum proteins in patients with toxemic glomerular lesion. *Am J Obstet Gynecol* 1971;111:580–590.
215. Studd JWW: Immunoglobulins in normal pregnancy, pre-eclampsia and pregnancy complicated by the nephrotic syndrome. *J Obstet Gynaecol Br Commonw* 1971;78:786–790.
216. Studd JWW, Shaw RW, Bailey DE: Maternal and fetal serum protein concentration in normal pregnancy and pregnancy complicated by proteinuric pre-eclampsia. *Am J Obstet Gynecol* 1972;114:582–588.
217. Honger PE: Albumin metabolism in preeclampsia. *Scand J Clin Lab Invest* 1968;22:177–184.
218. Kelly AM, McEwan HP: Proteinuria in pre-eclamptic toxaemia of pregnancy. *J Obstet Gynaecol Brit Commonw* 1973;80:520–524.
219. Horne CHW, Briggs JD, Howie PW, Kennedy AC: Serum α-macroglobulins in renal disease and preeclampsia. *J Clin Path* 1972;25:590–593.
220. Laakso L, Paasio J: Gastrointestinal protein loss in toxaemic patients. *Acta Obstet Gynecol Scandinav* 1969;48:357–361.
221. Conrad KP, Benyo DF: Placental cytokines and the pathogenesis of preeclampsia. *Am J Reprod Immunol* 1997;37:240–249.
222. Brown MA. The physiology of pre-eclampsia. *Clin Exp Pharmacol Physiol* 1995;22:781–791.
223. Leven CW: Case of puerperal convulsions. *Guys Hosp Rep* 1843;1:995.
224. National High Blood Pressure Education Program (NHBPEP). *Working Group Report on High Blood Pressure in Pregnancy. Am J Obstet Gynecol* 1990;163:1689–1712.
225. Fisher KA, Ahuja S, Luger A, et al: Nephrotic proteinuria with pre-eclampsia. *Am J Obstet Gynecol* 1977;129:643–646.
226. Parviainen S, Soiva K, Ehrnrooth CA: Electrophoretic study of proteinuria in toxemia of late pregnancy. *Scand J Clin Lab Invest* 1951;3:282–287.
227. Lorincz AB, McCartney CP, Pottinger RE, Li KH: Protein excretion patterns in pregnancy. *Am J Obstet Gynecol* 1961;82:252–259.
228. Buzanowski Z, Chojnowska I, Myszkowski L, Sadowski J: The electrophoretic pattern of proteinuria in cases of normal labor and in the course of toxemia of pregnancy. *Polish Med J* 1966;V:217–221.
229. McEwan HP: Investigation of proteinuria in pregnancy by immuno-electrophoresis. *J Obstet Gynaec Br Commonw* 1968;75:289–294.
230. McEwan HP: Investigation of proteinuria associated with hypertension in pregnancy. *J Obstet Gynaec Br Commonw* 1969;76:809–812.
231. Simanowitz MD, MacGregor WG, Hobbs JR: Proteinuria in pre-eclampsia. *J Obstet Gynaecol Br Commonw* 1973;80:103–108.
232. Katz M, Berlyne GM: Differential renal protein clearance in toxaemia of pregnancy. *Nephron* 1974;13:212–220.
233. Kumar S, Muchmore A: Tamm–Horsfall protein—uromodulin (1950–1990). *Kidney Intl* 1990;37:1395–1401.
234. MacLean PR, Paterson WG, Smart GE, et al: Proteinuria in toxaemia and abruptio placentae. *J Obstet Gynaecol Br Commonw* 1972;79:321–326.
235. Robson JS: Proteinuria and the renal lesion in preeclampsia and abruptio placentae. In: Lindheimer MD, Katz AI, Zuspan FP: *Hypertension in Pregnancy*. New York: John Wiley & Sons; 1976:61–73.
236. Simanowitz MD, MacGregor WG: A critical evaluation of renal protein selectivity in pregnancy. *J Obstet Gynaecol Br Commonw* 1974;81:196–200.
237. Wood SM, Burnett D, Studd J: Selectivity of proteinuria during pregnancy assessed by different methods. In: Lindheimer MD, Katz AI, Zuspan FP: *Hypertension in Pregnancy*. New York: John Wiley & Sons; 1976:75–83.
238. Chesley LC: The variability of proteinuria in the hypertensive complications of pregnancy. *J Clin Invest* 1939;18:617–620.
239. Anderson S, Kennefick TM, Brenner BM: Renal and systemic manifestations of glomerular disease. In: Brenner BM, ed. *The Kidney*, ed 5. Philadelphia: WB Saunders Co.; 1996:1981–2010.

240. Naicker T, Randeree IGH, Moodley J: Glomerular basement membrane changes in African women with early-onset preeclampsia. *Hyptens Pregnancy* 1995;14:371–378.

241. Naicker T, Randeree IGH, Moodley J, et al: Correlation between histological changes and loss of anionic charge of the glomerular basement membrane in early-onset pre-eclampsia. *Nephron* 1997;75:201–207.

242. Weise M, Prüfer D, Neubüser D: β_2-Microglobulin and other proteins in serum and urine during preeclampsia. *Klin Wschr* 1978;56:333–336.

243. Jackson DW, Sciscione A, Hartley TL, et al: Lysosomal enzymuria in preeclampsia. *Am J Kidney Dis* 1996;27:826–833.

244. Shaarawy M, El Mallah SY, El-Yamani AAE: Clinical significance of urinary human tissue non-specific alkaline phosphatase (hTNAP) in pre-eclampsia and eclampsia. *Ann Clin Biochem* 1997;34:405–411.

245. Nakagawa Y, Sirivongs D, Maikranz, P, et al: Excretion of Tamm–Horsfall glycoprotein (THP) during pregnancy: A defense against nephrolithiasis. *Kidney Int* 1987;31:56A.

246. Freidman EA, Neff RK: *Pregnancy and Hypertension. A Systemic Evaluation of Clinical Diagnostic Criteria.* Littleton, MA: PSG Publishing; 1977.

247. Page EW, Christianson R: The impact of mean arterial pressure in the middle trimester upon the outcome of pregnancy. *Am J Obstet Gynecol* 1976;125:740–746.

248. Lang RM, Pridjian G, Feldman T, et al: Left ventricular mechanics in preeclampsia. *Am Heart J* 1991;121:1768–1775.

249. Wallenburg HCS: Hemodynamics in hypertensive pregnancy. In: Rubin PC, ed. *Handbook of Hypertension. Vol 10: Hypertension in Pregnancy.* New York: Elsevier Science Publishers; 1988:66–101.

250. Sibai BM, Mabie WC: Hemodynamics of preeclampsia. *Clin Perinatol* 1991;18:727–747.

251. Visser W, Wallenburg HCS: Central hemodynamic observations in untreated preeclamptic patients. *Hypertension* 1991;17:1072–1077.

252. Groenendijk R, Trimbos JBMJ, Wallenburg HCS: Hemodynamic measurements in preeclampsia: Preliminary observations. *Am J Obstet Gynecol* 1984;150:232–236.

253. Easterling TR, Benedetti TJ, Schmucker BC, Millard SP: Maternal hemodynamics in normal and preeclamptic pregnancies: A longitudinal study. *Obstet Gynecol* 1990,76:1061–1069.

254. Messerli FH, De Carvalho JGR, Christie B, Frohlich ED: Systemic and regional hemodynamics in low, normal and high cardiac output borderline hypertension. *Circulation* 1978; 58:441–448.

255. Moutquin JM, Rainville C, Giroux L, et al: A prospective study of blood pressure in pregnancy: Prediction of pre-eclampsia. *Am J Obstet Gynecol* 1985;151:191–196.

256. Reiss RE, O'Shaughnessy RW, Quilligan TJ, Zuspan FP: Retrospective comparison of blood pressure course during preeclamptic and matched control pregnancies. *Am J Obstet Gynecol* 1987;156:894–898.

257. Villar MA, Sibai BM: Clinical significance of elevated mean arterial blood pressure in second trimester and threshold increase in systolic or diastolic blood pressure during third trimester. *Am J Obstet Gynecol* 1989;160:419–423.

258. Kyle PM, Clark SJ, Buckley D, et al: Second trimester ambulatory blood pressure in nulliparous pregnancy: A useful screening test for pre-eclampsia? *Br J Obstet Gynaecol* 1993;100:914–919.

259. Sibai BM, Gordon T, Thom E, et al and the National Institute of Child Health and Human Development Network of Maternal–Fetal Medicine Units: Risk factors for preeclampsia in healthy nulliparous women: A prospective multicenter study. *Am J Obstet Gynecol* 1995;172:642–648.

260. Atterbury JL, Groome LJ, Baker SL: Elevated midtrimester mean arterial blood pressure in women with severe preeclampsia. *Appl Nurs Res* 1996;9:161–166.

261. Hall JE: Renal and cardiovascular mechanisms of hypertension in obesity. *Hypertension* 1994;23:381–394.

262. Boslo P, O'Herlihy C, Conroy R, McKenna P: Maternal central hemodynamics in hypertensive disorders of pregnancy—a longitudinal study. *Am J Obstet Gynecol* 1998;178:S6.

263. Schobel HP, Fischer T, Heuszer K, et al: Preeclampsia—a state of sympathetic overactivity. *N Engl J Med* 1996;335:1480–1485.

264. Brust AA, Assali NS, Ferris EB: Evaluation of neurogenic and humoral factors in blood pressure maintenance in normal and toxemic pregnancy using tetraethylammonium chloride. *J Clin Invest* 1948;27:717–726.
265. Assali NS, Prystowsky H: Studies on autonomic blockade: I. Comparison between the effects of tetraethylammonium chloride (TEAL) and high selective spinal anesthesia on blood pressure of normal and toxemic pregnancy. *J Clin Invest* 1950;29:1354–1366.
266. Easterling TR, Benedetti TJ: Preeclampsia: A hyperdynamic disease model. *Am J Obstet Gynecol* 1989;160:1447–1453.
267. Gant NF, Worley RJ, Everett RB, MacDonald PC: Control of vascular responsiveness during human pregnancy. *Kidney Int* 1980;18:253–258.
268. Magness RR, Gant NF: Control of vascular reactivity in pregnancy: The basis for therapeutic approaches to prevent pregnancy-induced hypertension. *Semin Perinatol* 1994;18:45–69.
269. Gant NF, Daley GL, Chand S, et al: A study of angiotensin II pressor response throughout primigravid pregnancy. *J Clin Invest* 1973;52:2682–2689.
270. Nisell H, Hjemdahl P, Linde B: Cardiovascular responses to circulating catecholamines in normal pregnancy and in pregnancy-induced hypertension. *Clin Physiol* 1985;5:479–493.
271. Williams DJ, Vallance PJT, Neild GH, et al: Nitric oxide-mediated vasodilation in human pregnancy. *Am J Physiol* 1997;272:H748–H752.
272. Anumba DOC, Ford GA, Boys RJ, Robson SC: The role of nitric oxide in the modulation of vascular tone in normal pregnancy. *Br J Obstet Gynaecol* 1996;103:1169–1170.
273. Graves SW, Moore TJ, Seely EW: Increases in platelet angiotensin II receptor number in pregnancy-induced hypertension. *Hypertension* 1992;20:627–632.
274. Baker PN, Pipkin FB, Symonds EM: Comparative study of platelet angiotensin II binding and the angiotensin II sensitivity test as predictors of pregnancy-induced hypertension. *Clin Sci* 1992;83:89–95

9

Alterations in Volume Homeostasis

Eileen D.M. Gallery and Marshall D. Lindheimer

Hemoconcentration has been recognized as a central feature of preeclampsia throughout the 20th century, dating from Zangemeister's original description of increased hematocrit and plasma specific gravity in women with preeclampsia and eclampsia.[1] Subsequent authors extended his observations to show that the degree of hemoconcentration is an index of severity. Dieckmann described rapid changes in the hematocrit during the progress of eclampsia, which he attributed to variable hemoconcentration. He went on to show the associated plasma volume contraction,[2] and several authors have subsequently shown clinical improvement with hemodilution.[3-7]

Perusal of the older literature in this area also stresses the importance of recognizing the clinical significance of this volume contraction. Liley[8] emphasized the danger of accepting a normal hemoglobin as an indication of fitness for surgical procedures in this complicated situation. Chesley, in the first edition of this text,[9] reminded the reader of the old clinical observation that eclamptic women are particularly prone to shock because of unmasking of their underlying severe volume contraction. He pointed out that there is a sharp increase in blood viscosity as the hematocrit rises, augmenting resistance to blood flow, and increasing the susceptibility to end-organ damage in preeclampsia–eclampsia. He hypothesized that this may be a major predisposing factor to the circulatory failure characteristic of many eclamptic deaths.

Understanding of volume homeostasis in normal pregnancy and its disturbances in preeclampsia are essential to logical management. Volume homeostasis in normal pregnancy is discussed in detail in Chapter 4. The changes will be summarized only briefly here, to enhance appreciation of the changes of disorders such as preeclampsia in context. This chapter will focus on abnormalities in volume homeostatic mechanisms related to the development of preeclampsia and related disorders. Emphasis will be placed on the mechanisms of development of abnormalities, rather than on the ultimate causes, which again will be discussed elsewhere.

BODY FLUID VOLUMES

Normal Pregnancy (see also Chap. 4)

Pregnancy is a physiologic process in which repeated adjustment must occur in the steady state, and in which there are marked alterations in both intracellular and extracellular composition, normally held within relatively narrow limits. These changes are sensed as normal and "defended" in the face of variation in fluid/sodium intake. There is a significant increase in total extracellular fluid (ECF) volume, with gains in both extravascular (interstitial) and intravascular compartments. As noted in Chapter 4, plasma volume, ECF volume, and total body water all increase sequentially, often in association with peripheral edema.[10] The maximum plasma volume expansion is reached late in the second trimester, while total ECF volume and total body water continue to increase through the third trimester. Average increases of the order of 30 to 40% are found, but with wide variability; some healthy pregnant women experience increases in excess of 50%. Although there is a concomitant increase in total red cell mass, the magnitude of the increase is smaller (~25%), resulting in the "physiological anemia" of pregnancy, marked by a lower hematocrit (average ~34%), and in reality a form of dilutional hypervolemia. A well-documented fall in serum sodium concentration of ~5 mmol/L, indicating a greater increase in total body water than in ECF volume also occurs, with a resetting of osmoreceptor threshold and sensitivity.

Extracellular Fluid Volume in Preeclampsia

Women who develop preeclampsia can be divided into two subgroups—those with an abnormal shift of ECF from the vascular to the extravascular compartment (who have low plasma volume and normal or increased interstitial fluid volume), and those with a total reduction in ECF volume (who have low plasma and interstitial fluid volumes). It is possible that the two subgroups have different underlying disturbances in volume homeostatic mechanisms.

Preeclampsia with Peripheral Edema

Peripheral edema is generally seen as a manifestation of excessive accumulation of interstitial ECF. It is clear that the frequency of occurrence of peripheral edema, in both normal and preeclamptic pregnancy, is directly related to the assiduity with which it is sought. In the latter half of pregnancy, pedal and pretibial edema is seen in the majority of women. It occurs more commonly as the day proceeds, and usually disappears in recumbency. In addition to this dependant edema, many women develop edema of the hands and/or face as pregnancy advances, often associated with weight gain. Again, the frequency of this occurrence depends on the care with which it is sought, an incidence of > 60% described by Dexter and Weiss.[11] Even women who do not have visible edema have an increase in lower limb volume,[10] indicating subclinical fluid accumulation.

As summarized by Chesley in the initial edition of this text,[9] the primary reason for the increase in peripheral edema in normal pregnancy may be reduced plasma oncotic pressure. Values fall from an average of ~370 mm water (27 mm Hg) in nonpregnant individuals to ~345 (25 mm Hg) in early pregnancy and ~300 (22 mm Hg) in late pregnancy. Mean values adapted from Chesley's[9] summary of the earlier literature, and data added by Zinaman et al.[12] are shown in Figure 9–1, for both normal and preeclamptic women. The lowest values are reached in the hours following delivery, the period of time when women with preeclampsia are most at-risk of the development of pulmonary edema if fluid balance is not managed with extreme care.

Krogh et al.[13] showed that a reduction in plasma oncotic pressure of the order of that encountered in normal pregnancy can be associated with a significant increase in the rate of fluid extravasation from capillaries. The reduction in plasma oncotic pressure of normal pregnancy in turn is related to the overall increase in plasma volume and the lowered plasma level of sodium, with a dilutional fall in the plasma–albumin concentration. In normal pregnancies, women with peripheral edema, who also have the greatest weight gain and plasma volume expansion, have bigger babies with lower perinatal mortality rates than those with less fluid accumulation.[14]

There may well be two sorts of edema, one normal and related to a combination of intravascular and interstitial ECF volume expansion, and the other abnormal and related to a shift of ECF volume from vascular to interstitial space, but at

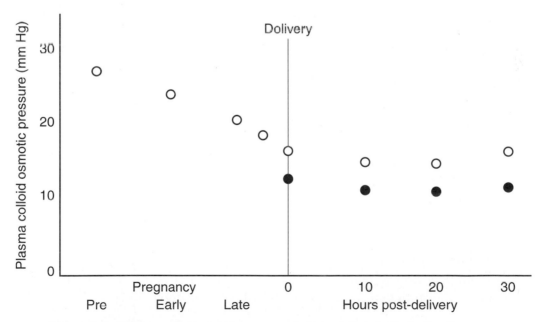

Figure 9–1. Plasma colloid oncotic pressure before, during, and shortly after pregnancy in normotensive (○) and preeclamptic (●) women. Mean values are shown. (*Data from Chesley LC:* Hypertensive Disorders in Pregnancy. *New York: Appleton Century Crofts; 1978 and Zinaman M, Rubin J, Lindheimer MD: Serial plasma oncotic pressure levels and echoencephalography during and after delivery in severe preeclampsia.* Lancet *1985;i:1245–1247.*)

present there is no way to distinguish them. In the latter circumstance, the total ECF may be normal or even increased, and patients may experience rapid increases in weight and peripheral edema. Support for this hypothesis was first provided in the early studies of Freis and Kenny,[15] who made simulataneous measurements of plasma volume and ECF volume (as assessed by thiocyanate space) in preeclamptic women, and showed a concomitant reduction in plasma volume and increase in ECF volume. This fluid shift is clearly not due to changes in vascular permeability for water and electrolytes, as the vessel wall is freely permeable to small molecules. It may, however, be related to an increase in capillary permeability to large molecules such as protein (capillary leak syndrome), as suggested by Friedberg and Lutz's finding[16] of increased disappearance rate of protein-bound markers from the circulation in preeclamptic rather than in normal pregnant subjects—a finding which has subsequently been confirmed by others.

When it has been measured,[9,12] (Fig. 9–1) the plasma oncotic pressure of women with preeclampsia has been found to be significantly lower (~250 mm water, ~18 mm Hg) than that of normal pregnant women, the lowest values being encountered in eclampsia (~240 mm water, ~17 mm Hg). Preeclamptic women with peripheral edema appear to be at particular risk of development of interstitial or frank pulmonary edema,[17] a risk increased by the administration of intravenous fluid challenges, particularly with crystalloid solutions, and this can present a major problem in fluid management around the time of delivery and in the early postpartum period. Benedetti and Carlson[18] have suggested that the risk of pulmonary edema can be predicted by measurement of colloid osmotic pressure, a suggestion supported by the finding that the lowest values are measured in the early postpartum period,[12,19] the time of greatest risk for this complication. Given that levels are already low in women with preeclampsia–eclampsia, these groups are at the greatest risk of this life-threatening complication. However, most authorities agree with Hytten's[20] conclusion that edema is so common in pregnancy that it is not a useful diagnostic criterion to use in individual patients for the diagnosis of preeclampsia.

Preeclampsia without Peripheral Edema

Women with preeclampsia, but with no peripheral edema, referred to in some of the older literature as "dry" preeclampsia, appear to have a total deficit of ECF volume. The absence of edema was used in the older literature on preeclampsia–eclampsia as an index of severity, as this group of women had the highest rates of complications, and mortality rates.[21] The reasons for the absence of edema are speculative, but they may be related to inappropriate renal fluid loss at an earlier stage of pregnancy, resulting in significant total ECF volume depletion.

Plasma Volume in Preeclampsia

Both edematous and nonedematous preeclamptic women have reduced plasma volume, the most clinically significant component of the ECF, as it is a major determinant of organ perfusion. The degree of plasma volume contraction is an index of severity, and in severe preeclampsia the plasma volume may decrease by as much as 30 to 40%. This explains, at least in part, the old clinical observation that eclamptic women are predisposed to shock. Table 9–1 is a summary of the major published data for plasma volume in preeclampsia–eclampsia, with the references from which the data were acquired.

In serial studies, the fall in plasma volume has been demonstrated several weeks prior to the rise in blood pressure, and appearance of other clinical manifestations of preeclampsia, as shown in Figure 9–2. Following appearance of the clinical features of preeclampsia, further volume contraction, proportional to the severity of the clinical disorder, occurs as shown in Figure 9–3. In the study from which these data were extracted,[7] there was a clear relationship among signs of severity of preeclampsia—plasma volume, blood pressure, and proteinuria. The presence or absence of edema shows no obvious relationship to the plasma volume level, but is associated with appropriate alterations in interstitial fluid volume (calculated from simultaneously measured plasma volume and total ECF volume). Preeclamptic women with edema had significantly higher than normal interstitial volumes, while those without edema had interstitial volumes not different from normotensive women. This finding has subsequently been confirmed by others.[34]

Although the mechanism of the plasma volume contraction may be different in edematous and nonedematous women, the effect is similar. Many authors have shown the significant and direct relationship referred to above between the extent of plasma volume expansion and intrauterine fetal growth, thought to be related to uteroplacental blood flow, a relationship common among normal pregnancy, pregnancy complicated by chronic hypertension, and preeclampsia. Severe preeclamp-

TABLE 9–1. PLASMA VOLUMES IN NORMAL PREGNANT WOMEN AND THOSE WITH PREECLAMPSIA[a]

Author (Reference No.)	Normal Pregnancy		Preeclampsia		
	Cases	Mean (mL)	Cases	Mean (mL)	% Change
Werko et al.[22]	4	3865	9	3145	−18
Freis & Kenny[15]	7	4287	5	3045	−29
Rottger[23,24]	20	3383	18	2890	−15
Cope[25]	29	3470	14	2820	−19
Friedberg & Lutz[16]	10	3104	17	3257	+5
Kolpakova[26]	20	3309	15	2918	−12
Honger[27]	20	3800	19	3300	−13
Haering et al.[28]	18	3721	21	3148	−15
Brody & Spetz[29]	46	4245	34	4010	−5
MacGillivray[30]	18	4040	35	3535	−12
Blekta et al.[31]	55	3133	14	2590	−17
Gallery et al.[32]*	199	3878	37	3383	−13
MacGillivray[33]	55	3763	29	3524	−6
Brown et al.[34]*	54	3912	49	3260	−17
Silver et al.[34a]	20	4070	20	3416	−16

Mean values are shown except for those marked with *, where median values were used. Values were listed as shown, or have been calculated from data in the publications listed.

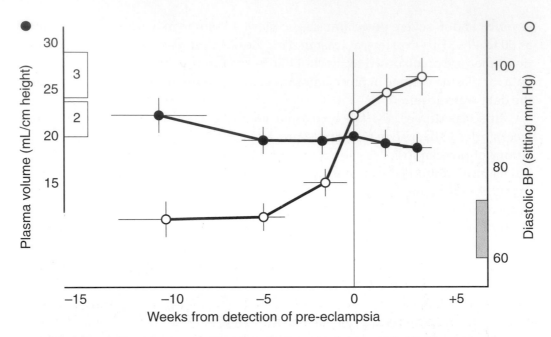

Figure 9–2. Time course of alterations in plasma volume and in blood pressure in women who develop preeclampsia. On the ordinates are also shown normal diastolic BP (± 95% confidence intervals) and normal 2nd and 3rd trimester plasma volume levels (± 95% CI). (*Data from Gallery EDM, Hunyor SN, Gyory AZ: Plasma volume contraction: A significant factor in both pregnancy-associated hypertension (pre-eclampsia) and chronic hypertension in pregnancy. Quart J Med 1979;48: 593–602.*)

sia is characterized also by reduced perfusion of several maternal organs, and often by reduced cardiac output, even though the heart is intrinsically normal. Lang et al.[35] have shown that volume-independent contractility is quite normal in preeclampsia. As well as the increased afterload due directly to hypertension and arteriolar constriction, the reduction in cardiac output is thought by some to be caused by reduced preload (i.e., reduced "effective" circulating volume). (See Chapter 4 for discussion and critique of this concept.) The increment in plasma volume in pregnancies destined for preeclampsia is normal or near normal in the second trimester, but plasma volume contraction precedes the development of frank hypertension and other clinical signs of preeclampsia by several weeks.[32] The reasons for this fall in plasma volume are not known. It appears to be different from the so-called "pressure natriuresis" seen in those with chronic hypertension pursuing an accelerated course, where the increment in pressure is deemed responsible for the decrement in plasma volume.

Plasma Volume Expansion as Therapy for Preeclampsia

Because of the early and significant change in plasma volume in preeclampsia, there have been a number of studies of the effect of infusing plasma volume expanders. Although Chesley[9] described this maneuver as "perhaps a form of imitative magic," he gave an excellent summary in the first edition of this book of the

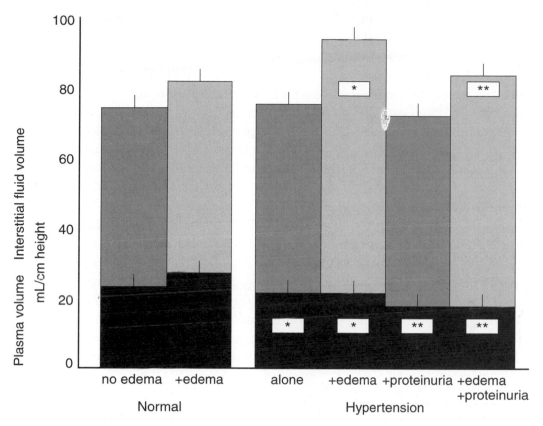

Figure 9–3. Plasma volumes (in lower half of diagram) and interstitial fluid volumes in normal pregnancy and in preeclampsia of varying severity (*P < 0.05, ** P < 0.01, compared with normal subjects). (*Data from Gallery EDM, Mitchell MD, Redman CWG: Fall in blood pressure in response to volume expansion in pregnancy-associated hypertension: Why does it occur? J Hypertens 1984;2:177–182.*)

early history of attempts to employ infusion of plasma volume expanders in the treatment of preeclampsia–eclampsia. He also stressed the fact that

> the use of plasma expanders is to be greatly preferred over the use of diuretic drugs, which aggravate the abnormality. Phlebotomy has been largely abandoned in the management of eclampsia, largely because of our recognition of the hypovolemia; the same reasoning applies to the use of potent diuretic drugs. (p. 340)

It has become clear that there is little place for the infusion of large quantities of crystalloid solutions; as discussed earlier, there is free vascular permeability to water and electrolyte solutions, and the expected effect therefore would be the appearance of edema, or its aggravation in women with preexisting edema. It would also lower plasma oncotic pressure further, and in many preeclamptics as outlined above, values prior to infusion are already near those associated with pulmonary and cerebral edema in nongravid populations.

However, the infusion of colloid solutions, which should remain within the vascular space and raise the colloid osmotic pressure of plasma, has attractions. It may ameliorate peripheral edema, and allow transfer of interstitial fluid back into the vessels. If vasoconstriction, thought to be central to the hypertension, is aggravated by hypovolemia, partial relief of this may allow the blood pressure to fall, and thus result in some improvement in cardiac function and organ perfusion. Cloeren et al.[5,6] reported, in addition to normalization of the low central venous pressure in women with preeclampsia in response to infusion of colloid volume expanders, the occurrence of a diuresis, a salutary effect on maternal blood pressure, as well as augmentation of uterine blood flow. Examining further the effects of volume expanders, Gallery et al.[7] described the effects of infusion of 500 mL of a 5% albumin-containing solution in women with preeclampsia and those with chronic hypertension. There was a universal fall in both systolic and diastolic blood pressure, the duration of effect being inversely proportional to the severity of the underlying preeclampsia, and lasting for up to 72 hours. There were no significant effects on weight, total ECF volume, or calculated interstitial fluid volume, but there was a significant increase in plasma volume (Fig. 9–4), most marked in preeclamptic women with preexisting peripheral edema. As pointed out by these and other authors, there is an ever-present risk of precipitating interstitial or frank pulmonary edema with the injudicious administration of intravenous fluid to women with un-

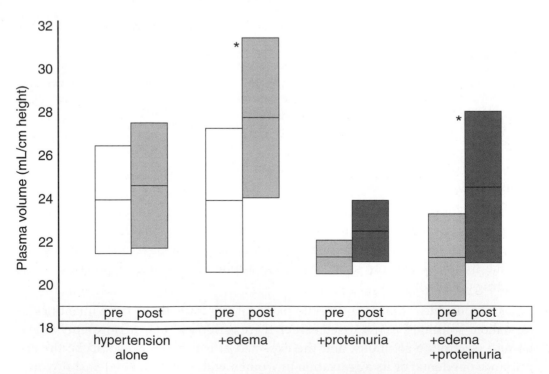

Figure 9–4. Plasma volume response to plasma volume expander in preeclampsia. Values shown are median/interquartile range (* $P < 0.05$, pre-post volume expander infusion). (*Data from Gallery EDM, Mitchell MD, Redman CWG: Fall in blood pressure in response to volume expansion in pregnancy-associated hypertension: Why does it occur? J Hypertens 1984;2:177–182.*)

stable fluid balance, and a possible capillary leak syndrome. That there is a maldistribution of ECF is particularly evident in preeclamptic women with peripheral edema. Attempts to correct the plasma volume contraction with crystalloid solutions could be expected to increase the peripheral edema significantly. As shown in Figure 9–4, the administration of colloid solutions is more likely to improve the fluid maldistribution, perhaps by increasing plasma colloid osmotic pressure, in turn causing a shift of interstitial fluid back to the intravascular space. While it is probably safe and of value to administer small volumes of intravenous colloid solutions to shift the balance in an appropriate direction, overenthusiastic administration of large quantities of intravenous fluid of any type may result in circulatory overload, particularly in the patient with severe preeclampsia and impairment of renal function.

As with other forms of treatment, limited value can be expected in women with accelerated disease, for whom the logical course is resuscitation and rapid delivery. However, for women with less severe disease, in whom temporization may have something to offer in achieving greater fetal maturity prior to delivery, there may be a place for judicious infusion of plasma volume expanders, provided that the patient's fluid balance is closely monitored.

Sodium Balance

Sodium is the principal cation of the extracellular space, and changes in total ECF volume are related primarily to sodium handling, the body content of which is primarily the result of a balance between factors promoting renal retention and excretion. In normal pregnancy, the expansion of plasma and interstitial fluid volumes is due to gradual net sodium retention, and in late pregnancy there is a marked effect of the gravid uterus, which results in a sharp fall in urinary sodium excretion when the woman turns from her side to her back, sits, or stands.[36] The disturbances seen in preeclampsia describe a more complicated set of interactions, as yet poorly understood. There have been a number of studies examining the ability of the normal and preeclamptic woman to cope with extremes of sodium intake.

Sodium Loading/Deprivation Studies

Normal pregnant women given a low salt diet will come into balance after 3 to 5 days, with significant weight loss but very little change in plasma volume, indicating interstitial fluid loss, while they tolerate increased sodium intake well, with little change in either weight or plasma volume. Administration of an acute sodium load is handled appropriately for the prior sodium balance, with rapid excretion if already sodium replete, and slower excretion if previously sodium depleted. Nonpregnant subjects with chronic essential hypertension respond to acute saline loading with an exaggerated natriuresis. There was early controversy about the capacity of pregnant women with chronic hypertension to excrete an acute intravenous sodium load, perhaps related to failure to standardize pretest sodium intake, and also reflecting the variable response to hypotonic, isotonic, and hypertonic solutions. Sarles et al.[37] studied pregnant women on a fixed sodium intake prior to saline infusions, and found that pregnancy did not abolish the exaggerated natriuresis of chronically hypertensive women whose peak natriuretic rate was double that of normotensive women.

Women destined to develop preeclampsia have an exaggerated natriuresis in response to oral and intravenous sodium loading in the second trimester of pregnancy, while they are still normotensive (Fig. 9–5A). This holds at all levels of prior sodium intake. Conversely, these women are slower to retain sodium when challenged with sodium deprivation. Following the development of clinical disease (Fig. 9–5B), they behave like sodium-depleted subjects, with avid retention of sodium, and slow excretion of additional sodium loads. If this represented a primary defect in renal tubular sodium handling, the fractional excretion of sodium (FENa) would be reduced. In the few studies that have been conducted, FENa was normal, and it was concluded that the slowness to excrete the sodium load was due to relative lack of increase in filtered sodium, suggesting that the reduced plasma volume was sensed by the kidney as a true reduction. This is shown clearly in Gallery and Brown.[38]

Renin–Angiotensin–Aldosterone Axis

The renin–angiotensin–aldosterone (RAA) axis is intimately involved in renal control of salt and water balance. All components of the RAA axis are increased in normal pregnancy.[39,39a]

Renin/Renin Substrate

Renin production involves both the maternal kidney and the uteroplacental unit, while angiotensinogen (renin substrate) is derived from the maternal liver,[39,39a] with an additional amount of high molecular weight angiotensinogen from the fetal circulation. Levels of prorenin increase quite early in pregnancy, probably partly accounting for the increase in measured levels of circulating total renin,[40,41] and active plasma renin concentration is also increased. The reset high levels include a "non-suppressible" component, unresponsive to physiologic stimulation and suppression, as well as the normally responsive portion. This portion falls in response to saline or colloid administration, and rises in response to sodium deprivation, diuretics, upright posture, and ambulation.[42] Renin substrate (angiotensinogen) also is increased, at least in part due to high levels of estrogen production, perhaps enhanced further by high molecular weight angiotensinogen from the fetal circulation. Plasma renin activity (a first order enzyme kinetic reaction, dependent on concentrations of both enzyme and substrate) is the most common renin measurement made in clinical practice, resulting in magnification of findings for renin concentration and substrate in normal pregnancy.

It has been shown, somewhat paradoxically in view of the well-documented plasma volume contraction of preeclampsia, that maternal plasma renin activity and active renin concentrations are lower than normal in this condition. In early

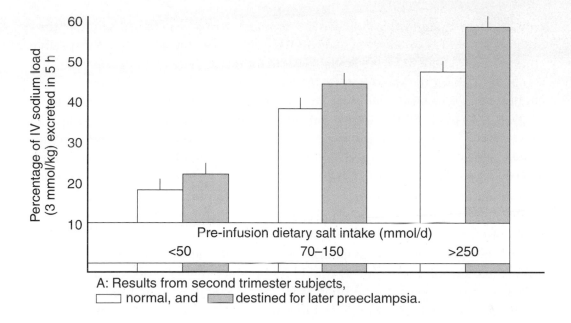

A: Results from second trimester subjects,
☐ normal, and ▨ destined for later preeclampsia.

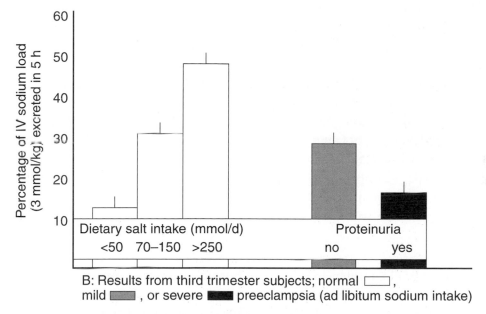

B: Results from third trimester subjects; normal ☐,
mild ▨, or severe ▦ preeclampsia (ad libitum sodium intake)

Figure 9–5. Responses of pregnant women to intravenous sodium loads. In the second trimester of pregnancy, women were studied at three levels of prior dietary sodium intake (< 50 mmol/d, 70–150 mmol/d, and > 250 mmol/d). In the third trimester, results from normal women at the same three levels of prior dietary sodium intake were compared with those from women with mild or severe preeclampsia. (*Data from Gallery EDM, Brown MA: Control of sodium excretion in human pregnancy.* Am J Kidney Dis *1987;9:290–295.*)

studies it was thought that this was a secondary change due to sodium retention, but subsequent researchers have uncovered a more complex situation. Prospective studies have shown that there is a fall prior to the development of hypertension, and probably at about the same time as the fall in plasma volume,[43,44] raising the possibility that lower levels were in part instrumental in causing the plasma volume contraction. However, this is also unlikely, because of the increase in total ECF in most women with preeclampsia, a disturbance that increases as the condition progresses. Since plasma–renin activity is lowered further in preeclampsia in response to physiologic challenges such as saline loading, and increased by maneuvers such as head-up tilt, renin secretion appears to be still appropriately responsive to physiologic demands. The reasons for lowered background levels are unknown, but it is of interest that there is a parallel fall in renal prostacyclin excretion. Since prostacyclin is known to stimulate renin release directly in the nonpregnant, these suppressed background renin levels could be secondary to low prostacyclin secretion in preeclampsia, a postulate supported by the finding of impaired renin release in response to the administration of furosemide. Total renin concentration is unchanged,[39,39a] and since the principal source of active renin is the maternal kidney, this suggests reduced renal activation and/or release of the activated molecule.

Within the fetoplacental circulation there appears to be divergence from the findings in the maternal circulation. There is recent evidence that the levels of components of the renin–angiotensin system in the placenta and fetal membranes are normal in preeclampsia.[45] In 1993, Ward et al. described the presence of a molecular variant of the angiotensinogen gene in preeclamptic women,[46] although overall angiotensinogen levels are not altered in the clinical disorder. The same group[47] has subsequently described elevated expression of this molecular variant in decidual spiral arteries in preeclampsia, and raised the possibility that this change may be associated with the development of atherotic changes in this vascular bed, a common feature of preeclampsia.

Angiotensin II

The elevated maternal angiotensin II levels of normal pregnancy are due to the increased renin and angiotensinogen production, with no evidence for increased angiotensin-converting enzyme levels in pregnancy. Increased aldosterone production occurs in response to this. Angiotensin II levels are reduced in preeclampsia, with a relative increase in AII receptors in platelets and possibly in other tissues. This may also explain the increased maternal sensitivity to pressor effects of AII described by Gant et al.[48] over 20 years ago. Within the placental villi, there are also AII-binding sites, inversely related to vessel size, with the characteristics of the AT1 class of receptor.[49] The capacity and affinity of these binding sites is lower than normal in preeclamptic placentas, in contradiction to maternal findings. The significance of this finding is as yet uncertain, but it has been interpreted as down-regulation secondary to activation of the placental renin–angiotensin system.

Aldosterone

Plasma and urinary aldosterone are increased in normal pregnancy, and there appears to be partial dissociation of the normally close relationship between renin and aldosterone. The ratio of aldosterone:renin is increased in the third trimester of pregnancy in comparison to that found in nonpregnant women, although the slope of the relationship across differing levels of sodium balance remains similar[42,50,51] (Fig. 9–6). This suggests a background stimulation of secretion not closely related to sodium or volume homeostasis. Certainly, direct stimulation of aldosterone secretion has been shown in response to progesterone and adrenocorticotrophic hormone (ACTH) in both normal and preeclamptic pregnancies, with direct suppression by dopamine and atrial natriuretic peptide (ANP). It should be noted that at the elevated setpoint of aldosterone levels, responses to physiologic manipulation are unimpaired.

Although a reduction in plasma and urinary aldosterone is well described in preeclampsia, there appears to be further dissociation from renin levels, and, as shown in Figure 9–6, the aldosterone:renin ratio is increased above that of normal

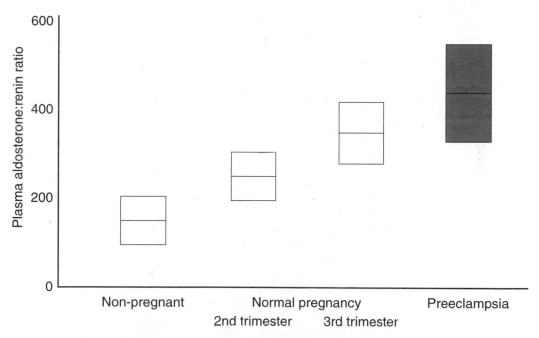

Figure 9–6. Changes in plasma aldosterone–renin ratio in normal pregnancy and in preeclampsia. Values shown are median and interquartile range. The ratio is increased in 3rd compared to 2nd trimester. Highest values were found in women with preeclampsia. (*Data from Gordon RD, Symonds EM, Wilmshurst EG, et al: Plasma renin activity, plasma angiotensin and plasma and urinary electrolytes in normal and toxaemic pregnancy, including a prospective study.* Clin Sci Molec Med 1973;45:115–127; *Brown MA, Nicholson E, Ross MR, et al: Progressive resetting of sodium-renin-aldosterone relationships in human pregnancy.* Clin Exper Hypertens 1986;B5:249–260; *and Brown MA, Zammit VC, Mitar DM, et al: Control of aldosterone in normal and hypertensive pregnancy: Effects of metoclopramide.* Hypertens Pregnancy 1993;12:37–51.)

pregnancy. Again, the reasons for this are not clear but it could represent increased adrenal sensitivity to AII, analogous to the increased pressor effect, or it could be due to the other direct stimuli listed above, bypassing the classical renin–angiotensin axis partly or wholly. A greater degree of inhibition of aldosterone release by dopamine in preeclampsia has been suggested by the studies of Brown et al.,[51] while ANP, known to inhibit aldosterone secretion directly, is increased in preeclampsia.

It is probable that both AII and aldosterone have a central role in determining the kidney's contribution to sodium balance, although there are surprisingly few data regarding their direct effect on renal function in the pregnant woman.

Atrial Natriuretic Peptide

In normal pregnancy, a moderate but variable increase in plasma atrial natriuretic peptide (ANP) levels has been described by some, but not all authors.[52-54] Castro et al.[55] in a meta-analysis of a number of previous publications concluded that there was a modest increase in normal pregnancy in the third trimester of pregnancy, the 95% confidence limits of pregnant and nonpregnant values still overlapping significantly. It is of great importance to account for both sodium intake and posture in analysis of values in pregnancy, and Lowe et al., in a very carefully conducted prospective study,[54] found that when these factors were accounted for, there was not a significant intrinsic increase in circulating ANP levels in normal pregnancy. Prolonged lateral recumbency causes an increase, perhaps because of mobilization of interstitial fluid into the vascular space. Sodium and volume loading also result in an increase in plasma ANP levels without any significant alteration in plasma volume, and sodium deprivation causes a decrease in these levels in normal human pregnancy.[54,56] In the nonpregnant state, its synthesis is stimulated by sodium administration and volume expansion, in response to atrial stretch, and it results in natriuresis. However, in pregnancy, the ANP system appears to be regulated differently; the increased levels are not related to changes in maternal atrial size or plasma volume.

Levels are even higher in preeclampsia,[57,58] where there is volume contraction rather than expansion, as in normal pregnancy. Preeclamptic women still have intact ANP responses to physiologic manipulations, suggesting that factors other than volume/sodium status are responsible for the elevated values (e.g., AII, arginine vasopressin, endothelin). The reasons for this further increase are not known; it has been speculated that it is to counteract endothelin- or angiotensin-induced vasoconstriction. An exaggerated increase in ANP levels has been described in response to intravenous volume loading in preeclampsia, correlated closely with a rise in central venous pressure.[59] It has also been suggested that atrial natriuretic peptide-mediated fetoplacental vasodilation is augmented in preeclampsia as a compensatory mechanism in the presence of increased vascular resistance within the fetoplacental unit.[60]

Prostaglandins

Prostaglandins, whose production is increased in normal pregnancy, may well play a central role in control of vascular tone, blood pressure, and sodium balance.

Prostaglandin E2 synthesis in the renal medulla is increased markedly in late pregnancy.[61] It is known to be natriuretic in the nonpregnant state, and presumed to have similar effects in pregnancy. Prostacyclin, the principal prostaglandin of endothelium, also secreted by myometrium, is also increased in late pregnancy.[62] While the most evident effect of prostacyclin is on blood pressure and coagulation, renal synthesis stimulates local renin secretion, and this may be one factor in the increased renin levels of normal pregnancy. There is indirect evidence that prostacyclin may induce resistance to the pressor effects of angiotensin, another characteristic feature of normal pregnancy.[61,63] This concept is supported by the finding that administration of cyclooxygenase inhibitors to pregnant women causes an increase in AII sensitivity.

Several authors have described a decrease in the ratio of prostacyclin/thromboxane in maternal urine and/or blood in preeclampsia,[61,62,64] but not in uncomplicated chronic essential hypertension.[62] In a prospective study, Smith et al.[65] were not able to detect a difference in women who remained continuously normotensive and those who developed hypertension, although it is possible that this was related to dilution of the preeclamptic population with subjects with less severe disease. Postulated reasons for an abnormal ratio have included endothelial cell damage resulting in a fall in prostacyclin production, and platelet activation resulting in an increase in circulating thromboxane levels. Such a change could be instrumental in causing increased AII sensitivity. When maternal endothelial cells from preeclamptic women have been examined directly in vitro[66] there has not been any apparent defect in their secretion of prostacyclin, and examination of the effect of preeclamptic maternal serum/plasma on endothelial cells from various sources, including maternal decidua, has shown stimulation of prostacyclin secretion rather than inhibition.[67,68] These findings are not in keeping with a primary role for the maternal endothelium in causing the prostanoid abnormalities of preeclampsia, or initiating the vasoconstriction or coagulation activation of the disorder. One more recent report[69] indicates that platelets from women with preeclampsia are resistant to the effect of prostaglandin E1 in inhibiting platelet aggregatory responses, an abnormality which would partly explain the increased platelet reactivity seen in preeclampsia. Platelet prostacyclin receptor affinity has been shown to be reduced in preeclampsia,[70] a defect which if generalized to other cell types might explain a lack of response to prostacyclin even if it were secreted in adequate amounts from endothelial cells. Consideration of the many other aspects of endothelial cell function which might contribute to the development or acceleration of preeclampsia is dealt with in more detail in Chapter 12.

Recent studies have examined production of prostanoids by placental villi,[71] and subsequently by cultured pure trophoblast cell populations from preeclamptic pregnancies, and there is general agreement that thromboxane secretion by tro-phoblasts from affected women is increased several-fold.[72-74] It is possible that the placental trophoblast is the source of the abnormal blood findings in the mother, as villous trophoblasts, bathed in maternal blood, have free access to the maternal circulation.

Cellular Sodium Handling/Transport

Cellular cation handling, especially in the kidney, plays an important role in both volume homeostasis and blood pressure control. In nonpregnant individuals with essential hypertension, cation transport abnormalities have been described in vascular tissues. Changes have been described in normal human pregnancy in the ouabain-sensitive Na/K ATPase sodium/potassium pump, in the sodium/potassium cotransport system, in the sodium/lithium countertransporter, and in the sodium/hydrogen exchanger. Most investigators have used the erythrocyte as the model cell system for study.

Sodium electrochemical gradients across cell membranes are maintained primarily by the ouabain-sensitive $Na+$, $K+$ ATPase-dependent pump. In circulating cells, this pump maintains low intracellular sodium and high intracellular potassium concentrations, while in the kidney, the same enzyme system implements tubular sodium reabsorption. Pregnancy is characterized by increased numbers of enzyme sites, both on circulating and on renal cells, and the resultant increase in function results in lowered intracellular sodium concentration, and aids in gradual renal sodium retention.[75-77] In preeclampsia, there is evidence for a circulating inhibitor of this pump, with a reduction in pump function and increase in intracellular sodium, which could in turn stimulate an increase in intracellular calcium concentrations.[78-81] If this occurred in vascular smooth muscle cells, it could result in vasoconstriction. This area is not entirely clear, as such a substance within the maternal kidney would result in a reduction in sodium reabsorption, not the net sodium retention so commonly seen.

Sodium/Hydrogen Exchange

A recent study of sodium/hydrogen exchange (NaHE)[82] described a gestational age-related increase in NaHE in platelets, parallelling findings for $Na+$, $K+$ ATPase function in normal pregnancy, but no alteration which could be attributed to preeclampsia.

Sodium/Potassium Cotransport

Furosemide-sensitive sodium/potassium cotransport is also increased, by about 30%, in pregnancy.[83] No specific changes have been described in preeclampsia by most authors, but one report suggests a reduction in transport by this pathway,[84] although it is not certain from this publication whether account was taken of prior intracellular sodium concentrations.

Sodium/Lithium (Na/Li) Countertransport

Another pathway of sodium transport across the cell membrane is Na/Li countertransport, first reported by Canessa et al.[84] to be faster than normal in subjects with essential hypertension. Erythrocyte Na/Li countertransport is increased significantly in normal pregnancy,[85,86] with some evidence that levels higher than normal are associated with an increased risk of developing hypertension.

CONCLUSION

Normal pregnancy is characterized by expansion of both extracellular fluid and plasma volume, while preeclampsia is associated with early and significant plasma volume contraction, largely but not entirely due to a shift from intravascular to extravascular space. Sodium is the principal component of extracellular fluid, and control of sodium balance is altered significantly in normal pregnancy to allow the physiologic fluid retention. Women with preeclampsia have abnormal control of sodium balance at several levels, including renin, aldosterone, angiotensin, and atrial natriuretic peptide secretion, prostaglandin production, renin–prostaglandin interactions, and cellular sodium transport pathways. The roles of each of these in producing the clinical disturbances seen in preeclamptic women have been described. Sodium restriction is likely to aggravate the preexisting plasma volume contraction and is not routinely recommended for women with preeclampsia. Active volume expansion by the infusion of colloid solutions does improve hypertension and the maldistribution of fluid between intra- and extravascular space in a proportion of patients, but carries with it a risk of volume overload and pulmonary edema.

REFERENCES

1. Zangemeister W: Untersuchungen über die Blutbeschaffenheit und die Harnsekretion bei Eklampsia. *Z Geburtsh Gynaekol* 1903;50:385–467.
2. Dieckmann WJ: Blood and plasma changes in eclampsia. *Am J Obstet Gynecol* 1936;32:927–936.
3. Vara P: Observations on the use of 10 percent salt-free Macrodex (dextran) in toxaemia of late pregnancy. *Acta Obstet Gynecol Scand* 1950;30(suppl 6):5–32.
4. Schwarz R, Retzke U: Kardiovasculare Wirkung von niedermolekularem Dextran mit Mannitol bei hypertensiven Spätschwangeren. *Zentralbl Gynaekol* 1971;93:657–662.
5. Cloeren SE, Lippert TH: Effect of plasma expanders in toxemia of pregnancy. *N Engl J Med* 1972;287:1356.
6. Cloeren SE, Lippert TH, Hinselmann M: Hypovolemia in toxemia of pregnancy: Plasma expander therapy with surveillance of central venous pressure. *Arch Gynaekol* 1973;215:123–132.
7. Gallery EDM, Mitchell MD, Redman CWG: Fall in blood pressure in response to volume expansion in pregnancy-associated hypertension: Why does it occur? *J Hypertens* 1984;2:177–182.
8. Liley AW: Clinical and laboratory significance of variations in maternal plasma volume in pregnancy. *Int J Gynaecol Obstet* 1970;8:358–362.
9. Chesley LC: *Hypertensive Disorders in Pregnancy.* New York: Appleton-Century-Crofts; 1978.

10. Robertson EG: The natural history of oedema during pregnancy. *J Obstet Gynaecol Br Commonw* 1971;78:520–529.

11. Dexter L, Weiss S: *Pre-eclamptic and Eclamptic Toxemia of Pregnancy*. Boston: Little & Brown; 1941.

12. Zinaman M, Rubin J, Lindheimer MD: Serial plasma oncotic pressure levels and echoencephalography during and after delivery in severe pre-eclampsia. *Lancet* 1985;i:1245–1247.

13. Krogh A, Landis EM, Turner AH: The movement of fluid through the human capillary wall in relation to venous pressure and to the colloid osmotic pressure of the blood. *J Clin Invest* 1932;11:63–95.

14. Thomson AM, Hytten FE, Billewicz WZ: The epidemiology of oedema during pregnancy. *J Obstet Gynaecol Br Commonw* 1967;74:1–10.

15. Freis ED, Kenny JF: Plasma volume, total circulating protein and "available fluid" abnormalities in pre-eclampsia and eclampsia. *J Clin Invest* 1948;27:283–289.

16. Friedberg V, Lutz J: Untersuchungen über die Capillarpermeabilität in der Schwangerschaft (ein Beitrag zur Ursache der Proteinurie bei Gestosen). *Arch Gynaekol* 1963;199:96–106.

17. Goodlin RC, Cotton DB, Haesslein HC: Severe edema-proteinuria-hypertension gestosis. *Am J Obstet Gynecol* 1978;132:595–598.

18. Benedetti TJ, Carlson RW: Studies of colloid osmotic pressure in pregnancy-induced hypertension. *Am J Obstet Gynecol* 1979;135:308–313.

19. Goodlin R, Kurpershoek C, Haesslein H: Colloid osmotic pressure changes during hypertensive pregnancy. *Clin Exper Hypertens Bull* 1982;1:49–56.

20. Hytten FE: Oedema in pregnancy. In: Rippman ET, ed: *Die Spätgestose*. Basel: Schwabe; 1970.

21. Eden TW: Eclampsia: A commentary on the reports presented to the British Congress of Obstetrics and Gynaecology, June 29, 1922. *J Obstet Gynaecol Br Emp* 1922;29:386–401.

22. Werkö L, Bucht H, Lagerlöf H, Holmgren A: Cirkulationen vid graviditet. *Nord Med* 1948;40:1868–1869.

23. Röttger H: Über den Wasserhaushalt in der physiologischen und toxischen Schwangerschaft. I. Der Wasserhaushalt in der physiologischen Schwangerschaft. *Arch Gynaekol* 1953;184: 59–85.

24. Röttger H: Über den Wasserhaushalt in der physiologischen und toxischen Schwangerschaft. II. Der Wasserhaushalt bei Schwangerschaftsspattoxikosen. *Arch Gynaekol* 1954;184:629–642.

25. Cope I: Plasma and blood volume changes in pregnancies complicated by pre-eclampsia. *J Obstet Gynaecol Br Commonw* 1961;68:413–416.

26. Kolpakova LL: Changes of the plasma volume and serum protein composition in late toxaemia of pregnancy. *Akush Ginecol* 1965;1:130–133.

27. Honger PE: Intravascular mass of albumin in pre-eclampsia and normal pregnancy. *Scand J Lab Clin Invest* 1967;19:283–287.

28. Haering M, Werners PH, Hemmerling J: Über das Verhalten des Gesamthämoglobins bei schweren Praeklampsien. *Z Geburtsh Gynaekol* 1967;166:271–279.

29. Brody S, Spetz S: Plasma, extracellular and interstitial fluid volumes in pregnancy complicated by toxaemia. *Acta Obstet Gynecol Scand* 1967;46:138–150.

30. MacGillivray I: The significance of blood pressure and body water changes in pregnancy. *Scot Med J* 1967;12:237–245.

31. Blekta M, Hlavaty V, Trnkova M, et al: Volume of whole blood and absolute amount of serum proteins in the early stage of late toxemia of pregnancy. *Am J Obstet Gynecol* 1970;106:10–13.

32. Gallery EDM, Hunyor SN, Gyory AZ: Plasma volume contraction: A significant factor in both pregnancy-associated hypertension (pre-eclampsia) and chronic hypertension in pregnancy. *Quart J Med* 1979;48:593–602.

33. MacGillivray I: Pre-eclampsia. *The Hypertensive Disease of Pregnancy*. London, Philadelphia, Toronto: WB Saunders Pty. Ltd., 1983.

34. Brown MA, Zammit VC, Mitar DM: Extracellular fluid volumes in pregnancy-induced hypertension. *J Hypertens* 1992;10:61–68.

34a. Silver HM, Seebeck MA, Carlson R: Comparison of total volume in normal, preeclamptic, and nonproteinuric gestational hypertensive pregnancy by subcutaneous measurement of red blood cell and plasma volume. *Am J Obstet Gynecol* 1998;179:87–93.

35. Lang RM, Pridjian G, Feldman T, et al: Left ventricular mechanics in preeclampsia. *Am Heart J* 1991;121:1768–1775.
36. Lindheimer MD, Weston P: Effect of hypotonic expansion on sodium, water and urea excretion in late pregnancy: The influence of posture on these results. *J Clin Invest* 1969;48:947–956.
37. Sarles HE, Hill SS, Le Blanc AL, et al: Sodium excretion patterns during and following intravenous sodium loads in normal and hypertensive pregnancies. *Am J Obstet Gynecol* 1968;102:1–7.
38. Gallery EDM, Brown MA: Control of sodium excretion in human pregnancy. *Am J Kidney Dis* 1987;9:290–295.
39. Broughton-Pipkin F: The renin–angiotensin system in normal and hypertensive pregnancies. In: Rubin PC, ed. *Handbook of Hypertension. Vol 10. Hypertension in Pregnancy.* Amsterdam: Elsevier; 1988:118–167.
39a. Baylis C, Beinder E, Suto T, August P: Recent insights into the roles of nitric oxide and renin–angiotensin in the pathophysiology of preeclamptic pregnancy. *Sem Nephrol* 1998;18:208–230.
40. Nicholson EC, Gallery EDM, Brown MA, et al: Renin activation in normal and hypertensive pregnancy. *Clin Exp Hypertens Pregnancy* 1988;6:453–464.
41. Sealey JE, von Lutterolti N, Rubattu S, et al: The greater renin system. *Am J Hypertens* 1991;4:972–977.
42. Brown MA, Gallery EDM: Volume homeostasis in normal pregnancy and preeclampsia: Physiology and clinical implications. *Clin Obstet Gynaecol (Baillière)* 1994;8:287–310.
43. Gordon RD, Symonds EM, Wilmshurst EG, et al: Plasma renin activity, plasma angiotensin and plasma and urinary electrolytes in normal and toxaemic pregnancy, including a prospective study. *Clin Sci Molec Med* 1973;45:115–127.
44. Gallery EDM, Hunyor SN, Györy AZ: Plasma renin activity in normal human pregnancy and in pregnancy-associated hypertension, with reference to cryoactivation. *Clin Sci* 1980;59:49–53.
45. Kalenga MK, Thomas K, deGasparo M, deHertogh R: Determination of renin, angiotensin converting enzyme and angiotensin II levels in human placenta, chorion and amnion from women with pregnancy induced hypertension. *Clin Endocrinol* (Oxf) 1996;44:429–433.
46. Ward K, Hata A, Jeunemaitre X, et al: A molecular variant of angiotensinogen associated with pre-eclampsia. *Nature Genetics* 1993;4:59–61.
47. Morgan T, Craven C, Nelson L, et al: Angiotensinogen T235 expression is elevated in decidual spiral arteries. *J Clin Invest* 1997;100:1406–1415.
48. Gant NF, Daley GL, Chand S, et al: A study of angiotensin II pressor response throughout primigravid pregnancy. *J Clin Invest* 1973;52:2682–2689.
49. Knock GA, Sullivan MH, McCarthy A, et al: Angiotensin II (AT1) vascular binding sites in human placentae from normal-term, preeclamptic and growth retarded pregnancies. *J Pharmacol Exp Ther* 1994;271:1007–1015.
50. Brown MA, Nicholson E, Ross MR, et al: Progressive resetting of sodium-renin-aldosterone relationships in human pregnancy. *Clin Exper Hypertens* 1986;B5:249–260.
51. Brown MA, Zammit VC, Mitar DM, et al: Control of aldosterone in normal and hypertensive pregnancy: Effects of metoclopramide. *Hypertens Pregnancy* 1993;12:37–51.
52. Fournier A, El Esper GN, Lalau JD, et al: Atrial natriuretic factor in pregnancy and pregnancy-induced hypertension. *Cana J Physiol Pharmacol* 1991;69:1601–1608.
53. Steegers EAP, Van Lakwijk HPJM, Fast JH, et al: Atrial natriuretic peptide and atrial size during normal pregnancy. *Br J Obstet Gynaecol* 1991;98:202–206.
54. Lowe SA, MacDonald GJ, Brown MA: Acute and chronic regulation of atrial natriuretic peptide in human pregnancy. *J Hypertens* 1992;10:821–829.
55. Castro LC, Hobel CJ, Gornbein J: Plasma levels of atrial natriuretic peptide in normal and hypertensive pregnancies: A meta-analysis. *Am J Obstet Gynecol* 1994;171:1642–1651.
56. Steegers EAP, Benraad TJ, Jongsma HW, et al: Effects of dietary sodium restriction or posture on plasma levels of atrial natriuretic peptide, aldosterone and free aldosterone in normal human pregnancy. *J Endocrinol* 1990;124:507–513.
57. Fievet P, Fournier A, DeBold A, et al: Atrial natriuretic factor in pregnancy-induced hyper-

tension and preeclampsia: Increased plasma concentrations possibly explain these hypovolemic states with paradoxical hyporeninism. *Am J Hypertens* 1988;1:16–21.

58. Lowe SA, Zammit VC, Mitar DM, et al: Atrial natriuretic peptide and plasma volume in
pregnancy-induced hypertension. *Am J Hypertens* 1991;4:897–903.

59. Pouta A, Karinen J, Vuolteenaho O, Laatikainen T: Pre-eclampsia: The effect of intravenous
preload on atrial natriuretic peptide secretion during caesarean section under spinal anaes-
thesia. *Acta Anaesthesiol Scand* 1996;40:1203–1209.

60. Kingdom JC, McQueen J, Ryan G, et al: Fetal vascular atrial natriuretic peptide receptors in
human placenta: Alteration in intrauterine growth retardation and preeclampsia. *Am J Obstet Gynecol* 1994;170:142–147.

61. Friedman SA: Preeclampsia: A review of the role of prostaglandins. *Obstet Gynecol* 1988;71:
122–137.

62. Goeschen K, Henkel E, Behrens O: Plasma prostacyclin and thromboxane concentrations in
160 normotensive, hypertensive and preeclamptic patients during pregnancy, delivery and
the postpartum period. *J Perinat Med* 1993;21:481–489.

63. Moutquin JM, Lindsay C, Arial N, et al: Do prostacyclin and thromboxane contribute to the
protective effect of pregnancies with chronic hypertension—a preliminary prospective longitudinal study. *Am J Obstet Gynecol* 1997;177:1483–1490.

64. Barden A, Beilen LJ, Ritchie J, et al: Plasma and urinary endothelin 1, prostacyclin metabolites and platelet consumption in preeclampsia and essential hypertensive pregnancy. *Blood
Pressure* 1994;3:38–46.

65. Smith AJ, Walters WAW, Buckley NA, et al: Hypertensive and normal pregnancy: A longitudinal study of blood pressure, distensibility of dorsal hand veins and the ratio of the stable metabolites of thromboxane A2 and prostacyclin in plasma. *Br J Obstet Gynaecol* 1995;102:
900–906.

66. Gallery EDM, Rowe J, Campbell S, Hawkins T: Secretion of prostaglandins and endothelin-
1 by decidual endothelial cells from normal and pre-eclamptic pregnancies. *Am J Obstet Gynecol* 1995;173:1557–1562.

67. Gallery EDM, Rowe J, Campbell S: Alteration of in vitro human decidual endothelial cell
growth, endothelin 1 and prostaglandin secretion, by growth factors and intracellular calcium. *Prostaglandins, Leukocytes, Essential Fatty Acids* 1996;54:411–418.

68. Wellings RP, Brockelsby JC, Baker PN: Activation of endothelial cells by plasma from
women with preeclampsia—differential effects on four endothelial cell types. *J Soc Gynecol
Invest* 1998;5:31–37.

69. Torres PJ, Escolar G, Palacio M, et al: Platelet sensitivity to prostaglandin E1 inhibition is
reduced in preeclampsia but not in nonproteinuric gestational hypertension. *Br J Obstet
Gynaecol* 1996;103:19–24.

70. Klockenbusch W, Hohlfeld T, Wilhelm M, et al: Platelet PGI2 receptor affinity is reduced in
preeclampsia. *Br J Pharmacol* 1996;41:616–618.

71. Walsh SW, Wang Y: Trophoblast and placental villous core production of lipid peroxides, thromboxane and prostacyclin in preeclampsia. *J Clin Endocrinol Metab* 1995;80:
1888–1893.

72. Ding ZQ, Rowe J, Sinosich MJ, et al: In vitro secretion of prostanoids by placental villous trophoblasts in preeclampsia. *Placenta* 1996;17:407–411.

73. Cervar M, Kainer F, Jones CJ, Desoye G: Altered release of endothelin 1, 2 and thromboxane
B2 from trophoblastic cells in preeclampsia. *Eur J Clin Invest* 1996;26:30–37.

74. Johnson RD, Sadovsky Y, Graham C, et al: The expression and activity of prostaglandin H
synthase 2 is enhanced in trophoblast from women with preeclampsia. *J Clin Endocrinol
Metab* 1997;82(abstr):3059–3062.

75. Lindheimer MD, Katz AI: Kidney function in the pregnant rat. *J Lab Clin Med* 1971;
78:633–641.

76. Gallery EDM, Rowe J, Brown MA, Ross MA: Effect of changes in dietary sodium on active
electrolyte transport by erythrocytes at different stages of human pregnancy. *Clin Sci* 1988;
74:145–150.

77. Tranquilli AL, Mazzanti L, Bertoli E, et al: Sodium/potassium-adenosine triphosphatase on

erythrocyte ghosts from pregnant women and its relationship to pregnancy-induced hypertension. *Obstet Gynecol* 1988;71:627–630.

78. Kaminski K, Rechberger T: Concentration of digoxin-like immunoreactive substance in patients with preeclampsia and its relation to severity of pregnancy-induced hypertension. *Am J Obstet Gynecol* 1991;165:733–736.

79. Miyamoto S, Makino N, Shimokawa H, et al: The characteristics of erythrocyte Na+ transport systems in normal pregnancy and pregnancy-induced hypertension. *J Hypertens* 1992;10: 367–372.

80. Seely EW, Williams GH, Graves SW: Markers of sodium and volume homeostasis in pregnancy-induced hypertension. *J Clin Endocrinol Metab* 1992;74:150–156.

81. Graham D, Kingdom JC, McDonald J, et al: Platelet sodium/hydrogen ion exchange in normal pregnancy and non-proteinuric preeclampsia. *J Human Hypertens* 1997;11:453–458.

82. Gallery EDM, Esber RP, Brown MA, et al: Alterations in erythrocyte Na+, K+-cotransport in normal and hypertensive human pregnancy. *J Hypertens* 1988;6:153–158.

83. Heilmann L, vonTempelhoff GF, Ulrich S: The Na^+/K^+ co-transport system in erythrocytes from pregnant patients. *Arch Gynecol Obstet* 1993;253:167–174.

84. Canessa M, Adragna N, Solomon HS, et al: Increased sodium-lithium countertransport in red cells of patients with essential hypertension. *N Engl J Med* 1980;302:772–776.

85. Worley RJ, Hentschel WM, Cormier C, et al: Increased sodium-lithium countertransport in erythrocytes of pregnant women. *N Engl J Med* 1982;307:412–416.

86. Yoshimura T, Okazaki T, Suzuki A: Increased red-cell sodium-lithium countertransport activity and urinary 11-dehydrothromboxane B2 during pregnancy. *Nippon-Sanka-Fujinka-Gakkai-Zashi* 1992;44:153–158.

10

Platelet and Coagulation Abnormalities

Philip N. Baker and F. Gary Cunningham

A major difficulty in compiling any review concerning preeclampsia is the use of variable or imprecise criteria for its diagnosis by different investigators (see Chap. 1). Accordingly, in this chapter, "preeclampsia" implies significant hypertension and proteinuria, although myriad different thresholds have been used. This caveat must be considered even when comparing more recent studies.

Only a minority of women with preeclampsia develop thrombocytopenia defined by a platelet count below 150,000/μL. Even less common are significant alterations in coagulation assays such as prothrombin, activated partial thromboplastin, and bleeding times.[1,2] Nevertheless, findings in preeclampsia of fibrin and platelet thromboses in the placental and systemic microcirculation[3] suggest that platelet and coagulation abnormalities are of fundamental significance. Fibrin deposits and thromboses in vessels of various organs of women who died from eclampsia were described over 100 years ago, and in 1912 it was first suggested that coagulation abnormalities were involved in the pathogenesis of preeclampsia (cited by Chesley[4]). In unusual cases, widespread activation of platelets and the coagulation cascade may occur, leading to clinically apparent disseminated intravascular coagulation.[2]

As basic knowledge and laboratory techniques concerning platelet and coagulation activity and function became available over the past two decades, a number of investigators applied these to the study of preeclampsia. Accordingly, much research in preeclamptic women has been directed to the study of platelet behavior—both in vivo and in vitro as well as to other aspects of the coagulation cascade.

PLATELETS

Guilio Bizzozero was probably the first person to observe platelets in the circulating blood of intact animals. In 1882, he coined the term *blut plattchen* and described changes that platelets undergo when exposed to a foreign surface.[5] Platelets are the smallest of the formed blood elements, with a diameter of 2 to 3 μm, and a lifespan in vivo of about 9 to 10 days. Platelets are considered to have three zones. The *peripheral zone* consists of three structural domains to include the exterior coat, unit membrane, and submembrane region. This zone includes an intricate system of channels which are continuous with the plasma membrane. The *Sol-gel zone* is the matrix of the platelet cytoplasm, while the *organelle zone* contains cytoplasm and several types of secretory granules.[6]

Platelets play an important role in hemostasis and clot formation. Various stimuli, including collagen, thrombin, serotonin, epinephrine, and adenosine diphosphate (ADP) can stimulate platelet aggregation. When endothelium is disrupted, platelets adhere to exposed subendothelial collagen. This process requires von Willebrand factor and results in platelet shape changes from a disk to a spiny sphere with fine filopodia. Most platelets that accumulate at a site of injury do not adhere directly to subendothelial surface, but rather to each other—a process termed *aggregation.* Such adherence results in the secretion of the contents of dense bodies and alpha-granules containing ADP, fibrinogen, calcium, 5-hydroxytryptamine, thromboxane, beta-thromboglobulin, and various other coagulation and platelet factors.

A number of changes that relate to platelets and their various functions are changed as a result of pregnancy. As perhaps expected, some of these changes are altered by preeclampsia (Table 10–1).

Platelets in Normal and Preeclamptic Pregnancies

With the introduction of automated counters, there have been several studies investigating platelet concentration and size in normal pregnancy and in preeclampsia. Most studies conclude that while there is little significant change in the platelet count during normal pregnancy, it does fall in preeclampsia.[1,4,7-12] The frequency and intensity of maternal thrombocytopenia vary between studies, and is apparently dependent upon severity of disease, the length of delay between the onset of preeclampsia and delivery, and the frequency with which the platelet counts are performed. Even with marked maternal thrombocytopenia that may be seen with severe preeclampsia and eclampsia, fetal or neonatal cord blood platelet counts are seldom affected.[13]

Redman et al.[7] demonstrated that the platelet count fell at an early stage in the evolution of preeclampsia as determined by a sustained rise in serum urate levels. Of considerable clinical significance are the findings of Leduc et al.,[14] who showed that in the absence of thrombocytopenia, women with severe preeclampsia did not have significant clotting abnormalities. More recently, Fitzgerald et al.[15] demonstrated minor abnormalities. Thus, studies of prothrombin and activated partial thromboplastin times and determination of plasma fibrinogen concentration can be reserved for women with platelet counts less than 100,000/μL.

In women with preeclampsia, there is an increase in mean platelet volume be-

TABLE 10–1. PLATELET CHANGES ASSOCIATED WITH PREECLAMPSIA COMPARED WITH NORMALLY PREGNANT WOMEN

Factor	Change—Preeclampsia vs. Normal Pregnancy	Comments
Circulating platelets		
Concentration	Decreased	Dependent on severity and duration
Volume	Increased	Younger, larger platelets
Lifespan	Decreased	
Platelet activation in vivo		
Beta-thromboglobulin	Increased (serum)	Associated with degranulation
Immune stimulation	Increased serum platelet-associated IgG	
Cell adherence molecule expression	Increased	Increased expression anti-P-selectin and anti-CD63
Thromboxane A_2	Urinary metabolites increased	Thromboxane generation also activates platelets
Platelets in vitro		
Aggregation	Decreased compared with increase of normal pregnancy	Reduced in response to ADP, arachidonic acid, vasopressin, and epinephrine
Release	Decreased	Reduced release of 5-hydroxytryptamine in response to epinephrine
Membrane microfluidity	Decreased	
Nitric oxide synthase	Decreased	
Platelet second messengers		
Intracellular free Ca^{++}	Increased over normal pregnancy increase	
cAMP	Reduced cAMP platelet response to prostacyclin	Causes platelet activation
	Magnesium increases cAMP levels via prostacyclin	
Platelet-binding sites		
Angiotensin II	Normal levels compared with decreased levels in normotensive pregnancy	Angiotensin II enhances platelet aggregation with ADP and epinephrine

351

yond the increase found in normal pregnancy.[1,4,8,10] There also is probably an increase in platelet distribution width,[10] and these together indicate a population of larger platelets in women with preeclampsia. Such size increases may be the result of increased peripheral platelet consumption or destruction causing an increased proportion of young platelets.[16] Other factors include complex changes in the pattern of platelet production and release by megakaryocytes.[16] With such evidence for platelet consumption, a reduced lifespan in preeclampsia would be anticipated. Because optimal studies require radiolabeling, platelet lifespan has been studied by measurement of platelet malondialdehyde production following the administration of a single dose of aspirin. In normal pregnancy, no significant reduction in platelet lifespan was demonstrated when this method was used.[17,18] Although one longitudinal study[18] did not show a significant reduction in platelet lifespan in preeclampsia, Rakoczi et al.[17] reported a significant diminution. Moreover, the demonstration of a shorter platelet production time is consistent with a shorter platelet half-life.[19]

Platelet Activation In Vivo

Circulating levels of factors stored within platelets reflect platelet activation, i.e., platelet aggregation and release of granule contents. Plasma levels of beta-thromboglobulin, the platelet alpha-granule protein, are higher in normal pregnant women than in nonpregnant women.[18-21] Several studies have demonstrated higher plasma levels of beta-thromboglobulin in preeclampsia compared with normal pregnant controls.[21-25] Janes and Goodall[24] reported that the increased beta-thromboglobulin concentrations were associated with degranulation, as evidenced by elevated levels of the lysosomal-granule membrane antigen, CD63. Socol et al.[23] found that this measure of platelet alpha-granule release correlated with levels of proteinuria and serum creatinine, suggesting a link between platelet activation and renal microvascular changes.

Elevation of beta-thromboglobulin levels precedes the clinical development of preeclampsia by at least 4 weeks.[25] In contrast with normal pregnancy, levels of beta-thromboglobulin were not found to correlate with increased fibrinopeptide A—a marker of thrombin generation—reported in preeclampsia.[19] These findings suggest that mechanisms other than thrombin-mediated platelet stimulation are responsible for platelet activation in preeclampsia. An immune mechanism may be a contributory factor. Burrows et al.[26] reported increased serum levels of platelet-associated immunoglobulin G which correlated with disease severity. In a prospective study,[27] platelet-bound and circulating platelet-bindable immunoglobulin was measured, and there was a higher frequency of abnormal platelet antiglobulin found in women with preeclampsia compared with normotensive pregnant women. Alterations in platelet-bound immunoglobulins could be caused by deposition of autoreactive antibodies or immune complexes caused by placental tissue antigens. Alternatively, platelet activation at sites of microvascular injury could lead to the externalization of IgG and other proteins in platelet alpha-granules.

Serum levels of platelet factor 4, another alpha-granule protein, are not significantly elevated in preeclampsia.[20] This factor is cleared by binding to the endothelium rather than by renal excretion, thus a contribution of impaired renal function to the changes in beta-thromboglobulin levels cannot be excluded. Serotonin is also released when platelets aggregate. Middelkoop et al.[28] found lower serotonin concentrations in platelet-poor plasma from preeclamptic women than in such plasma from normal pregnant women, a result consistent with platelet aggregation and consumption. Janes et al.[29] used a whole blood flow cytometric method to detect circulating-activated platelets in preeclamptic women. Activated platelets were identified by bound fibrinogen or by CD63 antigen expression, and were detected prior to the development of disease. These findings were confirmed by Konijnenberg et al.,[30] who also demonstrated enhanced expression of anti-P-selectin; a marker of alpha-granule secretion.

The most reliable method of assessing in vivo thromboxane production is by measurement of urinary metabolites of thromboxane A_2. Urinary excretion of 2,3-dinor-thromboxane B_2 and 11-dehydro-thromboxane B_2 is increased in normal pregnancy.[31] These urinary metabolites are further increased in women with preeclampsia, compared with normotensive pregnant women, and may increase before clinical signs develop.[32,33] These observations provide further evidence of increased platelet activation in preeclampsia; moreover, thromboxane generation activates platelets. Garzetti et al.[34] studied platelet membranes and found increased membrane fluidity and cholesterol concentration in women with preeclampsia. These changes are consistent with increased unsaturated fatty acid content, and unsaturated fatty acids are both a substrate for lipid oxidation and participate in thromboxane formation. Increased thromboxane production may thus reflect altered platelet membranes in preeclampsia.

Thus, there is ample evidence to indicate increased platelet activation in preeclampsia. These include reduced platelet concentrations, increased size, reduced lifespan, increased alpha-granule release, enhanced expression of cell adhesion molecules, and increased thromboxane production. This increased activation, which occurs early in the disease, may either result from an extrinsic factor such as endothelial damage with platelet activation, or it might be intrinsic and antedating pregnancy. Credence that intrinsic platelet alterations are at least partly responsible comes from findings of platelet binding site alterations. One example of this is increased platelet angiotensin II binding sites which are apparent in early gestation in some women who subsequently develop preeclampsia.[35,35a] Maki et al.[36] proposed an alternative mechanism caused by diminished circulating platelet-activating factor acetylhydrolase activity. This would lead to decreased platelet-activating factor in normal pregnant women compared with nonpregnant women, but not in those with preeclampsia. These authors hypothesized that this aspect of platelet behavior in preeclampsia represented a failure of adaptation to pregnancy.

Platelet Behavior In Vitro

Many studies have investigated platelet reactivity in vitro in preeclampsia; the majority of these have examined platelet aggregation. Results vary because of differences in patient selection, experimental technique, the parameter analyzed, and the type and concentration of agonists employed. In addition, artifactual effects of differing hematocrits on platelet aggregation have been reported. Roberts et al.[37] found that the increased ability of epinephrine to potentiate aggregation by adenosine diphosphate (ADP) in pregnancy was eliminated by normalization of the increased citrate concentration which resulted from the lower hematocrit normal for pregnancy. In normal pregnancy, platelet aggregation has been found to be increased.[38] In preeclampsia, however, there is a consensus that platelet aggregation in platelet-rich plasma is reduced in response to ADP,[11,39] arachidonic acid,[38,40] and vasopressin.[40] Similarly reduced responses to ADP in preeclampsia were found in whole blood,[41] again contrasting with elevated whole blood platelet aggregation in normal pregnancy.[42] Louden et al.[43] reported a significantly diminished response in whole blood when epinephrine was used to stimulate platelets from women with preeclampsia as compared with those from normal pregnancy.

Platelet-release reaction in vitro in preeclampsia is less well characterized. A reduced response is consistently reported, whereas an increased response is found in normal pregnancy as compared with nonpregnant women. Horn et al.[44] demonstrated a diminished radiolabeled 5-hydroxytryptamine release in platelet-rich plasma in response to arachidonic acid in vitro when women with preeclampsia were compared with healthy third-trimester control subjects. In whole blood, platelets from women with preeclampsia release less 5-hydroxytryptamine in response to epinephrine than those from normal pregnant women. This mirrors the in vitro reduction in platelet aggregation in response to this agonist in preeclampsia. The platelet content of 5-hydroxytryptamine is reduced in preeclampsia,[45,46] suggesting that platelets have released their products prior to in vitro studies. In one of the few reports of a heightened in vitro platelet response in preeclampsia, Janes and Goodall[24] found that platelet responsiveness to ADP was increased in preeclampsia compared with normal pregnancy. Enhanced expression of the lysosomal-granule membrane antigen CD63 provided evidence of an increased degranulation response.

Further evidence of an in vitro reduction in platelet reactivity in preeclampsia is provided by studies of platelet membrane microfluidity. Microfluidity is a pivotal physical parameter which facilitates molecular linkages, accessibility of membrane-bound receptors, and stimulus-response coupling. Using fluorescence polarization, Tozzi-Ciancarelli et al.[47] demonstrated reduced platelet fluidity in preeclampsia. They suggested that an associated increase in lipid peroxidation might be responsible.

Nitric oxide is a potent vasodilator which may play an important role in the physiologic adaptation to normal pregnancy (see also Chaps. 3 and 8). There is some evidence that nitric oxide generation may be inappropriately low in preeclampsia, leading to enhanced vasoconstriction.[48,49] Platelets, like endothelial cells, contain a constitutive form of nitric oxide synthase. When platelet nitric oxide activity was measured, nitric oxide synthase activity was significantly lower in platelets from women with preeclampsia compared with normal pregnant women.[50] Platelet nitric oxide synthesis may contribute to the vasodilation of normal pregnancy. It is unclear whether lower activity in preeclampsia reflects platelet changes in the disease, or contributes to its pathogenesis.

Serum thromboxane B_2—the stable hydrolysis product of thromboxane A_2—reflects platelet thromboxane production under conditions of spontaneous clotting of whole blood in vitro. Serum levels of thromboxane B_2 have been found to correlate with thromboxane released from platelets during induced aggregation in platelet-rich plasma.[51] As discussed above, in vivo thromboxane production is increased in preeclampsia. In contrast, serum thromboxane B_2 levels are similar in pregnancies complicated by preeclampsia and normal pregnancies.[20,43,44] Wallenburg and Rotmans[52] measured malondialdehyde formation in platelet-rich plasma after thrombin stimulation as a measure of in vitro platelet thromboxane production. They reported that production was only increased in hypertensive pregnancies if there was fetal growth restriction.

Thus, in the majority of in vitro studies, there is reduced platelet reactivity in preeclampsia compared with normal pregnancy. Although many in vitro studies were performed in platelet-rich plasma, similar findings in whole blood suggest that activation during platelet preparation is unlikely to account for this reduction. A more feasible explanation is that preeclampsia leads to in vivo activation which results in the circulation of "exhausted" platelets which are hyporeactive when tested in vitro.

In vitro studies have been performed to elucidate mechanisms responsible for increased platelet activation in preeclampsia. There is some evidence that the inhibitory mechanisms that switch off platelet activation responses may be less effective in preeclampsia. Vascular endothelial cell production of prostacyclin, which acts via cyclic adenosine monophosphate (cAMP) to inhibit platelet aggregation, is diminished in preeclampsia compared with normal pregnancy.[53] The resulting tendency to vasoconstriction and platelet aggregation is accentuated by a diminution in platelet sensitivity to prostacyclin. Horn et al.[44] found that there was no alteration in sensitivity to prostacyclin—or other manipulators of cAMP such as thromboxane synthase inhibitors—when platelets from women with pregnancy-induced hypertension (some of whom had preeclampsia) were compared with platelets from normal pregnant women. In reports focusing on preeclampsia, however, pregnancy-induced diminished susceptibility to prostacyclin inhibition was significantly more marked—up to 50%—in preeclampsia.[54,55] The finding of increased numbers of platelet thromboxane A_2-receptors in women with preeclampsia[56] is also consistent with increased in vivo platelet activation. Arachidonic acid, ADP, and epinephrine all have a thromboxane-dependent component in their mechanism of action.[57,58] Finally, increased thromboxane receptor density should lead to increased in vivo reactivity.

Platelet Second Messengers

In an attempt to further elucidate mechanisms underlying in vivo and in vitro changes in platelet behavior, investigators have studied platelet second messenger systems in normal pregnancy and in preeclampsia. The majority of studies have been directed at the second messengers, intracellular free calcium ($[Ca^{+2}]_i$) and cAMP.

In the first study to investigate platelet $[Ca^{+2}]_i$, Barr et al.[59] found no differences in basal or ADP-stimulated platelet $[Ca^{+2}]_i$ in either normal pregnancy or preeclampsia. They used the calcium-sensitive indicator, quin-2, which is known to quench increases in platelet $[Ca^{+2}]_i$ resulting from platelet stimulation.[60] Moreover, the method used to prepare washed platelets probably led to a significant loss of the most active platelets. These authors did demonstrate reduced 5-hydroxytryptamine-stimulated platelet $[Ca^{+2}]_i$ in preeclampsia compared with normal pregnancy. It was previously shown[61] that 5-hydroxytryptamine responses were easily suppressed as a result of prior platelet activation.

The calcium-sensitive fluorophore, fura-2, has the advantage of weaker calcium-chelating properties than quin-2.[60] Using this indicator, Kilby et al.[62] found that basal platelet $[Ca^{+2}]_i$ levels were increased in normal pregnancy and further increased in preeclampsia but not in nonproteinuric pregnancy-induced hypertension. Whether this increase in platelet $[Ca^{+2}]_i$ reflects a population of partially activated platelets in preeclampsia, or is a cause of altered platelet reactivity is unclear. There is some evidence that alteration in stimulated platelet $[Ca^{+2}]_i$ precedes clinical signs of preeclampsia. In a prospective study of nulliparous women at risk, Zemel et al.[63] found that women who subsequently developed preeclampsia had higher levels of platelet $[Ca^{+2}]_i$ following stimulation with arginine vasopressin. These findings were detected as early as the first trimester, although basal levels were unaltered. While Zemel et al.[63] studied urban African-American women, racial differences in platelet $[Ca^{+2}]_i$ have been reported.[64,65] Indeed, Kyle et al.[64] did not find increased arginine vasopressin stimulation of platelet $[Ca^{+2}]_i$ levels with established preeclampsia in Caucasian women.

Basal cAMP levels do not appear to differ from the nonpregnant state in either normal pregnancy or preeclampsia.[43,66,67] Horn et al.[44] demonstrated reduced platelet production of cAMP in pregnancy in response to a range of adenylate cyclase stimulators. They used a sensitive assay based on prelabeling of the metabolic adenine nucleotide pool in platelets with hydrogen 3-adenine. These findings are consistent with the reduction in sensitivity of platelets during pregnancy to inhibition by prostaglandins and other agents which act via raising the level of the inhibitory second messenger, cAMP. In a cross-sectional study, no differences were found between normal and hypertensive pregnant women—a heterogenous group including those with both nonproteinuric pregnancy-induced hypertension and preeclampsia was studied. In a small longitudinal comparison of normal pregnant women with a group of pregnant women deemed at risk of developing preeclampsia, these same investigators[67] found that platelets from women at-risk accumulated less cAMP in response to adenylate cyclase stimulators during pregnancy.

Thus, relative deficiency of in vivo prostacyclin production, combined with reduced cAMP response to prostacyclin, could promote extensive platelet activation in preeclampsia. Interestingly, magnesium, which has been administered for many years in order to prevent eclampsia,[68] increases the prostacyclin-induced elevation of platelet cAMP levels.[69] It seems reasonable that the beneficial effects of magnesium therapy in preeclampsia may involve this action on platelets.

Cyclic guanosine monophosphate (cGMP) is another second messenger which inhibits platelet activation.[70] It is synthesized from GTP by the cytosolic-soluble guanylate cyclase enzyme, and in platelets, guanylate cyclase is stimulated by nitric oxide, a potent inhibitor of platelet activation.[71] Hardy et al.[72] investigated the hypothesis that platelet activation in preeclampsia resulted from underactivity of the inhibitory cGMP system. Chirkov et al.[73] had reported reduced platelet guanylate cyclase sensitivity to stimulation by nitric oxide donors in diabetes mellitus, another condition accompanied by platelet hyperreactivity. They found that both platelet cGMP response to nitric oxide donors, as well as the inhibitory effect of donors on platelet release, were increased in platelets from women with preeclampsia compared with normotensive pregnant and nonpregnant women. They speculated that upregulation of platelet guanylate cyclase activity may be a compensatory response to impaired nitric oxide production in preeclampsia.

Platelet Angiotensin II-Binding Sites

Specific angiotensin II-binding sites with the characteristics of receptors have been demonstrated on the surface of human platelets.[74] Their role is unclear, although it has been suggested that angiotensin II enhances the platelet aggregation response to ADP and epinephrine.[75,76] Moreover, in vitro studies suggest that angiotensin II increases platelet $[Ca^{+2}]_i$ levels and this increase is greater in platelets from women with preeclampsia compared with normal pregnancy.[77]

Platelets have many of the structural and biochemical characteristics of smooth muscle cells, and similarities between catecholamine-induced changes in both platelet behavior and vascular tone have been described.[78] Measurement of platelet angiotensin II-binding sites has been suggested as an alternative to the invasive angiotensin II sensitivity test to predict preeclampsia and pregnancy-induced hypertension.[35] Platelets from normotensive pregnant women exhibit reduced angiotensin II-binding sites,[35a,79] whereas binding site concentrations revert toward nonpregnant levels in preeclampsia.[80] These results mirror the pressor sensitivity of vascular smooth muscle to intravenously infused angiotensin II, while in normal pregnancy there is a reduced pressor response to infused angiotensin II, but there is an increased pressor effect prior to clinical preeclampsia.[81]

COAGULATION

Activation of a cascade of coagulation factors leads to fibrin formation. Classically, this enzyme sequence is divided into two separate pathways, illustrated in Figure 10–1. The *intrinsic pathway* is initiated by activation of factor XII by collagen and involves factors VIII, IX, XI, XII, high-molecular weight kinogen, platelet factor 3, and prekallikrein. In the *extrinsic pathway*, thromboplastin release activates factor VII which then involves factors X and thromboplastin. Both systems converge as a common pathway that involves activated factor X, platelet-bound factor V, conversion of prothrombin to thrombin, and factor XIII. Regulation of the mechanisms involved in coagulation is by the fibrinolytic system (Fig. 10–1), composed primarily of plasminogen and regulatory proteins that include antithrombin III and proteins S and C.

Coagulation Cascade Factors

In normal pregnancy, the coagulation cascade appears to be in an activated state. Evidence of activation includes increased concentrations of all the clotting factors except factors XI and XIII, with increased levels of high-molecular weight fibrinogen complexes.[39,82,83] Considering the substantive physiologic increase in plasma volume in normal pregnancy, such increased concentrations represent a marked increase in production of these procoagulants.

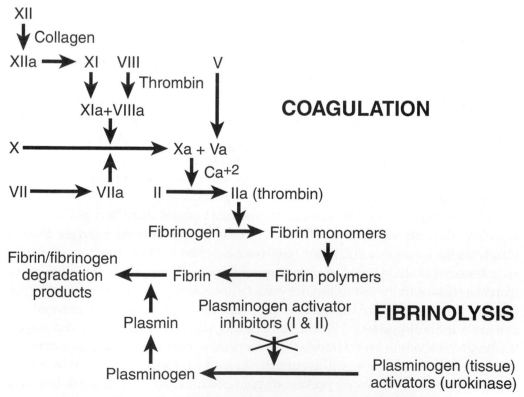

Figure 10–1. The coagulation and fibrinolysis cascades.

There is considerable evidence that preeclampsia is accompanied by a number of coagulopathic changes when compared with normal pregnant women (Table 10–2). Despite this, unless preeclampsia is complicated by overt clinical disseminated intravascular coagulation, routine coagulation tests are usually normal.[84] Clinical tests commonly used are relatively insensitive to minor changes in the coagulation system. There have been reports, however, of covert activation of both the intrinsic and extrinsic coagulation pathways in preeclampsia.[85,86] Vaziri et al.[86] found changes in plasma coagulation activity of all intrinsic pathway factors in preeclampsia and suggested that such activation was fundamental to the pathogenesis of preeclampsia. The mechanism for such an activation is unclear, although endothelial injury and exposure of subendothelial tissue would facilitate activation of factor XII.

One of the most definitive tests of coagulation activity is factor VIII consumption. The test depends on simultaneous measurement of factor VIII clotting activity and factor VIII-related antigen. When the clotting system is activated, circulating levels of both factors increase rapidly as a secondary response, but because factor VIII clotting activity is destroyed by thrombin, its final level is lower than that of the related antigen and the difference between the two is a reflection of factor VIII consumption. During normal pregnancy the levels of factor VIII coagulation activity and factor VIII-related antigen show a proportional rise, thus their ratio remains constant.[87,88] In preeclampsia, there is an early rise in the factor VIII-related antigen : coagulation activity ratio which correlates with severity of the disease and the degree of hyperuricemia.[89-91] While this increased ratio was initially thought to be due to factor VIII consumption, Scholtes et al.[91] found it to be almost entirely due to increased factor VIII-related antigen. This was most marked in cases of preeclampsia associated with fetal growth restriction. Because factor VIII-related antigen is synthesized by endothelial cells and megakaryocytes and is released by aggregating platelets, it is possible that increased levels result from endothelial damage and platelet aggregation rather than increased thrombin action.

During normal pregnancy, plasma fibrinogen concentration substantively increases. Although fibrinogen levels are the same or only slightly increased in women with preeclampsia compared with normal pregnant women,[11,84] the turnover of radiolabeled fibrinogen is increased in preeclamptic women.[92] Because increased fibrinogen turnover returned to normal with low-dose heparin therapy, it was concluded that it was thrombin-mediated.

The action of thrombin on fibrinogen is a crucial step in the coagulation cascade. Thrombin cleaves two pairs of peptides—fibrinopeptides A and B—from fibrinogen to produce soluble fibrin monomer which rapidly polymerizes to fibrin. Determination of free fibrinopeptides in blood is used to measure thrombin activity; indeed, fibrinopeptide concentrations are felt by many to be the best markers of accelerated thrombosis or coagulopathy. Levels of fibrinopeptide A have been reported to be elevated or unchanged in normal pregnancy.[21,39,82,93] Most investigators, however, have reported increased fibrinopeptide levels in women with

TABLE 10–2. CHANGES IN THE COAGULATION SYSTEMS ASSOCIATED WITH PREECLAMPSIA AND COMPARED WITH NORMAL PREGNANCY

Factor	Change—Preeclampsia vs. Normal Pregnancy	Comments
Coagulation factors		
Factor VIII consumption	Increased	Caused either by increased consumption or released factor VIII-related antigen from damaged endothelial cells
Fibrinogen	Normal to slightly increased over normal pregnancy	Radiolabeled fibrinogen turnover is increased in preeclampsia
Fibrinopeptides A and B	Increased over normal pregnancy	
Regulatory proteins		
Antithrombin III	Decreased	Fluctuates with disease severity; low levels associated with placental infarctions, perinatal morbidity and mortality, maternal morbidity
Thrombin–antithrombin III complexes	Increased over normal pregnancy	Marker of coagulation activation and consumption of inhibitors
Protein C	Decreased	
Protein S	Decreased	
Fibrinolytic system		
Plasminogen	Decreased from increased values in normal pregnancy	Very complex system involving plasminogen concentration and a variety of activators and activator-inhibitors
Fibrin–fibrinogen degradation products	Normal to increased	Conflicting data; monoclonal antibody to detect D-dimer showed correlation with disease severity

preeclampsia compared with normal pregnant women.[21,39,93,94] Borok et al.[94] found that the increased serial total fibrinopeptide measurements in preeclampsia correlated with the clinical manifestations of the disease and persisted for 3 to 7 days postpartum.

After the release of fibrinopeptides, fibrin monomers bind to each other until the polymers precipitate as fibrin. Soluble fibrin monomer can be detected by various techniques, including cold precipitation (cryofibrinogen) and use of protamine sulfate and ethanol gel precipitation assays. While increased cryofibrinogen levels have been reported in preeclampsia compared with normal pregnancy,[11,95] no consistent results have been obtained using protamine sulfate and ethanol gel assays.[39,93,95]

Regulatory Proteins

Antithrombin III is a glycoprotein manufactured by the liver. It is an important physiologic inhibitor of coagulation and forms irreversible complexes with all activated factors except VIIIa.[96] There is increased antithrombin III synthesis associated with coagulation activation. Decreased antithrombin III activity indicates increased thrombin binding secondary to increased thrombin generation and is found after thromboembolic events, in disseminated intravascular coagulopathy, and after major surgery.

Antithrombin III activity levels appear to be unchanged in normal pregnancy, although marginal decreases have been described.[82,97,98] Decreased antithrombin III activity has been demonstrated in most women with preeclampsia, but not in pregnant women with chronic hypertension.[39,99-101a] Exacerbations and remissions of the disease were reflected in fluctuations of antithrombin III levels, and low antithrombin III concentrations were associated with placental infarctions as well as perinatal and maternal morbidity and mortality.[39,99-102] Changes in antithrombin III levels did not, however, correlate with clinical improvement during the puerperium.[101] Weiner and Brant[103] reported that antithrombin III activity began to decline as much as 13 weeks prior to the development of clinical manifestations in three women who were studied longitudinally and who developed preeclampsia. Diminished antithrombin III activity in preeclampsia is not a consequence of liver dysfunction, but is caused by increased consumption. This led Paternoster et al.[104] to suggest that administration of antithrombin III to women with preeclampsia to normalize the chronic coagulopathy may improve fetal outcome. This was supported by studies in which administration of antithrombin III prevented renal dysfunction and hypertension induced by enhanced intravascular coagulation in pregnant rats.[105]

The levels of thrombin–antithrombin III complexes have been studied by several investigators. Thrombin, which converts fibrinogen to fibrin, is inactivated by antithrombin III, thus the generation of thrombin–antithrombin III complexes is a marker of coagulation activation and consumption of coagulation inhibitors. A progressive increase in the concentration of thrombin–antithrombin III complexes has been reported in normal pregnancy, suggesting increased thrombin forma-tion.[106] The finding of increased concentrations of thrombin–antithrombin III com-plexes in preeclampsia compared with normal pregnancy[106-108] is consistent with reported diminution in antithrombin III levels. Although Koh et al.[109] failed to demonstrate any difference in the concentrations of thrombin–antithrombin III complexes between normal pregnant women and those with preeclampsia, they also found no difference in beta-thromboglobulin levels between the groups.

Protein C, a serine protease probably also synthesized by the liver, is activated by contact with thrombin and thrombomodulin on the surface of endothelial cells. It is a potent inhibitor of activated factor V and VIII, and is an activator of fibrino-lysis.[87,110] Protein C is highly sensitive to consumption and reduced levels are found after surgery, thromboembolic events, and in disseminated intravascular co-agulation. Protein C levels appear to be unchanged in normal pregnancy compared with the nonpregnant state.[111] Protein C levels have been found to be substantively reduced in preeclampsia compared with normal pregnancy.[103,106,112]

Protein S serves as a cofactor for activated protein C in the degradation of the activated factors V and VIII by binding to lipid and platelet surfaces.[2,104] Levels during pregnancy may decrease to those found in patients with congenital protein S deficiency.[113] Levels are further diminished in women with preeclampsia com-pared with normal pregnant women.[104] Dekker et al.[114] studied regulatory protein abnormalities in 101 women with a history of severe early-onset preeclampsia as-sociated with a tendency to vascular thrombosis, and found that almost one-fourth had protein S deficiency.

The half-life of activated protein C:alpha 1-antitrypsin complexes is longer than that of thrombin–antithrombin III complexes, and Espana et al.[115] investigated whether levels of activated protein C:alpha 1-antitrypsin complexes provided a more sensitive marker of prethrombotic states. In a variety of clinical conditions, including preeclampsia, concentrations of these complexes were increased above that of the normal controls, and showed relatively higher increases than levels of thrombin–antithrombin III complexes. A significant and positive correlation be-tween levels of the two complexes further supported their hypothesis.

In 1993, a hereditary limitation in anticoagulant response to activated protein C was reported. This condition was termed *resistance to activated protein C*. Affected families had a history of venous thromboses which was not explained by deficien-cies of protein C, protein S, or antithrombin III.[116] Subsequently, the cause was iden-tified as a point mutation on the gene coding for factor V which results in the synthesis of a factor V molecule which is not properly activated by protein C.[117] The resultant mutation has become known as *factor V Leiden* because the re-search was carried out in the Dutch town of Leiden. Both heterozygotes and homozygotes for the factor V Leiden mutation are affected, the defect being in-herited in an autosomal-dominant fashion.[116,118] Prevalence of the factor V Leiden mutation varies between populations, and ranges from 2 to 7%.[117,119,120] Measure-ment of activated protein C resistance in pregnancy is potentially confounded by physiologic changes in resistance levels as pregnancy progresses.[120] In pregnant women, DNA testing for factor V Leiden mutation is the most effective method of diagnosis.

The discovery and characterization of activated protein C resistance is relatively recent, and population-based studies upon which to draw an accurate picture of the increased risks for preeclampsia from factor V Leiden mutation are awaited. In a retrospective study of 50 women with a history of preeclampsia and 50 control subjects, activated protein C resistance was found in 22% of the former group compared with 10% of the controls. All but two of the affected women in the preeclampsia group were heterozygous for factor V Leiden mutation.[121] Rotmensch et al.[122] studied 7 Israeli women referred over an 18-month period for recurrent pregnancy loss, fetal growth restriction, and preeclampsia who had activated protein C resistance. All had the factor V Leiden mutation identified by polymerase chain reaction; one woman was homozygous and the remainder were heterozygous. One had had a prior thromboembolism, and another three had a family history of thromboembolic events. The described cohort of patients clearly suggests a strong link between factor V Leiden and adverse pregnancy outcome, but the investigators made no attempt to obtain an overview of the prevalence of this problem.

Preeclampsia can be associated with *antiphospholipid antibodies*. The two known major antiphospholipid antibodies are *lupus anticoagulant* and *anticardiolipin antibodies*. These are misleading terms, as not all patients with lupus anticoagulant have lupus disease, or indeed any recognized autoimmune condition, and anticardiolipin antibodies are not specific to cardiolipin but recognize all anionic phospholipids. The presence of either antiphospholipid antibody carried a fourfold increase of thrombosis or thrombocytopenia.[123] Early-onset preeclampsia has been reported in association with antiphospholipid antibodies, and their presence conveys a fourfold increased risk of developing the condition.[124,125] Pregnancy outcome may be improved by treatment for these women,[126] thus women with a history of early-onset preeclampsia should be investigated.

Fibrinolytic System

The end-product of the coagulation cascade is fibrin formation. The main function of the fibrinolytic system is to remove excess fibrin deposited as a consequence of thrombin activity (see Fig. 10–1). The inactive precursor plasminogen is activated by serine proteases which convert plasminogen into plasmin. Plasminogen activators are either the tissue or urokinase type. The activity of tissue-type plasminogen activator, released by endothelial cells, is dramatically increased by thrombin, thus all tissue plasminogen activation is in the fibrin clot. Urokinase-type plasminogen activator is found in plasma as a proenzyme and is converted to a two-chain molecule upon activation. The activity of plasminogen activators is balanced by plasminogen-activator inhibitors: (1) plasminogen-activator inhibitor-1, derived from endothelial cells and present in plasma and platelets; (2) plasminogen-activator inhibitor-2, placental type, identified in plasma from pregnant women; and

(3) plasminogen-activator inhibitor-3, which inhibits protein C and the protease nexin.

The proteolytic enzyme plasmin facilitates cleavage of the polymerized fibrin strands into fragments known as the fibrin degradation products X, Y, D, and E. By the action of thrombin, fibrinopeptides are released and fibrin is degraded into D-dimer. Many of the stimuli that activate coagulation also stimulate plasmin activity, and thus increased fibrinolytic activity indirectly suggests increased thrombin action.

Studies of the fibrinolytic system in pregnancy have produced conflicting results, although the majority of evidence suggests that fibrinolytic activity is reduced in normal pregnancy. Conversely, investigators have reported that plasma–plasminogen concentrations are increased in normal pregnancy.[127] At the same time, the release of plasminogen activator from veins after they are temporarily obstructed is diminished.[83] Moreover, fibrinolytic activity, as determined by the euglobin clot lysis time—an indirect measure of the concentration of plasminogen activator that is reduced in normal pregnancy—remains low during labor and delivery, returning to nonpregnant values within one hour after delivery.[127]

There does appear to be a consensus that while plasminogen activator(s) concentrations have been found to be either increased or unchanged,[109,128] both plasminogen-activator inhibitor-1 and plasminogen-activator inhibitor-2 appear to increase in normal pregnancy.[129] It appears that levels of serum fibrin degradation products are elevated in normal pregnancy.[119] These conflicting findings may reflect the difficulty in interpreting measures of fibrinolysis. While low levels of plasminogen and plasminogen activator may indicate altered fibrinolysis, low levels may result from consumption and absorption of fibrin caused by increased fibrinolysis elicited by enhanced intravascular fibrin deposition. Similarly, increased levels may reflect either impaired or increased fibrinolysis.

Plasminogen levels determined by various methods seem to be lower in women with preeclampsia than in normal pregnancy.[39,130] Determination of the concentration of plasminogen activator using the euglobulin clot lysis time has not produced consistent differences between normal pregnant women and those with preeclampsia.[39,86] Increased levels of circulating tissue-type plasminogen-activator and tissue-type, plasminogen-activator antigen have been reported.[109,128,131] Conversely, urokinase-type plasminogen activator is reduced.[101a,109] In addition, levels of plasminogen-activator inhibitors differ in preeclampsia compared with normal pregnancy. Plasminogen-activator inhibitor-1 specifically inhibits tissue-type plasminogen activator,[132] and levels are increased in plasma, serum, and platelet lysates of preeclamptic women. Plasminogen-activator inhibitor-1 activity and antigen levels are similarly elevated.[128,131,133,134]

Decreased levels of plasminogen-activator inhibitor-2 are found in preeclampsia,[102,109,133,135,136] and mirror the reduced levels of urokinase-type plasminogen activator. Reduced levels of plasminogen-activator inhibitor-2 have also been reported in pregnancies complicated by fetal growth restriction, with or without concomitant preeclampsia.[137] The complex nature of the changes in the fibrinolytic system in preeclampsia is emphasized by the work of Kanfer et al.[138] who found that placental levels of the inhibitor were increased in pregnancies complicated by preeclampsia compared with normotensive pregnancies.

While levels of fibrin–fibrinogen degradation products have been extensively studied in women with preeclampsia, the results are inconclusive. Some have reported higher serum concentrations in preeclampsia compared with normal pregnancy, but others have found normal levels.[39,95,129] Using radioimmunoassay, Gordon et al.[139] found that levels of fibrin degradation product E were increased in about one-third of women with preeclampsia. Urinary excretion of fibrin degradation products in preeclamptic women has been reported as increased[11] or normal[140] compared with normotensive pregnant women. Gaffney et al.[141] developed an assay for monoclonal antibodies to fibrin degradation products and found increased levels in all women with preeclampsia. In another study, Trofatter et al.[142] used monoclonal antibody to detect D-dimers and showed that their detection correlated with disease severity, hypertension, proteinuria, thrombocytopenia, abnormal liver function tests, and increased levels of fibrin degradation products. Finally, Schjetlein et al.[102] found that serum D-dimer concentrations were increased in severe, but not in mild preeclampsia compared with normotensive controls.

At this juncture, it is fair to conclude that assessment of the fibrinolytic system in preeclampsia is difficult to interpret. There have been reports of reduced fibrinogen levels, increases in tissue- but not urokinase-type plasminogen-activators, increases in plasminogen-activator inhibitor-1 but not plasminogen-activator inhibitor-2, and equivocal evidence of increased fibrin–fibrinogen degradation products. Also, it is difficult to establish whether any of these changes contribute to, or merely reflect changes induced by preeclampsia. Altered endothelial cell function in preeclampsia may result in increased release of both tissue-type plasminogen activator and plasminogen-activator inhibitor-1, although increased expression of plasminogen-activator inhibitor-1 in placentas from women with preeclampsia has been described. The reduced levels of type II plasminogen-activator inhibitor might reflect either impaired placental function or a disorder in the fibrinolytic mechanism.

PREDICTIVE VALUE TO DIAGNOSE PREECLAMPSIA

Many of the platelet and coagulation changes associated with preeclampsia have been advocated as predictive tests. Unfortunately, as discussed in Chapter 6, when investigated in a prospective manner, the results usually have been disappointing.

Redman et al.[7] found that a reduction in platelet count occurred early in the development of preeclampsia, being detectable about 7 weeks prior to delivery. Neither platelet count nor platelet volume, however, were found to be useful predictive tests in normal nulliparas; the variation in counts between women is such that no importance can be attached to a single value.[143] In a subgroup of women with essential hypertension or nonproteinuric pregnancy-induced hypertension, platelet size was found to increase at least 1 week before preeclampsia was clinically apparent.[143]

The use of flow cytometric detection of activated platelets as a predictive test of preeclampsia has been studied. In a prospective study, platelets in whole blood samples from pregnant women were labeled with different antibodies associated with platelet activation. Although use of anti-CD63, a marker of lysosome secretion, was found to be an independent risk factor for the development of the disease, the odds ratios were two- to fourfold lower than those obtained using a first trimester diastolic blood pressure.[144]

Massé et al.[144a] used a simplified assay to determine platelet angiotensin II-receptor density. They found no correlation with preeclampsia predictability in 801 women studied in each trimester.

The use of antithrombin III as a marker or predictor of preeclampsia is controversial. Paternoster et al.[104] and Savelieva et al.[145] found that a fall in antithrombin III levels preceded any other demonstration of coagulopathy in women who developed preeclampsia. In a larger study, Ballageer et al.[25] found that antithrombin III determinations early in pregnancy had no predictive value for subsequent development of preeclampsia.

Ballageer et al.[25] also studied the predictive use of plasminogen-activator inhibitor-1 and fibronectin levels. Although plasminogen-activator inhibitor-1 levels were of some value, these investigators concluded that increased levels of fibronectin were the best predictor of preeclampsia. Fibronectin concentration decreases in diseases characterized by increased intravascular thrombin and fibrin deposition. Normal pregnancy is associated with similar or slightly increased plasma fibronectin levels.[146,147] In preeclampsia there is at least a twofold increase in fibronectin levels compared with normal pregnancy. Pregnant women with chronic hypertension have normal fibronectin concentrations, so increased plasma fibronectin concentrations in preeclampsia are not simply due to hypertension.[146-148] The prospective study of Lockwood and Peters[149] concurred with the finding of increased fibronectin levels prior to clinical evidence of the disorder.

In a serial study of women who developed preeclampsia, there was a tendency for changes in the factor VIII-related antigen:coagulation activity ratio to precede other changes.[89] Such changes in the coagulation system, however, were not sensitive enough for accurate screening. The *coagulation index,* derived from fibrin–fibrinogen degradation products, factor VIII-related coagulation activity, and platelet counts, did not discriminate between women with preeclampsia and normal pregnant women when used prospectively.[150] Similarly, in a study of 400 nulliparous women at 28 weeks' gestation, a battery of tests, including thrombin time, fibrin–fibrinogen degradation products, fibrinopeptide A, platelet factor 4, and beta-thromboglobulin, failed to suggest any useful discriminators.[151]

CONCLUSION

Changes in platelet function and the coagulation system in normal pregnancy and preeclampsia are complex and often conflicting, as summarized in Tables 10–1 and

10–2. There is consistent evidence to indicate that increased in vivo platelet activation of normal pregnancy is amplified in preeclampsia. Indeed, reduced platelet counts, increased size, and reduced lifespan, as well as increased alpha-granule release and thromboxane production have all been demonstrated. The majority of in vitro studies have found reduced platelet reactivity in preeclampsia compared with normal pregnancy. The most likely explanation of this dichotomy is that preeclampsia leads to platelet activation which results in circulation of "exhausted" platelets that are hyporeactive when tested in vitro. Alterations in platelet second messengers are consistent with increased platelet activation in preeclampsia, although whether these alterations reflect a population of partially activated platelets in preeclampsia or cause the altered platelet reactivity is unclear.

Study of coagulation factors provides evidence that preeclampsia accentuates pregnancy-induced hypercoagulability. Reduced levels of the coagulation regulatory proteins in preeclampsia, namely antithrombin III, protein S, and protein C, further accentuates the tendency to coagulation. Assessment of the fibrinolytic system in preeclampsia is difficult. Compared with normal pregnancy, plasminogen concentrations are reduced, as are fibrinogen levels. There are increases in tissue- but not urokinase-type plasminogen activators, increases in endothelial but not placental plasminogen-activator inhibitors, and equivocal evidence of increased fibrin–fibrinogen degradation products. Again, it is difficult to establish whether these alterations contribute to, or merely reflect, changes caused by preeclampsia.

Page[152] proposed that disseminated intravascular coagulation is a prominent event in the pathogenesis of preeclampsia. Much more likely, and as stated by Chesley[4]: *Many women with the diagnosis of eclampsia and of preeclampsia, even of severe degree, show no detectable signs of increased coagulation and fibrinolysis. Disseminated intravascular coagulopathy, if it does occur, does not appear to be a fundamental feature of the disease.* Instead, the platelet and coagulation abnormalities of preeclampsia probably represent a microangiopathy, in which endothelial cell damage stimulates platelet activation.

REFERENCES

1. Giles C: Intravascular coagulation in gestational hypertension and pre-eclampsia: The value of haematological screening tests. *Clin Lab Haemat* 1982;4:351–358.
2. Cunningham FG, Macdonald PC, Gant NF: *Williams' Obstetrics,* ed 19. Norwalk, CT: Appleton & Lange; 1993:763–817.
3. McKay DG: Chronic intravascular coagulation in normal pregnancy and pre-eclampsia. *Contr Nephrol* 1983;25:108–119.
4. Chesley LC: *Hypertensive Disorders in Pregnancy.* New York: Appleton-Century-Crofts; 1978.
5. Bizzozero G, (1882) cited by Wintrole M: Discovery of the platelet. In: *Haematology, the Blossoming of a Science.* Philadephia: Lea and Febiger; 1985:28–31.
6. White JG, Clawson CC, Gerrard JM: Platelet ultrastructure. In: Bloom AL, Thomas DP, eds. *Haemostasis and Thrombosis.* Edinburgh; Churchill Livingstone; 1981:22–49.
7. Redman WG, Bonnar J, Beilin L: Early platelet consumption in pre-eclampsia. *Br Med J* 1978;1:467–469.

8. Giles C: Thrombocytopenia and macrothrombocytosis in gestational hypertension. *Br J Obstet Gynaecol* 1981;88:1115–1119.

9. Fay RA, Bromham DR, Brooks JA, Gebski VJ: Platelets and uric acid in the prediction of preeclampsia. *Am J Obstet Gynecol* 1985;152:1038–1039.

10. Stubbs TM, Lazarchick J, Van Dorsten P, et al: Evidence of accelerated platelet production and consumption in nonthrombocytopenic preeclampsia. *Am J Obstet Gynecol* 1986;155: 263–265.

11. Howie PW, Prentice CRM, McNicol GP: Coagulation, fibrinolysis and platelet function in pre-eclampsia, essential hypertension and placental insufficiency. *J Obstet Gynaecol Br Commonw* 1971;78:992–1003.

12. Burrows RF: Thrombocytopenia in the hypertensive disorders of pregnancy. *Clin Exp Hypertens* 1990;B9:199–210.

13. Pritchard JA, Cunningham FG, Pritchard SA, Mason RA: How often does maternal preeclampsia–eclampsia incite thrombocytopenia in the fetus? *Obstet Gynecol* 1987;69: 292–297.

14. Leduc L, Wheeler JM, Kirshon B, et al: Coagulation profile in severe preeclampsia. *Obstet Gynecol* 1992;79:14–18.

15. Fitzgerald MP, Floro C, Siegel J, Hernandez E: Laboratory findings in hypertensive disorders of pregnancy. *J Natl Med Assoc* 1996;88:794–798.

16. Paulus J-M: Platelet size in man. *Blood* 1975;46:3–36.

17. Rakoczi I, Tallian F, Bagdany S, Gatai I: Platelet lifespan in normal pregnancy and pre-eclampsia as determined by a non-radioisotope technique. *Throm Res* 1979;15:553–556.

18. Pekonen F, Rasi V, Ammala M, et al: Platelet function and coagulation in normal and preeclamptic pregnancy. *Thromb Res* 1986;43:553–560.

19. Inglis TCM, Stuart J, George AJ, Davies AJ: Haemostatic and rheological changes in normal pregnancy and pre-eclampsia. *Br J Haematol* 1982;50:461–465.

20. Pekonen F, Rasi V, Ammala M, et al: Platelet function and coagulation in normal and preeclamptic pregnancy. *Thromb Res* 1986;43:553–560.

21. Douglas JT, Shah M, Lowe GDO, et al: Plasma fibrinopeptide A and betathromboglobulin in pre-eclampsia and pregnancy hypertension. *Thromb Haemostas* 1982;47:54–55.

22. Arocha-Pinago CL, Lopez AOG, Garcia L, Linares J: Beta-thromboglobulin (β-TG) and platelet factor 4 (PF4) in obstetrical cases. *Acta Obstet Gynecol Scand* 1995;64:115–120.

23. Socol ML, Weiner CP, Louis G, et al: Platelet activation in pre-eclampsia. *Am J Obstet Gynecol* 1985;151:494–497.

24. Janes SL, Goodall AH: Flow cytometric detection of circulating activated platelets and platelet hyper-responsiveness in pre-eclampsia and pregnancy. *Clin Sci* 1994;86: 731–739.

25. Ballegeer VC, Spitz B, De Baene LA, et al: Platelet activation and vascular damage in gestational hypertension. *Am J Obstet Gynecol* 1992;166:629–633.

26. Burrows RF, Hunter DJS, Andrew M, Kelton JG: A prospective study investigating the mechanism of thrombocytopenia in pre-eclampsia. *Obstet Gynecol* 1987;70:334–338.

27. Samuels P, Main EK, Tomaski A, et al: Abnormalities in platelet antiglobulin tests in preeclamptic mothers and their neonates. *Am J Obstet Gynecol* 1987;157:109–113.

28. Middelkoop CM, Dekker GA, Kraayenbrink AA, Popp-Snijders C: Platelet-poor plasma serotonin in normal and preeclamptic pregnancy. *Clin Chem* 1993;39:1675–1678.

29. Janes SL, Kyle PM, Redman C, Goodall AH: Flow cytometric detection of activated platelets in pregnant women prior to the development of pre-eclampsia. *Thromb Haemost* 1995;74: 1059–1063.

30. Konijnenberg A, Stokkers EW, van der Post JA, et al: Extensive platelet activation in preeclampsia compared with normal pregnancy: Enhanced expression of cell adhesion molecules. *Am J Obstet Gynecol* 1997;176:461–469.

31. Fitzgerald DJ, Mayo G, Catella F, et al: Increased thromboxane biosynthesis in normal pregnancy is mainly derived from platelets. *Am J Obstet Gynecol* 1987;157:325–330.

32. Fitzgerald DJ, Rocki W, Murray R, et al: Thromboxane A2 synthesis in pregnancy induced hypertension. *Lancet* 1990;335i:751–754.

33. Van Geet C, Spitz B, Vermylen J, Van Assche FA: Urinary thromboxane metabolites in pre-eclampsia. *Lancet* 1990;335i:1168–1169.
34. Garzetti GG, Tranquilli AL, Cugini AM, et al: Altered lipid composition, increased lipid peroxidation, and altered fluidity of the membrane as evidence of platelet damage in pre-eclampsia. *Obstet Gynecol* 1993;81:337–340.
35. Baker PN, Broughton Pipkin F, Symonds EM: Comparative study of platelet angiotensin II binding and the angiotensin II sensitivity test as predictors of pregnancy-induced hypertension. *Clin Sci* 1992;83:89–95.
35a. Pouliot L, Forest J-C, Montquin J-M, et al: Platelet angiotensin II binding sites and early detection of preeclampsia. *Obstet Gynecol* 1998;91:591–595.
36. Maki N, Magness RR, Miyaura S, et al: Platelet-activating factor-acetylhydrolase activity in normotensive and hypertensive pregnancies. *Am J Obstet Gynecol* 1993;168:50–54.
37. Roberts JM, Lewis V, Mize N, et al: Human platelet alpha-adrenergic receptors and responses during pregnancy: No change except that with differing hematocrit. *Am J Obstet Gynecol* 1986;154:206–210.
38. Morrison R, Crawford J, Macpherson M, Heptinstall S: Platelet behaviour in normal pregnancy, pregnancy complicated by essential hypertension and pregnancy-induced hypertension. *Thromb Haemostas* 1985;54:607–611.
39. Maki M: Coagulation, fibrinolysis, platelet and kinin-forming systems during toxaemia of pregnancy. *Bio Res Preg* 1983;4:152–154.
40. Whigham KAE, Howie PW, Drummond AH, Prentice CRM: Abnormal platelet function in pre-eclampsia. *Br J Obstet Gynaecol* 1978;85:28–32.
41. Splawinski B, Skret A, Palczak R, et al: Whole blood aggregation in normal pregnancy and pre-eclampsia. *Clin Exper Hyper* 1987;B6:311–319.
42. Leuschen PM, Davis RB, Boyd D, Goodlin RC: Comparative evaluation of antepartum and postpartum platelet function in smokers and nonsmokers. *Am J Obstet Gynecol* 1986;155: 1276–1280.
43. Louden KA, Broughton Pipkin F, et al: Platelet reactivity and serum thromboxane B2 production in whole blood in gestational hypertension and pre-eclampsia. *Br J Obstet Gynaecol* 1991;89:1239–1244.
44. Horn EH, Cooper J, Hardy E, et al: A cross-sectional study of platelet cyclic AMP in healthy and hypertensive pregnancy. *Clin Sci* 1991;80:549–558.
45. Howie PW: The haemostatic mechanisms of pre-eclampsia. *Clin Obstet Gynecol* 1977;4: 595–609.
46. Ahmed Y, Sullivan MHF, Elder MG: Detection of platelet desensitization in pregnancy-induced hypertension is dependent on the agonist used. *Thromb Haemostas* 1991;65:474–477.
47. Tozzi-Ciancarelli MG, Di Massimo C, D'Alfonso A, et al: Pregnancy-induced hypertension: Evidence for altered functional features of platelets. *Hypertens Pregnancy* 1994;13:33–42.
48. Pinto A, Sorrentino R, Sorrentino P: Endothelial-derived relaxing factor released by endothelial cells of human umbilical vessels and its impairment in pregnancy-induced hypertension. *Am J Obstet Gynecol* 1991;164:507–513.
49. Davidge ST, Stranko CP, Roberts JM: Urine but not plasma nitric oxide metabolites are decreased in women with preeclampsia. *Am J Obstet Gynecol* 1996;174:1008–1013.
50. Delacretaz E, de Quay N, Waeber B, et al: Differential nitric oxide synthase activity in human platelets during normal pregnancy and pre-eclampsia. *Clin Sci* 1995;88:607–610.
51. Ylikorkala O, Viinikka L: Thromboxane A2 in pregnancy and puerperium. *Br Med J* 1980;281: 1601–1602.
52. Wallenburg HCS, Rotmans N: Enhanced reactivity of the platelet thromboxane pathway in normotensive and hypertensive pregnancies with insufficient fetal growth. *Am J Obstet Gynecol* 1982;144:523–528.
53. Bussolino F, Benedetto C, Massobrio M, Camussi G: Maternal vascular prostacyclin activity in pre-eclampsia. *Lancet* 1980;ii:702.
54. Briel RC, Kieback DG, Lippert TH: Platelet sensitivity to a prostacyclin analogue in normal and pathological pregnancy. *Prost Leuk Med* 1984;13:335–340.
55. Dadak CH, Kefalides A, Sinzinger H: Prostacyclin-synthesis stimulating plasma factor and platelet sensitivity in pre-eclampsia. *Biol Res Preg Perinatol* 1985;6:65–69.

56. Liel N, Nathan I, Yermiyahu T, et al: Increased platelet thromboxane A2/prostaglandin H2 receptors in patients with pregnancy-induced hypertension. *Thromb Res* 1993;70:205–210.

57. Charo IF, Feinman RO, Detwiler TC: Interrelations of platelet aggregation and secretion. *J Clin Invest* 1977;60:866–873.

58. Moncada S, Vane JR: Pharmacology and endogenous roles of prostaglandin endoperoxides, thromboxane A2 and prostacyclin. *Pharmacol Rev* 1979;30:293–331.

59. Barr SM, Lees KR, Butters L, et al: Platelet intracellular free calcium concentration in normotensive and hypertensive pregnancies in the human. *Clin Sci* 1989;76:67–71.

60. Rao GHR, Peller JD, White JG: Measurements of ionised calcium in blood platelets with a new generation calcium indicator. *Biochem Biophys Res Comm* 1985;132:652–657.

61. Erne P, Mittelholzer E, Burgisser E, et al: Measurement of receptor-induced changes in intracellular free calcium in human platelets. *J Receptor Res* 1984;4:605–629.

62. Kilby MD, Broughton Pipkin F, et al: A cross-sectional study of basal platelet intracellular free calcium concentration in normotensive and hypertensive primigravid pregnancies. *Clin Sci* 1990;78:75–80.

63. Zemel MB, Zemel PC, Berry S, et al: Altered platelet calcium metabolism as an early predictor of increased peripheral vascular resistance and preeclampsia in urban black women. *New Engl J Med* 1990;323:434–439.

64. Kyle PM, Jackson MC, Buckley DC, et al: Platelet intracellular free calcium response to arginine vasopressin is similar in preeclampsia and normal pregnancy. *Am J Obstet Gynecol* 1995;172:654–660.

65. Cho JH, Nash F, Fekete Z, et al: Increased calcium stores in platelets from African Americans. *Hypertension* 1995;25:377–383.

66. Roberts JM, Lewis V, Mize N, et al: Human platelet alpha-adrenergic receptors and responses during pregnancy: No change except that with differing haematocrit. *Am J Obstet Gynecol* 1986;154:206–210.

67. Horn EH, Cooper JA, Hardy E, et al: Longitudinal studies of platelet cyclic AMP during healthy pregnancy and pregnancies at risk of pre-eclampsia. *Clin Sci* 1995;89:91–99.

68. Pritchard JA, Cunningham FG, Pritchard SA: The Parkland Memorial Hospital for treatment of eclampsia: Evaluation of 245 cases. *Am J Obstet Gynecol* 1984;148:951–960.

69. Hardy E, Glenn J, Heptinstall S, et al: Magnesium modifies the responses of platelets to inhibitory agents which act via cAMP. *Thromb Haemostat* 1995;74:1132–1137.

70. Mellion T, Ignarro LJ, Ohlstein EH, et al: Evidence for the inhibitory role of guanosine 3′,5′-monophosphate in ADP-induced human platelet aggregation in the presence of nitric oxide and related vasodilators. *Blood* 1981;57:946–955.

71. Hogan JC, Lewis MJ, Henderson AH: In vivo EDRF activity influences platelet function. *Br J Pharmacol* 1988;94:1020–1022.

72. Hardy E, Rubin PC, Horn EH: Effects of nitric oxide donors in vitro on the arachidonic acid-induced platelet release reaction and platelet cyclic GMP concentration in preeclampsia. *Clin Sci* 1994;85:195–202.

73. Chirkov YY, Tyschuck IA, Severina IS: Guanylate cyclase in human platelets with different aggregability. *Experimentia* 1990;46:697–699.

74. Moore TJ, Williams GH: Angiotensin II receptors on human platelets. *Circ Res* 1981;51:314–320.

75. Ding Y-A, MacIntyre E, Kenyon CJ, Semple PF: Angiotensin II effects on platelet function. *J Hypertens* 1985;3:S251–S253.

76. Poplawski A: The effect of angiotensin II on the platelet aggregation induced by adenosine-diphosphate epinephrine and thrombin. *Experimentia* 1970;26:86–89.

77. Haller H, Oeney T, Hauck U, et al: Increased intracellular free calcium and sensitivity to angiotensin II in platelets of preeclamptic women. *Am J Hypertens* 1989;2:238–243.

78. Cameron HA, Ardlie NG: The facilitating effects of adrenaline in platelet aggregation. *Prost Leuk Med* 1982;9:117–128.

79. Baker PN, Broughton Pipkin F, Symonds EM: Platelet angiotensin II binding and plasma renin substrate and plasma angiotensin II in human pregnancy. *Clin Sci* 1990;79:403–408.

80. Baker PN, Broughton Pipkin F, Symonds EM: Platelet angiotensin II binding in normotensive and hypertensive pregnancy. *Br J Obstet Gynecol* 1991;98:436–440.

81. Gant NF, Daley GL, Chand S, et al: A study of angiotensin II pressor response throughout primigravid pregnancy. *J Clin Invest* 1973;52:2682–2689.
82. Stirling Y, Woolf L, North WR, et al: Haemostasis in normal pregnancy. *Thromb Haemost* 1984;52:176–182.
83. Fletcher AP, Alkjaersig NK, Burstein R: The influence of pregnancy upon blood coagulation and plasma fibrinolytic enzyme function. *Am J Obstet Gynecol* 1979;134:743–745.
84. Davies JA, Prentice CRM: Coagulation changes in pregnancy-induced hypertension and growth retardation. In: Greer IA, Turpie AGG, Forbes CD, eds. *Haemostasis and Thrombosis in Obstetrics and Gynaecology.* London: Chapman and Hall; 1992:143–162.
85. Lox CD, Dorestt MM, Hampton RM: Observations on clotting activity during pre-eclampsia. *Clin Exp Hypertens* 1983;B2:179.
86. Vaziri ND, Toohey J, Powers D, et al: Activation of intrinsic coagulation pathway in pre-eclampsia. *Am J Med* 1986;80:103–107.
87. Brant JT: Current concepts of coagulation. *Clin Obstet Gynecol* 1985;28:3–14.
88. Fournie A, Monrozies M, Pontonnier G, et al: Factor VIII complex in normal pregnancy, pre-eclampsia and fetal growth retardation. *Br J Obstet Gynaecol* 1981;88:250–254.
89. Redman CWG, Denson KWE, Beilin LJ, et al: Factor VIII consumption in pre-eclampsia. *Lancet* 1977;2:1249–1252.
90. Thornton CA, Bonnar J: Factor VIII-related antigen and factor VIII coagulant activity in normal and pre-eclamptic pregnancy. *Br J Obstet Gynaecol* 1977;84:919–923.
91. Scholtes MCW, Gerretsen G, Haak HL: The factor VIII ratio in normal and pathological pregnancies. *Eur J Obstet Gynec Reprod Biol* 1983;16:89–95.
92. Wallenburg HCS: Changes in the coagulation system and platelets in pregnancy-induced hypertension and pre-eclampsia. In: Sharp F, Symonds EM, eds. *Hypertension in Pregnancy.* Proceedings of the 16th Study Group on RCOG. Ithaca, NY: Perinatology Press; 1986:227–248.
93. Wallmo L, Karlsson K, Teger-Nilsson AC: Fibrinopeptide A and intravascular coagulation in normotensive and hypertensive pregnancy and parturition. *Acta Obstet Gynecol Scand* 1984;63:637–640.
94. Borok Z, Wetz J, Owen J, et al: Fibrinogen proteolysis and platelet alpha-granule release in pre-eclampsia/eclampsia. *Blood* 1984;63:525–531.
95. Gibson B, Hunter D, Neame PB, Kelton JG: Thrombocytopenia in pre-eclampsia and eclampsia. *Semin Thromb Haemostas* 1982;8:234–247.
96. Seegers WH: Antithrombin III: Theory and clinical applications. *Am J Clin Pathol* 1978;69:299–359.
97. Weenink GH, Treffers PE, Kahle LH, ten Cate JW: Antithrombin III in normal pregnancy. *Thromb Res* 1982;26:281–287.
98. Weiner CP: Evaluation of clotting disorders during pregnancy. In: Sciarra JJ, Eschenbach DA, Depp R, eds. *Gynecology and Obstetrics.* 1990, Vol 3:1.
99. Weiner CP, Brant J: Plasma antithrombin III activity: An aid in the diagnosis of pre-eclampsia–eclampsia. *Am J Obstet Gynecol* 1982;142:275–281.
100. Weenink GH, Borm JJ, ten Cate JW, Treffers PE: Antithrombin III levels in normotensive and hypertensive pregnancy. *Gynecol Obstet Invest* 1983;16:230–242.
101. Saleh AA, Bottoms SF, Welch RA, et al: Preeclampsia, delivery, and the hemostatic system. *Am J Obstet Gynecol* 1987;157:331–336.
101a. Yin KH, Koh SC, Malcus P, et al: *J Obstet Gynaecol Res* 1998;24:231–238.
102. Schjetlein R, Haugen G, Wisloff F: Markers of intravascular coagulation and fibrinolysis in preeclampsia: Association with intrauterine growth retardation. *Acta Obstet Gynecol Scand* 1997;76:541–546.
103. Weiner CP, Brant J: Plasma antithrombin III activity in normal pregnancy. *Obstet Gynecol* 1982;56:601–603.
104. Paternoster D, Stella A, Simioni P, et al: Clotting inhibitors and fibronectin as potential markers in pre-eclampsia. *Int J Gynaecol Obstet* 1994;47:215–221.
105. Shinyama H, Akira T, Uchida T, et al: Antithrombin III prevents renal dysfunction and hypertension induced by enhanced intravascular coagulation in pregnant rats. *J Cardiovasc Pharmacol* 1996;27:702–711.

106. de Boer K, ten Cate JW, Sturk A, et al: Enhanced thrombin generation in normal and hypertensive pregnancy. *Am J Obstet Gynecol* 1989;160:95–100.

107. Kobayashi T, Terao T: Preeclampsia as chronic disseminated intravascular coagulation. *Gynecol Obstet Invest* 1987;24:170–178.

108. Reinthaller A, Mursch-Edlmayr G, Tatra G: Thrombin-antithrombin III complex levels in normal pregnancy with hypertensive disorders and after delivery. *Br J Obstet Gynaecol* 1990;97:506–510.

109. Koh SC, Anandakumar C, Montan S, Ratnam SS: Plasminogen activators, plasminogen activator inhibitors and markers of intravascular coagulation in pre-eclampsia. *Gynecol Obstet Invest* 1993;35:214–221.

110. Comp PC, Jacocks RM, Ferrell GL, Esmon CT: Activation of protein C in vivo. *J Clin Invest* 1982;70:127–134.

111. Gonzalez R, Alberca I, Vincente V: Protein C levels in late pregnancy, postpartum and in women on oral contraceptives. *Thromb Res* 1985;39:637–641.

112. Anzar J, Gilibert J, Estelles A, Espana F: Fibrinolytic activity and protein C in pre-eclampsia. *Thromb Haemostas* 1986;55:314–317.

113. Fernandez JA, Estelles A, Gilabert J: Functional and immunologic protein S in normal pregnant women and in full term neonates. *Thromb Haemostasis* 1989;61:474–478.

114. Dekker GA, de Vries JI, Doelitzsch PM, et al: Underlying disorders associated with severe early-onset preeclampsia. *Am J Obstet Gynecol* 1995;173:1042–1048.

115. Espana F, Gilabert J, Vicente V, et al: Activated protein C: alpha 1-antitrypsin (APC:alpha 1 AT) complex as a marker for in vitro diagnosis of prethrombotic states. *Thromb Res* 1992;66:499–508.

116. Dahlback B, Carlsson M, Svensson PJ: Familial thrombophilia due to a previously unrecognized mechanism characterized by poor anticoagulant response to activated protein C. *Proc Natl Acad Sci USA* 1993;90:1004–1008.

117. Bertina RM, Koeleman BPC, Koster T, et al: Mutation in blood coagulation factor V associated with resistance to activated protein C. *Nature* 1994;369:64–67.

118. Svensson PJ, Dahlback B: Twenty novel families with thrombophilia and inherited resistance to activated protein C. *Thromb Haemostat* 1993;69:(abstr)1252.

119. Lee DH, Henderson PA, Blajchman MA: Prevalence of factor V Leiden in a Canadian blood donor population. *Can Med Assoc J* 1996;155:285–289.

120. Walker MC, Garner PR, Keely EJ, et al: Changes in activated protein C resistance during normal pregnancy. *Am J Obstet Gynecol* 1997;177:162–169.

121. Lindoff C, Ingemarsson I, Martinsson G, et al: Preeclampsia is associated with a reduced response to activated protein C. *Am J Obstet Gynecol* 1997;176:457–460.

122. Rotmensch S, Liberati M, Mittelman M, Ben-Rafael Z: Activated protein C resistance and adverse pregnancy outcome. *Am J Obstet Gynecol* 1997;177:170–173.

123. McNeil HP, Chesterman CN, Krills SA: Immunology and clinical importance of phospholipid antibodies. *Adv Immunol* 1991;49:193–280.

124. Allen JY, Tapia-Santiago C, Kutteh WH: Antiphospholipid antibodies in patients with preeclampsia. *Am J Reprod Immunol* 1996;36:81–85.

125. Alsulyman OM, Castro MA, Zuckerman E, et al: Preeclampsia and liver infarction in early pregnancy associated with antiphospholipid syndrome. *Obstet Gynecol* 1996;88:644–646.

126. Cowchock FS, Reece EA, Balaban D: Repeated fetal losses associated with antiphospholipid antibodies: A collaborative randomized trial comparing prednisolone with low-dose heparin treatment. *Am J Obstet Gynecol* 1992;166:1318–1323.

127. Bonnar J, Daly L, Sheppard BL: Changes in the fibrinolytic system during pregnancy. *Semin Thromb Hemost* 1990;16:221.

128. Ho CH, Yang ZL: The predictive value of the hemostasis parameters in the development of preeclampsia. *Thromb Haemostas* 1992;67:214–218.

129. Thorburn J, Drummond MM, Whigham KA, et al: Blood viscosity and haemostatic factors in late pregnancy, pre-eclampsia and fetal growth retardation. *Br J Obstet Gynaecol* 1982;89:117–122.

130. Spencer JA, Smith MJ, Cederholm-Williams SA, Wilkinson AR: Influence of pre-eclampsia on concentrations of haemostatic factors in mother and infants. *Arch Dis Child* 1983;58:739–741.

131. Friedman SA, Schiff E, Emeis JJ, et al: Biochemical corroboration of endothelial involvement in severe preeclampsia. *Am J Obstet Gynecol* 1995;172:202–203.

132. Estelles A, Gilabert J, Keeton M, et al: Altered expression of plasminogen activator inhibitor type 1 in placentas from pregnant women with preeclampsia and/or intrauterine fetal growth retardation. *Blood* 1994;84:143–150.

133. Estelles A, Gilabert J, Anzar J, et al: Changes in the plasma levels of type 1 and type 2 plasminogen activator inhibitors in normal pregnancy and in patients with severe preeclampsia. *Blood* 1989;74:1332–1338.

134. Gilabert J, Estelles A, Anzar J, et al: Contribution of platelets to increased plasminogen activator inhibitor type 1 in severe preeclampsia. *Thromb Haemost* 1990;63:361–366.

135. de Boer K, Lecander I ten Cate JW, et al: Placental-type plasminogen activator inhibitor in preeclampsia. *Am J Obstet Gynecol* 1988;158:518–522.

136. Nakashima A, Kobayashi T, Terao T: Fibrinolysis during normal pregnancy and severe preeclampsia: Relationships between plasma levels of plasminogen activators and inhibitors. *Gynecol Obstet Invest* 1996;42:95–101.

137. Estelles A, Gilabert J, Espana F, et al: Fibrinolytic parameters in normotensive pregnancy with intrauterine fetal growth retardation and in severe preeclampsia. *Am J Obstet Gynecol* 1991;165:138–142.

138. Kanfer A, Bruch JF, Nguyen G, et al: Increased placental antifibrinolytic potential and fibrin deposits in pregnancy-induced hypertension and preeclampsia. *Lab Invest* 1996;74:253–258.

139. Gordon YB, Ratky SM, Baker LRI, et al: Circulating levels of fibrin/fibrinogen degradation fragment E measured by radioimmunoassay in preeclampsia. *Br J Obstet Gynaecol* 1976;83:287–291.

140. Naish P, Clark AD, Winston RML, Peters DK: Serum and urine fibrinogen derivatives in normal pregnancy and pre-eclampsia. *Obstet Gynecol* 1973;42:861–867.

141. Gaffney PJ, Creighton LJ, Callus M, Thorpe R: Monoclonal antibodies to crosslinked fibrin degradation products (XL-FDP): II. Evaluation in a series of clinical conditions. *Br J Haematol* 1988;68:91–96.

142. Trofatter KF Jr, Howell ML, Greenberg CS, Hage ML: Use of fibrin D-dimer in screening for coagulation abnormalities in pre-eclampsia. *Obstet Gynecol* 1989;73:435–439.

143. Walker JJ, Cameron AD, Bjornsson S, et al: Can platelet volume predict progressive hypertensive disease in pregnancy? *Am J Obstet Gynecol* 1989;161:676–679.

144. Konijnenberg A, van der Post JA, Mol BW, et al: Can flow cytometric detection of platelet activation early in pregnancy predict the occurrence of preeclampsia? *Am J Obstet Gynecol* 1997;177:434–442.

144a. Massé J, Forest J-C, Montquin J-M, et al: A prospective longitudinal study of platelet angiotensin II-receptors for the prediction of preeclampsia. *Clin Biochem* 1998;31:251–255.

145. Savelieva GM, Efimov VS, Grishin VL, et al: Blood coagulation changes in pregnant women at risk of developing preeclampsia. *Int J Gynaecol Obstet* 1995;48:3–8.

146. Eriksen HO, Hansen PK, Brocks V: Plasma fibronectin concentration in normal pregnancy and in severe preeclampsia. *Am J Obstet Gynecol* 1991;164:1310–1316.

147. Dekker GA, Kraayenbrink AA: Oxygen free radicals in preeclampsia. *Am J Obstet Gynecol* 1991;S164:273.

148. Taylor RN, Crombleholme WR, Friedman SA, Roberts JM: High plasma cellular fibronectin levels correlate with biochemical and clinical features of preeclampsia but cannot be attributed to hypertension alone. *Am J Obstet Gynecol* 1991;165:895–901.

149. Lockwood CJ, Peters JH: Increased plasma levels of ED1+ cellular fibronectin precede the clinical signs of pre-eclampsia. *Am J Obstet Gynecol* 1990;162:358–362.

150. Dunlop W, Hill LM, Landon MJ, et al: Clinical relevance of coagulation and renal changes in pre-eclampsia. *Lancet* 1978;ii:346–349.

151. Thornton JG, Molloy BJ, Vinall PS, et al: A prospective study of haemostatic tests at 28 weeks gestation as predictors of pre-eclampsia and growth retardation. *Thromb Haemost* 1989;61:243–245.

152. Page EW: On the pathogenesis of pre-eclampsia and eclampsia. *J Obstet Gynaecol Br Commonw* 1972;79:883–894.

V

The Etiology
of Preeclampsia

11

Defects in Placentation and Placental Perfusion

Susan J. Fisher and James M. Roberts

The placenta received little attention in the first edition of this book. Buried in a chapter entitled "Structural Lesions" were five-and-a-half pages of discussion of the placenta and no micrographs (in contrast to thirteen-and-a-half pages for the kidney including a table and two micrographs). Still, Leon Chesley had read and noted the publications of Robertson and colleagues[1,2] which implied problems of implantation, and their potential to explain the lesions termed acute atherosis by Zeek and Assali[3] two decades earlier. He further cited the work of MacLennan et al.,[4] who were among the first to suggest that exposing placental explants to hypoxic conditions could produce preeclampsia-like changes.

This chapter focuses on the unique process by which the human placenta normally forms, and how changes in this process can lead to serious pregnancy complications such as preeclampsia. Special emphasis will be placed on the role of oxygen tension in regulating normal and abnormal placental development, and the remarkable finding that invasive cytotrophoblasts acquire an endothelial cell adhesion phenotype as they invade uterine blood vessels. Next, observations that preeclampsia is associated with shallow placentation will be reviewed. The remainder of the chapter will elaborate on how these morphologic observations prompted the principal author's laboratory to use a combination of in vitro modeling and in situ immunolocalization techniques to gain insights into the molecular bases of normal placentation and how these mechanisms go awry in preeclampsia.

NORMAL HUMAN PLACENTATION

The human placenta's unique anatomy (Figs. 11–1 and 11–2) is due in large part to differentiation of its epithelial stem cells, termed cytotrophoblasts.[5] How these cells differentiate determines whether chorionic villi, the placenta's functional units,

A.

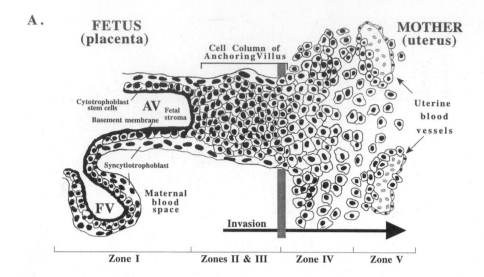

B.

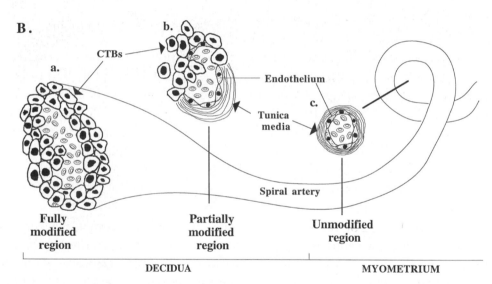

Figure 11–1. A. Diagram of a longitudinal section of an anchoring chorionic villus (AV) at the fetal–maternal interface at about 10 weeks' gestation. The anchoring villus (AV) functions as a bridge between the fetal and maternal compartments, whereas floating villi (FV) are suspended in the intervillous space and are bathed by maternal blood. Cytotrophoblasts (CTB) in AV (Zone I) form cell columns (Zones II and III). The CTB then invade the uterine interstitium (decidua and first third of the myometrium: Zone IV) and maternal vasculature (Zone V), thereby anchoring the fetus to the mother and accessing the maternal circulation. Zone designations mark areas in which CTB have distinct patterns of stage-specific antigen expression. **B.** Diagram of a uterine (spiral) artery in which endovascular invasion is in progress (10–18 weeks' gestation). Endometrial and then myometrial segments of spiral arteries are modified progressively. a. In fully modified regions, the vessel diameter is large. CTB are present in the lumen and occupy the entire surface of the vessel wall. A discrete muscular layer (tunica media) is not evident. b. Partially modified vessel segments. CTB and maternal endothelium occupy discrete regions of the vessel wall. In areas of intersection, CTB appear to lie deep to the endothelium and in contact with the vessel wall. c. Unmodified vessel segments in the myometrium. Vessel segments in the superficial third of the myometrium will become modified when endovascular invasion reaches its fullest extent (by 22 weeks), while deeper segments of the same artery will retain their normal structure.

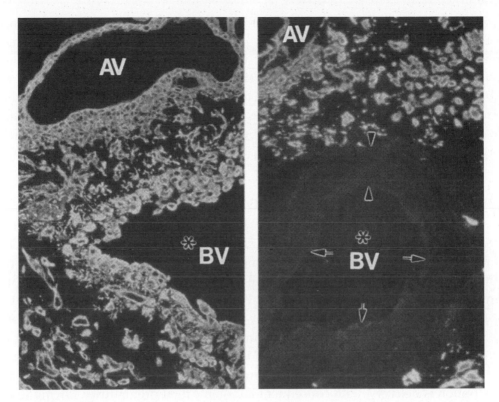

Figure 11–2. In normal pregnancy (left) fetal cytotrophoblasts (stained with anticytokeratin) from the anchoring villi (AV) of the placenta invade the maternal uterine blood vessels (BV). In preeclampsia (right) fetal cells fail to penetrate the uterine vasculature (arrows and arrowheads).

float in maternal blood or anchor the conceptus to the uterine wall. In floating villi, cytotrophoblasts differentiate by fusing to form multinucleate syncytiotrophoblasts whose primary function—transport—is ideally suited to their location at the villus surface. In anchoring villi, cytotrophoblasts also fuse, but many remain as single cells that detach from their basement membrane and aggregate to form cell columns. Cytotrophoblasts at the distal ends of these columns attach to, then deeply invade, the uterus (interstitial invasion) and its arterioles (endovascular invasion). As a result of endovascular invasion, the cells replace the endothelial and muscular linings of uterine arterioles, a process that initiates maternal blood flow to the placenta and greatly enlarges the vessel diameter. Paradoxically, the cells invade only the superficial portions of uterine venules. How this unusual behavior is regulated is unknown.

Cells that participate in endovascular invasion have two types of interactions with maternal arterioles. In the first, large aggregates of these fetal cells are found primarily inside the vessel lumen. These aggregates can either lie adjacent to the apical surface of the resident endothelium or replace it such that they appear directly attached to the vessel wall. In the second type of interaction, cytotrophoblasts are found within the vessel wall rather than in the lumen. In this position, they colonize the smooth muscle layer of the vessel and lie subjacent to the endothelium. These different types of interactions may be progressive stages in a single process, or indicative of different strategies by which cytotrophoblasts accomplish endovascular invasion. In either case, the stage in which fetal cytotrophoblasts cohabitate with maternal endothelium in the spiral arterioles is transient. By late second trimester these vessels are lined exclusively by cytotrophoblasts, and endothelial cells are no longer visible in either the endometrial or the superficial portions of their myometrial segments.

ABNORMAL HUMAN PLACENTATION IN PREECLAMPSIA

Preeclampsia is a disease that adversely affects 7 to 10% of first pregnancies in the United States,[6] with the mother-to-be demonstrating signs and symptoms that suggest widespread alterations in endothelial function (e.g., high blood pressure, proteinuria, and edema).[7] In some cases fetal growth slows, which leads to intrauterine growth retardation. The severity of the disease varies greatly. In its mildest form the signs/symptoms appear near term and resolve after birth, with no lasting effects on either the mother or the child. In its severest form the signs/symptoms often occur in the second or early third trimesters. If they cannot be controlled, the only option is delivery, with consequent iatrogenic fetal prematurity. Owing to the latter form of the disease, preeclampsia and hypertensive diseases of pregnancy are leading causes of maternal death and contribute significantly to premature deliveries in the United States.[7]

Although the cause of preeclampsia is unknown, the accumulated evidence strongly implicates the placenta.[8] Anatomic examination shows that the area of the placenta most affected by this syndrome is the fetal–maternal interface (see Fig. 11–2). Cytotrophoblast invasion of the uterus is shallow, and endovascular invasion does not proceed beyond the terminal portions of the spiral arterioles.[1] The effect of preeclampsia on endovascular invasion is particularly evident when interactions between fetal cytotrophoblasts and maternal endothelial cells are studied in detail.[9,10] Serial sections through placental bed biopsies of all the patients we have studied show that few of the spiral arterioles contain cytotrophoblasts. Instead, most cytotrophoblasts remain at some distance from these vessels. Where endovascular cytotrophoblasts are detected, their invasion is limited to the portion of the vessel that spans the superficial decidua. Thus, there is little difference between cytotrophoblast interactions with veins and arterioles in the uterus. Even if the cytotrophoblasts gain access to the lumen, they usually fail to form tight aggregates among themselves, or to spread out on the vessel wall, as is observed for cytotrophoblasts in control samples matched for gestational age. Instead they tend to remain as individual rounded cells, suggesting that they are poorly anchored to the vessel wall. Thus, cytotrophoblasts in preeclampsia not only have a limited capacity for endovascular invasion but also display an altered morphology in their interactions with maternal arterioles.

Because of these alterations in endovascular invasion, the maternal vessels of preeclamptic patients do not undergo the complete spectrum of physiologic changes that normally occur (e.g., loss of endothelial lining and muskuloelastic tissue); the mean external diameter of the myometrial vessels is less than half that of similar vessels from uncomplicated pregnancies.[2,11,12] In addition, not as many vessels show evidence of cytotrophoblast invasion.[2,11,13] Thus, the architecture of these vessels precludes an adequate response to gestation-related fetal demands for increased blood flow.

Human Cytotrophoblast Proliferation and Differentiation In Vitro

Information about the morphologic aspects of cytotrophoblast invasion in normal pregnancy and in preeclampsia has been used to formulate hypotheses about the regulatory factors involved. Specifically, in normal pregnancy cytotrophoblasts invade large-bore arterioles, where they are in contact with well-oxygenated maternal blood. But in preeclampsia, invasive cytotrophoblasts are relatively hypoxic. Another important consideration is that placental blood flow changes dramatically during early pregnancy. During much of the first trimester there is little endovascular invasion, so maternal blood flow to the placenta is at a minimum. The oxygen pressures of the intervillous space (that is, at the uterine surface) and within the endometrium are estimated to be approximately 18 mm Hg and 40 mm Hg, respectively, at 8 to 10 weeks' gestation.[14] Afterward, endovascular invasion proceeds rapidly; cytotrophoblasts are in direct contact with blood from maternal spiral arterioles, which could have a mean oxygen pressure as high as 90 to 100 mm Hg. Thus, as cytotrophoblasts invade the uterus during the first half of pregnancy, they encounter a steep, positive oxygen tension gradient. These observations, together with the results of our own experiments conducted on isolated cytotrophoblasts,[15] suggested that oxygen tension might regulate cytotrophoblast proliferation and differentiation along the invasive pathway.[16]

We used immunolocalization techniques to study the relationship between cytotrophoblast proliferation and differentiation in situ. Cytotrophoblasts in columns (i.e., cells in the initial stages of differentiation) reacted with an antibody against the Ki67 antigen,[16] which is indicative of DNA synthesis.[17] Distal to this region, anti-Ki67 staining abruptly stopped, and the cytotrophoblasts intricately modulated their expression of stage-specific antigens, including integrin cell-adhesion molecules,[18] matrix metalloproteinase-9,[19] HLA-G (a cytotrophoblast class Ib major histocompatibility complex molecule),[20,21] and human placental lactogen.[22] These results suggested that during differentiation along the invasive pathway, cytotrophoblasts first undergo mitosis, then exit the cell cycle and modulate their expression of stage-specific antigens.

As an in vitro model system for testing this hypothesis, we used organ cultures of anchoring villi explanted from early gestation (6–8 weeks) placentas onto an extracellular matrix substrate. Some of the anchoring villi were cultured for 72 hours in a standard tissue culture incubator (20% O_2 or 98 mm Hg). Figure 11–3A shows

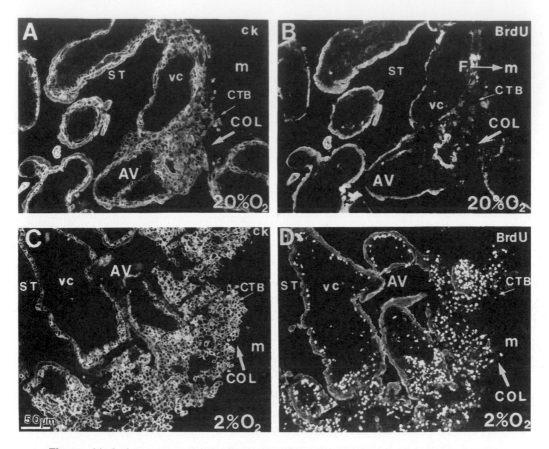

Figure 11–3. Low oxygen (2% O$_2$) stimulates cytotrophoblast bromodeoxyuridine (BrdU) incorporation in vitro. Anchoring villi (AV) from 6- to 8-week placentas were cultured on Matrigel (m) for 72 hours in either 20% O$_2$ (A, B) or 2% O$_2$ (C, D). By the end of the culture period, fetal cytotrophoblasts migrated into the Matrigel (F → m). To assess cell proliferation, BrdU was added to the medium. Tissue sections of the villi were stained with anticytokeratin (ck; A, C), which recognizes syncytiotropho-blasts (ST) and cytotrophoblasts (CTB) but not cells in the villus core (vc); and with anti-BrdU (B, D), which detects cells in S phase. Villus explants maintained in 2% O$_2$ (C) formed much more prominent columns (COL) with a larger proportion of CTB nuclei that incorporated BrdU (D) than explants cultured in 20% O$_2$ (A, B). (*Reprinted, with permission, from Genbacev O, Zhou Y, Ludlow JW, Fisher SJ: Regulation of human placental development by oxygen tension.* Science *1997;277:1669–1672. Copyright 1977 American Association for the Advancement of Science.*)

a section of one such control villus that was stained with an antibody that recognizes cytokeratin to demonstrate syncytiotrophoblasts and cytotrophoblasts. The attached cell columns were clearly visible. To assess the cells' ability to synthesize DNA, the villi were incubated with bromodeoxyuridine (BrdU). Incorporation was detected in the cytoplasm but not the nuclei of syncytiotrophoblasts. Few or none of the cells in columns incorporated BrdU (Fig. 11–3B). Other anchoring villi were maintained in an hypoxic atmosphere (2% O$_2$ or 14 mm Hg). After 72 hours, cytokeratin staining showed prominent cell columns (Fig. 11–3C), and the nuclei of many of the cytotrophoblasts in these columns incorporated BrdU (Fig. 11–3D).

Because cytotrophoblasts were the only cells that entered S phase, we also compared the ability of anchoring villus explants cultured under standard and hypoxic conditions to incorporate [^{3}H] thymidine. Villus explants cultured under hypoxic conditions (2% O_2) incorporated 3.3 ± 1.2 times more [^{3}H] thymidine than villi cultured under standard conditions (20% O_2). In contrast, [^{3}H] thymidine incorporation by explants cultured in a 6% O_2 atmosphere (40 mm Hg) was no different than in control villi. Taken together, these results suggest that a hypoxic environment, comparable to that encountered by early gestation cytotrophoblasts in the intervillous space, stimulates the cells to enter S phase.

Cytokeratin staining also showed that the cell columns associated with anchoring villi cultured under hypoxic conditions were larger than cell columns of control villi cultured under standard conditions (compare Figs. 11–3A and 11–3C). To quantify this, we made serial sections of villus explants maintained in either 20% or 2% O_2, and then counted the number of cells in columns. Under hypoxic culture conditions, the columns contained triple the number of cells present in columns maintained in 20% oxygen. These results indicate that hypoxia stimulates cytotrophoblasts in cell columns to proliferate.[15,16]

The next series of studies we conducted were based on the hypothesis that the hypoxia-induced changes in the cells' proliferative capacity would be reflected by changes in their expression of proteins that regulate passage through the cell cycle (Fig. 11–4). With regard to the G2 to M transition, we were particularly interested in their cyclin B expression, since threshold levels of this protein are required for cells to enter mitosis.[23] Immunoblotting of cell extracts showed that after 3 days in culture, anchoring villi maintained in 2% O_2 contained 3.1 times more cyclin B than did villi maintained in 20% O_2 (Fig. 11–4A). Immunolocalization experiments confirmed that cyclin B was primarily expressed by cytotrophoblasts (not shown). Since p21$^{\text{WF1/CIP1}}$ abundance has been correlated with cell-cycle arrest,[24] we also examined the effects of oxygen tension on cytotrophoblast expression of this protein. Very little p21$^{\text{WF1/CIP1}}$ expression was detected in cell extracts of anchoring villi maintained for 72 hours in 2% O_2, but expression increased 3.8-fold in anchor-

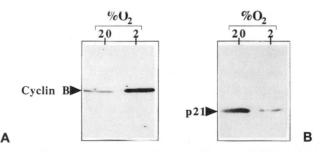

Figure 11–4. Hypoxia induces changes in cytotrophoblast expression of proteins that regulate progression through the cell cycle. **A.** Villus explants cultured for 72 hours in 2% O_2 contained 3.1 times more cyclin B than did villi maintained under standard culture conditions (20% O_2) for the same length of time. **B.** Expression of p21 increased 3.8-fold in anchoring villi cultured for 72 hours in 20% O_2 as compared to 2% O_2. (*Reprinted, with permission, from Genbacev O, Zhou Y, Ludlow JW, Fisher SJ: Regulation of human placental development by oxygen tension. Science 1997;277:1669–1672. Copyright 1997 American Association for the Advancement of Science*)

ing villi maintained for the same time period in 20% O_2 (Fig. 11–4B). Immunolocalization experiments confirmed that p21$^{WF1/CIP1}$ was primarily expressed by cytotrophoblasts. These results, replicated in five separate experiments, confirm that culturing anchoring villi in 20% O_2 induces cytotrophoblasts in the attached cell columns to undergo cell-cycle arrest, whereas culturing them in 2% O_2 induces them to enter mitosis.[15,16]

Changes in proliferative capacity are often accompanied by concomitant changes in differentiation. Accordingly, we investigated the effects of hypoxia on the ability of cytotrophoblasts to differentiate along the invasive pathway (Fig. 11–5). Under standard tissue culture conditions, cytotrophoblasts migrated from the cell columns and modulated their expression of stage-specific antigens, as they do during uterine invasion in vivo.[18] For example, they began to express integrin α1, a laminin-collagen receptor that is required for invasiveness in vitro.[25] Both differentiated cytotrophoblasts and villus stromal cells expressed this antigen (Fig. 11–5B). When cultured under hypoxic conditions, cytotrophoblasts failed to stain for integrin α1, but stromal cells continued to express this molecule, suggesting the observed effects were cell-type specific (Fig. 11–5E). Hypoxia also reduced cytotrophoblast staining for human placental lactogen, another antigen that is expressed once the cells differentiate. However, lowering the O_2 tension did not change cytotrophoblast expression of other stage-specific antigens, such as HLA-G (Figs. 11–5C and 11–5F) and integrins α5β1 and αVβ3 (not shown). These results suggest that hypoxia produces selective deficits in the ability of cytotrophoblasts to differentiate along the invasive pathway.

The effects of oxygen tension on the proliferative capacity of cytotrophoblasts could help explain some of the interesting features of normal placental development. Before cytotrophoblast invasion of maternal vessels establishes the uteroplacental circulation ($\leq$ 10 weeks), the conceptus is in a relatively hypoxic environment. During this period, placental mass increases much more rapidly than that of the embryo proper. Histologic sections of early-stage pregnant human uteri show bilaminar embryos surrounded by thousands of trophoblast cells.[26] The fact that hypoxia stimulates cytotrophoblasts, but not most other cells,[27] to undergo mitosis could help account for the discrepancy in size between the embryo and the placenta which continues well into the second trimester of pregnancy.[28] Although this phenomenon is poorly understood at a mechanistic level, we have recently shown (as will be discussed below) that cytotrophoblasts within the uterine wall mimic a vascular adhesion molecule phenotype.[29] In other tissues hypoxia induces vascular endothelial growth factor production, which stimulates endothelial cell proliferation.[30] This raises the possibility that similar regulatory pathways operate during placental development.

The effects of oxygen tension on cytotrophoblast differentiation/invasion could also have important implications. Relatively high oxygen tension promotes cytotrophoblast differentiation and could help explain why these cells extensively invade the arterial rather than the venous side of the uterine circulation. Conversely, if cytotrophoblasts do not gain access to an adequate supply of maternal ar-

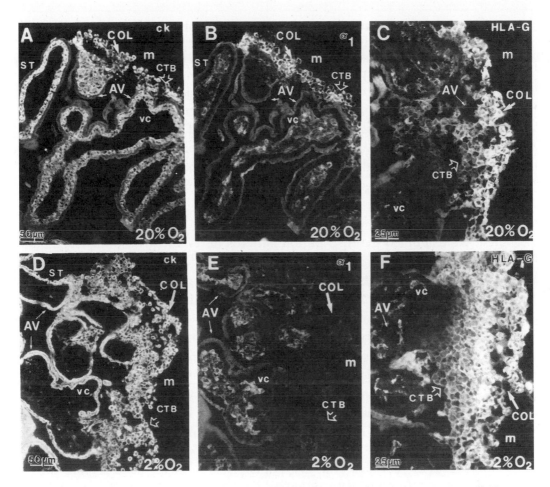

Figure 11–5. Some aspects of cytotrophoblast differentiation/invasion are arrested in hypoxia. Anchoring villi (AV) from 6- to 8-week placentas were cultured on Matrigel (m) for 72 hours in either 20% O_2 (A–C) or 2% O_2 (D–F). Tissue sections of the villi were stained with anticytokeratin (ck; A, D), anti-integrin $\alpha 1$ (B, E), or anti-HLA-G (C, F). Cytotrophoblasts (CTB) that composed the cell columns (COL) of villus explants cultured in 20% O_2 up-regulated both integrin $\alpha 1$ (B) and HLA-G expression (C). In contrast, cytotrophoblasts in anchoring villus columns maintained in 2% O_2 failed to express integrin $\alpha 1$, although constituents of the villus core continued to express this adhesion molecule (E). Not all aspects of differentiation were impaired; the cells up-regulated HLA-G expression normally (F). ST = syncytiotrophoblast; vc = villus core. (*Reprinted, with permission, from Genbacev O, Zhou Y, Ludlow JW, Fisher SJ: Regulation of human placental development by oxygen tension. Science 1997;277: 1669–1672. Copyright 1997 American Accociation for the Advancement of Science.*)

terial blood, their ability to differentiate into fully invasive cells may be impaired. We suggest that the latter scenario could be a contributing factor to pregnancy-associated diseases, such as preeclampsia, which are linked to abnormally shallow cytotrophoblast invasion and faulty differentiation, as evidenced by their inability to upregulate integrin $\alpha 1$ expression.[9] These results also prompted us to consider the possibility that the profound effects of oxygen on invasive cytotrophoblasts might be indicative of their ability to assume a vascular-like phenotype.

During Normal Pregnancy, Invasive Cytotrophoblasts Modulate Their Adhesion Molecule Repertoire to Mimic That of Vascular Cells

Recently, we tested the hypotheses that invasive cytotrophoblasts mimic broadly the adhesion phenotype of the endothelial cells they replace, and that these changes in adhesion phenotype have the net effect of enhancing cytotrophoblast motility and invasiveness.[29] To test these hypotheses, we first stained tissue sections of the fetal–maternal interface for specific integrins, cadherins, and immunoglobulin-family adhesion receptors that are characteristic of endothelial cells and leukocytes. Subsequent experiments tested the functional consequences for cytotrophoblast adhesion and invasion of expressing the particular adhesion receptors that were upregulated during cytotrophoblast differentiation.

First, we examined the distribution patterns of αV integrin family members. These molecules are of particular interest because of their regulated expression on endothelial cells during angiogenesis and their upregulation on some types of metastatic tumor cells.[31,32] Alpha-V family members displayed unique and highly specific spatial staining patterns on cytotrophoblasts in anchoring villi and the placental bed. An antibody specific for the $\alpha V \beta 5$ complex stained the cytotrophoblast monolayer in chorionic villi. Staining was uniform over the entire cell surface. The syncytiotrophoblast layer and cytotrophoblasts in cell columns and the placental bed did not stain for $\alpha V \beta 5$. In contrast, anti-$\alpha V \beta 6$ stained only those chorionic villus cytotrophoblasts that were at sites of column formation. The cytotrophoblast layer still in contact with basement membrane stained brightly, while the first layer of the cell column showed reduced staining. The rest of the cytotrophoblasts in chorionic villi, cytotrophoblasts in more distal regions of cell columns, and cytotrophoblasts within placental bed and vasculature did not stain for $\alpha V \beta 6$, documenting a specific association of this integrin with initiation of column formation. In yet a different pattern, staining for $\alpha V \beta 3$ was weak or not detected on villus cytotrophoblasts or on cytotrophoblasts in the initial layers of cell columns. However, strong staining was detected on cytotrophoblasts within the uterine wall and vasculature. Thus, individual members of the αV family, like those of the $\beta 1$ family,[18] are spatially regulated during cytotrophoblast differentiation. Of particular relevance is the observation that $\alpha V \beta 3$ integrin, whose expression on endothelial cells is stimulated by angiogenic factors, is prominent on cytotrophoblasts that have invaded the uterine wall and maternal vasculature.

Since blocking $\alpha V \beta 3$ function suppresses endothelial migration during angiogenesis, we determined whether perturbing its interactions also affects cytotrophoblast invasion in vitro. Freshly isolated first trimester cytotrophoblasts were plated for 48 hours on Matrigel-coated Transwell filters in the presence of control mouse IgG or the complex-specific anti-$\alpha V \beta 3$ IgG, LM609. Cytotrophoblast invasion was evaluated by counting cells and cellular processes that had invaded the Matrigel barrier and extended through the holes in the Transwell filters. LM609 reduced cytotrophoblast invasion by more than 75% in this assay, indicating that this receptor, like the α1β1 integrin,[25] contributes significantly to the invasive phenotype of cytotrophoblasts.

Next, we examined cadherin switching during cytotrophoblast differentiation in vivo (Fig. 11–6). The cytotrophoblast epithelial monolayer stained strongly for the ubiquitous epithelial cadherin, E-cadherin, in a polarized pattern (Fig. 11–6A). Staining was strong on the surfaces of cytotrophoblasts in contact with one another and with the overlying syncytiotrophoblast layer, and was absent at the basal surface of cytotrophoblasts in contact with basement membrane. In cell columns, E-cadherin-staining intensity was reduced on cytotrophoblasts near the uterine wall and on cytotrophoblasts within the decidua. This reduction in staining was particularly pronounced in second trimester tissue. At this stage, E-cadherin staining was also very weak or undetectable on cytotrophoblasts that had colonized maternal blood vessels and on cytotrophoblasts in the surrounding myometrium. All locations of reduced E-cadherin staining were areas in which invasion is active during the first half of gestation. Interestingly, the staining intensity of E-cadherin was

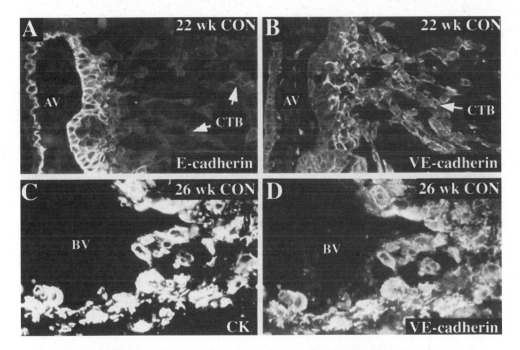

Figure 11–6. E-cadherin staining is reduced and VE-cadherin staining is upregulated in normal, differentiating second trimester cytotrophoblasts (CTB). Sections of second trimester placental bed tissue were stained with antibody against E-cadherin (A), VE-cadherin (B and D), or cytokeratin (CK, 7D3; C). **A.** E-cadherin staining was strong on anchoring villus (AV) CTB and on CTB in the proximal portion of cell columns (Zone II). Staining was sharply reduced on CTB in the distal column (Zone III) and in the uterine interstitium (Zone IV). Staining was not detected on CTB within maternal vessels (Zone V). **B.** VE-cadherin was not detected on CTB in AV (although fetal blood vessels in villus stromal core are stained). VE-cadherin was detected on column CTB (B) and on interstitial and endovascular CTB (D). VE-cadherin is also detected on maternal endothelium in vessels that have not been modified by CTB.

strong on cytotrophoblasts in all locations in term placentas, at which time cytotro-phoblast invasive activity is poor. Taken together, these data are consistent with the idea that cytotrophoblasts transiently reduce E-cadherin function at times and places of their greatest invasive activity.

Cadherin switching occurs frequently during embryonic development when significant morphogenetic events take place. Therefore, we stained sections of first and second trimester placental tissue with antibodies to other classic cadherins. These tissues did not react with antibodies against P-cadherin, but did stain with three different monoclonal antibodies that recognize the endothelial cadherin, VE-cadherin (Fig.11–6B). In chorionic villi, antibody to VE-cadherin did not stain villus cytotrophoblasts, although it stained the endothelium of fetal blood vessels within the villus stroma. In contrast, anti-VE-cadherin stained cytotrophoblasts in cell columns and in the decidua, the very areas in which E-cadherin staining was reduced. VE-cadherin staining was stronger in these areas in second trimester tissues. In maternal vessels that had not yet been modified by cytotrophoblasts, anti-VE-cadherin stained the endothelial layer strongly. Following endovascular invasion, cytotrophoblasts lining maternal blood vessels also stained strongly for VE-cadherin (Fig. 11–6D). Thus, cytotrophoblasts that invade the uterine wall and vasculature express a cadherin characteristic of endothelial cells.[29]

Next, we used function-perturbing anticadherin antibodies, in conjunction with the Matrigel invasion assay, to assess the functional consequences of cadherin modulation for cytotrophoblast invasiveness. We plated isolated second trimester cytotrophoblasts for 48 hours on Matrigel-coated filters in the presence of control IgG or function-perturbing antibodies against VE-cadherin or E-cadherin. By 48 hours, significant invasion was evident in control cytotrophoblasts. In cultures treated with anti-E-cadherin, cytotrophoblast invasiveness increased more than threefold, suggesting that E-cadherin normally has a restraining effect on invasiveness. In contrast, antibody against VE-cadherin reduced the invasion of cytotro-phoblasts to about 60% of control. This suggests that the presence of VE-cadherin normally facilitates cytotrophoblast invasion. Taken together, these functional data suggest that as they differentiate, the cells modulate their cadherin repertoire to one that contributes to their increased invasiveness.

Our data presented thus far indicate that, as they differentiate, cytotro-phoblasts down-regulate adhesion receptors highly characteristic of epithelial cells (integrin $\alpha6\beta4$[18] and E-cadherin) and up-regulate analogous receptors that are ex-pressed on endothelial cells (integrins $\alpha1\beta1$[18] and $\alpha V\beta3$, and VE-cadherin). These observations support our hypothesis that normal cytotrophoblasts undergo a com-prehensive switch in phenotype so as to resemble the endothelial cells they replace during endovascular invasion.

We hypothesize that this unusual phenomenon plays an important role in the process whereby these cells form vascular connections with the uterine vessels. Ul-timately, these connections are so extensive that the spiral arterioles become hybrid structures in which fetal cytotrophoblasts replace the maternal endothelium and much of the highly muscular tunica media. As a result, the diameter of the spiral arterioles increases dramatically, allowing blood flow to the placenta to keep pace with fetal growth. Circumstantial evidence suggests that several of the adhesion molecules whose expression we studied could play an important role in forming these novel vascular connections. In the mouse, for example, targeted disruption of either vascular cell adhesion molecule (VCAM)-1 or α4 expression results in failure of chorioallantoic fusion. It is very interesting to find that cytotrophoblasts are the only cells, other than the endothelium, that express VE-cadherin. In addition, VE-cadherin and platelet–endothelial cell adhesion molecule (PECAM)-1 are the first adhesion receptors expressed by differentiating endothelial cells during early development. The expression of αVβ3 is up-regulated on endothelial cells during angiogenesis by soluble factors that regulate this process. Thus, adhesion receptors that play vital roles in differentiation and expansion of the vasculature are up-regulated as normal cytotrophoblasts differentiate/invade.

In Preeclampsia, Invasive Cytotrophoblasts Fail to Switch Their Adhesion Molecule Repertoire to Mimic That of Vascular Cells

The next hypothesis tested was that preeclampsia impairs the ability of cytotrophoblasts to express the adhesion molecules that are normally modulated during the unique epithelial-to-vascular transformation that occurs in normal pregnancy.[10] First, we compared cytotrophoblast expression of three members of the αV family (αVβ5, αVβ6, and αVβ3) in placental bed biopsies obtained from control and preeclamptic patients that were matched for gestational age. Preeclampsia changed cytotrophoblast expression of all three αV-family members. When samples were matched for gestational age, fewer preeclamptic cytotrophoblast stem cells were stained with an antibody that recognized integrin β5. In contrast, staining for β6 was much brighter in preeclamptic tissue and extended beyond the column to include cytotrophoblasts within the superficial decidua. Of greatest interest, staining for β3 was weak on cytotrophoblasts in all locations; cytotrophoblasts in the uterine wall of preeclamptic patients failed to show strong staining for β3, as did cytotrophoblasts that penetrated the spiral arterioles. Thus, in preeclampsia, differentiating/invading cytotrophoblasts retain expression of αVβ6, which is transiently expressed in remodeling epithelium, and fail to up-regulate αVβ3, which is characteristic of angiogenic endothelium. Therefore, as was the case for integrin α1,[9] our analyses of the expression of αV-family members suggest that in preeclampsia, cytotrophoblasts start to differentiate along the invasive pathway but cannot complete this process.[10]

Preeclampsia also had a striking effect on cytotrophoblast cadherin expression (Fig. 11–7). In contrast to control samples, cytotrophoblasts in both the villi and decidua showed strong reactivity with anti-E-cadherin (Fig. 11–7A), and staining remained strong even on cytotrophoblasts that had penetrated the superficial portions of uterine arterioles (data not shown). Interestingly, in preeclampsia cytotrophoblasts within the uterine wall tended to exist as large aggregates, rather

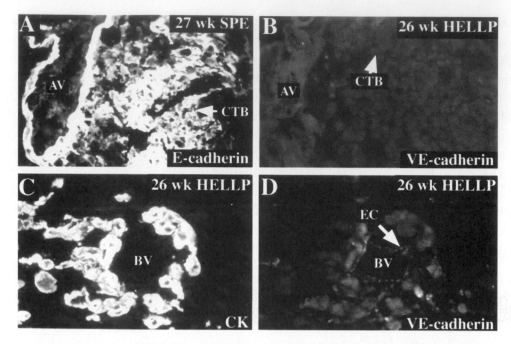

Figure 11–7. In preeclampsia, E-cadherin staining is retained on the placental bed CTB and VE-cadherin staining is not detected. Sections of 27-week severe preeclamptic (SPE: A) and 26-week HELLP tissue (B, C, D) were stained with antibody against E-cadherin (A), VE-cadherin (B and D), or cytokeratin (CK, 7D3; C). **A.** E-cadherin staining was strong on CTB in almost all locations. CTB also appeared to be in large aggregates. VE-cadherin was not detected on CTB in cell columns (B) or near blood vessels (D). But the EC that line the vessel did stain (arrows).

than as smaller clusters and single cells, as is the case in normal pregnancy. This observation is in accord with the likelihood that E-cadherin mediates strong intercellular adhesion between cytotrophoblasts, as it does in all other normal epithelia examined.

Strikingly, no VE-cadherin staining was detected on cytotrophoblasts in any location in placental bed specimens obtained from preeclamptic patients; neither cytotrophoblasts in the cell columns (Fig. 11–7B) nor the few cells that were found in association with vessels in the superficial decidua expressed VE-cadherin (Fig. 11–7D). However, staining for this adhesion molecule was detected on maternal endothelium in the unmodified uterine vessels in preeclamptic placental bed biopsy specimens. Thus, cadherin modulation by cytotrophoblasts in preeclampsia was defective, as shown by the persistence of strong E-cadherin staining and the absence of VE-cadherin staining on cytotrophoblasts in columns and in the superficial decidua.

The results summarized above raise the interesting possibility that the failure of preeclamptic cytotrophoblasts to express vascular-type adhesion molecules, as normal cytotrophoblasts do, impairs their ability to form connections with the uterine vessels. This failure ultimately limits the supply of maternal blood to the placenta and fetus, an effect thought to be closely linked to the pathophysiology of the disease. We also hypothesize that the failure of preeclamptic cytotrophoblasts to make a transition to a vascular cell adhesion phenotype might be part of a broader-spectrum defect in which the cells fail to function properly as endothelium. Such a failure would no doubt have important effects on the maintenance of vascular integrity at the maternal–fetal interface. Clearly, in preeclampsia, undifferentiated cytotrophoblasts that fail to mimic the adhesion phenotype of endothelial cells are present in the termini of maternal spiral arterioles. Whether their presence affects the phenotype of maternal endothelium in deeper segments of the same vessels and/or is linked to the maternal endothelial pathology that is a hallmark of this disease remains to be investigated.

CONCLUSION

We now understand a great deal about cytotrophoblast defects in the placentas of patients whose pregnancies are complicated by preeclampsia. In a landmark study published nearly 30 years ago,[2] Brosens and Robertson first described the abnormally shallow cytotrophoblast invasion that is observed in preeclampsia and a substantial proportion of pregnancies complicated by intrauterine growth retardation. These investigators considered the lack of invasion of the spiral arterioles to be particularly significant. Building on this foundation, our recent studies have shown that cytotrophoblast invasion of the uterus is actually a unique differentiation pathway in which the fetal cells adopt certain attributes of the maternal endothelium they normally replace. In preeclampsia, this differentiation process goes awry.

Currently, we are very interested in using these findings as a point of departure for studies of the disease process from its inception to the appearance of the maternal signs. With regard to its inception, understanding the nature of the phenotypic alterations that are characteristic of cytotrophoblasts in preeclampsia offers us the exciting opportunity to test hypotheses about the causes. From a reductionist viewpoint, preeclampsia can be considered as a two-component system in which the two parts—the placenta and the mother—fail to connect properly. In theory, this failure could be due to either component. For example, it is inevitable that cytotrophoblast differentiation must sometimes go awry. The high frequency of spontaneous abortions that are the results of chromosomal abnormalities is a graphic illustration of the consequences of catastrophic failure of cytotrophoblast differentiation. But the observation that confined placental mosaicism can be associated with intrauterine growth restriction (IUGR)[33] is especially relevant to the studies described in this chapter. Conversely, there is interesting evidence that in certain cases the maternal environment may not permit normal trophoblast invasion. For example, patients with preexisting medical conditions, such as lupus erythematosus and diabetes mellitus, or with increased maternal weight,[34] are prone to developing pregnancy complications, including preeclampsia.[35] Finally, the mother's genotype may also play a role; expression of an angiotensinogen genetic variant has been associated with the predisposition to develop preeclampsia.[36]

An equally interesting area of study is how the faulty link between the placentaand the uterus leads to the fetal and maternal signs of the disease. It is logical that a reduction in maternal blood flow to the placenta could result in fetal IUGR, a fact that has been confirmed in several animal models.[37] But how this scenario also leads to the maternal signs is much less clear. Since the latter signs rapidly resolve once the placenta is removed, most investigators believe that this organ is the source of factors that drive the maternal disease process. Another important consideration is that the local placental abnormalities eventually translate into maternal systemic defects. Thus, it is likely that the causative agents are probably widely distributed in the maternal circulation. But their identities are not yet known. Candidates include macromolecular entities such as fragments of the syncytiotrophoblast microvillous membrane that are shed from the surface of floating villi and can damage endothelial cells.[38] Molecular candidates include the products of hypoxic trophoblasts, whose in vitro vascular effects mimic in vivo blood vessel alteration in patients with preeclampsia.[39]

In summary, studies of the placenta's role in preeclampsia have reached a very exciting point. We are on the verge of unraveling the series of events that leads from abnormally shallow placentation to this intriguing and potentially catastrophic pregnancy syndrome. Once the connections are clarified, we will be in an excellent position to devise strategies for early diagnosis, and perhaps even treatment, of this condition. In doing so we will also gain vital information about how the normal placenta functions, and about the critical checkpoints in placental development that govern pregnancy outcome.

REFERENCES

1. Robertson WB, Brosens I, Dixon HG: The pathological response of the vessels of the placental bed to hypertensive pregnancy. *J Pathol Bacteriol* 1967;93:581–592.
2. Brosens IA, Robertson WB, Dixon HG: The role of the spiral arteries in the pathogenesis of preeclampsia. *Obstet Gynecol Ann* 1972;1:177–191.
3. Zeek PM, Assali NS: Vascular changes in the decidua associated with eclamptogenic toxemia. *Am J Clin Pathol* 1950;20:1099–1109.
4. MacLennan AH, Sharp F, Shaw-Dunn J: The ultrastructure of human trophoblast in spontaneous and induced hypoxia using a system of organ culture. A comparison with ultrastructural changes in pre-eclampsia and placental insufficiency. *J Obstet Gynaecol Br Commonw* 1972;79:113–121.
5. Cross JC, Werb Z, Fisher SJ: Implantation and the placenta: Key pieces of the development puzzle. *Science* 1994;266:1508–1518.
6. Roberts JM, Taylor RN, Friedman SA, Goldfien A: In: Dunlop W, ed. *Fetal Medical Review.* London: Edward Arnold Publishers; 1993.
7. Roberts JM, Taylor RN, Musci TJ, et al: Preeclampsia: An endothelial cell disorder. *Am J Obstet Gynecol* 1989;161:1200–1204.
8. Redman CW: Current topic: Pre-eclampsia and the placenta. *Placenta* 1991;12:301–308.
9. Zhou Y, Damsky CH, Chiu K, et al: Preeclampsia is associated with abnormal expression of adhesion molecules by invasive cytotrophoblasts. *J Clin Invest* 1993;91:950–960.

10. Zhou Y, Damsky CH, Fisher SJ: Preeclampsia is associated with failure of human cytotrophoblasts to mimic a vascular adhesion phenotype. One cause of defective endovascular invasion in this syndrome? *J Clin Invest* 1997;99:2152–2164.

11. Gerretsen G, Huisjes HJ, Elema JD: Morphological changes of the spiral arteries in the placental bed in relation to pre-eclampsia and fetal growth retardation. *Br J Obstet Gynaecol* 1981;88:876–881.

12. Moodley J, Ramsaroop R: Placental bed morphology in black women with eclampsia. *S Afr Med J* 1989;75:376–378.

13. Khong TY, De Wolf F, Robertson WB, Brosens I: Inadequate maternal vascular response to placentation in pregnancies complicated by pre-eclampsia and by small-for-gestational age infants. *Br J Obstet Gynaecol* 1986;93:1049–1059.

14. Rodesch F, Simon P, Donner C, Jauniaux E: Oxygen measurements in endometrial and trophoblastic tissues during early pregnancy. *Obstet Gynecol* 1992;80:283–285.

15. Genbacev O, Joslin R, Damsky CH, et al: Hypoxia alters early gestation human cytotrophoblast differentiation/invasion in vitro and models the placental defects that occur in preeclampsia. *J Clin Invest* 1996;97:540–550.

16. Genbacev O, Zhou Y, Ludlow JW, Fisher SJ: Regulation of human placental development by oxygen tension. *Science* 1997;277:1669–1672.

17. Schwarting R (editorial): Little missed markers and Ki-67. *Lab Invest* 1993;68:597–599.

18. Damsky CH, Fitzgerald ML, Fisher SJ: Distribution patterns of extracellular matrix components and adhesion receptors are intricately modulated during first trimester cytotrophoblast differentiation along the invasive pathway, in vivo. *J Clin Invest* 1992;89:210–222.

19. Librach CL, Werb Z, Fitzgerald ML, et al: 92-kD type IV collagenase mediates invasion of human cytotrophoblasts. *J Cell Biol* 1991;113:437–449.

20. McMaster MT, Librach CL, Zhou Y, et al: Human placental HLA-G expression is restricted to differentiated cytotrophoblasts. *J Immunol* 1995;154:3771–3778.

21. McMaster MT, Zhou Y, Shorter S, et al: HLA-G isoforms produced by placental cytotrophoblasts and found in amniotic fluid are due to unusual glycosylation. *J Immunol* 1998;160:5922–5928.

22. Kurman RJ, Young RH, Norris HJ, et al: Immunocytochemical localization of placental lactogen and chorionic gonadotropin in the normal placenta and trophoblastic tumors, with emphasis on intermediate trophoblast and the placental site trophoblastic tumor. *Int J Gynecol Pathol* 1984;3:101–121.

23. King RW, Jackson PK, Kirschner MW: Mitosis in transition. *Cell* 1994;79:563–571.

24. Gartel AL, Serfas MS, Tyner AL: p21—negative regulator of the cell cycle. *Proc Soc Exp Biol Med* 1996;213:138–149.

25. Damsky CH, Librach C, Lim KH, et al: Integrin switching regulates normal trophoblast invasion. *Development* 1994;120:3657–3666.

26. Hertig AT: On the eleven-day pre-villous human ovum with special reference to the variations in its implantation site. *Anat Rec* 1942;82:420.

27. Graeber TG, Osmanian C, Jacks T, et al: Hypoxia-mediated selection of cells with diminished apoptotic potential in solid tumours. *Nature* 1996;379:88–91.

28. Boyd JD, Hamilton WJ: Development and structure of the human placenta from the end of the 3rd month of gestation. *J Obstet Gynaecol Br Commonw* 1967;74:161–226.

29. Zhou Y, Fisher SJ, Janatpour M, et al: Human cytotrophoblasts adopt a vascular phenotype as they differentiate. A strategy for successful endovascular invasion? *J Clin Invest* 1997; 99:2139–2151.

30. Stone J, Itin A, Alon T, et al: Development of retinal vasculature is mediated by hypoxia-induced vascular endothelial growth factor (VEGF) expression by neuroglia. *J Neurosci* 1995;15:4738–4747.

31. Hayashi K, Madri JA, Yurchenco PD: Endothelial cells interact with the core protein of basement perlecan through $\beta 1$ and $\beta 3$ integrins: An adhesion modulated by glycosaminoglycan. *J Cell Biol* 1992;119:945–959.

32. Hynes RO, George EL, Georges EN, et al: Toward a genetic analysis of cell-matrix adhesion. *Cold Spring Harb Symp Quant Biol* 1992;57:249–258.

33. Kalousek DK, Vekemans M: Confined placental mosaicism. *J Med Genet* 1996;33:529–533.
34. Cnattingius S, Bergstrom R, Lipworth L, Kramer MS: Pregnancy weight and the risk of adverse pregnancy outcomes. *N Engl J Med* 1998;338:147–152.
35. Ness RB, Roberts JM: Heterogeneous causes constituting the single syndrome of preeclampsia: A hypothesis and its implications. *Am J Obstet Gynecol* 1996;175:1365–1370.
36. Ward K, Hata A, Jeunemaitre X, et al. A molecular variant of angiotensinogen associated with preeclampsia. *Nat Genet* 1993;4:59–61.
37. Combs CA, Katz MA, Kitzmiller JL, Brescia RJ: Experimental preeclampsia produced by chronic constriction of the lower aorta: Validation with longitudinal blood pressure measurements in conscious rhesus monkeys. *Am J Obstet Gynecol* 1993;169:215–223.
38. Cockell AP, Learmont JG, Smarason AK, et al: Human placental syncytiotrophoblast microvillous membranes impair maternal vascular endothelial function. *Br J Obstet Gynaecol* 1997;104:235–240.
39. Gratton MD, Gandley RE, Genbacev O, et al: Conditioned medium from hypoxic trophoblasts alters arterial functions (submitted).

12

Endothelial Cell Dysfunction

Robert N. Taylor and James M. Roberts

As detailed by Chesley in the first edition of this text and reported in Chapter 1, the clinical manifestations of preeclampsia–eclampsia have been recognized since antiquity, but for nearly two millennia the pathophysiology of this syndrome remained completely obscure. Only after the introduction of critical deductive and experimental principles in post-Napoleonic Europe was a scientific conceptualization of cellular pathology developed. In the mid-19th century, alterations in the renal handling of nitrogen and water were reported in eclamptic women, leading to the categorization of eclampsia as a form of "dropsy."[1] At that time, proteinuria also was identified as "a precursor of puerperal convulsions" establishing a preconvulsive phase of eclampsia, or "preeclampsia." In the early 20th century the term "toxemia" was introduced to describe a growing belief that the syndrome reflected "autointoxication" by noxious agents accumulating within the maternal organism. Also, the sphygmomanometer was used to determine that eclampsia and preeclampsia were associated with hypertension.[2] Recognition of the importance of the placenta in the etiology of this disorder began with identification of multiple placental infarcts in cases of preeclampsia and eclampsia[3] which led some to search for toxic products of placental decomposition, in particular, thromboplastin.[4]

The 20th century witnessed the recognition of renal changes in preeclampsia–eclampsia that predominantly involved the glomerular cells[5,6] and recent studies (reviewed below) indicate that the endothelia of several maternal and fetal vascular beds also are affected in preeclampsia.

Endothelial cells are strategically positioned at the interface between circulating blood and vascular smooth muscle or the extravascular space where they occupy a surface area of more than 1000 m^2. These cells secrete a variety of signaling molecules directly into the circulation, potentially providing access to every cell in the body.[7] In turn, endothelial cells are themselves targets for cellular and soluble plasma constituents (e.g., cytokines, lipoproteins, platelets, leukocytes, placental membranes, antibodies, and other circulating peptides). Endothelial cells modulate the regulation of vascular tone, coagulation, permeability, and the targeting of immune cells. Under normal physiologic conditions, the endothelium maintains a homeostatic balance. Vascular tone is controlled by vasoconstrictors (e.g., endothelin and thromboxane A_2) and vasodilators (e.g., nitric oxide [NO] and prostacyclin [PGI_2]). Hemostasis is maintained in equilibrium by procoagulant and anticoagulant influences and vascular permeability is controlled by endothelial tight junctions. Finally, maternal endothelial cell activation or injury may result in vasospasm, microthombosis, and vascular permeability.

This chapter is divided into four major sections: the hypothesis that endothelial cell dysfunction is pivotal to the pathogenesis of preeclampsia; evidence for this by the evaluation of preeclamptic women; effects of plasma or serum-derived factors on in vitro culture systems; and molecular candidates that mediate endothelial cell dysfunction in preeclamptic pregnancies in vivo. The chapter concludes with a summary integrating these findings, as well as speculations about future diagnostic and therapeutic approaches to preeclampsia, and suggestions for new studies into this enigmatic condition.

ENDOTHELIAL CELL OVERVIEW

Over the past decade attention has focused on the triad of impaired trophoblast invasion, uteroplacental ischemia, and generalized maternal endothelial cell activation or injury as mechanistic factors in preeclampsia pathogenesis.[8,9] The etiology(ies) underlying the development of this syndrome remains unknown, but as described in Chapter 11 by Fisher and Roberts, failure of normal placental invasion, trophoblast differentiation, and vascular remodeling of the placental bed are believed to be important initiating factors in the development of this syndrome. This chapter focuses on circulating factors elaborated in response to uteroplacental ischemia, which are postulated to alter maternal and fetal endothelial cell phenotypes.

ENDOTHELIAL CELL "ACTIVATION" IN PREECLAMPSIA

Endothelial cell "activation" is a term used to define an altered state of endothelial cell differentiation, typically induced as a result of cytokine stimulation.[10] It often represents a response to sublethal injury and is proposed to play a major role in the pathophysiology of atherosclerosis.[11] Endothelial cell dysfunction in preeclampsia may result from a variety of factors, including physical shear forces, hypoxia, or reactive oxygen products or their metabolites and other circulating constituents.[8] These factors may be of particular importance in the placental bed of preeclamptic women. For example, increased endovascular shear force, perhaps generated by vasospasm or failure of spiral arterial remodeling is known to affect endothelial cell morphology and function.[12] Hypoxia, a plausible result of reduced placental perfusion, is a known stimulator of endothelin and vascular endothelial growth factor synthesis and secretion in other vascular beds.[13] Certain oxygen species are highly reactive and, if generated within the vascular space, can alter endothelial cell function. Antiphospholipid and anti-endothelial cell antibodies and cytokines such as tumor necrosis factor-α and interleukin-6 also could be responsible for endothelial cell dysfunction in preeclampsia, and will be discussed further below.

Endothelial activation or damage is manifest biochemically by the synthesis and secretion of a variety of endothelial cell products including prostanoids, endothelin-1, platelet-derived growth factor, fibronectin, selectins, and other molecules that influence vessel tone and remodeling.[14,15] Such responses to acute mechanical or biochemical endothelial cell damage facilitate efficient wound healing. However, when activated by a chronic pathological process, such as preeclampsia, these responses can provoke a vicious cycle of vasospasm, microthrombosis, disruption of vascular integrity, and serious physiologic disturbances which persist until the inciting factor(s) is eliminated.

Insights into the vascular pathophysiology of preeclampsia are derived from clinical experience with thrombotic microangiopathic disorders occurring during pregnancy. These diseases are rare, but pregnancy appears to predispose or exacerbate their development.[16] Also, thrombotic thrombocytopenic purpura (TTP), characterized by thrombocytopenia, microangiopathic hemolytic anemia, renal involvement, neurological symptoms, and fever, like preeclampsia, most commonly manifests in the late second trimester.[17,18]

Atherosis

The endothelium lining the uterine spiral arterioles, which normally undergoes denudation and replacement by invading endovascular cytotrophoblasts, may manifest the first pathological changes associated with preeclampsia.[19,20] The failure of trophoblasts to assume an "endothelial" phenotype in preeclampsia has been discussed in Chapter 11 by Fisher and Roberts.

Abnormal trophoblast invasion and impaired placental perfusion are considered by some as requisite in the development of preeclampsia. If we accept that the placenta is where the disease originates, this is where we should initially look for evidence of endothelial cell injury. Lesions in the spiral arteries at placental sites, called acute atherosis, were first described by Zeek and Assali.[21] More descriptive ultrastructural studies are those by Nadji and Sommers[22] and DeWolf et al.,[23] who noted endothelial cell vacuolization, myointimal proliferation, and foam cell infiltration of the tunica media, all histologic changes that occur in the vascular pathology of atherosclerosis.[24] The similarity of the latter changes to those observed in atherosclerosis led us to propose that endothelial cell injury might be a mechanism responsible for diffuse vascular disease manifest in patients with preeclampsia.[25]

In the studies of Brosens et al.[26] and Kitzmiller and Benirschke,[27] histologic changes in the placental beds of women with preeclampsia were noted to bear resemblance to vascular pathology associated with allograft rejection. While not all spiral arterioles are affected in cases of preeclampsia, the extent and severity of the vascular lesions seem to parallel the clinical severity of this syndrome. In some cases of preeclampsia, immunohistochemical studies of affected blood vessels have demonstrated immunoglobulin, fibrin, and complement protein deposits. Despite these observations and epidemiologic evidence that support an immunologic etiology of preeclampsia, the hypothesis of an immune basis for vascular dysfunction in preeclampsia remains controversial.[28]

In a proportion (14%) of primigravid women undergoing voluntary first trimester pregnancy termination, Lichtig et al.[29] observed decidual vascular atherosis and heavy deposition of complement by immunofluorescence. Although the potential clinical outcomes of these patients can only be surmised, this observation was more common than in multiparae (3%) and supports early vascular injury in a minority of pregnancies that are at increased risk of developing preeclampsia. More recently, noninvasive Doppler ultrasound studies suggest decreased spiral artery flow and reduced placental perfusion during early pregnancy in groups of women destined to develop clinically evident preeclampsia.[30]

Glomeruloendotheliosis

Evidence of endothelial cell injury distant from the placental bed is well documented. Renal glomerular capillary endotheliosis, swelling of endothelial cytoplasm, and obliteration of endothelial fenestrae, detailed in Chapter 7, as pathognomonic features of preeclampsia, are the best characterized examples of such a lesion.[5,6] Investigators have documented morphologic and functional vascular injury in other organs of preeclamptic women. Sheehan and Lynch[31] described hepatic periportal vascular lesions in fatal cases of preeclampsia and eclampsia. These lesions were characterized by arterial media infiltration and capillary thrombosis, but specific abnormalities of the vascular endothelium were not noted. Shanklin and Sibai[32] observed ultrastructural defects in the mitochondria of uterine and extrauterine tissues in women with preeclampsia, further supporting a systemic metabolic disorder in this syndrome.

FUNCTIONAL EVIDENCE OF ENDOTHELIAL CELL ACTIVATION

In recent years, many clinical studies have added support to the hypothesis of endothelial cell dysfunction in preeclampsia. In retrospect, however, the first clues to this mechanism were data demonstrating abnormal vascular responses in women with this syndrome. In their now classic longitudinal study, Gant et al.[33] demonstrated that the refractoriness of normal pregnant women to infusions of angiotensin II was lost as early as 22 weeks' gestation in primigravid women destined to develop preeclampsia. It now appears that this loss of angiotensin II-resistance is a result of impaired expression of endothelium-derived vasodilator activities. Unfortunately, the clinical utility of sensitivity to infused angiotensin II to predict preeclampsia has recently been questioned.[34]

Ultrasonographic evidence of reduced cerebrovascular and retinal artery blood flow in preeclamptic women has been demonstrated, and treatment with magnesium sulfate has been shown to improve vascular flow in the middle cerebral artery.[35] The possible role of the endothelium in this response is suggested by the in vitro experiments of Watson et al.[36] who demonstrated that 2 to 3 mM $MgSO_4$ increased human endothelial cell PGI_2 production. Other groups, however, have not confirmed this finding.[37]

Myograph experiments using isolated resistance vessels from pregnant women have demonstrated resistance to pharmacologic inhibition of endothelium-dependent vasodilatation compared to vessels from nonpregnant women.[38] Arteries obtained from preeclamptic women show evidence of endothelial dysfunction by their failure to relax in response to some endothelium-dependent vasodilators[39] or to flow-induced shear stress.[40,41] Syncytiotrophoblast microvillous membranes[42] impair endothelium-dependent vasodilation of normal vessels mounted on the myograph and induce ultrastructural evidence of endothelial cell injury. In similar experiments, maternal plasma from preeclamptic women inhibited endothelium-mediated relaxation of myometrial arteries.[43] Plasma from matched, normal pregnant women did not have this effect.

CIRCULATING MARKERS OF ENDOTHELIAL CELL ACTIVATION IN VIVO

Multiple markers of vascular endothelial cell activation have been reported in preeclampsia,[43a] including decreased systemic levels of prostacyclin[44,45] and elevated circulating concentrations of endothelin-1[46,47] cellular fibronectin,[48,49] and thrombomodulin.[50] These data complement the morphologic[33,51] and functional[34,40] evidence of endothelial alterations in preeclampsia.

Prostaglandins

Prostaglandins are among the primary vasoactive products of endothelial cells. These bioactive lipids have profound regulatory effects on subjacent vascular smooth muscle cells and play an important role in the physiologic and pathophysiologic modulation of vascular tone. Their role as markers of endothelial cell activation is reviewed immediately below, and how they mediate vascular function is discussed further in this chapter. The major eicosanoid product produced by endothelial cells is reported to be prostacyclin (PGI_2).[52] Discovered in 1976,[53] PGI_2, is a potent vasodilator and inhibitor of platelet aggregation. This compound is remarkably unstable chemically, and it is its metabolite 6-keto-$PGF_{1\alpha}$ that is generally measured in vivo. Prostacyclin is not stored in endothelial cells but is released rapidly from these cells following a cascade of enzymatic transformations of its fatty-acid precursor, arachidonic acid. Plasma concentrations and urinary excretion of PGI_2 metabolites are decreased in women with preeclampsia,[44] and low urinary excretion of PGI_2 metabolites may predict development of preeclampsia by as early as 20 weeks' gestation.[45]

The reason for altered prostaglandin production during preeclampsia is unknown. Reduction in PGI_2 may simply be a nonspecific marker of endothelial cell dysfunction while increased thromboxane may indicate platelet activation by this endothelium. Another element may be the interaction between products of oxidative stress, lipid peroxides (discussed in Chapter 14), and the cyclooxygenase enzyme. Lipid peroxides can activate cyclooxygenase and stimulate thromboxane synthesis.[54] Placental perfusion with aspirin significantly blocked peroxide-induced vasoconstriction and secretion of prostaglandins. Walsh and Wang[55] compared the production of lipid peroxides, thromboxane, and PGI_2 in different compartments within the placentas of preeclamptic and normal pregnant women. Their data demonstrated that lipid peroxides and thromboxane primarily originated from trophoblast cells, whereas PGI_2 was primarily produced by vascular tissue in the villous core. Placentas from preeclamptic women produced more lipid peroxides and thromboxane than those from normal gravidas, whereas PGI_2 production was not different between the two patient sources. Trophoblast cells could be a site of increased lipid peroxide and thromboxane entry into the maternal circulation of women with preeclampsia. The evanescent nature of thromboxanes and lipid peroxides raises questions about this concept and the observation is more compatible with altered local effects.

Procoagulant Proteins and Plasminogen Activators

Preeclampsia is characterized by a maternal hypercoagulable state, intravascular coagulation, microthromboses in several organs, and impairment of the uteroplacental circulation (see Chap. 11). Excessive fibrin deposition occurs in the placenta, suggesting that disorders of placental coagulation and fibrinolysis may play a role in activation of hemostasis. The hypercoagulable state may be due, in part, to diffuse endothelial cell activation. The reduced expression of several relevant endothelial cell-associated anticoagulant proteins has been shown in preeclampsia, including antithrombin III, protein C, and protein S. The significance of these proteins as markers of maternal endothelial cell dysfunction is reviewed below.

Resistance to activated protein C is an inherited mutation of the coagulation factor V gene. The presence of the factor V Leiden mutation predisposes to thromboembolic events. The prevalence of this mutation is increased in patients with severe preeclampsia compared to women with normal pregnancies.[56,57] In a series of pregnancies complicated by severe, early-onset preeclampsia, 25% of the women had functional protein S deficiency, 18% demonstrated hyperhomocysteinemia, and 29% had detectable anticardiolipin IgG and IgM antibodies.[58]

Increased endothelial expression of other procoagulant proteins, including tissue factor, von Willebrand factor, platelet-activating factor, β-thromboglobulin, cellular fibronectin, and thrombomodulin also have been reported. The latter two endothelial cell markers have been shown to differentiate preeclampsia from other forms of hypertension in pregnancy.[49,59] Similarly, inhibitors of fibrinolytic or antithrombotic proteins also appear to play a role in the imbalance of the coagulation cascade. Plasminogen-activator inhibitor type 1 (PAI-1), whose synthesis during pregnancy is predominantly placental in origin, was observed by ourselves[60] and others to be increased in the plasma of women with preeclamptic pregnancies.[61,62] Increased decidual and amniotic fluid concentrations of PAI-1 also have been reported in preeclampsia.[63] The content of type 2 plasminogen-activator inhibitor (PAI-2) antigen was higher in preeclamptic placentas than in controls.[64] Circulating levels of PAI-1, thrombomodulin, and fibronectin were found to correlate directly with severity of the syndrome.[65]

Endothelial Cell Adhesion Molecules

In response to injury or activation, endothelial cells express extracellular matrix glycoproteins with procoagulant activities. Two examples are fibronectin and von Willebrand factor.[66] Both of these proteins are predominantly localized to the abluminal extracellular matrix of human endothelium,[67] but as discussed below, they can be actively secreted from endothelial cells under conditions of cellular activation. Immunoperoxidase techniques demonstrate a characteristic fibrillar morphology of fibronectin within the extracellular matrix surrounding endothelial cells. When endothelial monolayers are activated by interleukin-1, there is loss from the fibronectin molecule of a chymotryptic protease-sensitive epitope. Degraded fibronectin is stimulatory for neutrophils, and this is likely to induce further fibronectin breakdown. This sequence has the potential to set up a feed-forward inflammatory loop. Alteration of fibronectin architecture is a useful marker of endothelial injury, and has important pathophysiologic consequences.[68]

The majority of plasma fibronectin is shed into the circulation by hepatocytes,[66] where it constitutes a significant fraction of the total plasma protein. Elevated concentrations of this glycoprotein in women with preeclampsia have now been recognized for over a decade.[69] In an in vivo model of human endothelial cell dysfunction, the induction of venostasis in healthy volunteers, plasma fibronectin and von Willebrand factor were observed to increase.[70] Hypoxia also appears to enhance the expression of fibronectin.[71]

A specific isoform of fibronectin, cellular fibronectin (cFN), expresses two extra domains (ED-A and ED-B) generated by differential mRNA splicing in endothelial cells. The ED-A cellular fibronectin is nonhepatic in origin and almost exclusively localized to the endothelium of blood vessels in healthy nonpregnant women. In vitro studies have demonstrated that in addition to being incorporated into extracellular matrix, a soluble form of ED-A cFN is secreted into the medium, potentially reflecting intravascular release of this protein by human endothelial cells in vivo.[72] Cellular fibronectin plays a central role in the adhesion, morphology, and migration of endothelial cells. While it is a major component of the endothelial extracellular matrix, cFN is normally only a minor component of circulating fibronectin and thus is a more precise marker of endothelial cell injury than total fibronectin.[49]

Lockwood and Peters[48] used a cross-sectional study design to show that ED-A fibronectin levels were increased in the plasma of women who later developed preeclampsia. We used a monoclonal antibody that recognizes a conformational epitope near the ED-B region of cFN, and showed in a longitudinal study that plasma cFN concentrations were increased statistically at term and as early as the second trimester in women destined to develop preeclampsia.[49] In addition we observed that women with transient hypertension, a hypertensive condition of pregnancy without proteinuria and without the maternal or neonatal morbidity associated with preeclampsia, could be readily distinguished from those with preeclampsia according to their cFN level.

The concentrations of other endothelial cell adhesion molecules, including vascular cell adhesion molecule-1 (VCAM-1) and P-selectin, are elevated in cases of preeclampsia.[73] Intravascular cell adhesion molecule-1 (ICAM-1) and VCAM-1 appear to be predictive of the development of preeclampsia as early as the mid-trimester of pregnancy.[74]

Mitogenic Activities and Growth Factors

Endothelial cells respond to injury or activation with the release or secretion of mitogenic proteins or peptides. With acute vascular trauma, this response teleologically encourages the proliferation of vascular smooth muscle, allowing vessel remodeling and repair. However, in illnesses such as atherosclerosis or preeclampsia, release of mitogenic factors might exacerbate reduced blood flow by promoting vessel wall hypertrophy. Taylor et al.[75] postulated that in preeclampsia diffuse maternal endothelial cell injury or activation might result in the release of mitogenic proteins into the circulation. Indeed, they demonstrated increments in the mitogenic activity of plasma obtained from women with preeclampsia. The increased activity could be shown in women destined to develop preeclampsia as early as the first trimester but returned to normal by 6 to 12 weeks postpartum (Fig. 12–1). The increased mitogenic activity, however, did not promote endothelial cell proliferation. Further characterization of this mitogenic factor indicated it to be protease-, heat-, and acid-labile and to have an apparent molecular mass of ~150,000.[75]

Growth Factor-Binding Proteins in Preeclampsia

On the basis of these biochemical characteristics, we tested if the plasma mitogenic activity was attributable to insulin growth factor-binding protein-3, an acid-labile insulin growth factor binding protein complex. However, circulating concentrations of this protein complex were not found to be higher in cases of preeclampsia.[76] In other studies, maternal serum insulin growth factors (IGFs) and insulin growth factor-binding proteins (IGFBPs) were found to be similar in normal and preeclamptic pregnancies.[77] In a longitudinal study comparing 20 primiparous

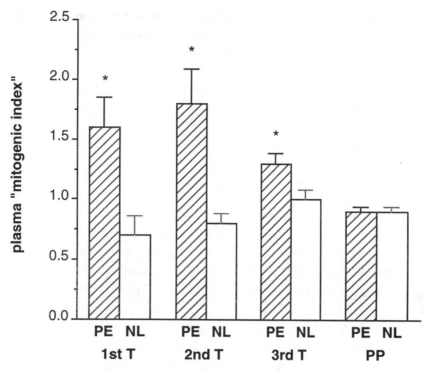

Figure 12–1. Mitogenic activity in pregnancy plasma. The ratios of plasma mitogenic activity in specimens obtained predelivery at each pregnancy trimester (T) and again at > 6 weeks postpartum (PP) were normalized to each patient's immediate (− 48 hours) postpartum plasma activity. Mitogenic activity was quantified by ^{3}H-thymidine incorporation into nascent fibroblast DNA. The mean ± SE mitogenic index of six preeclamptic (PE, hatched bars) and six, matched normal (NL, open bars) pregnant women are shown. The asterisk (*) indicates a significant difference between the predelivery preeclamptic and the normal pregnant groups (P < 0.05). (*Data adapted from Taylor RN, Heilbron DC, Roberts JM: Growth factor activity in the blood of women in whom preeclampsia develops is elevated from early pregnancy. Am J Obstet Gynecol 1990;163:1839–1844.*)

women who developed preeclampsia with 20 matched, normal pregnant controls, de Groot et al.[78] found that midtrimester maternal plasma IGFBP-1 concentrations were significantly reduced in the group of women who developed preeclampsia approximately 20 weeks later.[78] It should be noted that some reports of third trimester maternal serum IGFBP-1 show elevations in women with active, symptomatic severe preeclampsia.[79,80] Our data,[78] however, are more compatible with reduced trophoblastic invasion of the maternal decidual stroma in the first half of pregnancies destined to develop preeclampsia.[20] Decreased plasma levels of IGFBP-1 (a protein that binds and inhibits the mitogenic actions of IGF) may explain, in part, the increased plasma mitogenic index observed in early pregnancy in women destined to develop preeclampsia.[81] The findings support the hypothesis that increased quantities of mitogenic proteins are released into the circulation quite early in pregnancy in women destined to develop preeclampsia. The precise cellular derivation of the mitogenic activity is still unknown, but maternal endothelial cells remain a plausible source.

Endothelial Cell Permeability Factors in Preeclampsia

Given the edema and proteinuria associated with the clinical preeclampsia syndrome, markers of increased endothelial cell permeability might be expected to be increased in women with this disorder. Studies to quantify plasma levels of vascular endothelial growth factor (VEGF), also known as vascular permeability factor,[82] have supported this hypothesis. Using immunofluorimetric[83] and competitive enzyme immunoassays, plasma VEGF concentrations were found to be significantly elevated in women with active preeclampsia. Considerably higher VEGF levels (10–64 ng/mL) were detected in preeclampsia plasma using the more sensitive "total VEGF" assay developed by the latter group.[84] However, in one study maternal serum levels were reported to be lower in women with preeclampsia.[73]

A study comparing the concentration of placental VEGF mRNA in normal and preeclamptic pregnancies found decreased placental VEGF mRNA levels in cases of preeclampsia.[85] These findings suggest that the placenta is not the source of increased VEGF protein in the maternal circulation during preeclamptic pregnancy, lending additional support to the hypothesis that VEGF is a marker of endothelial cell activation in this syndrome.

In vitro studies using retinal epithelial cells indicate that exposure to reactive oxygen intermediates (e.g., superoxide or hydrogen peroxide) caused a rapid increase in VEGF mRNA levels. Superoxide-associated mRNA increases were dose-dependent, blocked by antioxidants, and associated with elevated VEGF protein levels in the conditioned media of the cells.[86] As detailed below, lipid peroxides and oxidative stress are increased in preeclampsia. If similar mechanisms exist in maternal endothelial cells, this could explain the elevated VEGF concentrations reported in these women.

Endothelin

Another endothelial cell marker of interest in preeclampsia is the vasoactive peptide endothelin-1 (ET-1). The endothelins, a family of 21 amino-acid peptides, are the most potent vasoconstrictors yet identified.[87] Of the three isoforms, ET–1 is the predominant endothelin produced in endothelial cells.[88] It exerts its biological actions in a paracrine fashion on subjacent vascular smooth muscle cells. Under normal conditions, vascular endothelin is secreted in insufficient amounts to induce vasoconstriction.[89] However, the ability of this basal level to enhance contraction evoked by other vasoconstrictors has been demonstrated.[90] This would be especially relevant to preeclampsia, in which there is increased response to all pressor agents.[91] Moreover, ET-1 is a potent vasoconstrictor of the human uterine[92] and renal[93] vascular beds, both of which are affected in this syndrome. Elevated ET-1 concentrations are present in preeclampsia but not prior to clinically evident disease.[46]

The expression of ET-1 mRNA is increased in villous placenta from women with preeclampsia.[94] Recent immunolocalization experiments have suggested that ET-1 and its precursor are synthesized in villous endothelial cells and not trophoblasts.[95] Genbacev et al.[96] demonstrated that villi cultured under hypoxic conditions in vitro mimic the cellular changes noted in preeclampsia. Thus, low oxygen tension in the preeclamptic placenta might be a stimulus for enhanced villous ET-1 production as it is in the pulmonary vascular bed.[97] However, the data of Rust et al.,[98] who compared near simultaneous maternal uterine vein and antecubital vein concentrations of immunoreactive ET-1, indicate that the placenta is not the source of elevated ET-1 levels in plasma from severely preeclamptic women. Systemic maternal endothelial cell activation may be the best explanation of this observation.

Nitric Oxide As a Marker of Endothelial Activation

The discovery of nitric oxide (NO) production by endothelial cells in the mid-1980s provided substantial support for the functional importance of endothelial cells.[99] Nitric oxide has numerous functions, many of which are relevant to maintenance of normal vascular function and quite pertinent to the cardiovascular adaptation of pregnancy. It is a vasodilator and inhibits platelet aggregation as well as acting to inhibit mitogenesis.[100] Nitric oxide has an unpaired electron and as a free radical can accept electrons to act as an antioxidant.[101] Loss of these functions secondary to decreased NO could result in many of the pathophysiologic changes of preeclampsia.

Several efforts have been made to assess NO production in preeclampsia. There are inherent problems with this assessment. First, NO is very labile and the stable metabolites nitrite and nitrate (NO_x) are used as indicators of NO concentration in biological fluids. Since diet can also contribute to NO_x, assessment of NO production is most appropriately performed after a controlled NO_x diet. This is not usually practical in sick preeclamptic women and none of the published studies have controlled diet. Some investigators have reported blood NO_x concentrations in preeclamptic women.[102-105] In one study concentrations were reduced,[102] while in others they were similar in the blood of preeclamptic and normal pregnant women.[103-105] The measurement of circulating concentrations of NO_x as an indicator is problematic. Since NO_x are excreted by the kidney, NO production could be reduced but blood levels maintained within the normal ranges by the reduced renal function that accompanies preeclampsia.[106] In a study that measured the excretion of NO_x in urine, the amount of NO_x excreted daily estimated from the ratio of urinary NO_x to creatinine was reduced in preeclamptic women.[107] Excretion appeared to have been measured under steady-state conditions as it was the same over 2 days, the results suggesting reduced production of NO. This study, as the others, is limited by failure to control diet and by the use of NO_x/creatinine as a surrogate for 24-hour urines. This strategy has been suggested to be especially problematic for NO_x. Decrements in NO_x excretion were confirmed in one[108] but not in another study[109] (in the latter 24-hour urine NO_x excretion was measured but there was a smaller number of patients and preeclampsia was poorly defined; 13% of women, in fact, did not manifest proteinuria). Additionally, there are multiple sources of NO; thus, the possibility cannot be excluded that production of NO by other tissues or organs (such as placenta) are reduced, and that endothelial cell production is normal.

Several investigators have administered NO-synthesis inhibitors chronically to experimental animals and produced a syndrome resembling human preeclampsia.[110-113] Although the results are interesting, the possibility that any pressor agent might have the same effects has not yet been excluded.

In summary, NO has many functions which, if deficient, can lead to pathophysiologic changes present in preeclampsia. The vagaries of determining NO production from blood or urine concentrations of metabolites in sick women preclude definitive conclusions about the role of NO in the syndrome. Nonetheless, the reduced NO activity in response to agonists present in vessels of preeclamptic women examined in vitro supports a role for NO in preeclampsia, as well as provides further evidence for the role of endothelial dysfunction in the pathophysiology of the disorder.

"PREDICTIVE" BIOCHEMICAL MARKERS AS HARBINGERS OF PREECLAMPSIA RISK

Among the endothelial cell-related markers described above, very few have met the desired criteria that these would be sensitive, specific, and might provide clinically useful predictors of preeclampsia. Significant decreases in the urinary excretion of prostacyclin (PGI_2) metabolite were observed months before the onset of clinical signs of preeclampsia,[45] but cut-off levels were not determined to evaluate the sensitivity or specificity of this assay. Likewise, circulating concentrations of von Willebrand factor (factor VIII-related antigen) and cellular fibronectin (cFN) were demonstrably elevated from the second trimester of gestation. Unfortunately, formal evaluation of these as a predictive test was not undertaken.[49,114] However, the variation in the published data suggests that none of these is likely to have useful predictive value.

FETAL ENDOTHELIAL INVOLVEMENT IN PREECLAMPSIA

Whether the fetal circulation is affected by, or protected from, humoral factors present in preeclampsia appears to be controversial. Dadak et al.[115] reported morphologic and biochemical evidence of endothelial cell injury in the cords of infants whose mothers had preeclampsia. Evidence of fetal thrombocytopenia[116] also was reported. Davidge et al.[117] observed that mixed arteriovenous umbilical cord plasma from neonates of preeclamptic mothers had elevated cFN levels (see further discussion below). These plasma samples also stimulated more endothelial cell NO production that matched normal neonatal plasma specimens. However, another study that included premature infants as "normal controls" failed to observe increases in fetal cord plasma cFN concentrations.[118]

IN VITRO ACTIVATION OF ENDOTHELIAL CELLS BY PREECLAMPSIA PLASMA AND SERUM

In the preceding section, data were presented which demonstrate maternal endothelial cell dysfunction manifested by a variety of circulating marker molecules. Evidence will now be reviewed which supports the concept that activities present in the blood of preeclamptic women can alter human endothelial cell function in vitro and might be responsible for affecting systemic maternal endothelial cell function in vivo. As suggested previously, these activities might be placentally derived.[25]

Any model of a human pathological process is de facto an experimental substitute for the actual disease. This limitation is particularly true of clinical syndromes, such as preeclampsia, for which disease equivalents in lower animals do not exist. Interesting primate models of preeclampsia have been induced in pregnant baboons[119] and rhesus monkeys[120] by the surgical reduction of uteroplacental perfusion pressure. As an alternative to these expensive and technically difficult primate preparations, several laboratories have developed and characterized in vitro models of endothelial function using cultures of isolated endothelial cells. Caveats of such models are numerous. The synthesis and secretion of specific endothelial cell autacoids are dependent on the species and vascular bed location from which the isolated cells are derived.[121] Moreover, the surface substrate upon which the endothelial cells are grown can affect cell-cycle kinetics, extracellular matrix protein, and ET-1 gene expression.[122] Finally, extrapolation from in vitro findings to hypotheses of endothelial cell pathophysiology in women with preeclampsia must be made and interpreted with caution.

Generic Evidence of Endothelial Cell Injury

Our group initiated in vitro studies of preeclampsia with the hypothesis that blood-borne factors were responsible for generalized endothelial cell injury or activation. One series of experiments[123] established that dilutions of serum from women with active preeclampsia could perturb the function of human endothelial cells in vitro, increasing the release of chromium 51-chromate from cells preloaded with the isotope (Fig. 12–2), results confirmed and extended by Tsukimori et al.[124] The data indicated that the serum factors responsible for the stimulation of ^{51}Cr release were specific for preeclampsia, not being detectable in chronic or transient hypertension of pregnancy. Initially, we adopted the terminology of the immunologists who pio-

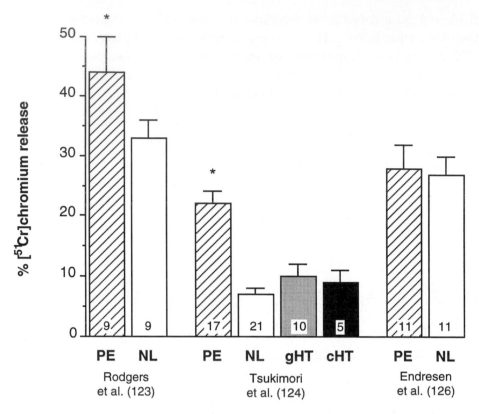

Figure 12–2. Chromium release as an indicator of endothelial cell activation. Human umbilical vein endothelial cells preloaded with ^{51}Cr-chromate were incubated with 10 to 30% serum from preeclamptic (PE, hatched bars), normal (NL, open bars), gestational hypertensive (gHT, stippled bar), and chronic hypertensive (cHT, solid bar), pregnant women. The mean ± SE chromium release expressed as a percentage of total cellular chromium is shown. The number of individual patients tested (N) is indicated at the base of each bar. Asterisks (*) indicate significant differences between the preeclamptic and the normal pregnant groups (P < 0.05). (*Data adapted from Rodgers GM, Taylor RN, Roberts JM: Preeclampsia is associated with a serum factor cytotoxic to human endothelial cells. Am J Obstet Gynecol 1988;159:908–914; Tsukimori K, Maeda H, Shingu M, et al: The possible role of endothelial cell in hypertensive disorders during pregnancy. Obstet Gynecol 1992;80:229–233; and Endresen MJ, Tosti E, Lorentzen B, et al: Sera of preeclamptic women are not cytotoxic to endothelial cells in culture. Am J Obstet Gynecol 1995;172:196–201.*)

neered these assays and referred to the observed release of intracellular ^{51}Cr as "cytotoxicity"[123] which has caused some conceptual confusion. More rigorous experiments, however, from our group[125] and by Endresen et al.,[126] indicated that endothelial cell viability and membrane integrity were not adversely affected under the conditions of our assays. The latter investigators, however, failed to observe increased ^{51}Cr release, but their endothelial cell culture conditions and pregnancy serum concentrations differed from those used in our protocols. Of interest, using a different assay based on intracellular calcium mobilization, Halim et al. also observed increased endothelial cell "cytotoxicity."[127] Summarizing the observed effects of preeclampsia serum on endothelial cell cultures, it is apparent that the perturbation is more consistent with cellular "activation" than toxicity per se.

Endothelial Cell Proteins As Markers of In Vitro Activation

The synthesis and secretion of specific endothelial cell gene products appear to be involved in the activation of human endothelial cell cultures by preeclampsia serum. Platelet-derived growth factor (PDGF) mRNA and protein expression were increased in human umbilical vein endothelial cells cultured with predelivery sera from preeclamptic women relative to postdelivery sera from the same patients.[128] Platelet-derived growth factor is known to have mitogenic and vasoconstrictive effects on vascular smooth muscle,[14] and is an indirect angiogenic factor.[129] Cellular fibronectin release also was specifically stimulated by preeclampsia serum.[130] Other markers of endothelial cell activation were stimulated by pregnancy plasma but did not differentiate between normal and preeclampsia specimens, including the expression of tissue factor, von Willebrand factor,[130] and intracellular cell adhesion molecule (Taylor, unpublished results). These findings imply that factors in preeclampsia serum induce selective markers of cellular activation and support the concept of endothelial activation rather than cytotoxicity in these in vitro experiments.

Prostanoid Production

There is precedent for the presence of circulating factors that alter endothelial cell function in vitro and in other disease states. Roles for endothelium-derived mitogens such as platelet-derived growth factor and ET-1 have been suggested in the preeclampsia-like pediatric disorder, hemolytic uremic syndrome.[131,132] Two other pathophysiologic examples of acute endothelial activation have been associated with increased prostacyclin (PGI_2) production in vivo. In Henoch–Schönlein purpura, a pediatric immune vasculitis, elevated plasma concentrations of PGI_2 metabolites correlate with the generalized endothelial activation observed in the acute phase of the disease.[133] In models of acute allograft rejection, where histopathologic similarities to preeclampsia have been noted previously,[134] the concentration of PGI_2 metabolite was increased 52%.[135] Thus, acute endothelial cell activation is accompanied by an increase in PGI_2 and other vasodilators (e.g., NO), while chronic endothelial cell disturbances are associated with predominantly vasoconstrictor responses.[136] Biphasic temporal patterns of PGI_2 production in response to endothelial activators have been described. Wang et al.[137] noted an initial increase followed by a persistent diminution of PGI_2 production when bovine endothelial cells were exposed to hyperlipidemic sera. Similar kinetics of PGI_2 release by human umbilical vein endothelial (HUVE) cells were reported by Baker et al.[138] after exposure to preeclampsia plasma. During the first 48 hours the secretion of PGI_2 was enhanced over baseline, whereas PGI_2 but not prostaglandin E_2 (PGE_2) production fell below basal values when the cultures were carried for > 72 hours.

More recent studies using high-performance liquid chromatography (HPLC) and thin layer chromatographic separation of [^{3}H] arachidonic acid metabolites indicate that the predominant eicosanoid synthesized by HUVE cells in the presence of human pregnancy plasma is the vasoconstrictor $PGF_{2\alpha}$.[139] Greater production of $PGF_{2\alpha}$ was observed after exposure to preeclampsia plasma compared to matched, normal pregnancy plasma. This finding suggests that circulating factors in the blood of preeclamptic women may contribute to an overall production of vasoconstrictor prostanoids by endothelial cells.

To gain insight into the molecular mechanism of increased prostaglandin production by HUVE cells in response to preeclampsia plasma, we examined the enzymes responsible for its synthesis. Although cyclooxygenase is thought to be the rate-limiting enzyme in prostaglandin biosynthesis, substrate availability plays a key role in the cascade. Multiple factors contribute to the regulation of free intracellular arachidonic acid concentration including hydrolysis of arachidonic acid at the sn (stereospecific number)–2 position of phospholipids and free fatty acid transport. Phospholipases A_2 (PLA_2) are a family of esterases that hydrolyze the sn–2–acyl ester bond in phospholipids and play a role in the regulation of intracellular arachidonic acid concentration. Both secretable and cytosolic forms exist. The cytosolic PLA_2 ($cPLA_2$) has a molecular weight of 85 kDa but can be phosphorylated and migrate at 110 kDa in SDS-PAGE gels.[140,141] It is believed that $cPLA_2$ has a greater selectivity for arachidonic acid and is more stable in the cytoplasm than the secretable form. The secretable PLA_2 (type II PLA_2) is a smaller molecule (14 kDa) and has very little homology to $cPLA_2$. The exact role of type II PLA_2 in the regulation of intracellular arachidonic acid concentration remains unclear. However, overexpression of type II PLA_2 has been associated with increased release of arachidonic acid in C127 mouse fibroblasts.[142] Furthermore, Murakami et al.[143] showed that increased PGI_2 production by HUVE cells in response to tumor necrosis factor-α stimulation could be partially blocked when antiserum against type II PLA_2 was used. These data suggest that both type II PLA_2 and $cPLA_2$ play roles in the regulation of intracellular arachidonic acid concentration.

Work from our laboratory suggests that PLA_2 activity may mediate the prostanoid activation of endothelial cells by preeclampsia plasma.[144] A PLA_2 antagonist, when added to cultured HUVE cells, abolished the differential PGI_2 production by these cells induced by exposure to preeclampsia plasma. In addition, we showed that the plasma levels of type II PLA_2 are elevated in severe preeclampsia (Fig. 12–3).[145] However, endothelial cells did not appear to increase their secretion of type II PLA_2 when stimulated with preeclampsia plasma. Although there are a number of enzymes involved in the cleavage of arachidonic acid from membrane phospholipids, such as phospholipases C and D, these studies suggest that the increased PGI_2 production by HUVE cells in response to preeclampsia plasma is also mediated by PLA_2.

Nitric Oxide Generation by Endothelial Cells in Response to Plasma of Preeclamptic Women

Endothelial cells exposed to plasma from preeclamptic women or their infants released greater amounts of NO than when exposed to plasma from normal preg-

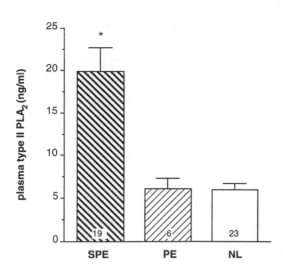

Figure 12–3. Type II phospholipase A_2 concentrations in pregnancy. Third trimester plasma levels of type II phospholipase A_2 (PLA_2) were determined by enzyme immunoassay. The mean ± SE plasma type II PLA_2 concentrations (ng/mL) in severe preeclampsia (SPE, heavy hatched bar), mild preeclampsia (PE, light hatched bar), and normal pregnancy (NL, open bar) are shown. The number of individual patients sampled (N) is indicated at the base of each bar. Asterisk (*) indicates significant differences between the severe preeclamptic and the other pregnant groups ($P < 0.05$). (*Data adapted from Lim KH, Rice GE, de Groot CJ, et al: Plasma type II phospholipase A2 levels are elevated in severe preeclampsia. Am J Obstet Gynecol 1995;172:998–1002.*)

nant women or their infants.[83,117] This release was associated with increased NO-synthase activity and mass.[146] This is paradoxical considering the postulated role of NO in preeclampsia, which predicts reduced NO release. Also, despite limitations of measuring excretion of NO_x, the changes reported in maternal fluids suggest reduced NO production.[102-104] Is there a potential explanation? Unlike the effect of plasma from preeclamptic women upon endothelial cells, which is consistent with what seems to occur in vivo, there is no change in NO production with time.[83] It is possible that artifactual in vitro conditions differ enough from the in vivo situation to render the results incomparable. This speculation is supported by the observation that exposure of endothelial cells to shear stress in vitro, the major stimulus for endothelial NO release in vivo, eliminates the unique effect of preeclampsia plasma on NO production.[138] However, there is another more physiologic possibility. Davidge et al. demonstrated that the component of plasma responsible for NO release is the low density lipoprotein (LDL) fraction.[147] It is now known that lysophosphatidyl choline, a component of oxidatively modified LDL, up-regulates nitric oxide synthase (NOS).[148] NO has also been demonstrated to act as an antioxidant in neutralizing lipid peroxides.[149] It is possible that in the in vitro setting with dilute (2%) plasma, the predominant effect is an increase in NO production resulting from NOS up-regulation. However, in vivo with "undiluted plasma," the predominant effect is the removal of NO and its neutralization of free radicals. Regardless of the physiologic relevance, the findings provide clear evidence that differences exist in the LDL fractions of plasma from normal and preeclamptic women.

Candidate Molecules Responsible for In Vitro Activation of Endothelial Cells

Our initial presumption when we found that serum or plasma from preeclamptic women altered endothelial cell function was that a single factor was responsible.

Further investigation into this hypothesis has shown this not to be the case. Preliminary characterization of the effects of plasma from preeclamptic women to increase either prostaglandins or NO indicate that at least two different activities are present. The activity responsible for stimulating PGI_2 in bovine microvascular endothelial cells persisted after charcoal stripping or lipoprotein removal, partitioned to the aqueous fraction, and had an approximate molecular weight of 50 kDa. In contrast, the factors stimulating NO production in these cells were extractable by charcoal, partitioned to lipid extracts and lipoprotein fractions, and had an apparent molecular weight greater than 1.5 million Da.[147] Attempts to further purify and identify these factors are in progress. The question of how these activities relate to altered endothelial function in vivo also remains to be answered.

CANDIDATE PLASMA FACTORS RESPONSIBLE FOR ENDOTHELIAL CELL ACTIVATION IN VIVO

Efforts to identify the putative circulating toxic factors responsible for endothelial cell dysfunction in preeclampsia have been ongoing for the past decade. While specific candidates have been identified, little data support a single molecular species accounting for endothelial injury. Because of their direct contact with the vascular endothelial cell monolayer in vivo, a variety of plasma constituents are likely candidates for endothelial cell activation in preeclampsia. Soluble proteins (e.g., anti-endothelial antibodies and cytokines), lipids and lipid peroxides, formed blood elements (e.g., platelets and neutrophils), placental membrane microvesicles, and some heavy metals all have been identified in the plasma of women with preeclampsia. In the following sections, we discuss postulated mediators of endothelial cell activation in preeclampsia.

IMMUNE COMPLEXES: ANTIPHOSPHOLIPID AND ANTI-ENDOTHELIAL CELL ANTIBODIES

As preeclampsia occurs more commonly in primigravidas[150] and in women with underlying collagen–vascular diseases[151] an immunologic component has long been suspected. The studies of Brosens et al.[26] and Kitzmiller and Benirschke[27] demonstrated histologic changes in the placental beds of women with preeclampsia that resemble those of acute allograft rejection, a concept consistent with an immunologic role in the pathogenesis, and supported by the results of several epidemiologic studies.[28,152-157]

Elevated levels of IgG or IgM antibodies to cardiolipin and phosphatidylserine were detected in 11 of 100 women diagnosed with preeclampsia in the third trimester compared to only 3 of 100 controls ($P < 0.05$). These findings suggest that antiphospholipid antibodies may play a pathogenic role in some women with preeclampsia.[158] In a recent case-control study, the prevalence of antineutrophil cytoplasmic autoantibodies was significantly increased in preeclamptic and eclamptic subjects compared to normal controls.[159]

Of the antiphospholipid antibodies noted in preeclampsia, those associated with beta-2-glycoprotein I appear to be the most relevant. In a study involving 1125 pregnant women, 50% of the beta-2-glycoprotein I-dependent anticardiolipin-positive patients and 4% of the anticardiolipin-negative patients experienced preeclampsia ($P < 0.001$). By contrast, beta-2-glycoprotein I-independent anticardiolipin antibodies did not show any significant association with adverse pregnancy outcomes.[160]

Rodgers et al.[123] postulated that immune complexes might be involved in this process, but were unsuccessful in detecting specific endothelial cell antigens by Western blotting with sera from preeclamptic women. However, using a more sensitive ELISA, Rappaport et al.[161] observed elevated serum concentrations of antiendothelial cell antibodies more commonly in women with severe preeclampsia than in normal controls. Subsequent studies have confirmed the presence of antiphospholipid antibodies and lupus anticoagulant in some women with preeclampsia.[57,159-161] Recent data suggest that anticardiolipin antibodies may be directed against oxidized phospholipids or beta-2-glycoprotein I, which calls into question their ability to directly alter cellular function.[162]

CYTOKINES

Tumor Necrosis Factor-Alpha as a Mediator of Endothelial Cell Activation in Preeclampsia

Prime candidates for the putative circulating endothelium-activating molecules in preeclampsia are the soluble, immunoactive proteins known as cytokines. Among these, tumor necrosis factor-alpha (TNF-α) fulfills several criteria as a mediator of endothelial cell dysfunction in preeclampsia. It was shown by Dr. Susan Fisher and her colleagues at the University of California, San Francisco, that this cytokine is a major secretory product of purified cytotrophoblast cells exposed to hypoxic conditions in vitro (personal communication), and this observation has been confirmed in villous explants.[163] Elevated concentrations of immunoactive TNF-α have been observed in the blood of women with preeclampsia.[164-166] Biological activities of TNF-α are relevant to prior observations in preeclampsia, including activation of endothelial cells, stimulation of platelet-derived growth factor production and mitogenic activity,[81,128] and the induction of glomerular endothelial damage in the rabbit.[167]

Tumor necrosis factor-α also has been shown to activate type II phospholipase A_2 (PLA_2) and prostanoid biosynthesis in a variety of cultured cells.[168,169] Thus, increased concentrations of PLA_2 in placental homogenates from women with preeclampsia[170] and elevated plasma concentrations of type II PLA_2 in severe preeclamptics[145] may be responses to increased TNF-α action in these women. Complicating these observations are recent reports that concentrations of soluble, p55 TNF-α receptor, a TNF-α binding protein and potential inhibitor of TNF-α action, also are increased in preeclampsia serum.[165,171]

Interleukin (IL)-2, a pleiotropic cytokine produced by activated T-lymphocytes, has potent autocrine and paracrine effects. Its ability to stimulate T cell, B cell, and natural killer cell mitogenesis and activity have led investigators to believe that excessive IL-2 action may be involved in the pathogenesis of preeclampsia. Normal maternal serum inhibits IL-2 production during pregnancy.[172] In a preliminary report, decidua from 3 of 3 primiparous preeclamptics showed intense IL-2 immunostaining, while decidua from 5 of 5 control primiparas had negative IL-2 signals. These data suggest enhanced immune activation in cases of preeclampsia.[173]

Circulating plasma concentrations of IL-1 receptor antagonist, an inhibitor of IL-1 action, and IL-6 were increased in concentration by 77% and 24%, respectively, in preeclamptics compared to normal pregnant controls.[15] It was suggested that these increased cytokine concentrations might contribute to the endothelial damage associated with preeclampsia. Other cytokines, including granulocyte-macrophage colony stimulating factor (GM-CSF), granulocyte colony stimulating factor (G-CSF), IL-1, and IL-8 in maternal blood and amniotic fluid have been associated with preeclampsia with intrauterine growth restriction (IUGR).[174]

CIRCULATING LIPIDS AND LIPOPROTEINS

An association between maternal obesity and increased risk of developing preeclampsia was confirmed in a large, prospective, NIH-sponsored clinical study of preeclampsia.[150] The overall incidence of preeclampsia in an otherwise healthy, nulliparous population whose prepregnancy weight was less than 20% above the desired body weight was 4.0%, whereas the incidence in patients whose body weight was greater than 20% above the desired body weight was 9.7%. The physiologic hyperlipidemia of pregnancy is reflected in elevated concentrations of several lipid and lipoprotein components.[175] Preeclamptic women manifest further elevations of plasma lipids.[176] An alternative mechanism to the increased production of lipoproteins in preeclampsia is a reduction in the clearance of these particles. Murata et al.[177] observed that the steady-state levels of mRNA encoding very low density lipoprotein (VLDL)-receptor and LDL-receptor were significantly lower in third trimester placentas from preeclamptic pregnancies compared to placentas from normal pregnancies. However, this finding may reflect end-stage placental dysfunction rather than a primary placental synthetic deficiency in preeclampsia.

Although total serum polyunsaturated fatty acid concentrations in normal pregnant women are not different from those in nonpregnant women, nonesterified fatty acid (NEFA) concentrations are elevated in preeclamptic pregnancies; in some studies this has been observed months before the clinical recognition of disease.[178,179]

Due to their intrinsic toxicity and the ability of unsaturated NEFA to form free radicals, evolution has directed the development of a variety of tight regulatory controls of NEFA concentrations. While tissue and blood levels of NEFA are normally very low, a marked increase in intracellular fatty acid flux is observed in some inborn errors of mitochondrial fatty oxidation. One of these syndromes, associated with a hemizygous G to C point mutation at nucleotide 1528 of the α-subunit of the long-chain hydroxyacyl dehydrogenase gene, is associated with acute fatty liver of pregnancy.[180] Preliminary studies from the University of California at San Francisco indicate that the prevalence of heterozygous carriers of this mutation is not more common in preeclampsia.[181]

Increased serum lipolytic activity may be one of the causes of higher concentrations of NEFA in preeclamptic patients. Endresen et al.[182] identified increased lysophospholipase activity in preeclampsia. This enzyme catalyzes the cleavage of a second fatty acid from a phospholipid that already has released one fatty acid moiety. Preliminary evidence indicates that deported placental syncytiotrophoblast microvillous membranes may be a source of lysophospholipase in the maternal circulation.[183] Sattar et al.[184] detected increased concentrations of hepatic lipase in the blood of women with preeclampsia compared to normal pregnant women.

Another relevant activity of known placental origin is the pregnancy hormone human placental lactogen (hPL). This hormone is reported to have lipolytic activities on maternal adipose cells[185] and is believed to liberate free fatty acids via growth hormone-receptor activation and enhanced sensitivity to endogenous catecholamines.[186] In a nested case-control study of matched preeclamptic and normal pregnant women, maternal and fetal modulators of lipid metabolism were associated with pregnancy outcome. Maternal body mass index, triglyceride, and NEFA concentrations all were increased significantly in women who developed preeclampsia ($P < 0.01$). Human placental lactogen also was found to be elevated in women with preeclampsia ($P < 0.01$). By contrast, hemoglobin levels were not statistically different between the two groups of women, indicating that the increased plasma lipids and hPL were not a result of hemoconcentration in the preeclamptic patients.[187] Elevated concentrations of hPL in primiparous preeclamptic women confirm the findings of Obiekwe et al.[188]

The role of sympathetic tone also may be important in lipolysis and the generation of circulating free fatty acids. A recent study demonstrated that sympathetic nerve activity in skeletal muscle blood vessels was increased more than threefold in women with preeclampsia relative to normal pregnant and nonpregnant controls.[189]

We, along with others, have suggested that endothelial cell toxicity may be caused by circulating VLDL particles[190] or other lipids.[191] As emphasized by Dekker and van Geijn, the VLDL/toxicity preventing albumin (TxPA) hypothesis and the imbalance between free radicals and scavengers appear to be most amenable to clinical intervention.[192]

A family with two cases of severe preeclampsia–eclampsia was found to have very high levels of Lp(a) lipoprotein. As the serum concentration of Lp(a) lipoprotein is genetically determined and the Lp(a) apolipoprotein has a close homology to plasminogen, very high levels of Lp(a) lipoprotein might interfere with fibrinolytic/thrombolytic processes. Very high Lp(a) lipoprotein levels could represent a genetically determined risk factor for preeclampsia.[193]

The dyslipidemia of preeclampsia is quite similar to that present in atherosclerosis.[194] In addition to markedly elevated triglycerides and fatty acids and reduced high density lipoprotein (HDL),[195] preeclamptic women manifest higher concentrations of VLDL[190] and small, dense LDL.[184] The latter are posited to be an important target for oxidative modification with subsequent effects on endothelial function.

FREE RADICALS AS CAUSAL FACTORS OF ENDOTHELIAL CELL DYSFUNCTION IN PREECLAMPSIA

Free radicals have been implicated in the pathogenesis of several diseases including preeclampsia.[196-198] This concept is discussed in detail Chapter 14 by Hubel and Roberts.

The elevated concentrations of free fatty acids in the circulation of women with preeclampsia provide substrate for lipid peroxidation. As detailed below, the generation of lipid peroxides and reactive oxygen intermediates has been proposed as a mechanism inducing endothelial cell injury in preeclampsia. Products of lipid peroxidation also can serve as in vivo indicators of excessive lipid peroxidation in women with the syndrome. Isoprostanes are metabolic products of arachidonic acid that are generated by nonenzymatic oxidative catalysis in situ. These lipids are biologically active vasoconstrictors in vivo. Barden et al.[199] used 8-isoprostane as a biomarker of lipid peroxidation in vivo. Plasma free, total, and urinary 8-isoprostane levels were measured in 20 preeclamptic women and compared to 18 age- and gestation-matched pregnant control subjects. Plasma free 8-isoprostane was significantly elevated in the preeclamptic women before delivery, and fell to control levels postpartum. Urinary 8-isoprostane excretion was significantly lower in the preeclamptic women compared with control subjects during pregnancy, suggesting that renal clearance of 8-isoprostane is impaired in preeclampsia. The data are consistent with increased lipid peroxidation, increased phospholipase A_2 activity,[145] and/or a reduction in renal 8-isoprostane clearance in the pathogenesis of preeclampsia. Other evidence of oxidative stress in preeclampsia includes increased blood and tissue concentrations of stable metabolites of the reactive oxygen species, lipid peroxides. It is also well recognized that these highly reactive molecules can have striking adverse effects on lipids and proteins with which they come in contact.[197] The specific effect of oxidatively modified lipids is felt to be important in the pathogenesis of the endothelial alterations associated with atherosclerosis.[200] A major point is that there is precedence for alteration of endothelial cell function by oxidative stress and dyslipidemia identical to that occurring in preeclampsia. In addition, these effects are interrelated with other pathophysiologic changes present in preeclampsia. Thus, TNF-α, which is increased in the blood of preeclamptic women, acts synergystically with oxidized LDL to increase expression of endothelial antigens that recruit inflammatory cells and stimulate them to release free radicals.[201] These findings raise the exciting possibility that reactive oxygen species, which might be countered by antioxidant therapy, are responsible for the endothelial cell injury of preeclampsia. However, the complexity of oxidant–antioxidant interactions can potentially have adverse effects as cautioned in Chapter 14.

FORMED ELEMENTS IN BLOOD AS ACTIVATORS OF ENDOTHELIUM

Platelets

In vitro evidence of abnormal platelet aggregation has been described in women with preeclampsia[202] and is discussed in detail in Chapter 10. There is extensive evidence of altered platelet function in preeclampsia antedating clinically evident disease.[203] It is reasonable to posit that altered platelets may interact with vascular endothelium to alter endothelial cell function.

Attempts to modify platelet function with aspirin initially appeared to support a role of platelet abnormalities in the genesis of preeclampsia.[204] Unfortunately, with the exception of the study by Hauth et al.,[205] other large trials of unselected pregnant women indicate that this antiplatelet drug has minimal effects on the incidence of preeclampsia.[206,207] These included groups of women at similar risk to those who benefitted in the earlier studies. However, other pharmacologic approaches for reducing adverse platelet–endothelium interaction may have some promise. These include selective thromboxane-A_2 synthase and thromboxane-A_2 receptor antagonists, serotonin 2-receptor blockers, hirudin, and ticlopidine.[208]

The platelet-specific nitric oxide donor S-nitrosoglutathione was administered to 10 women with severe preeclampsia at 21 to 33 weeks' gestation. Significant, dose-dependent reductions in mean arterial pressure and uterine artery resistance indices were observed. Platelet activation, as measured by P-selectin expression, also was decreased by S-nitrosoglutathione treatment. Thus, platelet-specific nitric oxide donors may prove beneficial in the management of severe preeclampsia.[209] As well, activated platelets may be one of the circulating factors in preeclampsia that mediate maternal endothelial cell activation.

Neutrophils

Neutrophil activation was studied in 20 eclamptic and 10 preeclamptic patients and compared to 10 normotensive controls. Plasma concentrations of neutrophil elastase were increased significantly in eclamptic and preeclamptic women ($P < 0.01$). Elastase values in cases of eclampsia were highly correlated with mean blood pressures, serum ET-1 levels, and cytotoxicity, measured by fura-2 release from HUVE cell cultures.[127] Lactoferrin also has been used as an indicator of neutrophil activation in normal and preeclamptic pregnancy. A comparative study between 40 normal and 42 preeclamptic women in the third trimester of pregnancy demonstrated that predelivery ratios of lactoferrin per neutrophil were higher in preeclamptic than in normal women.[210]

These and other data suggest that neutrophil activation plays a role in this syndrome.[211] Using a sophisticated whole blood cytometric analysis, recent data support this hypothesis. Studena et al.[212] observed an increase in leukocyte surface-antigen expression in normal pregnancy relative to nonpregnant women, and a further increase in activation-antigen expression in cells from preeclamptic pregnancies. In contrast, eosinophils do not appear to play a compelling role in preeclampsia.[213] Activation of neutrophils could provide a link between oxidative stress in the placenta and the maternal systemic vasculature. Neutrophils, activated by oxidative stress, passing through the intervillous space could generate free radicals at the endothelial surface.

PLACENTAL MEMBRANE MICROVESICLES

Circulating syncytiotrophoblast microvesicles have been postulated as endothelial toxic factors derived from the placenta.[214] Syncytiotrophoblast vesicles alter endothelial cell function in vitro, and these same syncytiotrophoblast microvillous membranes have been shown to induce ultrastructural endothelial cell injury and abnormal vasotone in isolated human arteries.[42] Although vesicles prepared from placentas of preeclamptic and normal women had similar activity on endothelial function, the concentration of microvillous membranes is greater in the blood of preeclamptic women.[215]

HEAVY METALS AS ENDOTHELIAL CELL TOXINS?

A complex of cadmium and the metal-binding protein, metallothionein has been proposed as a toxic serum factor associated with preeclampsia. Metallothionein-bound cadmium can be mobilized from the liver into the serum during pregnancy. In other conditions, the manifestations of cadmium toxicity closely mimic the manifestations of toxemia (i.e., hypertension, proteinuria, edema, and endovasculitis).[216] Further investigations into this and other heavy metals may cast new light on the elusive "toxin(s)" associated with preeclampsia.

Deficiency of metal cations also has been implicated in the pathogenesis of preeclampsia. A number of studies suggests that calcium supplementation, particularly in populations with dietary insufficiency, can decrease the incidence of hypertension in pregnancy.[217] A recent, large-scale, randomized, placebo-controlled trial was conducted by the NIH and enrolled > 4500 US nulliparas between 11 and 21 weeks' gestation. The findings showed no effects of 2 g/day of supplemented elemental calcium on the incidence of preeclampsia or other adverse pregnancy outcomes at delivery.[218]

CONCLUSION

Current evidence suggests that the pathogenesis of preeclampsia involves circulating plasma constituents that can induce endothelial cell activation and/or dysfunction. Given our understanding of the epidemiology of this disease, it is highly probable that the placenta contributes to the plasma factors responsible for endothelial cell dysfunction (Fig. 12–4). In addition, considerable evidence suggests that maternal constitutional factors also are involved. It is possible that interactions between initiating events (e.g., relative placental ischemia, secretion of cytokines, and embolization of syncytiotrophoblast membranes) and maternal constitutional factors (e.g., genetic disposition, antioxidant reserves, total body fat, and circulat-

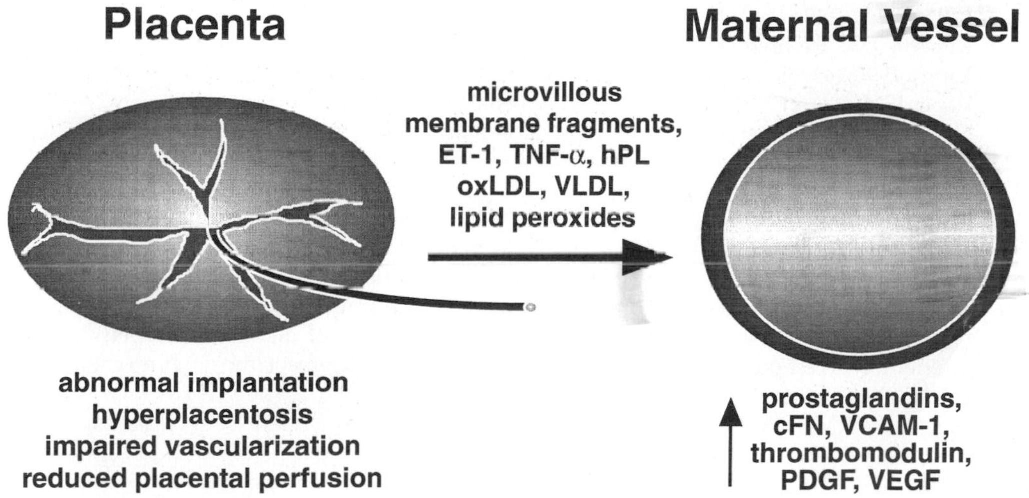

Placenta   **Maternal Vessel**

microvillous
membrane fragments,
ET-1, TNF-α, hPL
oxLDL, VLDL,
lipid peroxides

abnormal implantation
hyperplacentosis
impaired vascularization
reduced placental perfusion

prostaglandins,
cFN, VCAM-1,
thrombomodulin,
PDGF, VEGF

Figure 12–4. Proposed model of preeclampsia pathogenesis. We propose that compromised implantation, hyperplacentosis, and/or impaired placental bed vascularization result in the functional reduction of placental perfusion. In response to this ischemic and/or hypoxic state, these placentae secrete or elaborate into the maternal circulation factors that directly or indirectly cause systemic vascular endothelial cell dysfunction. Possible candidates for such translational factors include placental microvillous membrane fragments, endothelin-1 (ET-1), tumor necrosis factor-α (TNF-α), human placental lactogen (hPL), oxidized LDL (oxLDL), VLDL, and lipid peroxides. Activation of the systemic maternal vascular endothelium appears to result in increased secretion of vasopressors, procoagulants, cell adhesion molecules, and growth and permeability factors (e.g., prostaglandins [PGs], fibronectin [cFN], VCAM-1, thrombomodulin, PDGF, and VEGF). This model provides a framework for the development of experimentally testable hypotheses for future investigations into the preeclampsia syndrome.

ing lipoproteins) ultimately give rise to endothelial cell dysfunction, culminating in the maternal syndrome of preeclampsia. Effective treatment and prevention of this syndrome ultimately will require a fuller understanding of the etiology of preeclampsia.

REFERENCES

1. Lever JCW: Cases of puerperal convulsions, with remarks. *Guy's Hosp Reports* 1843;1: 495–517.
2. Cook HW, Briggs JB: Clinical observations on blood pressure. *Johns Hopkins Hosp Rep* 1903;11:452–534.
3. Young J: Recurrent pregnancy toxaemia and its relation to placental damage. *Trans Edinburgh Obstet Soc* 1927;47:61–76.
4. Schneider CL: The active principle of placental toxin: Thromboplastin; and its inactivator in blood: Antithromboplastin. *Am J Physiol* 1947;149:123–129.
5. Bell ET: Renal lesions in the toxemias of pregnancy. *Am J Pathol* 1932;8:1–42.
6. Spargo BH, Lichtig C, Luger AM, et al: The renal lesion in preeclampsia: Examination by light-, electron- and immunofluorescence-microscopy. In: Lindheimer MD, Katz AI, Zuspan FP, eds. *Hypertension in Pregnancy.* New York: Wiley; 1976:129–137.
7. Jaffe EA: Cell biology of endothelial cells. *Hum Pathol* 1987;18:234–239.
8. de Groot CJ, Taylor RN: New insights into the etiology of pre-eclampsia. *Ann Med* 1993;25:243–249.
9. Roberts JM, Redman CW: Pre-eclampsia: More than pregnancy-induced hypertension. *Lancet* 1993;341:1447–1451.
10. Pober JS, Cotran RS: Cytokines and endothelial cell biology. *Physiol Rev* 1990;70:427–451.
11. Nachman RL, Silverstein R: Hypercoagulable states. *Ann Intern Med* 1993;119:819–827.
12. Resnick N, Gimbrone MAJ: Hemodynamic forces are complex regulators of endothelial gene expression. *FASEB J* 1995;9:874–882.
13. Namiki A, Brogi E, Kearney M, et al: Hypoxia induces vascular endothelial growth factor in cultured human endothelial cells. *J Biol Chem* 1995;270:31189–31195.
14. Berk BC, Alexander RW, Brock TA, et al: Vasoconstriction: A new activity for platelet-derived growth factor. *Science* 1986;232:87–90.
15. Greer IA, Lyall F, Perera T, et al: Increased concentration of cytokines interleukin-6 and interleukin-1 receptor antagonist in plasma of women with preeclampsia: A mechanism for endothelial dysfunction? *Obstet Gynecol* 1994;84:937–940.
16. Bukowski RM: Thrombotic thrombocytopenic purpura: A review. *Prog Hemostat Thromb* 1982;6:287–337.
17. Weiner CP: Thrombotic microangiopathy in pregnancy and the postpartum period. *Semin Hematol* 1987;24:119–129.
18. Chen YC, McLeod B, Hall ER, et al: Accelerated prostacyclin degradation in thrombotic thrombocytopenic purpura. *Lancet* 1981;2:267–269.
19. Khong TY, Sawyer IH, Heryet AR: An immunohistologic study of endothelialization of uteroplacental vessels in human pregnancy: Evidence that endothelium is focally disrupted by trophoblast in preeclampsia. *Am J Obstet Gynecol* 1992;167:751–756.
20. Zhou Y, Damsky CH, Fisher SJ: Preeclampsia is associated with failure of human cytotrophoblasts to mimic a vascular adhesion phenotype. One cause of defective endovascular invasion in this syndrome? *J Clin Invest* 1997;99:2152–2164.
21. Zeek PM, Assali NS: Vascular changes in the decidua associated with eclamptogenic toxemia. *Am J Clin Pathol* 1950;20:1099–1109.
22. Nadji P, Sommers SC: Lesions of toxemia in first trimester pregnancies. *Am J Clin Pathol* 1973;59:344–348.
23. De Wolf F, Robertson WB, Brosens I: The ultrastructure of acute atherosis in hypertensive pregnancy. *Am J Obstet Gynecol* 1975;123:164–174.

24. Raines EW, Ross R: Smooth muscle cells and the pathogenesis of the lesions of atherosclerosis. *Br Heart J* 1993;69:S30–S37.

25. Roberts JM, Taylor RN, Musci TJ, et al: Preeclampsia: An endothelial cell disorder. *Am J Obstet Gynecol* 1989;161:1200–1204.

26. Brosens IA, Robertson WB, Dixon HG: The role of the spiral arteries in the pathogenesis of preeclampsia. *Obstet Gynecol Annu* 1972;1:177–191.

27. Kitzmiller JL, Benirschke K: Immunofluorescent study of placental bed vessels in preeclampsia of pregnancy. *Am J Obstet Gynecol* 1973;115(2):248–251.

28. Taylor RN: Review: Immunobiology of preeclampsia. *Am J Reprod Immunol* 1997;37:79–86.

29. Lichtig C, Deutsch M, Brandes J: Immunofluorescent studies of the endometrial arteries in the first trimester of pregnancy. *Am J Clin Pathol* 1985;83:633–636.

30. Bower S, Schuchter K, Campbell S: Doppler ultrasound screening as part of routine antenatal scanning: Prediction of pre-eclampsia and intrauterine growth retardation. *Br J Obstet Gynaecol* 1993;100:989–994.

31. Sheehan HL, Lynch JB: *Pathology of Toxaemia of Pregnancy.* London: Churchill, 1973.

32. Shanklin DR, Sibai BM: Ultrastructural aspects of preeclampsia. II. Mitochondrial changes. *Am J Obstet Gynecol* 1990;163:943–953.

33. Gant NF, Daley GL, Chand S, et al: A study of angiotensin II pressor response throughout primigravid pregnancy. *J Clin Invest* 1973;52:2682–2689.

34. Kyle PM, Buckley D, Kissane J, et al: The angiotensin sensitivity test and low-dose aspirin are ineffective methods to predict and prevent hypertensive disorders in nulliparous pregnancy. *Am J Obstet Gynecol* 1995;173:865–872.

35. Belfort M: Doppler assessment of retinal blood flow velocity during parenteral magnesium treatment in patients with preeclampsia. *Magnesium Res* 1993;6:239–246.

36. Watson KV, Moldow CF, Ogburn PL, et al: Magnesium sulfate: Rationale for its use in preeclampsia. *Proc Natl Acad Sci USA* 1986;83:1075–1078.

37. Branch DW, Dudley DJ, LaMarche S, et al: Sera from preeclamptic patients contain factor(s) that stimulate prostacyclin production by human endothelial cells. *Prostaglandins Leuko Essen Fatty Acids* 1992;45:191–195.

38. Pascoal I, Umans J: Effect of pregnancy on mechanisms of relaxation in human omental microvessels. *Hypertens* 1996;28:183–187.

39. McCarthy AL, Woolfson RG, Raju SK, et al: Abnormal endothelial cell function of resistance arteries from women with preeclampsia. *Am J Obstet Gynecol* 1993;168:1323–1330.

40. Pascoal IF, Lindheimer MD, Nalbantian-Brandt C, Umans JG: *J Clin Invest* 1998;101:464–470.

41. Cockell AP, Poston L: Flow-mediated vasodilation is enhanced in normal pregnancy but reduced in preeclampsia. *Hypertension* 1997;30:247–251.

42. Cockell AP, Learmont JG, Smarason AK, et al: Human placental syncytiotrophoblast microvillous membranes impair maternal vascular endothelial function. *Br J Obstet Gynaecol* 1997;104:235–240.

43. Ashworth JR, Baker PN, Warren AY, et al: Plasma from pre-eclamptic women induces a functional change in myometrial resistance arteries. *J Soc Gynecol Invest* 1997;4(suppl 1):71.

43a. Roberts JM: Endothelial dysfunction in preeclampsia. *Sem Repro Endocrinol* 1998;16:5–15.

44. Remuzzi G, Marchesi D, Zoja C, et al: Reduced umbilical and placental vascular prostacyclin in severe pre-eclampsia. *Prostaglandins* 1980;20:105–110.

45. Fitzgerald DJ, Entman SS, Mulloy K, et al: Decreased prostacyclin biosynthesis preceding the clinical manifestation of pregnancy-induced hypertension. *Circulation* 1987;75:956–963.

46. Taylor RN, Varma M, Teng NNH, et al: Women with preeclampsia have higher plasma endothelin levels than women with normal pregnancies. *J Clin Endocrinol Metab* 1990;71:1675–1677.

47. Nova A, Sibai BM, Barton JR, et al: Maternal plasma level of endothelin is increased in preeclampsia. *Am J Obstet Gynecol* 1991;165:724–727.

48. Lockwood CJ, Peters JH: Increased plasma levels of ED1+ cellular fibronectin precede the clinical signs of preeclampsia. *Am J Obstet Gynecol* 1990;162:358–362.

49. Taylor RN, Crombleholme WR, Friedman SA, et al: High plasma cellular fibronectin levels

correlate with biochemical and clinical features of preeclampsia but cannot be attributed to hypertension alone. *Am J Obstet Gynecol* 1991;165:895–901.

50. Hsu CD, Iriye B, Johnson TR, et al: Elevated circulating thrombomodulin in severe preeclampsia. *Am J Obstet Gynecol* 1993;169:148–149.

51. Kincaid-Smith P: Participation of intravascular coagulation in the pathogenesis of glomerular and vascular lesions. *Kidney Internat* 1975;7:242–253.

52. Spector AA: Lipid and lipoprotein effects on endothelial eicosanoid formation. *Semin Thromb Hemost* 1988;14:196–201.

53. Moncada S, Gryglewski R, Bunting S, et al: An enzyme isolated from arteries transforms prostaglandin endoperoxides to an unstable substance that inhibits platelet aggregation. *Nature* 1976;263:663–665.

54. Walsh SW, Wang Y, Jesse R: Peroxide induces vasoconstriction in the human placenta by stimulating thromboxane. *Am J Obstet Gynecol* 1993;169:1007–1012.

55. Walsh S, Wang Y: Trophoblast and placental villous core production of lipid peroxides, thromboxane, and prostacyclin in preeclampsia. *J Clin Endocrinol Metab* 1995;80:1888–1893.

56. Dizon-Townson DS, Nelson LM, Easton K, et al: The factor V Leiden mutation may predispose women to severe preeclampsia. *Am J Obstet Gynecol* 1996;175:902–905.

57. Lindoff C, Ingemarsson I, Martinsson G, et al: Preeclampsia is associated with a reduced response to activated protein C. *Am J Obstet Gynecol* 1997;176:457–460.

58. Dekker GA, de Vries JI, Doelitzsch PM, et al: Underlying disorders associated with severe early-onset preeclampsia. *Am J Obstet Gynecol* 1995;173:1042–1048.

59. Hsu CD, Copel JA, Hong SF, et al: Thrombomodulin levels in preeclampsia, gestational hypertension, and chronic hypertension. *Obstet Gynecol* 1995;86:897–899.

60. Paidas MJ, Taylor RN, Schwartzman H, et al: Third trimester type 1 and type 2 plasminogen activator inhibitor (PAI 1, PAI 2) levels are associated with preeclampsia. *Soc Gynecol Invest* 1994;148(abst).

61. Estelles A, Gilabert J, Espana F, et al: Fibrinolytic parameters in normotensive pregnancy with intrauterine fetal growth retardation and in severe preeclampsia. *Am J Obstet Gynecol* 1991;165:138–142.

62. Friedman SA, Schiff E, Emeis JJ, et al: Biochemical corroboration of endothelial involvement in severe preeclampsia. *Am J Obstet Gynecol* 1995;172:202–203.

63. Gao M, Nakabayashi M, Sakura M, et al: The imbalance of plasminogen activators and inhibitor in preeclampsia. *J Obstet Gynaecol Res* 1996;22:9–16.

64. Kanfer A, Bruch JF, Nguyen G, et al: Increased placental antifibrinolytic potential and fibrin deposits in pregnancy-induced hypertension and preeclampsia. *Lab Invest* 1996;74:253–258.

65. Shaarawy M, Didy HE: Thrombomodulin, plasminogen activator inhibitor type 1 (PAI-1) and fibronectin as biomarkers of endothelial damage in preeclampsia and eclampsia. *Int J Gynaecol Obstet* 1996;55:135–139.

66. Hynes RO: *Cell Biology of the Extracellular Matrix*. New York: Plenum Press; 1981:295–334.

67. Aznar-Salatti J, Bastida E, Buchanan MR, et al: Differential localization of von Willebrand factor, fibronectin and 13-HODE in human endothelial cell cultures. *Histochemistry* 1990; 93:507–511.

68. Forsyth KD, Levinsky RJ: Fibronectin degradation; an in-vitro model of neutrophil mediated endothelial cell damage. *J Pathol* 1990;161:313–319.

69. Lazarchick J, Stubbs TM, Romein L, et al: Predictive value of fibronectin levels in normotensive gravid women destined to become preeclamptic. *Am J Obstet Gynecol* 1986; 154:1050–1052.

70. Letowska M, Bykowska K, Sablinski J, et al: Venostasis but not DDAVP infusion provokes the plasma fibronectin increase. *Thrombos Haemostas* 1990;64:294–296.

71. Ogawa S, Shreeniwas R, Butura C, et al: Modulation of endothelial function by hypoxia: Perturbation of barrier and anticoagulant function, and induction of a novel factor X activator. *Adv Exp Med Biol* 1990;281:303–312.

72. Peters JH, Sporn LA, Ginsberg MH, et al: Human endothelial cells synthesize, process, and secrete fibronectin molecules bearing an alternatively spliced type III homology (ED1). *Blood* 1990;75:1801–1808.

73. Lyall F, Greer IA, Boswell F, et al: Suppression of serum vascular endothelial growth factor

immunoreactivity in normal pregnancy and in pre-eclampsia. *Br J Obstet Gynaecol* 1997; 104:223–228.

74. Krauss T, Kuhn W, Lakoma C, et al: Circulating endothelial cell adhesion molecules as diagnostic markers for the early identification of pregnant women at risk of developing preeclampsia. *Am J Obstet Gynecol* 1997;177:443–449.

75. Taylor RN, Musci TJ, Kuhn RW, et al: Partial characterization of a novel growth factor from the blood of women with preeclampsia. *J Clin Endocrinol Metab* 1990;70:1285–1291.

76. Varma M, de Groot C, Lanyi S, et al: Evaluation of plasma insulin-like growth factor-binding protein-3 as a potential predictor of preeclampsia. *Am J Obstet Gynecol* 1993;169: 995–999.

77. Lewitt MS, Scott FP, Clarke NM, et al: Developmental regulation of circulating insulin-like growth factor-binding proteins in normal pregnancies and in pre-eclampsia. *Prog Growth Factor Res* 1995;6:475–480.

78. de Groot CJM, O'Brien TJ, Taylor RN: Biochemical evidence of impaired trophoblastic invasion of decidual stroma in women destined to have preeclampsia. *Am J Obstet Gynecol* 1996;175:24–29.

79. Howell RJ, Economides D, Teisner B, et al: Placental proteins 12 and 14 in pre-eclampsia. *Acta Obstet Gynecol Scand* 1989;68:237–240.

80. Giudice LC, Martina NA, Crystal RA, et al: Insulin-like growth factor binding protein-1 at the maternal–fetal interface and insulin-like growth factor-I, insulin-like growth factor-II, and insulin-like growth factor binding protein-1 in the circulation of women with severe preeclampsia. *Am J Obstet Gynecol* 1997;176:751–757.

81. Taylor RN, Heilbron DC, Roberts JM: Growth factor activity in the blood of women in whom preeclampsia develops is elevated from early pregnancy. *Am J Obstet Gynecol* 1990;163: 1839–1844.

82. Dvorak HF, Brown LF, Detmar M, et al: Vascular permeability factor/vascular endothelial growth factor, microvascular hyperpermeability, and angiogenesis. *Am J Pathol* 1995;146: 1029–1039.

83. Baker PM, Krasnow J, Roberts JM, et al: Elevated serum levels of vascular endothelial growth X factor in patients with preeclampsia. *Obstet Gynecol* 1995;86:815–821.

84. Sharkey AM, Cooper JC, Balmforth JR, et al: Maternal plasma levels of vascular endothelial growth factor in normotensive pregnancies and in pregnancies complicated by pre-eclampsia. *Eur J Clin Invest* 1996;26:1182–1185.

85. Cooper JC, Sharkey AM, Charnock-Jones DS, et al: VEGF mRNA levels in placentae from pregnancies complicated by pre-eclampsia. *Br J Obstet Gynaecol* 1996;103:1191–1196.

86. Kuroki M, Voest EE, Amano S, et al: Reactive oxygen intermediates increase vascular endothelial growth factor expression in vitro and in vivo. *J Clin Invest* 1996;98:1667–1675.

87. Yanagisawa M, Kurihara H, Kimura S, et al: A novel potent vasoconstrictor peptide produced by vascular endothelial cells. *Nature* 1988;332:411–415.

88. Watanabe Y, Naruse M, Monzen C, et al: Is big endothelin converted to endothelin-1 in circulating blood? *J Cardiovasc Pharmacol* 1991;17:S503–S505.

89. Suzuki N, Matsumoto H, Kitada C, et al: A sensitive sandwich-enzyme immunoassay for human endothelin. *J Immunol Methods* 1989;118:245–250.

90. Molnár M, Hertelendy F: Pressor responsiveness to endothelin is not attenuated in gravid rats. *Life Sci* 1990;47:1463–1468.

91. Friedman SA, Taylor RN, Roberts JM: Pathophysiology of preeclampsia. *Clin Perinatol* 1991;18:661–682.

92. Bodelsson G, Sjoberg NO, Stjernquist M: Contractile effect of endothelin in the human uterine artery and autoradiographic localization of its binding sites. *Am J Obstet Gynecol* 1992;167:745–750.

93. Remuzzi G, Benigni A: Endothelins in the control of cardiovascular and renal function. *Lancet* 1993;342:589–593.

94. McMahon LP, Redman CW, Firth JD: Expression of the three endothelin genes and plasma levels of endothelin in pre-eclamptic and normal gestations. *Clin Sci* 1993;85: 417–424.

95. Wilkes BM, Susin M, Mento PF: Localization of endothelin-1-like immunoreactivity in human placenta. *J Histochem Cytochem* 1993;41:535–541.
96. Genbacev O, Joslin R, Damsky CH, et al: Hypoxia alters early gestation human cytotrophoblast differentiation/invasion in vitro and models the placental defects that occur in preeclampsia. *J Clin Invest* 1996;97:540–550.
97. Wiebke JL, Montrose-Rafizadeh C, Zeitlin PL, et al: Effect of hypoxia on endothelin-1 production by pulmonary vascular endothelial cells. *Biochim Biophys Acta* 1992;1134: 105–111.
98. Rust OA, Bofill JA, Zappe DH, et al: The origin of endothelin-1 in patients with severe preeclampsia. *Obstet Gynecol* 1997;89:754–757.
99. Ignarro LJ: Signal transduction mechanisms involving nitric oxide. *Biochem Pharmacol* 1991;195:485–490.
100. Davies MG, Fulton GJ, Hagen PO: Clinical biology of nitric oxide. *Br J Surg* 1995;82: 1598–1610.
101. Freeman BA, White CR, Gutierrez H, et al: Oxygen radical nitric oxide reactions in vascular diseases. *Adv Pharmacol* 1995;34:45–69.
102. Seligman SP, Buyon JP, Clancy RM, et al: The role of nitric oxide in the pathogenesis of preeclampsia. *Am J Obstet Gynecol* 1994;171:944–948.
103. Cameron IT, vanPapendorp CL, Palmer RMJ, et al: Relationship between nitric oxide synthesis and increase in systolic blood pressure in women with hypertension in pregnancy. *Hypertens Pregnancy* 1993;12:85–92.
104. Curtis NE, Gude NM, King RG, et al: Nitric oxide metabolites in normal human pregnancy and preeclampsia. *Hypertens Pregnancy* 1995;14:339–349.
105. Silver RK, Kupferminc MJ, Russell TL, et al: Evaluation of nitric oxide as a mediator of severe preeclampsia. *Am J Obstet Gynecol* 1996;175:1013–1017.
106. Roberts JM (letter): Plasma nitrites as an indicator of nitric oxide production: Unchanged production or reduced renal clearance in preeclampsia? *Am J Obstet Gynecol* 1997; 176:954–955.
107. Davidge S, Stranko C, Roberts J: Urine but not plasma nitric oxide metabolites are decreased in women with preeclampsia. *Am J Obstet Gynecol* 1996;174:1008–1013.
108. Begum S, Yamasaki M, Mochizuki M: Urinary levels of nitric oxide metabolites in normal pregnancy and preeclampsia. *J Obstet Gynaecol Res* 1996;22:551–559.
109. Brown MA, Tibben E, Zammit VC, et al: Nitric oxide excretion in normal and hypertensive pregnancies. *Hypertens Pregnancy* 1995;14:319–326.
110. Molnar M, Suto T, Toth T, et al: Prolonged blockade of nitric oxide synthesis in gravid rats produces sustained hypertension, proteinuria, thrombocytopenia, and intrauterine growth retardation. *Am J Obstet Gynecol* 1994;170:458–466.
111. Yallampalli C, Garfield RE: Inhibition of nitric oxide synthesis in rats during pregnancy produces signs similar to those of preeclampsia. *Am J Obstet Gynecol* 1993;169:1316–1320.
112. Buhimschi I, Yallampalli C, Chwalisz K, et al: Pre-eclampsia-like conditions produced by nitric oxide inhibition: Effects of L-arginine, D-arginine and steroid hormones. *Human Reprod* 1995;10:2723–2730.
113. Helmbrecht GD, Farhat MY, Lochbaum L: L-Arginine reverses the adverse pregnancy changes induced by nitric oxide synthase inhibition in the rat. *Am J Obstet Gynecol* 1996;175: 800–805.
114. Redman CWG, Beilin LJ, Denson KWE, et al: Factor-VIII consumption in pre-eclampsia. *Lancet* 1977;2:1249–1252.
115. Dadak C, Kefalides A, Sinzinger H, et al: Reduced umbilical artery prostacyclin formation in complicated pregnancies. *Am J Obstet Gynecol* 1982;144:792–795.
116. Huang SC, Chang FM: The adverse effect on fetal hemogram by preeclampsia: Marked anisocytosis with normocytic, normochromic erythrocythemia as well as thrombocytopenia. *Early Human Devel* 1994;37:91–98.
117. Davidge ST, Signorella AP, Lykins DL, et al: Evidence of endothelial activation and endothelial activators in cord blood of infants of preeclamptic women. *Am J Obstet Gynecol* 1996;175:1301–1306.

118. Friedman SA, Schiff E, Emeis JJ, et al: Fetal plasma levels of cellular fibronectin as a measure of fetal endothelial involvement in preeclampsia. *Obstet Gynecol* 1997;89:46–48.
119. Hennessy A, Phippard AF, Harewood WF, et al: Histomorphometry of the renal lesions in baboons with placental ischaemia. *Hypertens Pregnancy* 1993;12:302.
120. Combs CA, Katz MA, Kitzmiller JL, et al: Experimental preeclampsia produced by chronic reduction of uteroplacental pressure. *Am J Obstet Gynecol* 1993;169:215–223.
121. Glassberg MK, Nolop KB, Jackowski JT, et al: Microvascular and macrovascular endothelial cells produce different constrictor substances. *J Appl Physiol* 1992;72:1681–1686.
122. de Groot CJ, Chao VA, Roberts JM, et al: Human endothelial cell morphology and autacoid expression. *Am J Physiol* 1995;H1613–1620.
123. Rodgers GM, Taylor RN, Roberts JM: Preeclampsia is associated with a serum factor cytotoxic to human endothelial cells. *Am J Obstet Gynecol* 1988;159:908–914.
124. Tsukimori K, Maeda H, Shingu M, et al: The possible role of endothelial cells in hypertensive disorders during pregnancy. *Obstet Gynecol* 1992;80:229–233.
125. Roberts JM, Edep ME, Goldfien A, et al: Sera from preeclamptic women specifically activate human umbilical vein endothelial cells in vitro: Morphological and biochemical evidence. *Am J Reprod Immunol* 1992;27:101–108.
126. Endresen MJ, Tosti E, Lorentzen B, et al: Sera of preeclamptic women are not cytotoxic to endothelial cells in culture. *Am J Obstet Gynecol* 1995;172:196–201.
127. Halim A, Kanayama N, El Maradny E, et al: Correlated plasma elastase and sera cytotoxicity in eclampsia. A possible role of endothelin-1 induced neutrophil activation in preeclampsia–eclampsia. *Am J Hypertens* 1996;9:33–38.
128. Taylor RN, Musci TJ, Rodgers GM, et al: Preeclamptic sera stimulate increased platelet-derived growth factor mRNA and protein expression by cultured human endothelial cells. *Am J Reprod Immunol* 1991;25:105–108.
129. Folkman J: Clinical applications of research on angiogenesis. *N Engl J Med* 1995;333: 1757–1763.
130. Taylor RN, Casal DC, Jones LA, et al: Selective effects of preeclamptic sera on human endothelial cell procoagulant protein expression. *Am J Obstet Gynecol* 1991;165:1705–1710.
131. Siegler RL, Edwin SS, Christofferson RD, et al: Endothelin in the urine of chidren with the hemolytic uremic syndrome. *Pediatrics* 1991;88:1063–1066.
132. Levin M, Walters MDS, Waterfield MD, et al: Platelet-derived growth factor as possible mediators of vascular proliferation in the sporadic haemolytic uraemic syndrome. *Lancet* 1986;2:830–833.
133. Tonshoff B, Momper R, Schweer H, et al: Increased biosynthesis of vasoactive prostanoids in Schonlein–Henoch purpura. *Pediatr Res* 1992;32:137–140.
134. Redman CWG: Current topic: Pre-eclampsia and the placenta. *Placenta* 1991;12:301–308.
135. Suckfull MM, Pieske O, Mudsam M, et al: The contribution of endothelial cells to hyperacute rejection in xenogeneic perfused working hearts. *Transplantation* 1994;57: 262–267.
136. Vane JR, Botting RM: Formation by the endothelium of prostacyclin, nitric oxide and endothelin. *J Lipid Mediat* 1993;6:395–404.
137. Wang J, Zhen E, Guo Z, et al: Effect of hyperlipidemic serum on lipid peroxidation, synthesis of prostacyclin and thromboxane by cultured endothelial cells: Protective effect of antioxidants. *Free Rad Biol Med* 1989;7:243–249.
138. Baker PN, Davidge ST, Barankiewicz J, et al: Plasma of preeclamptic women stimulates and then inhibits prostacyclin. *Hypertens* 1996;27:56–61.
139. de Groot CJM, Murai JT, Vigne J-L, et al: Eicosanoid secretion by human endothelial cells exposed to normal pregnancy and preeclampsia plasma in vitro. *Prostaglandins Leuk Essen Fatty Acids* 1998;58:91–97.
140. Clark JD, Lin LL, Kriz RW, et al: A novel arachidonic acid-selective cytosolic PLA_2 contains a Ca(2+)-dependent translocation domain with homology to PKC and GAP. *Cell* 1991; 65:1043–1051.
141. Sharp JD, White DL: Cytosolic PLA_2: mRNA levels and potential for transcriptional regulation. *J Lipid Mediat* 1993;8:183–189.
142. Pernas P, Masliah J, Olivier JL, et al: Type II phospholipase A2 recombinant overexpression

enhances stimulated arachidonic acid release. *Biochem Biophys Res Commun* 1991;178: 1298–1305.

143. Murakami M, Kudo I, Inoue K: Molecular nature of phospholipases A2 involved in prostaglandin I2 synthesis in human umbilical vein endothelial cells. Possible participation of cytosolic and extracellular type II phospholipases A2. *J Biol Chem* 1993:268:839–844.

144. de Groot CJ, Davidge ST, Friedman SA, et al: Plasma from preeclamptic women increases human endothelial cell prostacyclin production without changes in cellular enzyme activity or mass. *Am J Obstet Gynecol* 1995;172:976–985.

145. Lim KH, Rice GE, deGroot CJ, et al: Plasma type II phospholipase A2 levels are elevated in severe preeclampsia. *Am J Obstet Gynecol* 1995;172:998–1002.

146. Davidge ST, Baker PN, Roberts JM: NOS expression is increased in endothelial cells exposed to plasma from women with preeclampsia. *Am J Physiol* 1995;269:1106–1112.

147. Davidge ST, Signorella AP, Hubel CA, et al: Distinct factors in plasma of preeclamptic women increase endothelial nitric oxide or prostacyclin. *Hypertens* 1996;28:758–764.

148. Hirata K, Miki N, Kuroda Y, et al: Low concentration of oxidized low-density lipoprotein and lysophosphatidylcholine upregulated constitutive nitric oxide synthase mRNA expression in bovine aortic endothelial cells. *Circ Res* 1995;76:958–962.

149. Rubbo H, Darley-Usmar V, Freeman BA: Nitric oxide regulation of tissue free radical injury. *Chem Res Toxicol* 1996;9:809–820.

150. Sibai BM, Gordon T, Thom E, et al: Risk factors for preeclampsia in healthy nulliparous women: A prospective multicenter study. The National Institute of Child Health and Human Development Network of Maternal–Fetal Medicine Units. *Am J Obstet Gynecol* 1995;172: 642–648.

151. Houser MT, Fish AJ, Tagatz GE, et al: Pregnancy and systemic lupus erythematosus. *Am J Obstet Gynecol* 1980;138:409–413.

152. Robillard PY, Hulsey TC, Alexander GR, et al: Paternity patterns and risk of preeclampsia in the last pregnancy in multiparae. *J Reprod Immunol* 1993;24:1–12.

153. Klonoff-Cohen HS, Savitz DA, Cefalo RC, et al: An epidemiologic study of contraception and preeclampsia. *JAMA* 1989;262:3143–3147.

154. Soderstrom-Anttila V, Hovatta O: An oocyte donation program with goserelin down-regulation of voluntary donors. *Acta Obstet Gynecol Scand* 1995;74:288–292.

155. Feeney JG, Tovey LA, Scott JS: Influence of previous blood-transfusion on incidence of pre-eclampsia. *Lancet* 1977;1:874–875.

156. Dekker GA: Oral tolarization to paternal antigens and preeclampsia. *Am J Obstet Gynecol* 1996;174:(abstr)450.

157. Robillard PY, Hulsey TC, Perianin J, et al: Association of pregnancy-induced hypertension with duration of sexual cohabitation before conception. *Lancet* 1994;344:973–975.

158. Allen JY, Tapia-Santiago C, Kutteh WH: Antiphospholipid antibodies in patients with preeclampsia. *Am J Reprod Immunol* 1996;36:81–85.

159. Shaarawy M, El-Mallah SY, El-Yamani AMA: The prevalence of serum antineutrophil cyto-plasmic autoantibodies in preeclampsia and eclampsia. *J Soc Gynecol Invest* 1997;4:34–39.

160. Katano K, Aoki A, Sasa H, et al: Beta 2-glycoprotein I-dependent anticardiolipin antibodies as a predictor of adverse pregnancy outcomes in healthy pregnant women. *Human Reprod* 1996;11:509–512.

161. Rappaport VJ, Hirata G, Yap HK, et al: Anti-vascular endothelial cell antibodies in severe preeclampsia. *Am J Obstet Gynecol* 1990;162:138–146.

162. Horkko S, Miller E, Branch DW, et al: The epitopes for some antiphospholipid antibodies are adducts of oxidized phospholipid and beta 2 glycoprotein 1 (and other proteins). *Proc Natl Acad Sci USA* 1997;94:10356–10361.

163. Benyo DF, Miles TM, Conrad KP: Hypoxia stimulates cytokine production by villous ex-plants from the human placenta. *J Clin Endocrinol Metab* 1997;82:1582–1588.

164. Meekins JW, McLaughlin PJ, West DC, et al: Endothelial cell activation by tumour necrosis factor-alpha (TNF-alpha) and the development of pre-eclampsia. *Clin Exp Immunol* 1994;98: 110–114.

165. Vince GS, Starkey PM, Austgulen R, et al: Interleukin-6, tumour necrosis factor and soluble

tumour necrosis factor receptors in women with pre-eclampsia. *Br J Obstet Gynaecol* 1995;102:20–25.

166. Kupferminc MJ, Peaceman AM, Wigton TR, et al: Fetal fibronectin levels are elevated in maternal plasma and amniotic fluid of patients with severe preeclampsia. *Am J Obstet Gynecol* 1995;172:649–653.

167. Bertani T, Abbate M, Zoja C, et al: Tumor necrosis factor induces glomerular damage in the rabbit. *Am J Pathol* 1989;134:419–430.

168. Jacobson PB, Schrier DJ: Regulation of CD11b/CD18 expression in human neutrophils by phospholipase A2. *J Immunol* 1993;151:5639–5652.

169. Pfeilschifter J, Schalkwijk C, Briner VA, et al: Cytokine-stimulated secretion of group II phospholipase A2 by rat mesangial cells. Its contribution to arachidonic acid release and prostaglandin synthesis by cultured rat glomerular cells. *J Clin Invest* 1993;92: 2516–2523.

170. Jendryczko A, Drózdz M: Increased placental phospholipase A_2 activities in pre-eclampsia. *Zentralbl Gynakol* 1990;112:889–891.

171. Opsjon SL, Novick D, Wathen NC, et al: Soluble tumor necrosis factor receptors and soluble interleukin-6 receptor in fetal and maternal sera, coelomic and amniotic fluids in normal and pre-eclamptic pregnancies. *J Reprod Immunol* 1995;29:119–134.

172. Domingo CG, Domenech N, Aparicio P, et al: Human pregnancy serum inhibits proliferation of T8-depleted cells and their interleukin-2 synthesis in mixed lymphocyte cultures. *J Reprod Immunol* 1985;8:97–110.

173. Hara N, Fujii T, Okai T, et al: Histochemical demonstration of interleukin-2 in decidua cells of patients with preeclampsia. *Am J Reprod Immunol* 1995;34:44–51.

174. Stallmach T, Hebisch G, Joller H, et al: Expression pattern of cytokines in the different compartments of the feto-maternal unit under various conditions. *Reprod Fertil Devel* 1995;7:1573–1580.

175. Potter JM, Nestel PJ: The hyperlipidemia of pregnancy in normal and complicated pregnancies. *Am J Obstet Gynecol* 1979;133:165–170.

176. Kaaja R, Tikkanen MJ, Viinikka L, et al: Serum lipoproteins, insulin, and urinary prostanoid metabolites in normal and hypertensive pregnant women. *Obstet Gynecol* 1995;85:353–356.

177. Murata M, Kodama H, Goto K, et al: Decreased very-low-density lipoprotein and low-density lipoprotein receptor messenger ribonucleic acid expression in placentas from preeclamptic pregnancies. *Am J Obstet Gynecol* 1996;175:1551–1556.

178. Lorentzen B, Drevon CA, Endresen MJ, et al: Fatty acid pattern of esterified and free fatty acids in sera of women with normal and pre-eclamptic pregnancy. *Br J Obstet Gynaecol* 1995;102:530–537.

179. Arbogast B, Leeper S, Merrick R, et al: Plasma factors that determine endothelial cell lipid toxicity in vitro correctly identify women with preeclampsia in early and late pregnancy. *Hypertens Pregnancy* 1996;15:263–279.

180. Sims HF, Brackett JC, Powell CK et al: The molecular basis of pediatric long chain 3-hydroxyacyl-CoA dehydrogenase deficiency associated with maternal acute fatty liver of pregnancy. *Proc Natl Acad Sci USA* 1995;92:841–845.

181. Burlingame J, Musci TJ, Taylor RN, et al: Long chain 3-acyl coA fatty acid dehydrogenase G1528C mutations: Association with acute fatty liver of pregnancy but not with preeclampsia. *J Soc Gynecol Invest* 1997;4 (suppl #1):667.

182. Endresen MJ, Lorentzen B, Henriksen T: Increased lipolytic activity of sera from pre-eclamptic women due to the presence of a lysophospholipase. *Scand J Clin Lab Invest* 1993;53: 733–739.

183. Endresen MJR, Morris J, Knight M, et al: Presence of lysophospholipase activity in placental syncytiotrophoblast microvillous membranes. *Int Soc Study Hypertens Pregnancy* 1997;21 (abstr).

184. Sattar N, Bendomir A, Berry C, et al: Lipoprotein subfraction concentrations in preeclampsia: Pathogenic parallels to atherosclerosis. *Obstet Gynecol* 1997;89:403–408.

185. Williams C, Coltart TM: Adipose tissue metabolism in pregnancy: The lipolytic effect of human placental lactogen. *Br J Obstet Gynaecol* 1978;85:43–46.

186. Marcus C, Bolme P, Micha-Johansson G, et al: Growth hormone increases the lipolytic sensitivity for catecholamines in adipocytes from healthy adults. *Life Sci* 1994;54:1335–1341.
187. Murai JT, Muzykanskiy E, Taylor RN: Maternal and fetal modulators of lipid metabolism correlate with the development of preeclampsia. *Metabolism* 1997;46:963–967.
188. Obiekwe B, Sturdee D, Cockrill BL, et al: Human placental lactogen in pre-eclampsia. *Br J Obstet Gynaecol* 1984;91:1077–1080.
189. Schobel HP, Fischer T, Heuszer K, et al: Preeclampsia: A state of sympathetic overactivity. *N Engl J Med* 1996;335:1480–1485.
190. Arbogast BW, Leeper SC, Merrick RD, et al: Which plasma factors bring about disturbance of endothelial function in pre-eclampsia? *Lancet* 1994;343:340–341.
191. Endresen MJ, Tosti E, Heimli H, et al: Effects of free fatty acids found increased in women who develop pre-eclampsia on the ability of endothelial cells to produce prostacyclin, cGMP and inhibit platelet aggregation. *Scand J Clin Lab Invest* 1994;54:549–557.
192. Dekker GA, van Geijn HP: Endothelial dysfunction in preeclampsia. Part I: Primary prevention. Therapeutic perspectives. *J Perinat Med* 1996;24:99–117.
193. Husby H, Roald B, Schjetlein R, et al: High levels of Lp(a) lipoprotein in a family with cases of severe pre-eclampsia. *Clin Genet* 1996;50:47–49.
194. Hubel CA, McLaughlin MK, Evans RW, et al: Fasting serum triglycerides, free fatty acids, and malondialdehyde are increased in preeclampsia, are positively correlated, and decrease within 48 hours postpartum. *Am J Obstet Gynecol* 1996;174:975–982.
195. Rosing U, Samsioe G, Olund A, et al: Serum levels of apolipoprotein A-I, A-II and HDL-cholesterol in second half of normal pregnancy and in pregnancy complicated by pre-eclampsia. *Horm Metab Res* 1989;21:376–382.
196. Sieron G, Jendryczko A, Drozdz M, et al: Plasma lipid peroxidation in pre-eclampsia. *Ginekol Pol* 1988;59:668–671.
197. Kehrer JP, Smith CV: Free radicals in biology: Sources, reactivities, and roles of etiology of human diseases. In: Frei B (ed.): *Natural Antioxidants in Human Health and Disease.* New York: Academic Press 1994.
198. Shatos MA, Doherty JM, Hoak JC: Alterations in human vascular endothelial cell function by oxygen free radicals. *Arterioscler Thromb* 1991;11:594–601.
199. Barden A, Beilin LJ, Ritchie J, et al: Plasma and urinary 8-iso-prostane as an indicator of lipid peroxidation in pre-eclampsia and normal pregnancy. *Clin Sci* 1996;91:711–718.
200. Segrest JP, Anantharamaiah GM: Pathogenesis of atherosclerosis. *Curr Opin Cardiol* 1994;9:404–410.
201. Haller H, Schaper D, Ziegler W, et al: Low-density lipoprotein induces vascular adhesion molecule expression on human endothelial cells. *Hypertension* 1995;25:511–516.
202. Ahlawat S, Pati HP, Bhatla N, et al: Plasma platelet aggregating factor and platelet aggregation studies in pre-eclampsia. *Acta Obstet Gynecol Scand* 1996;75:428–431.
203. Hutt R, Ogunniyi SO, Sullivan MH, et al: Increased platelet volume and aggregation precede the onset of preeclampsia. *Obstet Gynecol* 1994;83:146–149.
204. Collins R, Wallenburg HCS: Pharmacological prevention and treatment of hypertensive disorders in pregnancy. In: Chalmers I, Enkin M, Keirse MC, eds. *Effective Care in Pregnancy and Childbirth.* New York: Oxford University Press; 1992.
205. Hauth JC, Goldenberg RL, Parker CJ, et al: Low-dose aspirin therapy to prevent preeclampsia. *Am J Obstet Gynecol* 1993;168:1083–1091.
206. Sibai BM, Caritis SN, Thom E, et al: Prevention of preeclampsia with low-dose aspirin in healthy, nulliparous pregnant women. The National Institute of Child Health and Human Development Network of Maternal–Fetal Medicine Units. *N Engl J Med* 1993;329:1213–1218.
207. CLASP (Collaborative Low-Dose Aspirin Study in Pregnancy) Collaborative Group: A randomised trial of low-dose aspirin for the prevention and treatment of pre-eclampsia among 9364 pregnant women. *Lancet* 1994;343:619–629.
208. Dekker GA, van Geijn HP: Endothelial dysfunction in preeclampsia. Part II: Reducing the adverse consequences of endothelial cell dysfunction in preeclampsia; therapeutic perspectives. *J Perinat Med* 1996;24:119–139.
209. Lees C, Langford E, Brown AS, et al: The effects of S-nitrosoglutathione on platelet activa-

tion, hypertension, and uterine and fetal Doppler in severe preeclampsia. *Obstet Gynecol* 1996;88:14–19.

210. Rebelo I, Carvalho-Guerra F, Pereira-Leite L, et al: Comparative study of lactoferrin and other blood markers of inflammatory stress between preeclamptic and normal pregnancies. *Eur J Obstet Gynecol Reprod Biol* 1996;64:167–173.

211. Barden A, Graham D, Beilin LJ, et al: Neutrophil CD11b expression and neutrophil activation in pre-eclampsia. *Clin Sci* 1997;92:37–44.

212. Studena K, Sacks GP, Sargent IL, et al: Leucocyte phenotypic and functional changes in preeclampsia and normal pregnancy. Combined detection by whole blood flow cytometry. *J Soc Gynecol Invest* 1997;4(suppl):664(abstr).

213. Salafia CM, Ghidini A, Minior VK: Uterine allergy: A cause of preterm birth? *Obstet Gynecol* 1996;88:451–454.

214. Smarason AK, Sargent IL, Redman CWG: Endothelial cell proliferation is suppressed by plasma but not serum from women with preeclampsia. *Am J Obstet Gynecol* 1996;174: 787–793.

215. Smarason AK, Sargent IL, Starkey PM, et al: The effect of placental syncytiotrophoblast microvillous membranes from normal and pre-eclamptic women on the growth of endothelial cells in vitro. *Br J Obstet Gynaecol* 1993;100:943–949.

216. Chisolm JC, Handorf CR: Further observations on the etiology of pre-eclampsia: Mobilization of toxic cadmium-metallothionein into the serum during pregnancy. *Med Hypoth* 1996;47:123–128.

217. Carroli G, Duley L, Belizan JM, et al: Calcium supplementation during pregnancy: A systematic review of randomised controlled trials. *Br J Obstet Gynaecol* 1994;101:753–758.

218. Levine RJ, Hauth JC, Curet LB, et al: Trial of calcium to prevent preeclampsia. *N Engl J Med* 1997;337:69–76.

13

Genetic Factors

Kenneth Ward and Marshall D. Lindheimer

Current interest in the genetics of preeclampsia can be traced back to the signal study of Leon Chesley, who single-handedly followed the remote course of 267 women who survived eclampsia during the years 1931 through 1951. In the absence of a renal biopsy, a convulsion—especially in a primiparous hypertensive patient—strongly suggested that the clinical diagnosis of preeclampsia was correct. These patients were interviewed and reexamined periodically; the data from some women span more than 40 years after their eclamptic convulsion.[1] The parsimonious funding provided by the National Institutes of Health in the United States to complete the follow-up examinations would provoke smiles in relation to the research budgets for lesser projects in the 1990s. In the course of his evaluations, Dr. Chesley noted the increased occurrence of preeclampsia–eclampsia within families.[2] His observations and his reviews of other data that suggested familial factors are involved in the etiology of preeclampsia caught the attention of genetic investigators, who studied his original data set or who developed their own data to analyze the genetics of preeclampsia. With the advent of molecular genetics, this field is now advancing rapidly. This chapter, dedicated to the pioneering studies of Leon Chesley, summarizes research into the genetics of preeclampsia through 1998. A glossary of genetics terminology is provided in Table 13–1 for readers who are less familiar with genetic concepts.

BACKGROUND

Preeclampsia is familial. Some conditions "run in families" because of similar diet, habits, or environment, but published reports show that preeclampsia is a genetic disease. Analyses of affected families suggest that one or more relatively common alleles act as "major genes" conferring susceptibility to preeclampsia. It is unlikely that any particular genotype is necessary for the disease to occur; rather, these "preeclampsia genes" act as susceptibility loci that lower a woman's threshold for developing preeclampsia.

TABLE 13–1. GLOSSARY OF GENETIC TERMINOLOGY

Alleles: Alternative forms of a genetic locus; a single allele for each locus is inherited separately from each parent.

Centimorgan (cM): A unit of measure of recombination frequency. One centimorgan is equal to a 1% chance that a marker at one genetic locus will be separated from a marker at a second locus due to crossing over in a single generation. In humans, 1 centimorgan is equivalent, on average, to 1 million base pairs.

Gene expression: The process by which gene-coded information is converted into structural proteins and enzymes. Expressed genes are transcribed into mRNA and then translated into protein and those that are transcribed into RNA but not translated into protein (e.g., transfer and ribosomal RNAs).

Gene map: The linear arrangement (relative positions) of genetic sites (mutations, variants, polymorphisms, express sequence tags [ESTs]) on a chromosome as deduced from genetic recombination, fluorescence in situ hybridization [FISH], or physical mapping experiments. A gene map usually expresses the distance, in linkage units or physical units, between sites.

Haploid: A single set of chromosomes (half the full set of genetic material), as present in the egg and sperm cells.

Heterogeneity: The production of identical or similar phenotypes by different genetic mechanisms.

Heterozygosity: The presence of different alleles at one or more loci on homologous chromosomes.

Incomplete penetrance: The gene for a condition is present, but not obviously expressed in all individuals who carry the gene.

Linkage map: A map of the relative positions of genetic loci on a chromosome, determined on the basis of how often the loci are inherited together. Distance is measured in centimorgans (cM).

Locus (*pl.* loci): The position on a chromosome of a gene or other chromosome marker; also, the DNA at that position. The use of locus is sometimes restricted to mean regions of DNA that are expressed. See *Gene expression,* above.

LOD score: Logarithm of the odd score; a measure of the likelihood of two loci being within a measurable distance of each other.

Marker: An identifiable physical location on a chromosome (e.g., restriction enzyme cutting site, gene), the inheritance of which can be monitored. Markers can be expressed regions of DNA (genes) or some segment of DNA with no known coding function, the inheritance pattern of which can be determined. Markers must have a clearcut phenotype; they are used as a point of reference when mapping new mutants.

Multifactorial: A characteristic influenced in its expression by many factors, both genetic and environmental.

Mutation: Any heritable change in DNA sequence or the process by which genes undergo a structural change.

Nucleotide: One of the monomeric units from which DNA or RNA polymers are constructed; consists of a purine or pyrimidine base, a pentose sugar, and a phosphoric acid group.

Physical map: A map of the locations of identifiable landmarks on DNA (e.g., restriction enzyme cutting sites, genes), regardless of inheritance. Distance is measured in base pairs.

Polygenic disorders: Genetic disorders resulting from the combined action of alleles of more than one gene (e.g., heart disease, diabetes, and some cancers). Although such disorders are inherited, they depend on the simultaneous presence of several alleles; thus the hereditary patterns are usually more complex than those of single-gene disorders.

Polymerase chain reaction (PCR): A method of amplifying a DNA base sequence using a heat-stable polymerase and two short DNA primers (usually about 20 base pairs), one complementary to the $(+)$-strand at one end of the sequence to be amplified and the other complementary to the $(-)$-strand at the other end. Because the newly synthesized A strands can subsequently serve as additional templates for the same primer sequences, successive rounds of primer annealing, strand elongation, and dissociation produce rapid and highly specific amplification of the desired sequence. PCR can also be used to detect the existence of the defined sequence in a DNA sample.

TABLE 13–1. (Continued)

Polymorphism: Difference in DNA sequence among individuals. Genetic variations occurring in more than 1% of a population would be considered useful polymorphisms for genetic linkage analysis.

Predisposition: In this case, an increased likelihood, or an advanced tendency toward, a specific medical condition.

Probe: Single-stranded DNA labeled with radioactive isotopes or tagged in other ways for ease in identification.

Promoter: A site on DNA to which RNA polymerase will bind and initiate transcription.

Recessive: A gene that is phenotypically manifest in the homozygous state but is masked in the presence of a dominant allele.

Recombination: The process by which offspring derive a combination of genes different from that of either parent. In higher organisms, this can occur by crossing over.

Repeat sequences: The length of a nucleotide sequence that is repeated in a tandem cluster.

Sequence tagged site (STS): Short (200–500 base pairs) DNA sequence that has a single occurrence in the human genome, the location and base sequence of which are known. Detectable by polymerase chain reaction, STSs are useful for localizing and orienting the mapping and sequence data reported from many different laboratories and serve as landmarks on the developing physical map of the human genome.

Single-gene disorder: Hereditary disorder caused by a mutant allele of a single gene (e.g., cystic fibrosis, myotonic dystrophy, sickle-cell disease).

Transgenic organism: One into which a cloned genetic material has been experimentally transferred; a subset of those foreign genes express themselves in their offspring.

While the ultimate causes of preeclampsia remain unknown, it is perhaps obvious that genes should play a role. As discussed in other chapters of this book, many investigators feel that preeclampsia occurs when there is a mismatch between the maternal blood supply and the fetal or placental demands for nutrition and oxygen. Placental ischemia results and various circulating mediators are released directly into the maternal circulation. The maternal endothelium and arterioles respond, initially in an adaptive manner, but ultimately causing profound dysfunction of various major organs. If this hypothesis is correct, any number of disorders, many of which are genetically determined, might interfere with maternal vascular responses, affect trophoblast function, or increase the placental mass causing fetal demands to outpace the supply. Every ligand, every receptor, every amplification cascade, every aspect of the programmed responses which orchestrate the pathophysiologic response is under the control of either the genes of the mother or the fetus.

Regardless of the theory invoked, mutant genes in any of dozens of pathways could affect a woman's risk of developing preeclampsia. Indeed, as noted below, preeclampsia is best understood as a multifactorial, polygenic condition. Many of the aberrant genes will be "private" mutations, affecting one woman or only a handful of women; however, any mutation identified that affects a woman's risk may give us new insights into the pathophysiologic cascade or lead to a treatment that is applicable to all women. A more exciting outcome from genetic studies of preeclampsia would be the discovery of a gene that has a critical role and that is common enough in the population to have epidemiologic importance. A common predisposing mutation might allow predictive testing or suggest a treatment that is widely applicable. Fortunately, modern molecular techniques promise discovery of both rare and common alleles that contribute to this serious complication of pregnancy.

PROBLEMS WITH THE STUDY OF PREECLAMPSIA GENES

Unfortunately, preeclampsia is a difficult "phenotype" to study using genetic methodologies. The diagnostic signs are nonspecific. Although preeclampsia may be a fairly homogeneous entity when it is defined by glomerular endotheliosis—the unique histopathologic feature of the condition—we are forced to depend on other criteria. The blood pressure and proteinuria criteria in common use depend upon arbitrary cutoffs along a continuous distribution of values. The normal reference ranges for blood pressure and proteinuria also vary with respect to measurement protocols, gestational age, and ethnic background. Even if perfect diagnostic criteria existed, there is a great deal of debate about what the proper phenotype is for study, whether it is proteinuric hypertension, gestational hypertension, a placental phenotype such as reduced placental invasion, a renal phenotype such as glomerular endotheliosis, and so forth. As discussed elsewhere in this text, given the multisystem nature of the disease, perhaps too much attention has been focused on "hypertension;" alternative case definitions may prove highly informative for genetic and other etiologic investigations.

A major lesson of modern genetics is that syndromes defined on the basis of clustering of clinical symptoms often reveal marked heterogeneity once they are understood at a molecular level. In this respect, the boundaries around preeclampsia, gestational hypertension, and hemolysis, elevated liver enzymes, and low platelets ("HELLP" syndrome) are likely to be redrawn when genetic determinants can be examined directly. Proceeding from genes to biological or clinical manifestations or "phenotypes" constitutes a radical alternative in the logic of scientific inference.

Studies of the genetics of preeclampsia have been hampered by a number of factors. Pregnancy is obviously a sex-limited trait and the expression of any preeclampsia allele is further limited to women who become pregnant. Males presumably do not manifest a phenotype when they carry the susceptibility gene. The age of onset of the condition is delayed until the reproductive years. Prior to the last few generations, record-keeping in obstetrics was extremely limited; the shift to hospitalized birth in many developed countries being a recent phenomenon. Also, expression of the gene can be interrupted by appropriate medical care or early delivery. The gene may be extremely common with spouses bringing the gene into pedigrees frequently, and there is probably genetic heterogeneity. For most of human history, eclampsia was frequently a fatal disease for mother, child, or both. The available data suggest that eclampsia was probably as common as preeclampsia is today; therefore, a large percentage of cases must have been due to new mutations without a familial pattern. No convincing animal model of preeclampsia exists and there are numerous difficulties in identifying and collecting human families. Finally, genetic studies of pregnancy disorders have an additional complexity since either the genotype of the mother, or the fetus, or an interaction between the two can be important.

FAMILY REPORTS

The first suspicions that preeclampsia is a genetic disease came from reports of familial clustering. The numerous, early case series have been summarized by Chesley et al.[3] Elliott was the first to report familial incidence of eclampsia over 125 years ago in 1873. He reported a woman who died of eclampsia during her fifth pregnancy. Three of her four daughters subsequently died of eclampsia as well. The older reports discuss only eclampsia, since "pre-" eclampsia could not be recognized until roughly 150 years ago when it became possible to check for proteinuria. Indirect (clinical) blood pressure measurements have only been possible for the last 100 years, and the recognition that proteinuric, pregnancy-induced hypertension is preeclampsia occurred shortly thereafter. It was several decades after the familial nature of eclampsia was observed before it was recognized that preeclampsia is familial as well.

Perhaps the first systematic study of the genetics of preeclampsia was presented in 1960 by Humphries, who studied mother-daughter pairs delivering at the Johns Hopkins Hospital[4] (Table 13–2). The disease occurred in 28% of the daughters of the women who had preeclampsia compared with 13% of the comparison group. As noted above, Chesley's remarkable study was well underway in the 1960s: having already reported data on the pregnancies of the daughters, daughters in law, and sisters of the eclamptic probands, he was about to publish data on the granddaughters and granddaughters-in-law.[3] Remarkably persistent in this effort, Dr. Chesley was able to find information on 96% of all the daughters, greatly reducing the possibility of ascertainment bias. The index cases had all delivered at the Margaret Hague Hospital in New Jersey, but women in the subsequent generations delivered at hospitals throughout the United States. The quality

TABLE 13–2. FAMILY CLUSTERING IN PREECLAMPSIA

1st Author	Year	Comments
Humphries[4]	1960	Studied mother-daughter pairs
Adams F[5]	1961[a]	Noted increased preeclampsia in sisters of preeclamptics
Chesley[3]	1968	Compared pregnancies of daughters and granddaughters of eclamptics to daughters- and granddaughters-"in-law"
Cooper[6]	1979[a]	Focused on "severe" preeclampsia
Sutherland[7]	1981[a]	Noted increased preeclampsia in mothers and daughters of preeclamptics
Arngrimson[8]	1990	Noted increased rate of preeclampsia in mothers and daughters of preeclamptics

[a] These three groups studied the record from the Aberdeen Maternity Hospital in Scotland.

of the available records varied, so it is not certain that all of these patients had proteinuric hypertension. Chesley and his collaborators found that the rate of preeclampsia was higher in the mothers, sisters, daughters, and granddaughters of probands with preeclampsia. The rate of preeclampsia was not significantly increased in the in-laws of these probands.

Another large body of information comes from the Aberdeen Maternity Hospital in Scotland. Adams and Finlayson in 1961,[5] Cooper and Liston in 1979,[6] and Sutherland et al. in 1981,[7] studied this population. These studies were unique because of the consistent classification system and recording of births through several decades. Sisters of preeclamptic women had a 2.5- to 3.4-fold increase in the rate of preeclampsia compared with controls. Mothers of preeclamptic women were four times more likely to have had preeclampsia than mothers of controls. In one study, the rate of preeclampsia was 16% in mothers of probands, 4.4% in mothers-in-law, and 3.5% in mothers of controls.[7]

More recently, Arngrimsson et al. has studied the Icelandic population.[8] Because of the small population of this country, the emphasis on genealogic knowledge, and the concentration of maternity records at only one hospital, relatively complete information was available on the relatives of the index cases with preeclampsia. According to the Arngrimsson study, the recurrence risk for preeclampsia in the daughters of either eclamptic or preeclamptic mothers is in the 20 to 40% range; for sisters it is in the 11 to 37% range. Much lower rates are seen in relatives by marriage, such as daughters-in-law and mothers-in-law.

TWIN STUDIES

Once there is a suspicion that a disorder is genetic, twin studies can be used to measure the heritability of the condition (the proportion of the occurrence due to genetic factors as opposed to environmental factors). Interestingly, little such information has been published for eclampsia. The only two studies we could locate involve a total of only ten monozygotic twin pairs.[9,10] Sophisticated zygosity tests were not performed to prove the twins were monozygotic and it is not certain that both twins had the same opportunity to develop preeclampsia. These authors found that none of the ten twin pairs were concordant for the development of preeclampsia, suggesting very low heritability. These data are inconsistent with all the other segregation data. Alternatively, these twin studies imply that the penetrance of any preeclampsia gene must be less than 30%. Again, this is inconsistent with the family data. Clearly, there remains a need for a larger, carefully performed twin study.

CONSANGUINITY STUDIES

Another classic approach to estimating heritability is to examine consanguineous families. Unfortunately, few consanguinity studies have been published, and all suffer problems with methodology. In 1976, Stevenson et al. conducted a study in Turkey, where one-fifth of all the deliveries are consanguineous.[11] Using clinical definitions that are probably too inclusive, they found that the incidence of "toxemia" was decreased when the couple was consanguineous. In 1992, George et al. published a study examining pregnancy outcomes in 814 primigravida women in South India.[12] Twenty-six percent of these pregnancies were believed to be consanguineous. They studied all gestational hypertension, and not proteinuric preeclampsia specifically. Most of the marriages were either cousin–cousin or uncle–niece. They found the odds of preeclampsia were 1.12 in consanguineous couples compared to nonconsanguineous couples with a confidence interval of 0.72 to 1.75.

SEGREGATION ANALYSES

Segregation analyses attempt to fit the recurrence risk data from the family studies to a genetic model. Several segregation analyses have been published with varying conclusions. Some authors favor a recessive gene hypothesis, others suggest there is a maternal and fetal genotype interaction, while the most recent analysis suggests that preeclampsia is a polygenic trait with a strong maternal factor. All of these models predict that a very common allele is necessary to explain the observed inheritance of preeclampsia.

Liston and Kilpatrick examined six simple Mendelian models of inheritance and rejected all except the one in which both mother and fetus must express the same recessive gene to confer susceptibility.[13] They considered this model to be consistent with the putative association with HLA-DR4.

Based on segregation analysis, Cooper et al.[14] hypothesized that a single recessive gene can determine susceptibility to preeclampsia, but they could not determine whether the gene acts in the mother or in the fetus. The analysis by Sutherland et al. suggested that the fetal genotype played, at most, a minor role in the development of preeclampsia.[7] In the most extensive segregation study to date, Chesley and Cooper[15] analyzed data over a 50-year period on the incidence of preeclampsia and eclampsia in the sisters, daughters, granddaughters, and daughters-in-law of eclamptic probands. They felt their data were most consistent with a single-gene, autosomal-recessive model, with affected women being homozygous for a putative preeclampsia gene at a frequency of 0.25. They subsequently modified this hypothesis[14] to include a possible role for the fetal genotype.

Recently, Arngrimsson et al.[8] studied the segregation of preeclampsia in three- and four-generation families among the Icelandic population. The families were descended from index women who were delivered in the years 1931 through 1947 and who had either eclampsia or severe preeclampsia. Inheritance was followed through both sons and daughters. The authors were unable to distinguish between autosomal-recessive inheritance, which had a gene frequency of 0.31, and autosomal-dominant inheritance with 48% penetrance and a predicted gene frequency of 0.14. No model was rejected when the disease allele was allowed to be common. Because the number of granddaughters tested was small, precise inferences could not be drawn. The authors concluded that a major dominant gene model with a low penetrance or multifactorial inheritance are the best working hypotheses at present. Of course, segregation analyses can never prove a model, they can only reject an alternative model. Certainly, the available data reject the hypothesis that there are no genes involved.

In the aggregate, these segregation analyses are consistent with a relatively common allele acting as a "major gene" conferring susceptibility to preeclampsia. The marked increase in the incidence of preeclampsia in blood relatives but not in relatives by marriage implies that maternal genes are more important than fetal genes. It is possible that a maternal–fetal gene interaction is involved (analogous with rhesus incompatibility) as Kalmus[16] and Penrose[17] proposed over 50 years ago.

One alternative not adequately addressed in these models is a very high new mutation rate (as would be expected for a common but deadly condition). Chesley has reviewed the recorded history of eclampsia and it is clear that mortality from eclampsia was high until the last few generations. Given a high lethality, it is unclear how a preeclampsia gene would become so common in the population. With the exception of one report describing a gorilla pedigree with "preeclampsia," there seems to be no evidence that preeclampsia occurs in our recent primate ancestors.[18] Usually the only way a lethal gene will stay common in the population is if there are frequent new mutations or if the gene is positively selected for on some other basis. Both of these are possibilities in preeclampsia.

It is impossible to determine from segregation analyses whether every family has the same gene involved or a private mutation. Stated another way, it is unclear whether there are only a few preeclampsia-causing alleles common in the population, or whether new mutations are frequent, potentially creating thousands of disease-associated alleles in dozens of critical genes involved in the pathophysiologic cascade. To differentiate between these two models, we will need to find the genes involved.

ASSOCIATION STUDIES

A number of genetic-association studies have been published. These studies are relatively easy to perform: DNA samples are collected from cases and controls, then educated guesses are made about a gene which may be involved. Polymorphisms or, preferably, functional variants of the "candidate gene" are assayed in both populations and chi-square comparisons are tested. Unfortunately, these simple studies often lead to false conclusions as spurious associations can arise due to hidden biases. If performed carefully, positive data can point to a factor as being either a predisposing or causative gene, or a marker linked to such a gene (linkage disequilibrium). Association studies cannot prove biologic causation.

Associations with Maternal Genes (Table 13–3)

Methylenetetrahydrofolate Reductase

The 677T variant of the methylenetetrahydrofolate-reductase (MTHFR) gene has been identified as a risk factor for vascular disease. Sohda et al. tested whether the 677T polymorphism of the MTHFR gene is associated with preeclampsia.[19] They found an increased 677T allele frequency and a greater percentage of the 677T homozygous genotype in patients as compared with controls. Grandone et al. found a similar association; but the frequency of the 677T allele was higher in the Italian population than the Japanese.[20] Powers et al. and Ward et al. did not find an association with preeclampsia in either the Pittsburgh population or the Utah population, respectively (unpublished data).

Tumor Necrosis Factor-Alpha

Elevated concentrations of tumor necrosis factor-alpha (TNF-α) have been reported in both the plasma and amniotic fluid of patients with severe preeclampsia and intrauterine growth restriction. Recently, the TNF T2 mutation in the promoter region at position −308 in the TNF-α gene was shown to be associated with both higher constitutive and inducible levels of TNF-α gene transcription.[21] Chen et al. studied the TNF T1/T2 polymorphism and TNF-α expression in preeclampsia.[22] They evaluated TNF-α mRNA expression in 14 patients meeting "ACOG criteria" compared to 12 normal pregnant women and 15 normal nonpregnant women. First, they found 8/14 (57.1%) patients with preeclampsia were homozygous for the TNF T1 allele, 4/14 (28.6%) were heterozygous for TNF T1, and one (7.1%) was homozygous for the TNF T2 allele. Second, they observed that TNF-α mRNA expression was significantly higher ($P < 0.05$) in the group that was homozygous for the TNF T1 allele. The findings of an increase in the T1 allele associated with preeclampsia conflicts with the in vitro data showing an increased transcrip-

TABLE 13–3. ASSOCIATION OF PREECLAMPSIA WITH OTHER GENETIC CONDITIONS

1st Author	Year	Association
Brockhuizen[30]	1983	Triploidy (+)
Boyd J[29]	1987	Trisomy 13 (+)
Feinberg[31]	1991	Trisomy 13 (+)
Arngrimsson[24]	1994	Renin gene variant (−)
McCowan[32]	1994	Bechwith–Wiedemann syndrome (+)
Chen[22]	1996	Tumor necrosis factor-α polymorphism (+)
Dizon-Townson[23]	1996	Tumor necrosis factor polymorphism ( )
Folgero[25]	1996	Mitochondrial transfer ribonucleic acid genes (+)
Sohda[19]	1997	Methylenetetrahydrofolate reductase variant (+)[a]
Grandone[20]	1997	Methylenetetrahydrofolate (+)

(+) = association
(−) = no association
[a] Two groups including this chapter's first author have unpublished observations in variance with these associations (see text).

tion of the T2 allele. Dizon-Townson et al. did not find an allelic association in a larger series.[23]

Renin

Arngrimsson et al.[24] investigated linkage between a renin gene variant, and excluded this alteration of the renin gene in pregnancy as being directly responsible for the manifestations of preeclampsia or eclampsia in these families.

Mitochondrial

Folgero et al. studied two families with a high incidence of preeclampsia and eclampsia.[25] Several affected women in each pedigree had mitochondrial mutations in regions coding for transfer ribonucleic acids. Similar point mutations underlie other systemic diseases. Maternal inheritance would be observed in such pedigrees. Clearly, other families need to be examined for mitochondrial mutations.

Associations with Fetal Genes

As mentioned above, many investigators believe fetal genes, or an interaction between maternal and fetal genes, may be involved in the pathophysiology of preeclampsia. If fetal genes are involved, a paternal effect should be seen in families. There have been several reports of a paternal or fetal genetic effect.[26,27] For example, Astin et al., at the University of Utah, reported a man who lost two consecutive wives to eclampsia.[28] His third wife was also affected with severe preeclampsia. The observation that preeclampsia is extremely common in a molar pregnancy (in which all the fetal chromosomes are derived from the father) is considered further evidence of the role of paternal genes. In the segregation analyses described above, Cooper et al. found an increased rate of preeclampsia if the proband's own mother was eclamptic with their pregnancy.[14] Arngrimsson et al. found a small increase in the incidence of preeclampsia in the daughters-in-law of women who had gestational hypertension.[8]

A number of genetic conditions, when present in the fetus, have been associated with preeclampsia. Triploidy or complete hydatidiform mole, trisomy 13, long-chain 3-hydroxyacyl CoA dehydrogenase (LCAHD) deficiency, congenital adrenal hypoplasia, and Beckwith–Weidemann syndrome in the fetus have all been associated with an increased risk of preeclampsia or eclampsia in the mother.

Triploidy, although unusual in advanced gestations, frequently presents with preeclampsia.[29] The increase in paternal genetic material associated with the triploid-diandric placenta may support the role of paternal genes in the development of preeclampsia. As above, hydatidiform moles that also have two sets of paternal chromosomes can cause a preeclampsia-like illness.[30] Trisomy 13 is likely to cause abnormal trophoblastic invasion and suboptimal placental function. In at least one report, biopsy of the placental bed taken immediately after delivery of a trisomy 13 infant demonstrated inadequate trophoblastic remodeling of the maternal uterine vasculature, with an absence of normal physiologic changes in the spiral arteries.[31]

Beckwith–Weidemann Syndrome

This autosomal-recessive condition is due to mutations in the p57 gene on chromosome 11 that cause fetal and placental overgrowth. An association with preeclampsia has been described; it is postulated that fetal demands outstrip the normal maternal supply resulting in placental ischemia and ultimately, preeclampsia.[32]

Long Chain 3-Hydroxyacyl CoA Dehydrogenase (LCHAD) Deficiency

Treem et al. speculated that the hepatic pathology seen in acute fatty liver of pregnancy (AFLP) and HELLP syndrome is similar to that seen in inherited disorders of fatty acid oxidation LCHAD deficiency.[33] They evaluated 12 women previously diagnosed with AFLP or HELLP and found that 8 had reduced LCHAD activity consistent with the mother being heterozygous for an LCHAD deficiency allele.

LINKAGE ANALYSES

Several investigators are now studying the genetics of preeclampsia using powerful new approaches. Among those being tried are positional cloning using affected families and affected sibling pairs, examination of candidate genes in genetic association studies (as above), and substractive hybridization of placentas from preeclamptic and normal pregnant patients.

Linkage studies require an accurate diagnosis of the disease under study and precise histories of family relationships among the study participants. Furthermore, linkage analysis of pedigrees requires that the appropriate model is used in the logarithm of the odd (LOD) score analysis. Markers are tested in families studied to find any violations of Mendel's second law, which states that independent traits segregate independently. Whenever two independent traits are closely located on the same chromosome, Mendel's second law is violated. These aberrations from independent segregation can be used to map the chromosomal location of a disease gene by comparing these markers with the other chromosomes. Thus far, four linkage analyses have focused on candidate regions and two have taken a more general approach (Table 13–4). Wilton et al.[34] and Cooper et al.[35] excluded several candidate regions in the first reports of linkage studies.

In 1993, Arngrimsson et al.[36] typed 22 Icelandic preeclamptic pedigrees for a dinucleotide repeat marker at the angiotensinogen (AGT) locus. Using the affected pedigree method, they found significant allele sharing in family members, implying close linkage. Arngrimsson has followed up this finding with a genome-wide linkage search suggesting linkage on chromosome 1 (personal communication).

Hayward et al. were the first to perform a more generalized search; they looked at 35 two-generation families, ten of which only contained one affected individual.[37] Assuming that preeclampsia is due to a relatively common recessive

TABLE 13–4. LINKAGE ANALYSIS OF PATIENTS WITH PREECLAMPSIA

1st Author	Year	Model	Type	Results
Wilton[34]	1990, 1991	AR	Candidate	HLA region excluded
Cooper[35]	1993	AR	Candidate	1q32, 14q32–33 excluded
Hayward[37]	1992	AR	General	25% of genome excluded
Arngrinssom[36]	1993	NP	Candidate	Linkage with AGT
Harrison[38]	1997	Various	General	Linkage with 4q
Arngrinssom[39]	1997	Various	Candidate	Linkage with 7q36

AR = autosomal-recessive
NP = nonparametric

gene acting in the mother with complete penetrance, they examined 43 markers and published a preliminary exclusion map.

Harrison et al. published their results of a genome-wide linkage study of preeclampsia–eclampsia families.[38] There were 15 informative pedigrees used in this analysis. After typing 90 polymorphic DNA markers, they found a 2.8-cM candidate region between D4S450 and D4S610 on 4q. Because of uncertainties concerning inheritance and diagnosis, four different inheritance models were used to carry out LOD-score analysis. The maximum multipoint LOD score within this interval was barely significant at 2.9. Analysis of markers in the region using the affected pedigree member method also supported the possibility of a susceptibility locus in this region.

Most recently, Arngrinssom et al. examined markers on 7q36 in the region of the endothelial isoform of nitric oxide synthase (eNOS).[39] They reported an LOD score over 3 for this region. Follow-up studies are underway.

PROMISING CANDIDATE GENES

Factor V Leiden

Factor V Leiden is a missense mutation that prevents normal degradation of activated factor V.[40] Normally, inactivation of factor Va occurs through enzymatic cleavage (by activated protein C) at Arg506, which subsequently allows exposure and cleavage at Arg306. However, factor V Leiden molecules have a glutamine substituted for arginine at position 506, and they are, therefore, resistant to degradation in this way.[41] Because factor V Leiden molecules retain their procoagulant activity, patients are predisposed to thromboembolic disorders. Indeed, this mutation is associated with over 60% of thromboembolic complications which occur in pregnancy.[41,42]

Two to seven percent of the population carries the Leiden mutation. Dekker and Van Geijn studied the related phenotype (activated protein C [APC] resistance) and found that 16% of patients with severe, early-onset, pregnancy-induced hypertension show APC resistance.[43] They studied a Dutch population and used a very broad definition for the hypertensive disorder under study (i.e., 39% of their patients had chronic hypertension and 53% had the HELLP syndrome). Brenner et al. observed two patients with the HELLP syndrome who were heterozygous for the factor V Leiden mutation, suggesting that the pathogenesis of HELLP syndrome is associated with an underlying thrombophilia.[44]

In 1997, Rotmensch et al. reported on seven patients with recurrent early pregnancy losses, intrauterine fetal deaths, intrauterine growth restriction, and early severe preeclampsia.[45] All had resistance to APC. Six patients were heterozygous for the Leiden mutation, and one patient was homozygous. Dizon-Townson et al., using strict criteria for severe preeclampsia found that 14/158 (8.9%) gravidas with severe preeclampsia were heterozygous for the Leiden mutation, a rate double the carrier rate (4.2%) in the 403 normotensive gravid controls.[23]

How can a gene responsible for thrombophilia lead to preeclampsia? The primary author's group at the University of Utah hypothesizes that low-pressure intervillous blood flow in the presence of a maternal hypercoaguable state and trophoblast dysfunction may trigger excessive fibrin deposition in the placenta. In turn, trophoblast and placental infarction occur, frequent features of preeclamptic pathophysiology. Indeed, when Dizon-Townson et al. studied a series of placentas with large infarcts (greater than 10% of the placental mass), there was a greater than tenfold increase in the factor V Leiden carrier rate. The odds ratio (OR) with 95% confidence intervals (CI) calculated was 37.24 (10.98 < OR < 130.43).[46]

Grandone et al. also performed a case-control study to investigate whether the factor V Leiden mutation is associated with the occurrence of preeclampsia in 96 otherwise healthy preeclamptic women and 129 parous controls.[20] There were ten factor V Leiden carriers among the cases (10.5%), and three among the controls (2.3%) (OR = 4.9, [95%] CI – 1.3–18.3).

If this association is present in other populations, DNA analysis for the factor V Leiden mutation may serve as a component of a genetic screening test for a variety of obstetric complications, including preeclampsia. Carriers of this common thrombophilic mutation need to be identified, since they and their family members are at risk for thromboembolic disease with surgical procedures, immobilization, oral contraceptive use, future pregnancies, hormone replacement therapy, etc. Studies are underway to determine whether antithrombotic therapy can lower the risk of preeclampsia in women with the factor V Leiden mutation.

Angiotensinogen (Table 13–5)

By three sets of observations—genetic linkage, allelic associations, and differences in plasma angiotensinogen concentrations among AGT genotypes—Jeunemaitre et al. demonstrated involvement of the T235 variant of the AGT gene in essential hypertension.[47] It is uncertain whether the T235 variant directly mediates a predisposition to hypertension, or an unidentified risk factor is associated with the T235 haplotype.

If molecular variants of AGT predispose to essential hypertension, then several

TABLE 13–5. STUDIES OF FACTOR V LEIDEN AS A CANDIDATE GENE FOR PREECLAMPSIA

1st Author	Year	Approach
Dekker[43]	1992[a]	APC resistance, case control
Dizon-Townson[23]	1996	Case control
Rotmensch[45]	1997	Case series
Grandone[20]	1997	Case control
Dizon-Townson[46]	1997	Placental infarction

[a] 1992 citation in ref 43 (1995).

arguments can be advanced to postulate a similar implication in preeclampsia: (1) plasma angiotensinogen is elevated in estrogenic states; (2) the relative hypo-volemia of preeclampsia suggests an abnormality in the control of extracellular fluid volume; and, (3) the renin–angiotensin–aldosterone axis is frequently per-turbed in preeclamptic patients.

In a series of Caucasian women with carefully defined preeclampsia and eth-nically matched controls, Ward et al. observed significant association of preeclamp-sia with the M235T variant.[48] The finding was corroborated in a sample ascertained in Japan. Following this initial report, Arngrimsson et al. reported a sibling pair analysis on 22 multigeneration families from Iceland and Scotland in which they found that the tendency to develop preeclampsia is linked to the dinucleotide-repeat polymorphism in the AGT gene.[36] Significant allele sharing was observed in both the Icelandic (T = 3.16 P = 0.006) and the Scottish (T = 2.20 P = 0.026) preeclamptic families.

Hemolysis, elevated liver function tests, and low platelets (the HELLP syn-drome) is frequently associated with preeclampsia, but evidence is mounting that this syndrome is not a simple subset of severe preeclampsia. HELLP syndrome can occur without hypertension or proteinuria, and as a rule usually presents earlier in gestation than other forms of severe preeclampsia. Patients are more likely to be older, Caucasian, and multiparous. Laboratory abnormalities in HELLP syndrome tend to worsen for the first 24 to 48 hours postpartum, while the signs of preeclampsia improve rapidly. In fact, 20% of published HELLP syndrome cases have a postpartum onset. The T235 allele is not a risk factor for the HELLP syn-drome, so the primary author's group at the University of Utah excludes these pa-tients when studying the effects of angiotensinogen.

One interpretation of these data is that preeclamptic women simply have pre-clinical essential hypertension, a conclusion that would be a radical departure from conventional wisdom. Most investigators feel that preeclampsia and essential hy-pertension have different etiologies. This view is supported by remote, follow-up studies showing that women who had severe preeclampsia in their first pregnancy do not have an exceptionally high risk of developing essential hypertension.[49] In Chesley's study, the mean length of follow-up was 33 years after the diagnosis of eclampsia. Despite the fact that clinical misclassification is indeed common, studies with the most stringent definitions of preeclampsia show the lowest remote risk for essential hypertension.[2,50] MacGillivray et al.[51] came to similar conclusions.

Any genetic hypothesis of preeclampsia must explain the first pregnancy effect. It is widely known that most women will not have preeclampsia with future pregnancies unless another condition exists (twins, diabetes). This has suggested an immunogenetic mechanism to many investigators, but other explanations are feasible. For instance, certain enzymes in pregnancy are permanently induced and never go back to baseline levels after delivery.[52,53] Similarly, permanent changes occur in maternal blood volume and in the vascular architecture of the uterus after a term gestation. In addition, a greater volume expansion is achieved in normal pregnancies at later parities.[54]

The decreased incidence of preeclampsia after a first pregnancy may hold a clue as to why preeclamptic patients do not have a particularly high rate of developing essential hypertension. If T235 increases the risk for both preeclampsia and essential hypertension through a blood volume mechanism, sustained changes in baseline blood volumes that occur after delivery may explain both the first pregnancy effect and possible reduction in an affected woman's lifelong risk of essential hypertension. Although the published data remain inconclusive, a recent epidemiologic survey demonstrated a modest protective effect of parity on lifelong risk of essential hypertension, a protective effect which increased with the number of pregnancies.[55]

Further evidence that angiotensinogen is a reasonable candidate gene for preeclampsia comes from studies at the University of Utah, whose investigators observed a rare variant in a nulliparous 18-year-old woman who developed severe preeclampsia early in the third trimester.[56] The mutation consists of the substitution of a phenylalanine for a leucine at residue 10 of mature angiotensinogen (L10F). This nonconservative substitution occurs at a residue conserved in all species examined. It defines the amino-terminal side of the peptide bond at which renin cleaves angiotensinogen to release angiotensin I (scissile bond), residues 10 and 11 (Leu-Val in primates and Leu Leu in all other species), with residue 10 forming the amino-terminus of angiotensin I. It is well known that the specificity and the reaction rates of an endopeptidase for a substrate depends critically on the nature of the amino acids present in the vicinity of the scissile bond, with residues directly flanking it being of primary significance. Kinetic studies using synthetic peptides spanning the renin binding site show this substitution leads to a tenfold decrease in Km of the renin reaction and a fivefold decrease in kcat. As a result, the catalytic efficiency (kcat/Km) is increased by a factor of 2. In the reaction of angiotensin-converting enzyme on angiotensin decapeptides, the substitution has no effect on Km, it increases the catalytic efficiency more than twofold.

Negative studies have also been published with regard to angiotensinogen, but they have much less power to address the issue.[57,58]

In 1997, Guo et al. performed a population-based, case-control study in Australian and Chinese populations testing the AGT dinucleotide repeat polymorphism as well as the T235 variant.[59] The allele distributions of the microsatellite and the variant T235 of AGT were significantly different between the two ethnic groups. However, no significant allele associations were found with disease when comparing preeclamptic–eclamptic patients and controls in Australian or Chinese populations. This suggests that finding is not constant across populations.

One explanation for discrepant results in different ethnic groups is that the T235 variant is only a marker for the functional mutation. Inoue et al. found that a common variant in the proximal promoter of the AGT gene—an adenine instead of a guanine 6 bp (base pairs) upstream from the site of transcription initiation—is in very tight linkage disequilibrium with T235.[60] Tests of promoter function in vitro and studies of binding between AGT oligonucleotides and nuclear proteins strongly suggested that the substitution at nucleotide −6 affects specific interactions between at least one transacting nuclear factor and the promoter of AGT, increasing basal transcription of the gene.

As discussed elsewhere in this text, preeclampsia is characterized by a failure of physiologic change in the spiral arteries of the placental bed and by endothelial cell perturbation and damage termed "acute atherosis." Trophoblast invasion into the uterus is incomplete and fails to reach the myometrial segments of the spiral artery. Histologic signs of preeclampsia have been reported in placental samples from first trimester elective abortions.[61] Acute atherosis and "premature aging of chorionic villi" were found before 12 weeks' gestation in 14% of samples. The endometrium of 75 nonpregnant women showed none of these preeclamptic signs, suggesting that the pathophysiology of preeclampsia begins in the first trimester and not before pregnancy.[62,63]

In other tissues, AGT mediates vascular remodeling. Angiotensin II is a smooth muscle mitogen and high levels of AGT in the vessel wall lead to vascular smooth muscle hypertrophy. Morgan et al. recently showed that angiotensinogen is expressed in remodeling vessels in the first trimester uterus.[64] Using an allele-specific ligation assay and a single nucleotide primer extension assay, they showed that the T235 allele is expressed at higher levels than the M235 allele in heterozygous women. These observations suggest a biologic mechanism for the association between the T235 allele, lesions in the spiral arteries, and the development of preeclampsia. The Utah group theorizes that −6 A variant is associated with preeclampsia because local AGT expression is elevated in remodeling spiral arteries of women carrying this allele. Elevated local AGT expression would presumably lead to elevated local angiotensin II levels and an increased frequency of abnormal pregnancy-induced remodeling of the uterine spiral arteries. Alternatively, women who are homozygous for the M235 allele have normal local AGT expression, permitting normal spiral artery remodeling in enough vessels so that these women are less likely to develop preeclampsia.

Takimoto et al. provided additional support for this view by mating transgenic mice expressing components of the human renin–angiotensin system.[65] When transgenic females expressing angiotensinogen were mated with transgenic males expressing renin, the pregnant females developed elevated blood pressure in late pregnancy. Blood pressure returned to normal levels after delivery of the pups. Histopathologic examination revealed uniform enlargement of glomeruli associated with an increase in urinary protein excretion, myocardial hypertrophy, and necrosis and edema in the placenta. Although the model is incompletely character-ized, these mice may provide a means for testing the role of angiotensinogen in the pathophysiology of human preeclampsia.

Harvard biologist, David Haig, has theorized that there is a genetic conflict that exists between maternal and fetal genes.[66] He hypothesizes that fetal genes will be selected to increase the transfer of nutrients to their fetus, and maternal genes will be selected to limit transfers in excess of some maternal optimum. This conflict may have given rise to the phenomenon of genomic imprinting. This theory also predicts tremendous inefficiencies at the uteroplacental interface, and rapid evolu-tion of genes and alleles conferring an advantage. Lifton provided evidence that the T235 allele may have been the ancestral form of an allele present in all primates.[67] He speculates that increased salt and water retention associated with T235 may have been an advantage prior to the diaspora from salt-poor Africa to salt-rich ar-eas, but that subsequently M235 became the most prevalent allele in Caucasians be-cause it had "some advantage." Perhaps the M235 advantage is due to the im-proved physiologic change of spiral arteries and that M235 is an allele that protects women against preeclampsia and related pregnancy disorders.

IMMUNOGENETIC FACTORS

Circumstantial evidence suggests that immunologic factors are operative in preeclampsia. A number of immunologic disorders such as systemic lupus predis-pose women to preeclampsia. The histologic findings in many affected placentas are reminiscent of acute graft rejection. Disorders with very large placentas increase the risk of preeclampsia because they reflect a larger antigenic load. The first preg-nancy effect suggests to many investigators that desensitization or tolerance to pa-ternal antigens protects mothers in subsequent gestations. The observation that a change in paternity can increase the risk may be due to the new paternal antigens presented in the placenta. Limited evidence shows that couples who use condoms for contraception, who accept an ovum donation, or who have a shorter length of cohabitation prior to conception have an increased risk of preeclampsia. Couples who practice oral sex and women who have had multiple blood transfusions have a lower risk.

It has become fashionable to talk about the fetus as an allograft. Since graft re-jection is mediated by the HLA system, there have been many studies concerning the role of the HLA locus in preeclampsia.[35] In general, there are no consistent find-ings from these studies. Several show allelic associations or increasing sharing of a particular allele, but most of the studies suffer from small sample sizes that limit their power. This is especially true because the complexity of the HLA locus has in-creased dramatically as we move from serologic typing to DNA typing. Few stud-ies use statistical correction for the multiple comparisons inherent in most HLA studies. Future work will need to use molecular typing methods on much larger samples from diverse ethnic groups. Many immunologic assays have been performed, (usually after the mother is ill), suggesting various derangements. Taylor's recent review covers this field well.[68]

Simon et al. studied the frequency of HLA-DR antigens in 96 women, 50 with preeclampsia and 46 with gestational hypertension.[69] The DR4 antigen was increased in both hypertensive groups compared to controls. Kilpatrick et al. studied a group of 56 women who had had proteinuric preeclampsia and who had parous sisters.[70] Their sisters had a sixfold greater rate of preeclampsia than in the general maternity hospital population. The frequency of HLA-DR4 was higher in sisters with pregnancy-induced hypertension than in sisters with normotensive pregnancies, and more of these sisters shared HLA-DR4 with their spouses.

Schneider et al. studied HLA-antigen sharing and the development of preeclampsia (PE) in 48 women with PE and their partners.[71] In 8 of 15 primigravidae with PE (53%), the child shared at least two paternal antigens with the mother. An increased homozygosity at the HLA-B locus was also seen in the children of primigravidae with PE (40 vs. 4%, P = 0.01).

Takakuwa et al. studied the distribution of human leukocyte antigens in 35 patients with severe preeclampsia and compared these to Japanese controls.[72] The frequency of patients with HLA-CW7 and HLA-DR6 was significantly greater compared with the general population (P < 0.05, chi-square test), while the frequency of those with DR4 was significantly lower (P < 0.05, chi-square test). Spouses showed no significant difference.

HLA-G

Most of the classic, class I histocompatibility antigens are not expressed on the invading trophoblast. Instead, the minimally polymorphic HLA-G antigen is expressed, presumably protecting the trophoblast from maternal immune recognition. Initially, HLA-G was thought to be monomorphic; but a number of investigators have described polymorphisms in the gene. For instance, van der Ven and Ober found 25 sequence variations that change amino acids in 45 healthy African-American patients.[73] To date, variant alleles have not been associated with the development of preeclampsia.

A number of investigators have found decreased HLA-G expression on trophoblasts from preeclamptic women using immunohistochemical techniques. Colbern et al. used ribonuclease protection assays to determine levels of HLA-G expression, which was normalized for trophoblast content in the tissue by comparing cytokeratin levels.[74] HLA-G expression in placental tissue was reduced in preeclampsia. This decreased expression was related to reduced numbers of trophoblasts in placental tissue examined at term from patients with primary preeclampsia. When controlled for the number of trophoblast cells, HLA-G expression was similar to normal for all clinical groups except for intrauterine growth retardation, which was slightly increased.

CONCLUSIONS

Preeclampsia is a familial disorder and one or more major predisposing genes are likely to be characterized in the next several years. There is still a need for some rather simple twin and consanguinity studies. Multicenter efforts are needed to define clinical and pathologic subsets. Modern linkage studies, gene expression studies, and transgenic animals hold great promise. The search for a preeclampsia gene could lead to the development of blood tests for susceptibility to preeclampsia, a greater understanding of its primary physiology, and the development of rational treatment or preventive strategies. Clearly, the potential results warrant the variety and scope of current research.

REFERENCES

1. Chesley LC, Cosgrove RE: The remote prognosis of preeclamptic women; sixth periodic report. *Am J Obstet Gynecol* 1976;124:446–459.
2. Chesley LC: Hypertension in pregnancy: Definitions, familial factor, and remote prognosis. *Kidney Internat* 1980;18:234–240.
3. Chesley LC, Annitto JE, Cosgrove RA: The familial factor in toxemia of pregnancy. *Obstet Gynecol* 1968;32:303–311.
4. Humphries J: Occurrence of hypertensive toxemia of pregnancy in mother-daughter pairs. *Johns Hopkins Hosp Bull* 1960;107:271–277.
5. Adams E, Finlayson A: Familial aspects of pre-eclampsia and hypertension in pregnancy. *Lancet* 1961;ii:1375.
6. Cooper DW, Liston WA: Genetic control of severe pre-eclampsia. *J Med Gen* 1979;16:409–416.
7. Sutherland A, Cooper DW, Howie PW, et al: The incidence of severe pre-eclampsia amongst mothers and mothers-in-law of pre-eclamptics and controls. *Br J Obstet Gynaecol* 1981; 88:785–791.
8. Arngrimsson R, Bjornsson S, Geirsson RT, et al: Genetic and familial predisposition to eclampsia and pre-eclampsia in a defined population. *Br J Obstet Gynaecol* 1990;97:762–769.
9. Thornton JC, Onwulde JL: Pre-eclampsia: Discordance among identical twins. *Br Med J* 1991;303:1241–1242.
10. Thompson B, Fraser C: Some aspects of first births and heights of twin sisters of known zygosity. In: MacGillivray I CD, Thompson B, eds. *Twinning and Twins*. Chichester: Wiley, 1988.
11. Stevenson AC, Say B, Ustaoglu S, Durmus Z: Aspects of pre-eclamptic toxaemia of pregnancy, consanguinity, and twinning in Ankara. *J Med Gen* 1976;13:1–8.
12. George K, Vedamony J, Idikulla J, Rao PS: The effect of consanguinity on pregnancy-induced hypertension. *Aust N Z J Obstet Gynaecol* 1992;32:231–232.
13. Liston WA, Kilpatrick DC: Is genetic susceptibility to pre-eclampsia conferred by homozygosity for the same single recessive gene in mother and fetus? *Br J Obstet Gynaecol* 1991; 98:1079–1086.
14. Cooper DW, Hill JA, Chesley LC, Bryans CI: Genetic control of susceptibility to eclampsia and miscarriage. *Br J Obstet Gynaecol* 1988;95:644–653.
15. Chesley LC, Cooper DW: Genetics of hypertension in pregnancy: Possible single gene control of pre-eclampsia and eclampsia in the descendants of eclamptic women. *Br J Obstet Gynaecol* 1986;93:898–908.
16. Kalmus H: Genetical antigenic incompatibility as a possible cause of the toxaemias occurring late in pregnancy. *Ann Eugen* 1946;13:146–149.
17. Penrose L: On the familial appearances of maternal and foetal incompatibility. *Ann Eugen* 1946;13:141–145.

18. Thornton J, Onwude JL: Convulsions in pregnancy in related gorillas. *Am J Obstet Gynecol* 1992;167:240–241.
19. Sohda S, Arinami T, Hamada H, et al: Methylenetetrahydrofolate reductase polymorphism and pre-eclampsia. *J Med Gen* 1997;34:525–526.
20. Grandone E, Margaglione M, Colaizzo D, et al: Factor V Leiden, > T MTHFR polymorphism and genetic susceptibility to preeclampsia. *Thromb Haemost* 1997;77:1052–1054.
21. Wilson AG, di Giovine FS, Blakemore AIF, Duff GW: Single base polymorphism in the human tumor necrosis factor alpha (TNF-α) gene detectable by Nco1 restriction of PCR product. *Human Mol Gen* 1992;1:353.
22. Chen G, Wilson R, Wang SH, et al: Tumour necrosis factor-alpha (TNF-alpha) gene polymorphism and expression in pre-eclampsia. *Clin Exp Immuno* 1996;104:154–159.
23. Dizon-Townson D, Nelson LM, Easton K, Ward K: The factor V Leiden mutation may predispose women to severe preeclampsia. *Am J Obstet Gynecol* 1996;175:902–905.
24. Arngrimsson R, Geirsson RT, Cooke A, et al: Renin gene restriction fragment length polymorphisms do not show linkage with preeclampsia and eclampsia. *Acta Obstetr Gynecol Scand* 1994;73:10–13.
25. Folgero T, Storbakk N, Torbergsen T, Olan P: Mutations in mitochondrial transfer ribonucleic acid genes in preeclampsia. *Am J Obstet Gynecol* 1996;174:1626–1630.
26. Need J: Pre-eclampsia in pregnancies by different fathers: Immunological studies. *Br Med J* 1975;I:548.
27. Feeney JG, Scott JS: Preeclampsia and changed paternity. *Eur J Obstet Gynecol Reprod Biol* 1980;11:35–38.
28. Astin M, Scott JR, Worley RJ: Pre-eclampsia/eclampsia: A fatal father factor. *Lancet* 1981; 2:533.
29. Boyd PA, Lindenbaum RH, Redman C: Pre-eclampsia and trisomy 13: A possible association. *Lancet* 1987;2:425–427.
30. Broekhuizen FF, Elejalde R, Hamilton PR: Early-onset preeclampsia, triploidy and fetal hydrops. *J Reprod Med* 1983;29:223–226.
31. Feinberg RF, Kliman HJ, Cohen AW: Preeclampsia, trisomy 13, and the placental bed. *Obstet Gynecol* 1991;78:505–508.
32. McCowan L, Becroft DM: Beckwith–Wiedemann syndrome, placental abnormalities, and gestational proteinuric hypertension. *Obstet Gynecol* 1994;83:813–817.
33. Treem WR, Shoup ME, Hale DE, et al: Acute fatty liver of pregnancy, hemolysis, elevated liver enzymes, and low platelets syndrome, and long chain 3-hydroxyacyl-coenzyme A dehydrogenase deficiency. *Am J Gastroenter* 1996;91:2293–2300.
34. Wilton AN, Cooper DW, Brennecke SP, et al: Absence of close linkage between maternal genes for susceptibility to pre-eclampsia/eclampsia and HLA DR beta. *Lancet* 1990;336(8716): 653–657.
35. Cooper DW, Brennecke SP, Wilton AN: Genetics of preeclampsia. *Hypertens Pregnancy* 1993;12:1–23.
36. Arngrimsson R, Purandare S, Connor M, et al: Angiotensinogen: A candidate gene involved in preeclampsia? *Nat Gen* 1993;4:114–115.
37. Hayward C, Livingstone J, Holloway S, et al: An exclusion map for pre-eclampsia: Assuming autosomal recessive inheritance. *Am J Human Gen* 1992;50:749–757.
38. Harrison GA, Humphrey KE, Jones N, et al: A genomewide linkage study of preeclampsia/eclampsia reveals evidence for a candidate region on 4q. *Am J Human Gen* 1997;60: 1158–1167.
39. Arngrimsson R, Hayward C, Nadaud S, et al: Evidence for a familial pregnancy-induced hypertension locus in the eNOS-gene region. *Am J Human Genet* 1997;61:354–362.
40. Bertina RM, Koeleman BP, Koster T, et al: Mutation in blood coagulation factor V associated with resistance to activated protein C. *Nature* 1994;369:64–67.
41. Dahlback B: Inherited resistance to activated protein C, a major cause of venous thrombosis, is due to a mutation in the factor V gene. *Haemostasis* 1994;24:139–151.

42. Bonnar J: Venous thromboembolism and pregnancy. *Clin Obstet Gynecol* 1981;30:455–473.

43. Dekker GA, de Vries JI, Doelitzch PM, et al: Underlying disorders associated with severe early-onset preeclampsia. *Am Obstet Gynecol* 1995;173:1042–1048.

44. Brenner B, Lanier N, Thaler I: HELLP syndrome associated with factor V R506Q mutation. *Br J Haematol* 1996;92:999–1001.

45. Rotmensch S, Liberati M, Mittlemann M, Ben-Rafael Z: Activated protein C resistance and adverse pregnancy outcome. *Am J Obstet Gynecol* 1997;171:170–173.

46. Dizon-Townson DS, Meline L, Nelson LM, et al: Fetal carriers of the factor V Leiden mutation are prone to miscarriage and placental infarction. *Am J Obstet Gynecol* 1997;177:402–405.

47. Jeunemaitre X, Soublier F, Kotelevtsev YV, et al: Molecular basis of human hypertension: Role of angiotensinogen. *Cell* 1992;71:168–180.

48. Ward K, Hata A, Jeunemaitre X, et al: A molecular variant of angiotensinogen associated with pre-eclampsia. *Nat Gen* 1993;4:59–61.

49. Fisher K, Luger A, Spargo BH, Lindheimer MD: Hypertension in pregnancy: Clinical–pathological correlations and remote prognosis. *Medicine* 1981;60:267–276.

50. Arias F: Expansion of intravascular volume and fetal outcome in patients with chronic hypertension and pregnancy. *Am J Obstet Gynecol* 1975;123:610–616.

51. MacGillivray I, Rose GA, Rowe D: Blood pressure survey in pregnancy. *Clin Sci* 1969;37:395–407.

52. Brown MA: The physiology of pre-eclampsia. *Clin Exper Pharmacol Physiol* 1995;22:781–791.

53. Lunell NO, Nylund L, Lewander R, Sarby B: Uteroplacental blood flow in preeclampsia. Measurement with iridium-113m and a computer. Graded gamma camera. *Clin Exper Hyper* 1982;1:105–117.

54. Wallenburg HCS: Hemodynamics in hypertensive pregnancy. In Rubin PC (ed.): *Handbook of Hypertension* Amsterdam: Elsevier Vol 10; 1980:66–101. (Second edition in press 1999–2000.)

55. Ness RB, Kramer RA, Flegal KM: Gravidity, blood pressure, and hypertension among white women in the second National Health and Nutrition Examination Survey. *Epidemiology* 1993;4:303–309.

56. Inoue I, Rohrwasser A, Helin C, et al: A mutation of angiotensinogen in a patient with preeclampsia leads to altered kinetics of the renin–angiotensin system. *J Biol Chem* 1995;270:11430–11436.

57. Morgan L, Baker P, Pipkin FB, Kalsheker N: Pre-eclampsia and the angiotensinogen gene. *Br J Obstet Gynaecol* 1995;102:489–490.

58. Wilton AN, Guo G, Brennecke SP, Cooper DW: Is angiotensinogen a good candidate gene for preeclampsia? *Hypertens Pregnancy* 1995;14:251–260.

59. Guo G, Wilton AN, Fu Y, et al: Angiotensinogen gene variation in a population case-control study of preeclampsia/eclampsia in Australians and Chinese. *Electrophoresis* 1997;18:1646–1649.

60. Inoue I, Nakajima T, Williams CS, et al: A nucleotide substitution in the promoter of human angiotensinogen is associated with essential hypertension and affects basal transcription in vitro. *J Clin Invest* 1997;99:1786–1797.

61. Nadji P: Lesions of toxemia in first trimester pregnancies. *Am J Clin Path* 1973;59:344–349.

62. Lichtig C, Brandes J: Vascular changes of endometrium in early pregnancy. *Am J Clin Path* 1984;81:702–707.

63. Bandes JM, Abramovici H, Katz M, et al: The effect of postural changes on plasma–renin activity during normal and pathologic pregnancies. *Obstet Gynecol* 1978;52:530–532.

64. Morgan T, Craven C, Nelson L, et al: Angiotensinogen T235 expression is elevated in decidual spiral arteries. *J Clin Invest* 1997;100:1406–1415.

65. Takimoto E, Ishida J, Sugiyama F, et al: Hypertension induced in pregnant mice by placental renin and maternal angiotensinogen. *Science* 1996;274:995–998.

66. Haig D: Genetic conflicts in human pregnancy. *Quart Rev Biol* 1993;68:495–532.

67. Lifton R: Genetic factors in hypertension. *Curr Opin Nephrol Hyper* 1993;2:258–264.

68. Taylor R: Review: Immunology of preeclampsia. *Am J Reprod Immunol* 1997;37:79–86.

69. Simon P, Faucet R, Pilorge M, et al: Association of HLA DR4 with the risk of recurrence of pregnancy hypertension. *Kidney Int Suppl* 1988;25:S125–S128.
70. Kilpatrick DC, Liston WA, Gibson F, Livingstone J: Association between susceptibility to pre-eclampsia within families and HLA DR4. *Lancet* 1989;2:1063–1065.
71. Schneider K, Knutson F, Tamsen L, Sjoberg O: HLA antigen sharing in preeclampsia. *Gynecol Obstet Invest* 1994;37:87–90.
72. Takakuwa K, Arakawa M, Tamura M, et al: HLA antigens in patients with severe preeclampsia. *J Perinat Med* 1997;25:79–83.
73. van der Ven K, Ober C: HLA-G polymorphisms in African Americans. *J Immunol* 1994; 153:5628–5633.
74. Colbern GT, Chiang MH, Main EK: Expression of the nonclassic histocompatibility antigen HLA-G by preeclamptic placenta. *Am J Obstet Gynecol* 1994;170:1244–1250.

14

Lipid Metabolism and Oxidative Stress

Carl A. Hubel and James M. Roberts

There is substantial evidence to suggest that the protean pathologic and pathophysiologic manifestations of preeclampsia, including activation of the coagulation cascade, altered vascular reactivity, and discrete pathology in many organ systems, relate to widespread pathologic changes within the mother's vascular endothelium. This latter subject was detailed in Chapter 12, where it was noted that the mechanisms involved in inducing endothelial cell dysfunction are largely unknown. While abnormal placentation (see Chap. 11) appears to be the proximate cause of both fetal intrauterine growth restriction (IUGR) and preeclampsia,[1,2] the latter disorder further requires the development of pathogenic conditions which extend to the maternal vasculature.[3,4] For instance, it has been proposed that product(s) of the fetoplacental unit enter the circulation and then initiate the maternal pathophysiologic changes of preeclampsia.[5,6] There is, however, increasing evidence that both fetoplacental and maternal factors interact in manifesting endothelial cell dysfunction and its clinical manifestations, a theme that will be underscored in this chapter.[3,7,8]

One hypothesis receiving a great deal of attention is that placental and maternal factors converge to generate "oxidative stress" (an imbalance between oxidant and antioxidant forces in favor of oxidants), promoting a vicious cycle of events that compromise the "defensive" vasodilatory, antiaggregatory, and barrier functioning of the vascular endothelium.[9-11] Problems relating to maternal constitution, such as abnormal lipid metabolism and associated insulin resistance, may be particularly important in this regard.[8,12-14]

This chapter begins with a brief review of oxidant–antioxidant interactions. Then it focuses on the roles of oxidative stress in the pathogenesis and manifestations of preeclampsia stressing (1) evidence and mechanisms of oxidative stress in the placenta, (2) whether the placenta is the sole source of agents that alter maternal endothelial cell function, (3) possible contributions of maternal dyslipidemia to oxidative stress, (4) markers of oxidative stress in the maternal circulation, and (5) maternal and placental interactions that potentially amplify oxidative stress. A recurrent theme is that free radical reactions, promoted by "cross-talk" between the diseased placenta and maternal dyslipidemia, create positive feedback loops which make cause versus effect difficult to distinguish but likely contribute to the progression of preeclampsia. A final section will deal with the issue of antioxidant clinical trials.

OXIDANT–ANTIOXIDANT INTERACTIONS

Free Radicals and Reactive Oxygen Species

A free radical is any molecular species capable of independent, albeit brief, existence that contains one or more unpaired electrons.[15] Because they participate in transfer of single electrons, free radicals are highly reactive and some are capable of inducing cell and tissue damage. Most free radicals of biologic relevance fall under the category of reactive oxygen species (ROS), a term used to include oxygen-containing free radicals, such as hydroxyl radical (HO•), peroxyl radical (ROO•), and superoxide anion radical (O_2•$-$), and also reactive oxygen derivatives that do not contain unpaired electrons, such as hydrogen peroxide (H_2O_2), hypochlorous acid (HOCl), and peroxynitrite anion ($ONOO^-$).[16-18]

There are comprehensive reviews on interactions between reactive oxygen species and antioxidants in human health and disease.[19-25] A wide spectrum of reactive oxygen species function as signal transducers in normal physiology but their overproduction may result in, or be the result of, a number of human health problems. Overproduction of reactive oxygen species can arise from a variety of sources, both environmental and metabolic. Tissue ischemia/hypoxia followed by reperfusion is one established generator of reactive oxygen species and lipid peroxidation in vivo.[26] Systems altered to generate reactive oxygen species during postischemic reperfusion include mitochondrial respiration, neutrophil NADPH oxidase, xanthine oxidase, and cyclooxygenase.[26-29] Iron delocalized from its normal cellular compartments during ischemic damage will also promote reactive oxygen species generation upon reoxygenation.[26] As will be discussed, postischemic reperfusion generation of reactive oxygen species could be one source of oxidative injury in placentae of women with preeclampsia.

A diverse array of cellular and extracellular fluid antioxidants has evolved to control and compartmentalize, but not necessarily eliminate, the production of reactive oxygen species. Antioxidants examined in normal and preeclamptic pregnancies include the enzymatic antioxidants (superoxide dismutases [SOD], catalase, and glutathione peroxidase), and transition metal binding proteins (transferrin, caeruloplasmin, and ferritin).[10,30,31] There are also low molecular mass free radical scavengers which primarily protect against oxidative damage in the extracellular compartment. These include water-soluble forms (ascorbate [vitamin C], glutathione and protein thiols, uric acid) and lipoprotein- and cell membrane-soluble forms (including α-tocopherol [vitamin E]).[32,33]

Lipid Peroxidation

Lipid peroxidation has received a great deal of attention in preeclampsia. The process can be described as oxidative deterioration of polyunsaturated fatty acids. Lipid peroxidation can occur by a free radical chain process as shown in Figure 14–1, or alternatively by enzymes such as cyclooxygenase and lipoxygenase.[34] Formation of most reactive oxygen species that initiate and propagate the lipid peroxidation chain depends upon the presence of a catalytic, "low molecular mass pool" of iron or other transition metals (for example, OH• formed from H_2O_2 and $O_2•-$ by the "iron-catalyzed Haber–Weiss reaction").[16,35] However, peroxynitrite anion can initiate lipid peroxidation without requirement of transition metals.[36,37] The primary products of lipid peroxidation, lipid hydroperoxides, function in normal physiology. For example, activation of the cyclooxygenase component of prostaglandin H (PGH) synthase requires the presence of lipid hydroperoxides.[38] Reactive oxygen species/antioxidant imbalances can lead to uncontrolled lipid peroxidation. The subsequent detrimental activity ascribed to lipid hydroperoxides is primarily due to (1) the physical disruption of lipoproteins and cell membranes consequent to their production, (2) reactive intermediates (lipid peroxyl and

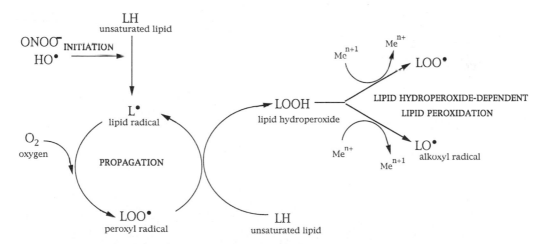

Figure 14–1. Free radical mechanism of lipid peroxidation. Peroxidation is initiated when a reactive oxygen species of sufficient power abstracts a methylene hydrogen from the unsaturated fatty acid (LH), forming a lipid radical (L•). The lipid radical reacts with molecular oxygen to form a lipid peroxyl radical (LOO•). The lipid peroxyl radical attacks another unsaturated lipid, forming another lipid radical (that enters the chain), and a lipid hydroperoxide (LOOH) (propagation). Once the lipid matrix is "seeded" with low concentrations of lipid hydroperoxides, peroxidation can be amplified by transition metal (Me^{n+}/Me^{n+1})-catalyzed conversion of lipid hydroperoxides to radical species (LOO• ; LO•) (lipid hydroperoxide-dependent lipid peroxidation). Bonding of two radical species or reaction with antioxidants such as vitamin E will slow the peroxidation process.

alkoxyl radicals) formed during the peroxidation process or during reaction of lipid hydroperoxides with transition metals, or (3) cytotoxic, more stable degradation products of lipid hydroperoxides such as malondialdehyde and 4-hydroxynonenal or by-products of lipid peroxidation such as lysophospholipids.[39-41]

Oxidative Stress and the Vascular Endothelium

Research focusing on atherosclerosis has aptly demonstrated that the vascular endothelium is prone to damage from reactive oxygen species. Because vascular endothelial cells interface with blood, they are exposed to a variety of prooxidants including heme compounds and reactive species from activated neutrophils and platelets.[42-44] Circulating lipids have diverse effects upon endothelial cell function, and dyslipidemia is associated with endothelial cell dysfunction.[45,46] In particular, there is a considerable interest in the role played by low density lipoprotein (LDL) oxidation in endothelial disturbances. LDL particles can undergo oxidation in vivo and such modification contributes to arterial lesions in atherosclerosis[47] and diabetes.[48] The LDL particles continuously enter and exit the artery wall. In the subendothelial interstitial matrix, LDL may be exposed more frequently to cell-derived oxidants and at the same time are less protected by antioxidants relative to circulating LDL.[22,47] This potential for prolonged contact between LDL and the cell makes the subendothelial space the likely site of LDL oxidation and is one reason the endothelium is a likely target for oxidized LDL-mediated disturbances.[49-51] As will be discussed later in this chapter, the appearance of hypertriglyceridemia followed by increased prevalence of smaller, more oxidation-susceptible LDL particles might contribute to endothelial dysfunction in preeclampsia.[8]

Minimally modified LDL (those containing low levels of lipid hydroperoxides but without substantial protein modification) induces the activation of nuclear transcription factor NFκB, and thus, endothelial mRNA and protein expression for a number of inflammatory cytokines, including monocyte chemoattractants.[22,52,53] Continued oxidation is facilitated (primed) by "feed-forward" interaction of lipid hydroperoxides in the LDL particle with cell-derived oxidants.[47,54,55] Lipid peroxidation can propagate to core lipids and ultimately result in modification and degradation of apolipoprotein B. These more extensive changes lead to recognition by the macrophage scavenger[56] and synthesis of oxidized LDL antibodies.[57]

The deleterious effects of lipid peroxidation (including peroxidation of LDL) on the vasculature include inhibition of endothelium-dependent relaxation.[22,47,58] Also, the "oxidative stress theory" of preeclampsia finds indirect support in that many of the endothelial abnormalities described in preeclampsia can be reproduced by lipid peroxidation in experimental systems. Examples are summarized in Table 14–1.[9]

Cause vs. Consequence

In many human diseases, oxidative stress and lipid peroxidation probably occur as a consequence of cell or tissue damage.[21,25,59] In such circumstances oxidative stress

TABLE 14–1. DYSFUNCTION IN PREECLAMPSIA MIMICKED BY EXPERIMENTAL LIPID PEROXIDATION

Dysfunction in Preeclampsia	Peroxidation in Experimental Models
1. Evidence of endothelial structural injury: • Glomerular capillary endothelium • Umbilical endothelium	1. Lipid peroxidation and/or acute exposure to lipid peroxides damages endothelial cells.[237,238]
2. Proteinuria	2. Intrarenal infusion of hydrogen peroxide induces reversible proteinuria in rats.[239]
3. Convulsions during eclampsia	3. Rats fed a diet deficient in vitamin E and containing lipid peroxides beginning on day 13 of gestation developed eclampsia-like convulsions and intravascular thrombosis at term.[240]
Endothelial Functional/Biochemical Changes	
4. Vasoconstriction and increased sensitivity to pressor agonists[241,242]	4. Lipid peroxides or oxidized LDL increase artery sensitivity to agonists in vivo and in vitro.[9,243-245]
5. Impaired endothelial-dependent relaxation of isolated arteries from women with preeclampsia[246]	5. Oxidized LDL inhibits endothelial-dependent vasodilatation.[247,248]
6. Reduced prostacyclin (PGI$_2$) production by vessels[249]	6. Increased lipid peroxidation via vitamin E deprivation decreases PGI$_2$ production.[250]
7. Increased circulating cellular fibronectin[251]	7. Peroxides induce tissue release of cellular fibronectin.[252]
Serum/Plasma from Preeclamptic Women Alters Endothelial Cell Function In Vitro	
8. Preeclampsia plasma increases endothelial production of nitric oxide.[253,254]	8. Oxidized LDL at low concentration increases nitric oxide production from endothelial cells in culture.[255,256]
9. Preeclampsia plasma induces biphasic release of PGI$_2$ from endothelial cells in culture (increased at 24 h; decreased at 72 h)[257]	9. Oxidized LDL or hyperlipidemic sera increase endothelial PGI$_2$ production at 24 h but inhibit during longer incubations (48–72 h).[258,259]
Functional Changes in Red Blood Cells	
10. Hemolysis and increased red cell osmofragility[260,261]	10. Lipid peroxidation promotes osmofragility and hemolysis.[262]
11. Decreased calcium-ATPase activity[263]	11. Lipid peroxides and other ROS inhibit calcium-ATPase via modification of protein thiols.[264]

ROS, reactive oxygen species.

may aggravate the disease and contribute to its progression. This is because feed-forward amplification loops occur during free radical reactions. For example, focal cell or tissue trauma with decompartmentalization can lead to interaction of oxidation accelerants (such as mobilized iron) with susceptible molecules (such as polyunsaturated fatty acids) resulting in lipid peroxidation. Lipid peroxidation can lead to further membrane disruption with expansion to outlying zones (⟶ cell damage ⟶ peroxidation ⟶ further cell damage ⟶ further peroxidation ⟶). Untangling cause and effect is confounded by the reactivity and, hence evanescence, of reactive oxygen species. Using lipid hydroperoxides again as an example, it is difficult to prove their presence in blood or other biologic material in vivo because these compounds are generated in blood or dying tissues exposed to oxygen ex vivo.[25] Another problem is insufficient sensitivity and specificity of tools to evaluate oxidative stress.[60-62] Although there is compelling evidence that oxidative stress occurs during preeclampsia, we lack clear evidence that it causes disease progression. This is partly due to unique difficulties in obtaining longitudinal blood and tissue samples in this low prevalence disorder and the lack of completely suitable animal models for preeclampsia.

During pregnancy, there are potential mechanisms in both the placental and maternal compartments to increase oxidative stress by increasing prooxidants and oxidation-susceptible lipids and perhaps decreasing antioxidants. Oxidative stress, in turn, may be the point at which multiple factors converge resulting in endothelial cell dysfunction and the consequent clinical manifestations of preeclampsia.

PLACENTAL OXIDATIVE STRESS

The hypothesis that the etiology of preeclampsia is related to deficient trophoblast invasion and failure of uterine artery remodeling is well founded[3,63] and is detailed in Chapter 11. Defective arterial remodeling in preeclampsia and in intrauterine growth restriction (IUGR) likely results in reduced uteroplacental perfusion which may predispose to episodes of placental hypoxia or ischemia.[3,64,65] Placental infarcts occur with increased frequency in preeclampsia, consistent with focal hypoxia/ischemia.[1,66] Many of the ultrastructural changes of preeclamptic placental tissue resemble alterations in placental tissue when placed in hypoxic organ culture.[67] Preeclampsia is more common at high altitude, suggesting that chronic hypoxia might be a predisposing factor.[68,69] Multiple gestation and hydrops fetalis predispose to preeclampsia and are associated with a larger than normal placenta which could lead to a relative reduction of placental perfusion.[7]

Placental Nitrotyrosine, Xanthine Oxidase, and the Issue of Reperfusion Damage

Tissue hypoxia/ischemia followed by reoxygenation can generate reactive oxygen species and lipid peroxidation in vivo.[26] If conjoined with vascular reperfusion, placental hypoxia/ischemia could result in oxidative damage and elaboration of cytotoxic reactive oxygen products into the circulation. However, it is unclear whether placental postischemic reoxygenation damage occurs in preeclampsia. Recent data showing that vascular endothelial growth factor (VEGF) mRNA is decreased in the placenta of preeclamptic pregnancies conflicts with the notions of hypoxia[70] and reactive oxygen species generation by postischemic reoxygenation.[71] As will be discussed, however, there are changes consistent with reperfusion oxidative damage in the preeclampsia placenta. Changes consistent with oxidative stress in the preeclampsia placenta are summarized in Table 14–2.

Peroxynitrite anion (ONOO$^-$) is capable of nitrating proteins and inducing

TABLE 14–2. SOME CHANGES CONSISTENT WITH OXIDATIVE STRESS IN THE PREECLAMPSIA PLACENTA

Marker or Activity	Location	Reference No.
Decreased total superoxide dismutase (SOD) activity	Placental homogenate, and mitochondrial and cytosolic fractions	92,93
Decreased Cu,Zn-SOD activity and mRNA expression	Placental cotyledons, excluding chorionic and basal plates	94
Decreased glutathione peroxidase activity	Placental tissue homogenate	102
Increased immunohistochemical staining for xanthine oxidase holoenzyme	Invasive cytotrophoblast	87
Increased xanthine oxidase holoenzyme and specific oxidase isoform activity	Placental bed curettings (containing cytotrophoblast)	87,88
Increased nitrotyrosine immunostaining (indicating protein nitration by ONOO⁻)	Villous vascular endothelium, surrounding smooth muscle and villous stroma	79
Increased lipid hydroperoxide levels	Placental tissue homogenate	102
Increased lipid hydroperoxide production	Trophoblast cells and villous tissue	108
Increased production of 8-isoprostane (produced by radical-catalyzed peroxidation of arachidonic acid)	Placental tissue pieces	111
Increased malondialdehyde (lipid peroxidation product)	Placental homogenate and mitochondrial and cytosolic fractions; syncytiotrophoblast plasma membranes	92,93,220
Increased membrane fluidity (possible indicator of lipid peroxidation)	Syncytiotrophoblast plasma membranes	222
Increased membrane susceptibility to lipid peroxidation in response to prooxidant challenge	Syncytiotrophoblast plasma membranes	220
Increased maximum amount of peroxidizable material	Placental homogenate	92
Presence of lipid laden macrophages (foam cells)	Decidual arterioles	112,114
Increased elastase-positive neutrophils (marker of neutrophil activation)	Decidua of the placental bed	128

lipid peroxidation.[71-74] Peroxynitrite formation is favored when nitric oxide (NO) is formed in high enough concentration to outcompete superoxide dismutase (SOD) for $O_2 \bullet -$.[73] Thus NO•, which in certain settings can behave as an antioxidant by inhibiting lipid peroxidation,[75,76] can also promote oxidative damage through ONOO⁻ formation. Nitrotyrosine is the stable reaction product of peroxynitrite attack on proteins and thus provides a "footprint" of oxidative damage. Extensive nitrotyrosine-specific immunostaining has been detected around foam cells in human atherosclerotic lesions[77] and in lung tissue of newborns with acute lung injury.[78] Greater nitrotyrosine immunostaining has been found in placental villous vascular endothelium, and surrounding vascular smooth muscle and villous stroma in preeclampsia and also in IUGR compared to normal pregnant controls.[79] These data provide evidence of oxidative stress and also suggest fetal involvement.

Placental trophoblast produce nitric oxide.[80] Preeclampsia and intrauterine growth restriction are associated with increased expression of the endothelial isoform of nitric oxide synthase (eNOS) in the villous vessel endothelium.[79] Macrophages, interstitial cells, and endothelial cells can be induced to produce both $O_2\bullet-$ and $NO\bullet$ (and consequently $ONOO^-$) by inflammatory stimuli or by post-ischemic reperfusion.[81-84] Increased nitrotyrosine immunoreactivity may reflect up-regulation of such pathways in preeclampsia.[79]

Changes in the enzyme xanthine oxidase in preeclampsia suggest ischemic injury and may favor increased production of $O_2\bullet-$ (and thus $ONOO^-$). The dehydrogenase (type D) form of xanthine oxidase requires NAD^+ and produces uric acid and NADH. During periods of hypoxia/ischemia, this form is increasingly converted to the oxidase (type O form) which requires oxygen and produces uric acid and $O_2\bullet-$ during reoxygenation.[26-28,85] There is considerable support for the role of xanthine oxidase in the genesis of tissue reperfusion injury.[26-28] However, the placenta was thought to be one of the few tissues in which xanthine oxidase activity could not be detected. Recent results show mRNA, immunoreactivity, and enzyme activity for the holoenzyme (combined D and O) in human placental trophoblast (although at low levels compared to liver), contradicting the earlier findings.[86] In addition, there is increased immunohistochemical staining for the holoenzyme in invasive, but not villous, trophoblast from preeclamptic pregnancies.[87] Thirdly, placental site curettings (which contain cytotrophoblast) from women with preeclampsia exhibit increased holoenzyme and increased type O activity compared to samples from normal controls. Increased type O activity is also associated with an increase in nitrotyrosine labeling on these cells consistent with in vivo interaction of $O_2\bullet-$ with $NO\bullet$.[88]

Placental generation of $O_2\bullet-$ and other ROS in preeclampsia might be facilitated by decreases in SOD expression and activity. Superoxide dismutase removes $O_2\bullet-$ by accelerating its conversion to H_2O_2. It acts in concert with peroxysomal catalase which converts H_2O_2 to water. One form containing manganese at its active site (Mn-SOD) is found in mitochondria and another with copper and zinc (Cu,Zn-SOD) is found mainly in the cytosol. An extracellular form (EC-SOD) has been reported which binds to the surface of endothelial cells.[89]

Superoxide dismutase activity in placental homogenates reportedly increases with gestational age.[90,91] Total activity is decreased in whole placental homogenates[92,93] and mitochondiral and cytosolic fractions[93] from women with preeclamptic compared to normal gestations. Placental tissue homogenate Cu,Zn-SOD activity and mRNA expression are also decreased in preeclampsia relative to normal pregnancy.[94] Immunohistochemistry on placental villous tissue has local-ized Cu,Zn-SOD to cells of the villous stroma and more weakly to syncytiotro-phoblast and villous endothelium, and Mn-SOD primarily to villous vessel en-dothelium and faintly to syncytiotrophoblast and some stromal cells.[95] Tissue from placentae of women with preeclampsia (with or without growth restricted fetuses), of women with IUGR alone, and of normal pregnancies did not differ with respect to SOD immunostaining except that villous stromal Cu,Zn-SOD was more diffuse in the pathologic pregnancies. Two other studies have shown that white and red blood cells from women with preeclampsia have decreased superoxide dismutase activity but not in the concentration of its mRNA, suggesting posttranscriptional reduction.[96,97] It is plausible that local NO• production coupled with increased xanthine oxidase generation of O_2•$-$ and decreased SOD promotes regional $ONOO^-$ production in the placenta in preeclampsia. As is typical in the free radi-cal field, paradoxes exist. One is that cellular SOD gene expression and enzyme ac-tivity are sometimes up-regulated by reactive oxygen species.[98,99] Another is that the primary product of xanthine oxidase, uric acid, is elevated in the plasma of women with preeclampsia and is an effective antioxidant.[100,101]

Placental Lipid Peroxidation

The lipid peroxidation degradation product, malondialdehyde, is reportedly in-creased in placental tissue along with decreases in SOD activity in preeclamp-sia.[92,93] In vitro data indicate a relative deficiency of glutathione peroxidase in pla-cental tissue from preeclamptic women in conjunction with increased tissue production of lipid hydroperoxides and thromboxane A_2.[10,102] The actions of this vasoconstrictive and proaggregatory prostaglandin, produced primarily by macro-phages and platelets, is normally opposed by the vasodilator prostacyclin. Chemi-cal inhibition of placental glutathione peroxidase resulted in increased production of lipid hydroperoxides and an increase in the placental thromboxane to prostacy-clin output ratio.[102] Lipid hydroperoxides can inhibit prostacyclin-synthase activity and simultaneously stimulate the cyclooxygenase component of prostaglandin H synthase.[103,104] Thromboxane-synthase activity is unchanged or even stimu-lated.[10,105] These effects of lipid hydroperoxides could be responsible for the re-ported decrease in the placental prostacyclin to thromboxane production ratio in preeclampsia, especially since expression of their synthases is not altered in the uteroplacental unit.[106] The consequences of this altered ratio might include va-sospasm with exacerbation of placental ischemia, increased cell damage, and in-creased lipid peroxidation (amplification loop).[9]

A study of isolated, perfused human placental cotyledons exposed to the oxi-dant, tert-butyl hydroperoxide showed more lipid hydroperoxides appearing in maternal- than fetal-side effluent samples.[107] From follow-up studies it was con-cluded that production of lipid hydroperoxides and thromboxane are increased in both trophoblast cells and villous tissues from women with preeclampsia.[108,109] The lipid hydroperoxide detection system used in these studies (glutathione peroxidase/glutathione reductase oxidation of NADPH) is not completely immune to interference.[110] However these findings were further bolstered in that production of 8-isoprostane, produced by free radical-catalyzed peroxidation of arachidonic acid, is increased in incubated placental tissue from women with preeclampsia compared to normal pregnancy.[111] Determination of predelivery arterial–venous differences in peroxidation metabolites would help to confirm the placental origin of lipid hydroperoxides.

In preeclampsia, the pathologic lesions of the decidual arterioles bear a striking resemblance to atherosclerotic lesions of coronary arteries, both showing fibrinoid necrosis of the vessel wall, aggregates of platelets, and accumulation of lipid-laden macrophages (foam cells).[1,112-114] This "acute atherosis" involves endothelial damage and is probably a true atherosclerosis-like change.[115] Interestingly, it is not specific to preeclampsia but can also occur in the placentae from pregnancies with IUGR without a "maternal syndrome."[115] The morphology of these vessels has interesting parallels with the atherogenic process of carotid arteries, in which LDL lipid peroxidation with foam cell formation has a paramount role.[47,57] However, there has been no direct demonstration of arterial oxidized products in preeclampsia.

Are Activated Neutrophils Purveyors of Oxidative Stress into the Maternal Circulation?

A continuing mystery is how the initial placental lesions are connected to the maternal syndrome. Circumstantial evidence supports the poorly perfused placenta as a source of agents contributing to bloodborne materials that, directly or indirectly, lead to endothelial cell dysfunction. One candidate factor is syncytiotrophoblast shed from the microvillous membrane into the maternal circulation.[1,116] Alternatively, placental hypoxia/ischemia per se could result in production of cytokines such as tumor necrosis factor-alpha (TNF-α) that activate maternal endothelial cells,[117] perhaps via free radical mechanisms.[118] In theory, stable peroxidation metabolites produced during placental oxidative stress could enter the maternal circulation and contribute to widespread endothelial dysfunction. Malondialdehyde and 4-hydroxynonenal, for example, are potential "second toxic messengers" of focal lipid peroxidation; exposure of cells in culture to pathophysiologically relevant concentrations of these agents has toxic effects.[40,41,119]

Activated neutrophils are also candidates. Activation of maternal neutrophils during their transit through the placenta could provide a pathway for transfer of oxidative disturbances into the maternal circulation in preeclampsia. The enzymatic production of $O_2\bullet-$ by NADPH oxidase present in the cell membrane of phagocytes is an important component of defense against infectious agents. However, phagocyte-derived reactive oxygen species can cause problems if increased by chronic infection or postischemic reperfusion. Postischemic reoxygenated cells release activators that induce neutrophils to discharge injurious oxidants ($O_2\bullet-$, H_2O_2, HOCl, Cl_2 gas).[26,120-122] Neutrophil adherence to endothelial cells and release of oxidants will occur in response to components of the complement cascade, adhesion molecules, TNF-α, and certain oxidized and nonoxidized fatty acids.[26,123-127] Elastase-positive neutrophils, a marker of neutrophil activation in vivo, are found in increased numbers in the decidua of the placental bed in women with preeclampsia compared with those experiencing normal pregnancies. This is seen at the same site as the "acute atherosis" mentioned earlier and correlates with plasma uric acid.[127,128]

Concentrations of neutrophil elastase are increased in the peripheral circulation of women with preeclampsia[129] well as in IUGR.[130] A significant correlation exists between plasma neutrophil elastase and von Willebrand factor, a marker of endothelial dysfunction.[131] According to one study, neutrophils isolated from normally pregnant women compared with nonpregnant women show no difference in $O_2\bullet-$ production in response to the chemotactic peptide, N-formyl-methionyl-leucyl-phenylalanine (fMLP). However, $O_2\bullet-$ production was markedly increased in neutrophils from women with preeclampsia compared with those experiencing normal pregnancy. In addition, preeclampsia sera potentiated $O_2\bullet-$ generation from isolated, fMLP-stimulated nonpregnancy neutrophils whereas normal pregnancy or nonpregnancy sera did not. The stimulatory factor was reportedly a heat-labile protein(s).[132] Neutrophil activation might result from endothelial dysfunction in preeclampsia. However, it seems logical to propose a role for neutrophils in progression of the disease.

Is the Placenta the Sole Source of Agents That Alter Endothelial Cell Function in Preeclampsia?

There are inconsistencies with the hypothesis that the poorly perfused placenta is the sole origin of factors altering endothelial function and causing preeclampsia. The failure of spiral artery transformation seen in preeclampsia is also seen in women with IUGR and no manifestations of preeclampsia.[1,133] Maternal constitutional problems, particularly gestational diabetes[134] and prepregnancy obesity,[135] are associated with larger babies, yet also predispose to preeclampsia. The interaction of underlying maternal disease (such as chronic hypertension and diabetes mellitus) with preeclampsia results in higher perinatal morbidity and mortality.[7] These and other lines of evidence suggest that maternally-derived factors, perhaps interacting with the placenta or placental factors, contribute to endothelial cell dysfunction and consequent clinical manifestations.[3,7,8] In particular, the role of "Syndrome X" (a cluster of metabolic abnormalities characterized by dyslipidemia and resistance to insulin-stimulated glucose uptake) in cardiovascular disease suggests intriguing parallels for the pathogenesis of preeclampsia.

DYSLIPIDEMIA AND OXIDATIVE STRESS IN PREECLAMPSIA

The dyslipidemia of preeclampsia is best understood in the context of lipid changes during normal pregnancy. Although the emphasis will be on promotion of oxidative stress by dyslipidemia, oxidative stress-independent mechanisms might also be involved.[46,136,137] Abnormal maternal systemic sensitivity or response to circulating lipids might also be important in preeclampsia.

Lipid Metabolism in Normal Pregnancy

Circulating lipids are carried primarily in lipoproteins, which are composed primarily of free and esterified lipids, proteins (apolipoproteins), and phospholipids. The two main triglyceride-carrying lipoproteins are chylomicrons and very low density lipoproteins (VLDL). The two main cholesterol-carrying lipoproteins are LDL and high density lipoproteins (HDL). During the first half of normal pregnancy, increased maternal adipose fat accumulation is presumed to be important for the subsequent physiologic hyperlipidemia of late gestation.[138] Circulating concentrations of VLDL and LDL increase progressively with gestational age and are reflected by marked increases in serum triglycerides and cholesterol (approximately 300% and 50% by term, respectively).[139,140] Increased triglyceride is found in all the lipoprotein fractions during late gestation. Mechanisms driving these changes include increased adipose tissue lipolytic activity secondary to the insulin-resistant condition of late gestation.[141] This presumably boosts free fatty acid and glycerol release into the circulation, increasing substrate for hepatic triglyceride (VLDL) synthesis. Estrogen-induced increases in hepatic output of VLDL coupled with enhanced conversion of VLDL to lipoproteins of higher density are also involved.[139,141] The triglyceride-enrichment of LDL and HDL contributing to hypertriglyceridemia may be due to increased cholesteryl ester transfer protein (CETP) activity during normal pregnancy.[141] This enzyme transfers triglycerides from VLDL to HDL and LDL in exchange for cholesteryl esters. Also, both adipose tissue lipoprotein lipase and hepatic lipase activities are decreased in normal pregnancy (effects primarily related to insulin resistance and increased estrogen, respectively). The latter changes probably impair removal of triglyceride-rich lipoproteins from the circulation.[141] These physiologic adaptations may maximize transfer of maternal essential fatty acids to the fetus.[139,142]

Dyslipidemia in Preeclampsia

Agents of primary importance to the pathogenesis of preeclampsia are likely to be present before the woman is overtly ill and decrease with resolution of the disorder postpartum. Disturbed lipid metabolism was noted to be a feature of preeclampsia as early as 1936 (and the manuscript includes a 1924 citation proclaiming that "lipid ratios were of significance in the toxemias of pregnancy and eclampsia").[143] Supernormal increases in serum triglyceride and free fatty acids develop as early as 10 weeks' gestation in women destined to develop preeclampsia.[13,144] The hypertriglyceridemia and increased free fatty acids in preeclamptic women are thus not a consequence of the clinical syndrome. These lipid differences maximize during clinically evident disease.[12-14] Nearly 50% of women with preeclampsia have triglyceride concentrations $\geq$ 400 mg/dL.[12] This concentration is greater than the 90th percentile measured in 553 randomly selected women at 36 weeks' gestation.[139] Total cholesterol[12-14,144] and LDL-cholesterol[12,14] concentrations are usually not different whereas HDL_2 cholesterol is decreased[14] in clinically evident preeclampsia. Serum triglyceride, cholesterol, and free fatty acid concentrations decrease sharply in preeclamptics and pregnant controls by 24 to 48 hours postpartum.[12] More gradual decreases in triglycerides and cholesterol may continue for more than 6 weeks.[140] Full triglyceride and cholesterol normalization has been documented postlactationally in normal pregnancy[141] but has not been adequately documented in preeclampsia.

Accentuated triglyceride and free fatty acid increases in preeclampsia are consistent with a metabolic pattern known as "syndrome X" (insulin-resistance syndrome). This phenotype includes resistance to insulin-stimulated glucose uptake and compensatory hyperinsulinemia, hyperuricemia, prevalence of obesity, and dyslipidemia (hypertriglyceridemia with profound increases in triglyceride-rich VLDL, predominance of smaller, denser LDL particles, and decreased plasma HDL [particularly HDL_2] despite normal or only moderately elevated LDL-cholesterol concentrations).[145-147] These metabolic abnormalities occur in up to 25% of the nonpregnant population and predispose to coronary artery disease.[145] Notably, *all* of these manifestations exist in preeclampsia relative to normal pregnancy.[12-14,134,135,148-151] Heightened insulin resistance in preeclampsia would increase fatty acid mobilization from visceral fat, promote overproduction of VLDL by the liver, and suppress activity of lipoprotein lipase, resulting in elevated serum free fatty acids and triglycerides.[152,153] In humans and animal models, increased tumor necrosis factor-alpha (TNF-α) production by adipose tissue is correlated with obesity, insulin resistance, and hypertriglyceridemia.[154,155] This factor decreases lipoprotein lipase activity, increases adipose tissue lipolysis, and may be a mediator of insulin resistance.[154,155] Hypothetically, increased production of this cytokine, either from placenta or adipose tissue, might contribute to insulin resistance and dyslipidemia and perhaps endothelial dysfunction in preeclampsia.

Potential Impact of Dyslipidemia on Oxidative Stress

Free fatty acid increases might contribute to endothelial dysfunction in preeclampsia by several means.[46,156] Free fatty acid-mediated endothelial dysfunction by facilitation of reactive oxygen species generation has been demonstrated in vitro and in vivo,[157-159] but it remains to be determined whether such pathways occur in preeclampsia.

There is growing recognition of hypertriglyceridemia as a major risk factor for coronary and atherosclerotic vascular disease.[145,160-162] Hypertriglyceridemia may compromise vascular function in several ways. For example, triglyceride-rich lipoproteins have prothrombotic activity.[162] In the realm of oxidative stress, monocytes isolated from individuals with hypertriglyceridemia show increased superoxide production and enhanced binding to endothelial cells.[124,163,164] One might speculate that hypertriglyceridemia predisposes to immune cell activation in vivo, but these relationships have not been explored in preeclampsia. An important consequence of hypertriglyceridemia relative to increased risk of cardiovascular disease is the shift in LDL toward smaller, denser, more atherogenic particles.[160,161] The pathogenic significance of small, dense LDL and the formation of small, dense LDL during normal and preeclamptic pregnancy are summarized in the next two sections.

Small, Dense LDL Phenotype and Its Vascular Consequences

Low density lipoproteins comprise a heterogeneous spectrum of particles which differ in density, size, and chemical composition. This LDL particle size is subject to both genetic and nongenetic influences.[160] The larger, more buoyant subclasses of LDL are elevated in healthy females of reproductive age, whereas an LDL of intermediate size represents the principal subclass in adult males.[165,166] Metabolic changes producing hypertriglyceridemia generally shift the spectrum of LDL subfractions toward a proportional increase of smaller, denser LDL.[160,166,167] Small, dense LDL particles are relatively depleted of cholesteryl esters, and enriched in protein.[166,167]

The small, dense LDL phenotype predicts the onset of coronary artery disease[168] and myocardial infarction.[169] Nonfasting triglycerides and predominant LDL diameter show a strong inverse correlation, probably because nonfasted triglycerides sufficiently reflect average 24-hour triglyceride levels.[168] A preponderance of small, dense LDL precedes the onset of noninsulin-dependent diabetes in elderly Finnish women.[170] There is also a cumulative association between the number of manifestations of syndrome X and the prevalence of small, dense LDL.[146,171]

Small, dense LDL particles are more likely to penetrate and adhere (by increased proteoglycan binding) to the subendothelium of the artery wall (the site of LDL oxidation).[166,167,172-174] In addition, smaller, denser LDL particles are intrinsically more susceptible to oxidation compared to the large buoyant variety.[175,176] Proportional increases in small, dense LDL with heightened susceptibility to oxidative modification may account for part of the increased cardiovascular risk in individuals with the small, dense LDL phenotype.[55,177,178] The reasons for increased oxidation susceptibility with decreasing particle size may include proportional polyunsaturated fatty acid increases[55,179] and decreased antioxidants (ubiquinol-10 and/or vitamin E)[180] per particle. Compared with more buoyant particles, small, dense LDLs show greater capacity to stimulate thromboxane synthesis by human umbilical vein endothelial cells[181] and to increase intracellular calcium in rat aorta smooth muscle.[182] These changes are consistent with a preferential effect of small, dense LDL on mechanisms promoting vasoconstriction.

Small, Dense LDL in Normal and Preeclamptic Pregnancy

The normal pregnancy rise in plasma triglyceride is associated with a shift from predominantly large and buoyant LDL (nonpregnancy) to intermediate and small, dense LDL (36 weeks' gestation), with partial reversal by 6 weeks postpartum.[183] The gestational progression of LDL particle diameter changes has been analyzed in plasma obtained serially from ten normally pregnant nonsmokers. The LDL peak particle diameter (predominant LDL size), corresponding to the major electrophoretic band, was measured by nondenaturing polyacrylamide gel electrophoresis.[184] LDL size correlated negatively with triglycerides (R = −0.61, P < 0.01). The within–individual decrease in LDL diameter from early (5–12 weeks) gestation to term (38–41 weeks) (mean angstroms [Å]: early 264; term 254), is unprecedented in normal physiology and substantial considering the usual size spectrum of LDL (about 270–240 Å) seen in large cross-sectional studies of nonpregnant populations.[146,185,186]

Hubel et al.[149] noted that LDL peak particle diameter is significantly decreased in preeclampsia relative to normal pregnancy plasma, correlating inversely with triglyceride concentrations. Sattar et al.[150] measured the mass of three LDL subfractions (LDL-I, II, and III) isolated on the basis of increasing density from plasma of women with preeclampsia and normal pregnancy. They observed that women with preeclampsia had lower concentrations of LDL I and II (the more buoyant, larger type), and markedly raised concentrations of LDL III (denser, smaller variant). Preheparin hepatic lipase activity was increased in preeclampsia plasma which, by hydrolysis of LDL triglycerides, could partially explain predominance of small, dense LDL in the syndrome.

It is evident that not all women with preeclampsia exhibit smaller, denser LDL relative to normal pregnancy. Apart from size differences, one component of pathophysiology in preeclampsia might be abnormal maternal or placental response to (or handling of) the small, dense LDL formed during pregnancy. Seemingly minor shifts to smaller, denser LDL may impart substantial increases in LDL oxidation susceptibility. The intrinsic susceptibility of isolated LDL to Cu^{2+}-mediated oxidation is increased in preeclampsia.[187] Whether this is a function of LDL size shift or some unrelated LDL difference is presently unclear.

The dyslipidemia and endothelial changes of preeclampsia have pathogenic parallels to atherosclerosis and diabetes, diseases in which oxidative stress is strongly implicated as a causal factor.[8,47,48] In preeclampsia, however, evidence for the interaction of plasma lipids, reactive oxygen species, and endothelial cell dysfunction is largely indirect. In contrast to atherosclerosis, for example, there are currently no positive or negative reports on isolation of oxidized lipids from vascular tissues in preeclampsia. Despite these gaps in our knowledge, other findings in the maternal circulation bolster the contention that oxidative stress exists in preeclampsia and is of pathogenic importance. Some data are summarized in the next section.

MARKERS OF OXIDATIVE STRESS IN THE MATERNAL CIRCULATION

Lipid Peroxidation Products

Scores of reports indicate that lipid peroxidation degradation products (especially as estimated by thiobarbituric acid-reactive substances, which include malondi-aldehyde) are increased in plasma/sera of women with preeclampsia relative to normal pregnancy.[12,30,188-194] (Articles cited in references 9 through 11 also support this information.) Increased lipid peroxidation products have been observed in platelets[195] and red blood cells[196] from women with preeclampsia. Since peroxidation metabolites in serum also appear to be increased above nonpregnant levels in pregnancy,[10,197] it is possible that normal pregnancy induces oxidative stress. One of the more compelling evidences of lipid peroxidation is the reported decrease in linoleic acid (expressed as percentage of total esterified fatty acids) in plasma phospholipid and triglyceride fractions from early to late pregnancy in women with preeclampsia compared to normal pregnancy. Progressive lipid peroxidation is a likely culprit in these changes as reviewed by the authors.[13]

High-pressure liquid chromatography can be used to separate authentic serum malondialdehyde from interfering chromogens. Use of this technique revealed that malondialdehyde concentrations are about 50% higher in sera from women with preeclampsia and decrease significantly within 48 hours postpartum. In comparison, no decrease was noted postpartum in normal controls. Predelivery serum triglycerides and free fatty acids (higher in preeclampsia) correlated positively with malondialdehyde ($R = 0.62$, $P < 0.02$) in both cases. Addition of antioxidants before assay did not substantially change the levels, suggesting a linkage of maternal dyslipidemia and lipid peroxidation in preeclampsia.[12]

Apart from platelets and red cells, evidence for increased lipid peroxidation in cells or tissues outside the placenta is sparse. Lipofuscin-like pigments indicative of lipid peroxidation have been reported in hepatocytes of women with preeclampsia although there was no control group.[198]

Circulating Anti-oxidized LDL Antibodies

During LDL modification, malondialdehyde and 4-hydroxynonenal are formed. These products react with lysine residues and become immunogenic. Low titers of antibodies directed against oxidized LDL are found in the serum of most people but are increased in disorders associated with oxidative stress and in individuals with the small, dense LDL phenotype.[190] Increased autoantibodies to an epitope of oxidized LDL have been described in women with preeclampsia relative to normal pregnancy, although a negative report also exists.[200,201] Kurki et al. found that antibodies to oxidized LDL and anticardiolipin were not increased in pregnant women who subsequently developed preeclampsia compared to women whose pregnancies remained normal.[202] The pathophysiologic implications of these circulating markers remain uncertain.

Do Lipid Hydroperoxides Circulate?

Plasma ascorbate (vitamin C) completely protects plasma lipoproteins from peroxidation during exposure to a wide spectrum of water- or lipid-soluble free radical generators in vitro. Lipid peroxidation does not begin in these assay systems until ascorbate concentrations reach virtually zero.[89,203] Thus, since ascorbate and other antioxidants are present in plasma, susceptible lipids are believed to be protected from significant oxidation in the circulation.[47,204] The existence of substantial lipid hydroperoxides in the circulation (as opposed to vascular wall) is debated at present.[205,206] A minimally oxidized form of LDL may escape recognition by scavenger receptors and thus persist longer in the circulation.[47] Single photon counting of lipid hydroperoxides in normal (nonpregnant) human plasma reveals very low concentrations (range 230–500 nM), but unveils artifactual peroxidation during isolation of LDL from plasma.[207,208] Pregnancy and preeclampsia are unique situations which might predispose to damaging increases in circulating lipid hydroperoxides. However, there is presently insufficient evidence for this. High circulating levels of malondialdehyde presumably originate from outside the plasma compartment and do not necessarily indicate higher circulating lipid hydroperoxides.

Lessons from Extracellular Antioxidants

Nonenzymatic, low molecular mass antioxidants are the primary protectants against oxidative damage in the extracellular compartment.[89] They protect by reacting with radicals faster than radicals can react with potential targets and because antioxidant radicals formed during electron transfer are usually less reactive than the initial inciting radical. Whether a molecule acts as an oxidant or reductant in any given interaction can often be predicted from tables of standard one-electron reduction potentials.[18,209] For example, α-tocopherol (α-TOH) slows lipid peroxidation by scavenging lipid peroxyl radicals (LOO•), thus breaking the peroxidation chain (LOO• + α-TOH• $\longrightarrow$ lipid hydroperoxide (LOOH + α-TO•). The tocopherol (chromanoxyl) radical (αTO•) formed is less reactive than the initial peroxyl radical. However, tocopherol radical produced as a "side effect" of initial protection can behave as an oxidant depending upon the availability of suitable reduced species.[210] One likely function of ascorbate is to regenerate α-TOH by reducing tocopherol radicals in membranes and lipoproteins at the water–lipid interface.[89] The resulting semidehydroascorbate anion radical (asc•−) is extremely unreactive. Ascorbate is thus a supreme antioxidant nutrient.[89,211]

Plasma ascorbate reserves decrease gradually throughout normal pregnancy.[212] Decreased plasma ascorbate concentrations in preeclampsia relative to normal pregnancy was reported in 1964.[213] In a more recent study, plasma ascorbate was decreased in mild and severe preeclampsia whereas α-TOH and beta-carotene were decreased only in severe disease compared to normal pregnant controls. The oxidized form of ascorbate, dehydroascorbic acid, was not decreased, suggesting that oxidative consumption of ascorbate occurred.[33] Table 14–3 is com-

TABLE 14–3. PLASMA ANTIOXIDANT RESERVES IN WOMEN WITH PREECLAMPSIA AND NORMAL PREGNANCY

	Ascorbate nmol/mL	Total Thiols nmol/mL	Vitamin E nmol/mL	Vitamin E nmol/μmol Lipid[a]
Preeclampsia (N = 12)	11.0 (9.2–15.3)	646 (518–794)	25.7 (21.8–30.6)	2.8 (2.4–2.9)
Normal pregnancy (N = 13)	21.1 (16.8–26.4)	516 (476–598)	21.3 (16.1–22.8)	2.4 (2.0–3.0)
Significance	$P < 0.002$	NS ($P = 0.05$)	NS ($P = 0.06$)	NS ($P = 0.53$)

Data are medians and interquartile ranges
NS = not significant
[a] Lpid corrected = vitamin E/(cholesterol + triglycerides) in nmol/μmol

piled from a recent study on concentrations of ascorbate, total thiols (glutathione + protein thiols), and α-TOH in plasma.[32] Ascorbate concentrations were 50% lower in preeclampsia relative to normal pregnancy plasma but thiols and α-TOH did not differ. These relationships were maintained in a subset of samples obtained at term and were independent of labor or magnesium sulfate.

Assessment of these data prompted experiments to determine whether endogenous factors in blood and plasma from women with preeclampsia escalate oxidative depletion of ascorbate in vitro. Freshly obtained, EDTA-anticoagulated whole blood samples from women with normal and preeclamptic pregnancies (prior to labor and $MgSO_4$) were incubated and plasma aliquots harvested at successive time intervals. Concentration changes in endogenous plasma ascorbate and total thiols were measured over time by electron paramagnetic resonance (EPR) spectroscopy. The median time interval required for half-consumption of ascorbate was markedly less in the case of preeclampsia (preeclampsia: 95 minutes [69–136 interquartile range]; normal pregnancy: 360 minutes [302–410 interquartile range]; $P < 0.04$).[32] No concomitant decrease in thiols was evident.

During its antioxidant action, ascorbate undergoes two consecutive one electron oxidations to dehydroascorbic acid with intermediate formation of the ascorbate radical. In contrast to ascorbate radical, ascorbate and dehydroascorbate are EPR-silent. The initial ascorbate radical signal amplitude is directly proportional to the overall rate of ascorbate oxidation, whereas the signal duration is inversely proportional. Ascorbate radical thus serves as a marker for the degree of ongoing oxidative stress in plasma,[211,214] and EPR spectroscopy was used to measure temporal changes in ascorbate radical signal amplitude in plasma after equalization of ascorbate concentrations by addition of exogenous ascorbate. Figure 14–2 illustrates that the initial ascorbate radical signal amplitude was greater in preeclampsia plasma and then, in contrast to normal pregnancy plasma, decreased progressively during the recording interval. These data demonstrate that an ascorbate-oxidizing activity is increased in blood from women with preeclampsia, at least a portion of which is present in the plasma (independent of blood cells). Iron chelators had no effect on the ascorbyl radical signal suggesting that free iron

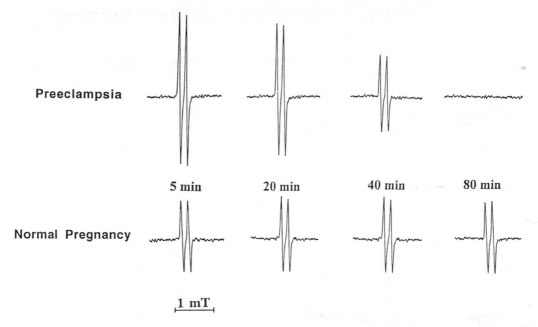

Figure 14–2. Representative electron paramagnetic resonance spectra of ascorbate radical in plasma from preeclamptic (top) and normal (bottom) pregnancies. The amplitude of the signal is proportional to the steady-state concentration of ascorbate radical. The initial ascorbate radical signal amplitude is higher in preeclampsia plasma and then, in contrast to normal plasma, decreases progressively indicating increased ascorbate oxidation. Method: Plasma containing added ascorbate (1 mmol/L final concentration) was drawn into a gas-permeable Teflon tube and ascorbate radical spectra were continuously recorded (postascorbate addition) at 25°C, g = 2.00, 335.5 mT center field, 10 mW power, 0.05 mT field modulation, 5 mT sweep width, 1600 receiver gain, and 1.0 second time constant. Spectra were collected using EPRMare software (Scientific Software Services, Bloomington, IL). No exogenous oxidation catalysts were added.

is not the catalyst for ascorbate oxidation.[32] The identity of the factor(s) is presently unknown.

Plasma vitamin E concentrations are increased in preeclampsia especially in severe cases.[215] An earlier study found increased serum α-TOH in severe, but not mild, preeclampsia, relative to normal pregnancy, but these differences were eliminated after normalization to cholesterol.[190] One likely explanation for the vitamin E increase is the marked hyperlipoproteinemia characterizing preeclampsia. Vitamin E is transported in plasma lipoproteins and thus elevated lipid concentrations generally result in elevated vitamin E.[216] Lipid-adjustment better reflects the number of α-TOH molecules per lipoprotein particle and thus, potential impact upon lipoprotein oxidative resistance. It is notable that Table 14–3 indicates no differences in lipid-corrected vitamin E concentrations. These patients reported daily intake of prenatal vitamins containing vitamins E and C during pregnancy, a factor likely to diminish the influence of diet.

DO INTERACTIONS OF MATERNAL AND PLACENTAL FACTORS AMPLIFY OXIDATIVE STRESS?

The interplay of placental and maternal components has the potential to amplify oxidative stress. For example, the progressively smaller, denser LDL formed during pregnancy should be increasingly susceptible to oxidation, and oxidation could occur during transit through the abnormal placenta in preeclampsia. In trophoblasts and macrophages of the normal placenta, scavenger receptor activity (uptake of modified LDL) greatly exceeds "native" LDL receptor activity.[217] Low density lipoprotein might be prone to oxidation during its relatively slow traversal through the intervillous space in direct contact with trophoblast cells.[217] Low density lipoprotein from retroplacental blood collected from the maternal surface of the human placenta shows increased electrophoretic mobility on agarose gel relative to LDL from maternal peripheral blood.[218] This change could be secondary to oxidation and would predict enhanced recognition by scavenger receptors.[58,219] More work is needed to explore these potential relationships.

Apart from the lack of conclusive evidence of oxidized placental lipids, there are indications of increased potential for lipid peroxidation in placentae of women with preeclampsia. Syncytiotrophoblast plasma membranes isolated from women with preeclampsia show increased concentrations of malondialdehyde and are intrinsically more susceptible to lipid peroxidation in response to the prooxidant, phenylhydrazine. An associated increase in availability of unsaturated fatty acids (the substrate for peroxidation) could account for susceptibility increases.[220] The maximum amount of peroxidizable material (normalized as per mg protein) is increased in homogenates of placentae from women with preeclampsia relative to normal pregnancy.[92] Increased unsaturated lipid availability or increased triglyceride content in preeclamptic placentae[221] could account for the latter finding. Syncytiotrophoblast membranes from preeclamptics have decreased fluidity suggesting the presence of lipid peroxidation products that may predispose to increased membrane shedding (deportation) into the circulation.[222] There are few details relating maternal lipid metabolism and placental membrane lipid composition.

Placental changes might contribute to maternal dyslipidemia. Expression of mRNA for LDL and VLDL receptors increase in the placenta late in normal pregnancy but to a lesser degree in preeclampsia, indicating reduced synthesis of the receptors. Decreased receptor concentrations would decrease placental receptor-mediated uptake of maternal plasma VLDL and thus reduce clearance of these lipoproteins.[223]

Hypoxia promotes excess production of placental TNF-α. Hypoxic placental release of the cytokine into the maternal circulation might promote endothelial dysfunction in preeclampsia.[117] Amplification of injurious effects of TNF-α by increased maternal lipids is possible. Unsaturated fatty acids and TNF-α cooperatively amplify endothelial oxidative stress and dysfunction in vitro.[158,159] The increased adipose production of TNF-α, characteristic of insulin resistance, could conjoin with placentally derived TNF-α to further raise circulating levels of this cytokine in a subset of women with preeclampsia. A vicious circle of further placental vasospasm and hypoxic production of TNF-α could be instigated by TNF-α stimulation of mitochondrial and neutrophil reactive oxygen species production.[118]

Neutrophil activation can be promoted by hyperlipidemia (particularly hypertriglyceridemia and increased free fatty acids).[123,124,164,224,225] Increased triglyceride and/or free fatty acid in the circulation of women with preeclampsia could combine with placental factors, such as TNF-α, to promote oxidative stress by neutrophil activation.

The multiple possible sources of oxidative stress in preeclampsia suggest mechanisms by which the maternal constitution (i.e., genetic predisposition and environmental influences) and reduced placental perfusion could converge. At one extreme, the generation of reactive oxygen species could be solely due to placental postischemic reperfusion/reoxygenation. Alternatively, in women with normal placental perfusion, qualitative and quantitative changes in circulating lipids consequent to genetically linked insulin resistance and obesity could increase susceptibility beyond the threshold for excessive lipid peroxidation. At another extreme, marked dietary deficiency or genetically decreased antioxidant protection alone could precipitate oxidative stress. More likely, combinations of these variables cross-amplify (or summate) to generate oxidative injury. Such interactions could contribute to the observed heterogeneity of preeclampsia.[7]

ANTIOXIDANT HAZARDS AND CLINICAL TRIALS

There has been increasing interest in clinical trials of antioxidants for prevention or treatment of preeclampsia. Reconstitution of the physiologic balance between reactive oxygen species generation and antioxidant protection may preserve the "defensive" activities of the vascular endothelium and thus restrict the pathophysiologic changes of the disorder. Therapeutic strategies against oxidative stress, however, should be mechanism-based. In this respect, antioxidants are not always "good" nor reactive oxygen species always "evil." Unwanted perturbation of the normal signal transduction role of various reactive oxygen species would be counterproductive. Certain antioxidants can cause damage in biologic systems different from those in which they exert protection; an antioxidant in one setting can behave as a prooxidant in another.[25,209,226] For example, the water-soluble vitamin E analog, Trolox C, shows both antioxidant and prooxidant properties in vitro, and caution has been recommended regarding its therapeutic use.[15] Another example is the concern regarding possible prooxidant effects of ascorbate in vivo under unusual circumstances. Ascorbate reduces ferric iron (Fe^{3+}) to the highly oxidizing ferrous form (Fe^{2+}) and iron-ascorbate mixtures are often used to stimulate lipid peroxidation in vitro. The combination of unsequestered, catalytic transition metal ions and administered vitamin C is associated with adverse clinical effects in hemochromatosis patients.[209]

It follows that no one antioxidant is effective in all circumstances. The heterogeneic function of antioxidants is exemplified by two different antioxidant bioassays used to study preeclampsia. Serum antioxidant activity, measured as the ability of serum to inhibit trace iron-catalyzed peroxidation of tissue homogenate lipids, is governed by apotransferrin and ceruloplasmin.[209,227-229] Serum ceruloplasmin and transferrin act in concert to effectively eliminate iron-catalyzed free radical activity in normal plasma. Ceruloplasmin converts Fe^{2+} to Fe^{3+} by its iron-oxidizing (ferroxidase) activity, and apotransferrin then sequesters Fe^{3+} with high affinity.[230] A substantial deficit in this serum antioxidant activity is observed in preeclampsia relative to normal pregnancy[231] because serum transferrin iron-binding reserve (apotransferrin) is decreased.[30] In contrast, antioxidant activity measured as the ability of plasma to scavenge water-soluble peroxyl radicals is increased in preeclampsia and this is largely a function of increased uric acid concentrations.[232] Xanthine oxidase produces uric acid (an antioxidant) but can also be a major source of local reactive oxygen species as previously discussed. In preeclampsia plasma, increased uric acid concentrations could be protective. However, reaction of uric acid with some reactive oxygen species, such as hydroxyl radical (OH•), can generate uric acid radicals that are themselves capable of causing cell damage.[230,233] It would not be surprising if the effects of a xanthine-oxidase inhibitor, such as allopurinol, are complex in preeclampsia.

In one trial, vitamin E supplementation failed to have a salutary effect on the course of already established preeclampsia,[234] but, as noted, plasma vitamin E deficiency is not a characteristic of the disorder. In another report, a randomized control trial in which a combination of antioxidants were orally administered (800 IU vitamin E, 1000 mg vitamin C, 200 mg allopurinol twice daily for 1–2 weeks) to women with established early-onset preeclampsia (usually severe), no changes in maternal placental thiobarbituric acid-reactive substances (an index of lipid peroxidation) and no alterations in glutathione concentration were noted. There was, however, a tendency for the treated group to deliver later.[235] Also, decreased concentrations of uric acid and increased concentrations of vitamin E, but no differences in thiobarbituric acid-reactive substances, were noted in the sera of these treated subjects.[236]

In essence, although the potential for administering antioxidants to prevent or treat preeclampsia is appealing, we suggest that their incorporation into clinical care be deferred until (1) appropriate antioxidants can be established and (2) clinical trials demonstrate safety and efficacy for both mother and baby.

CONCLUSION

Multiple lines of evidence implicate oxidative stress in the pathogenesis of preeclampsia. Abnormal placentation with reduced uteroplacental perfusion might lead primarily to intrauterine growth restriction. If further complicated by maternal dyslipidemia, and/or a primary or secondary decrease of antioxidants, preeclampsia might become increasingly likely. Differences in importance of placental defects relative to maternal oxidative stress risk factors in different subsets of women could account for the heterogeneity of preeclampsia. Work is needed regarding (1) definitive evidence of maternal oxidative injury in vivo, (2) the status, origin, and targets of specific reactive oxygen species, (3) whether observed decrements in antioxidant levels, including ascorbate, are a cause or consequence of oxidative stress, and (4) the role of reactive oxygen species, small, dense LDL, and abnormal lipids in endothelial dysfunction. Although emphasis has been placed on increased oxidative stress in preeclampsia, differences in maternal vascular response to a given oxidant burden in preeclampsia compared to intrauterine growth restriction or normal pregnancy may exist and be vitally important. The signal transduction role of reactive oxygen species in normal pregnancy progression deserves study. Longitudinal studies using new probes for antioxidant/reactive oxygen species interactions should be helpful.

REFERENCES

1. Redman CWG: Current topic: Pre-eclampsia and the placenta. *Placenta* 1991;12:301–308.
2. Zhou Y, Damsky CH, Chiu K, et al: Preeclampsia is associated with abnormal expression of adhesion molecules by invasive cytotrophoblasts. *J Clin Invest* 1993;91:950–960.
3. Cross JC: Trophoblast function in normal and preeclamptic pregnancy. *Fetal Maternal Med Rev* 1996;8:57–66.
4. Friedman SA, Taylor RN, Roberts JM: Pathophysiology of preeclampsia. *Clin Perinatol* 1991;18(4):661–682.
5. Roberts JM, Taylor RN, Musci TJ, et al: Preeclampsia: An endothelial cell disorder. *Am J Obstet Gynecol* 1990;163(1):1365–1366.
6. deGroot CJM, Taylor RN: New insights into the etiology of pre-eclampsia. *Ann Med* 1993; 25:243–249.
7. Ness RB, Roberts JM: Heterogeneous causes constituting the single syndrome of preeclampsia: A hypothesis and its implications. *Am J Obstet Gynecol* 1996;175:1365–1370.
8. Sattar N, Gaw A, Packard CJ, Greer IA: Potential pathogenic roles of aberrant lipoprotein and fatty acid metabolism in pre-eclampsia. *Br J Obstet Gynaecol* 1996;103:614–620.
9. Hubel CA, Roberts JM, Taylor RN, et al: Lipid peroxidation in pregnancy: New perspectives on preeclampsia. *Am J Obstet Gynecol* 1989;161:1025–1034.
10. Walsh SC: Lipid peroxidation in pregnancy. *Hypertens Pregnancy* 1994;13:1–25.
11. Zeeman GG, Dekker GA: Pathogenesis of preeclampsia. A hypothesis. *Clin Obstet Gynecol* 1992;35(2):317–337.
12. Hubel CA, McLaughlin MK, Evans RW, et al: Fasting serum triglycerides, free fatty acids, and malondialdehyde are increased in preeclampsia, are positively correlated, and decrease within 48 hours postpartum. *Am J Obstet Gynecol* 1996;174:975–982.
13. Lorentzen B, Drevon CA, Endressen MJ, Henriksen T: Fatty acid pattern of esterfied and free fatty acids in sera of women with normal and pre-eclamptic pregnancy. *Br J Obstet Gynaecol* 1995;102:530–537.
14. Kaaja R, Tikkanen MJ, Viinikka L, Ylikorkala O: Serum lipoproteins, insulin, and urinary prostanoid metabolites in normal and hypertensive pregnant women. *Obstet Gynecol* 1995; 85(3):353–356.
15. Halliwell B, Gutteridge JMC, Cross CE: Free radicals, antioxidants, and human disease: Where are we now? *J Lab Clin Med* 1992;119(6):598–620.
16. Halliwell B: Reactive oxygen species in living systems: Source, biochemistry, and role in human disease. *Am J Med* 1991;91:14S–22S.

17. Halliwell B: The biochemistry of oxygen free radicals. In: Aruoma O, ed. *Free Radicals in Tropical Diseases*. Chur, Switzerland: Harwood Academic Publishers; 1993:1–12.
18. Buettner GR: The pecking order of free radicals and antioxidants: Lipid peroxidation, α-toxopherol, and ascorbate. *Arch Biochem Biophys* 1993;300(2):535–543.
19. Sen CK, Packer L: Antioxidant and redox regulation of gene transcription. *FASEB J* 1996; 10:709–720.
20. Yu BP: Cellular defenses against damage from reactive oxygen species. *Physiol Rev* 1994;74(1):139–162.
21. Gutteridge JMC: Invited review free radicals in disease processes: A compilation of cause and consequence. *Free Rad Res Comm* 1993;19(3):141–158.
22. Berliner JA, Heinecke JA: The role of oxidized lipoproteins in atherogenesis. *Free Rad Biol Med* 1996;20:707–727.
23. Halliwell B: The role of oxygen radicals in human disease, with particular reference to the vascular system. *Haemostasis* 1993;23:118–126.
24. Halliwell B: Free radicals and vascular disease: How much do we know. *Br Med J* 1993; 307:885–886.
25. Halliwell B: Free radicals, antioxidants, and human disease: Curiosity, cause, or consequence? *Lancet* 1994;344:721–724.
26. Kirschner RE, Fantini GA: Role of iron and oxygen-derived free radicals in ischemia-reperfusion injury. *J Am Coll Surg* 1994;179(1):103–117.
27. Omar B, McCord J, Downey J: Ischaemia–reperfusion. In: Sies H, ed. *Oxidative Stress: Oxidants and Antioxidants*. New York: Academic Press; 1991:493–527.
28. Sussman MS, Bulkley GB: Oxygen-derived free radical in reperfusion injury. In: Packer L, ed. *Methods in Enzymology*. San Diego: Academic Press; 1990, vol 186:711–723.
29. Bulkley GB: Reactive oxygen metabolites and reperfusion injury: Aberrant triggering of reticuloendothelial function. *Lancet* 1994;344:934–936.
30. Hubel CA, Kozlov AV, Evans RW, et al: Decreased transferrin and increased transferrin saturation in sera of women with preeclampsia: Implications for oxidative stress. *Am J Obstet Gynecol* 1996;175:692–700.
31. Entman SS, Richardson LD, Killam AP: Elevated serum ferritin in the altered ferrokinetics of toxemia of pregnancy. *Am J Obstet Gynecol* 1982;144:418–422.
32. Hubel CA, Kagan VE, Kisin ER, et al: Increased ascorbate radical formation and ascorbate depletion in plasma from women with preeclampsia: Implications for oxidative stress. *Free Rad Biol Med* 1997;23(4):597–609.
33. Mikhail MS, Anyaegbunam A, Garfinkel D, et al: Preeclampsia and antioxidant nutrients: Decreased plasma levels of reduced ascorbic acid, α-tocopherol, and beta-carotene in women with preeclampsia. *Am J Obstet Gynecol* 1994;171:150–157.
34. Halliwell B, Chirico S: Lipid peroxidation: Its mechanism, measurement, and significance. *Am J Clin Nutr* 1993;57:715S–725S.
35. Wardman P, Candeias LP: Fenton chemistry: An introduction. *Radiat Res* 1996;145:523–531.
36. Radi R, Beckman JS, Freeman BS: Peroxynitrite-induced membrane lipid oxidation: The cytotoxic potential of superoxide and nitric oxide. *Arch Biochem Biophys* 1991;288:481–487.
37. Freeman BA, White CR, Gutierrez H, et al: Oxygen radical-nitric oxide reactions in vascular diseases. *Adv Pharmacol* 1995;34:45–69.
38. Smith WL, Marnett LJ, DeWitt DL: Prostaglandin and thromboxane biosynthesis. *Pharmacol Ther* 1991;49:153–179.
39. Cowan CL, Steffen RP: Lysophosphatidylcholine inhibits relaxation of rabbit abdominal aorta mediated by endothelium-derived nitric oxide and endothelium-derived hyperpolarizing factor independent of protein kinase C activation. *Arterioscler Thromb Vasc Biol* 1995;15: 2290–2297.
40. Esterbauer H, Schaur RJ, Zollner H: Chemistry and biochemistry of 4-hydroxynonenal, malonaldehyde and related aldehydes. *Free Rad Biol Med* 1991;11:81–128.
41. Esterbauer H: Cytotoxicity and genotoxicity of lipid-oxidation products. *Am J Clin Nutr* 1993;57:779S–786S.
42. Harlan JM: Neutrophil-mediated vascular injury. *Acta Med Scand* 1987;715:123–129.

43. Gorog P, Kovacs IB: Lipid peroxidation by activated platelets: A possible link between thrombosis and atherogenesis. *Atherosclerosis* 1995;115:121–128.
44. Aviram M: LDL-platelet interaction under oxidative stress induces macrophage foam cell formation. *Thromb Haemostat* 1995;74:560–564.
45. Stewart DJ, Monge JC: Hyperlipidemia and endothelial dysfunction. *Curr Opin Lipidol* 1993;4:319–324.
46. Endresen MJR: Preeclampsia and endothelial cell function. *Acta Obstet Gynecol Scand* 1995;74:667–669.
47. Witztum JL: The oxidation hypothesis of atherosclerosis. *Lancet* 1994;344:793–795.
48. Chisolm GM, Irwin KC, Penn MS: Lipoprotein oxidation and lipoprotein-induced cell injury in diabetes. *Diabetes* 1992;41(2):61–66.
49. Steinberg D, Parthasarathy S, Carew T, et al: Beyond cholesterol: Modifications of low-density lipoprotein that increase its atheogenicity. *N Engl J Med* 1989;320:915–924.
50. Yla-Herttuala S, Palinski W, Rosenfeld ME, et al: Evidence for the presence of oxidatively modified low density lipoprotein in atherosclerotic lesions of rabbit and man. *J Clin Invest* 1989;84:1086–1095.
51. Dabbagh AJ, Frei B: Human suction blister interstitial fluid prevents metal ion-dependent oxidation of low density lipoprotein by macrophages and in cell-free systems. *J Clin Invest* 1995;96:1958–1966.
52. Parhami F, Fang ZT, Fogelman AM, et al: Minimally modified low density lipoprotein-induced inflammatory responses in endothelial cells are mediated by cyclic adenosine monophosphate. *J Clin Invest* 1993;92:471–478.
53. Navab M, Berliner JA, Watson AD, et al: The yin and yang of oxidation in the development of the fatty streak. *Arterioscler Thromb Vasc Biol* 1996;16:831–842.
54. Frei B, Gaziano JM: Content of antioxidants, preformed lipid hydroperoxides, and cholesterol as predictors of the susceptibility of human LDL to metal ion-dependent and independent oxidation. *J Lipid Res* 1993;34:2135–2145.
55. Witztum JL: Susceptibility of low-density lipoprotein to oxidative modification. *Am J Med* 1993;94:347–349.
56. Haberland ME, Fong D, Cheng L: Malondialdehyde-altered protein occurs in atheroma of watanabe heritable hyperlipidemic rabbits. *Science* 1988;241:215–218.
57. Salonen JT, Yla-Herttuala S, Yamamoto R, et al: Autoantibody against oxidized LDL and progression of carotid atherosclerosis. *Lancet* 1992;339:883–887.
58. Steinberg D, Parthasarathy S, Carew TE, et al: Beyond cholesterol: Modifications of low-density lipoprotein that increase its atherogenicity. *N Engl J Med* 1989;320(14):915–924.
59. Spiteller G: Enzymic lipid peroxidation—A consequence of cell injury. *Free Rad Biol Med* 1996;21:1003–1009.
60. Janero DR: Malondialdehyde and thiobarbituric acid-reactivity as diagnostic indices of lipid peroxidation and peroxidative tissue injury. *Free Rad Biol Med* 1990;9:515–540.
61. Pryor WA, Godber SS: Noninvasive measures of oxidative stress status in humans. *Free Rad Biol Med* 1991;10:177–184.
62. Puhl H, Waeg G, Esterbauer H: Methods to determine oxidation of low-density lipoproteins. In: Packer L, ed. *Methods in Enzymology*. San Diego: Academic Press; 1994, vol 233:425–441.
63. Zhou Y, Damsky CH, Fisher SJ: Preeclampsia is associated with failure of human cytotrophoblasts to mimic a vascular adhesion phenotype. *J Clin Invest* 1997;99:2152–2164.
64. Lunell NO, Lewander R, Mamoun I, et al: Uteroplacental blood flow in pregnancy-induced hypertension. *Scand J Clin Lab Invest* 1984;44:28–35.
65. Trudinger BJ, Giles WD, Cook CM, et al: Fetal umbilical artery flow velocity waveforms and placental resistance: Clinical significance. *Br J Obstet Gynaecol* 1985;92:23–30.
66. Wigglesworth JS: Morphologic variations in the insufficient placenta. *J Obstet Gynecol Br Commonw* 1964;71:871–884.
67. Tominaga T, Page EW: Accommodation of the human placenta to hypoxia. *Am J Obstet Gynecol* 1966;94:679–685.
68. Zamudio S, Palmer SK, Dahms TE, et al: Alterations in uteroplacental blood flow precede hypertension in preeclampsia at high altitude. *Am Physiol Soc* 1995;79:15–22.

69. Zamudio S, Palmer SK, Regensteiner JG, Moore LG: High altitude and hypertension during pregnancy. *Am J Human Biol* 1995;7:183–193.

70. Cooper JC, Sharkey AM, Charnock-Jones DS, et al: VEGF mRNA levels in placentae from pregnancies complicated by pre-eclampsia. *Br J Obstet Gynecol* 1996;103:1191–1196.

71. Kuroki M, Voest EE, Amano S, et al: Reactive oxygen intermediates increase vascular endothelial growth factor expression in vitro and in vivo. *J Clin Invest* 1996;98:1667–1675.

72. Beckman JS: Oxidative damage and tyrosine nitration from peroxynitrite. *Chem Res Toxicol* 1996;9:836–844.

73. Beckman JS, Koppenol WH: Nitric oxide, superoxide, and peroxynitrite: The good, the bad, and the ugly. *Am J Physiol* 1996;271:C1424–C1437.

74. Vliet AVD, Smith D, O'Neill CA, et al: Interactions of peroxynitrite with human plasma and its constituents: Oxidative damage and antioxidant depletion. *Biochem J* 1994;303:295–301.

75. Goda N, Suematsu M, Mukai M, et al: Modulation of mitochondrion-mediated oxidative stress by nitric oxide in human placental trophoblastic cells. *Am J Physiol* 1996;271: H1893–H1899.

76. Rubbo H, Radi R, Trujillo M, et al: Nitric oxide regulation of superoxide and peroxynitrite-dependent lipid peroxidation. *J Biol Chem* 1994;269:26066–26075.

77. Beckmann JS, Ye YZ, Anderson PG, et al: Extensive nitration of protein tyrosines in human atherosclerosis detected by immunohistochemistry. *Biol Chem Hoppe-Seyler* 1994;375:81–88.

78. Kooy NW, Royall JA, Ye YZ, et al: Evidence for in vivo peroxynitrite production in human acute lung injury. *Am J Respir Crit Care Med* 1995;151:1250–1254.

79. Myatt L, Rosenfield RB, Eis ALW, et al: Nitrotyrosine residues in placenta: Evidence of peroxynitrite formation and action. *Hypertension* 1996;28:488–493.

80. Conrad KP, Vill M, McGuire PG, et al: Expression of nitric oxide synthase by syncytiotrophoblast in human placental villi. *FASEB J* 1993;7:1269–1276.

81. Kimura E, Kosaka H, Shiga T, et al: Elevation of plasma nitric oxide end-products during focal cerebral ischemia and reperfusion in the rat. *J Cereb Blood Flow Metab* 1994;14: 487–491.

82. Kooy NW, Royall JA: Agonist-induced peroxynitrite production from endothelial cells. *Arch Biochem Biophys* 1994;310(2):352–359.

83. Radi R, Cosgrove TP, Beckman JS, Freeman BA: Peroxynitrite-induced luminol chemiluminescence. *Biochem J* 1993;290:51–57.

84. Carreras MC, Pargament GA, Catz SD, et al: Kinetics of nitric oxide and hydrogen peroxide production and formation of peroxynitrite during the respiratory burst of human neutrophils. *FEBS Letters* 1994;341:65–68.

85. Many A, Hubel CA, Roberts JM: Hyperuricemia and xanthine oxidase in preeclampsia revisited. *Am J Obstet Gynecol* 1996;174:288–291.

86. Many A, Westerhausen-Larson A, Kanbour-Shakir A, Roberts JM: Xanthine oxidase/dehydrogenase is present in human placenta. *Placenta* 1996;17:361–365.

87. Many A, Friedman SA, Hubel CA, Roberts JM: Xanthine oxidase activity in preeclamptic women is higher in invasive but not villous trophoblast. *J Soc Gynecol Invest* 1996;3:36A.

88. Many A, Zhou Y, Hubel CA, et al: Invasive cytotrophoblast manifest evidence of oxidative stress in preeclampsia. *Submitted*. 1998.

89. Stocker R, Frei B: Endogenous antioxidant defences in human blood plasma. In: Sies H, ed. *Oxidative Stress: Oxidants and Antioxidants*. New York: Academic Press Ltd.; 1991:213–243.

90. Takehara Y, Yoshioka T, Sasaki J: Changes in the levels of lipoperoxide and antioxidant factors in human placenta during gestation. *Acta Med Okayama* 1990;44(2):103–111.

91. Sekiba K, Yoshioka T: Changes of lipid peroxidation and superoxide dismutase activity in the human placenta. *Am J Obstet Gynecol* 1979;135:368–371.

92. Poranen AK, Ekblad U, Uotila P, Ahotupa M: Lipid peroxidation and antioxidants in normal and pre-eclamptic pregnancies. *Placenta* 1996;17:401–405.

93. Pandey S, Gujrati VR, Chandravati, et al: Status of human placental lipid peroxidation, superoxide dismutase and catalase during pregnancy-induced hypertension (PIH). *Asia Pacific J Pharmacol* 1995;10:41–44.

94. Wang Y, Walsh SW: Antioxidant activities and mRNA expression of superoxide dismutase,

catalase, and glutathione peroxidase in normal and preeclamptic placentas. *J Soc Gynecol Invest* 1996;3:179–184.

95. Myatt L, Eis ALW, Brockman DE, et al: Differential localization of superoxide dismutase isoforms in placental villous tissue. *J Soc Gynecol Invest* 1996;3:226A.

96. Chen G, Wilson R, Boyd P, et al: Normal superoxide dismutase (SOD) gene in pregnancy-induced hypertension: Is the decreased SOD activity a secondary phenomenon? *Free Rad Res* 1994;21(2):59–66.

97. Wisdom SJ, Wilson R, McKillip JH, Walker JJ: Antioxidant systems in normal pregnancy and in pregnancy-induced hypertension. *Am J Obstet Gynecol* 1991;165:1701–1704.

98. Warner HR: Superoxide dismutase, aging, and degenerative disease. *Free Rad Biol Med* 1994;17:249–258.

99. Lu D, Maulik N, Moraru II, et al: Molecular adaptation of vascular endothelial cells to oxidative stress. *Am J Physiol* 1993;264:C715–C722.

100. Uotila J, Kirkkola AL, Rorarius M, et al: The total peroxyl radical-trapping ability of plasma and cerebrospinal fluid in normal and preeclamptic parturients. *Free Rad Biol Med* 1994;16:581–590.

101. Becker BF: Towards the physiological function of uric acid. *Free Rad Biol Med* 1993;14:615–631.

102. Walsh SW, Wang Y: Deficient glutathione peroxidase activity in preeclampsia activity in preeclampsia is associated with increased placental production of thromboxane and lipid peroxides. *Am J Obstet Gynecol* 1993;169:1456–1461.

103. Warso MA, Lands WEM: Lipid peroxidation in relation to prostacyclin and thromboxane physiology and pathophysiology. *Br Med Bull* 1983;39(3):277–280.

104. Hemler ME, Lands WEM: Evidence for a peroxide-initiated free radical mechanism of prostaglandin synthesis. *J Biol Chem* 1980;255:6253–6261.

105. Moncada S, Vane JR: The discovery of prostacyclin—A fresh insight into arachidonic acid metabolism. In: Kharasch N, Fried J, eds. *Biochemical Aspects of Prostaglandins*. New York: Academic Press; 1997:155–177.

106. Wetzka B, Charnock-Jones DS, Viville B, et al: Expression of prostacyclin and thromboxane synthases in placenta and placental bed after pre-eclamptic pregnancies. *Placenta* 1996; 17:573–581.

107. Walsh SW, Wang Y: Secretion of lipid peroxides by the human placenta. *Am J Obstet Gynecol* 1993;169:1462–1466.

108. Walsh SW, Wang Y: Trophoblast and placental villous core production of lipid peroxides, thromboxane, and prostacyclin in preeclampsia. *J Clin Endocrinol Metab* 1995;80(6):1888–1893.

109. Walsh SW, Wang Y, Jesse R: Placental production of lipid peroxides, thromboxane, and prostacyclin in preeclamppsia. *Hypertens Pregnancy* 1996;15:101–111.

110. Pryor WA, Castle L: Chemical methods for the detection of lipid hydroperoxides. In: Packer L, ed. *Methods Enzymol*. San Diego: Academic Press; 1984, vol 105:293–299.

111. Walsh SW, Wang Y, Vaughan JE: Placental production of 8 isoprostane is significantly increased in preeclampsia. *J Soc Gynecol Invest* 1997;4:96A.

112. DeWolf F, Robertson WB, Brosens I: The ultrastructure of acute atherosis in hypertensive pregnancy. *Am J Obstet Gynecol* 1975;123(2):164–174.

113. Haust MD, Heras JL, Harding PG: Fat-containing uterine smooth muscle cells in "toxemia:" Possible relevance to atherosclerosis? *Science* 1977;195:1353–1354.

114. Sheppard BL, Bonnar J: An ultrastructural study of uteroplacental spiral arteries in hypertensive and normotensive pregnancy and fetal growth retardation. *Br J Obstet Gynaecol* 1981;88:695–705.

115. Fox H: *Pathology of the Placenta*. London: WB Saunders; 1978:213–237.

116. Smarason AK, Sargent IL, Starkey PM, Redman CWG: The effect of placental syncytiotrophoblast microvillous membranes from normal and pre-eclamptic women on the growth of endothelial cells in vitro. *Br J Obstet Gynecol* 1993;100:943–949.

117. Benyo DF, Miles TM, Conrad KP: Hypoxia stimulates cytokine production by villous explants from the human placenta. *J Clin Endocrinol Metab* 1997;82(5):1582–1588.

118. Stark JM: Pre-eclampsia and cytokine induced oxidative stress. *Br J Obstet Gynecol* 1993; 100:105–109.

119. Zollner H, Schaur RJ, Esterbauer H: Biological activities of 4-hydroxyalkenals. In: Seis H, ed. *Oxidative Stress: Oxidants and Antioxidants.* San Diego: Academic Press; 1991:337–355.

120. Packer L: Oxidative stress, antioxidants, aging and disease. In: Cutler RG, Packer L, Bertram J, Mori A, eds. *Oxidative Stress and Aging.* Basel: Birkhauser Verlag; 1995:1–14.

121. Hazen SL, Hsu FF, Mueller DM, et al: Human neutrophils employ chlorine gas as an oxidant during phagocytosis. *J Clin Invest* 1996;98:1283–1289.

122. Hansen PR, Stawski G: Neutrophil mediated damage to isolated myocytes after anoxia and reoxygenation. *Cardiovasc Res* 1994;28:565–569.

123. Hardy SJ, Ferrante A, Poulos A, et al: Effect of exogenous fatty acids with greater than 22 carbon atoms (very long chain fatty acids) on superoxide production by human neutrophils. *J Immunol* 1994;153:1754–1761.

124. Pronai L, Hiramatsu K, Saigusa Y, Nakazawa H: Low superoxide scavenging activity associated with enhanced superoxide generation by monocytes from male hypertriglyceridemia with and without diabetes. *Atherosclerosis* 1991;90:39–47.

125. Gorog P: Activation of human blood monocytes by oxidized polyunsaturated fatty acids: A possible mechanism for the generation of lipid peroxides in the circulation. *Int J Exp Path* 1991;72:227–237.

126. Maeba R, Maruyama A, Tarutani O, et al: Oxidized low-density lipoprotein induces the production of superoxide by neutrophils. *FEBS Letter* 1995;377:309–312.

127. Lyall F, Greer IA: Pre-eclampsia: A multifaceted vascular disorder of pregnancy. *J Hypertens* 1994;12:1339–1345.

128. Butterworth BH, Green IA, Liston WA, et al: Immunocytochemical localization of neutrophil elastase in term placenta decidua and myometrium in pregnancy-induced hypertension. *Br J Obstet Gynecol* 1991;98:929–933.

129. Greer IA, Dawes J, Johnston TA, Calder AA: Neutrophil activation is confined to the maternal circulation in pregnancy-induced hypertension. *Obstet Gynecol* 1991;78:28–32.

130. Johnston TA, Greer IA, Dawes J, Calder AA: Neutrophil activation in small for gestational age pregnancies. *Br J Obstet Gynecol* 1989;98:978–982.

131. Greer IA, Leask R, Hodson BA, et al: Endothelin, elastase, and endothelial dysfunction in preeclampsia. *Lancet* 1991;337:558.

132. Tsukimori K, Maeda H, Ishida K, et al: The superoxide generation of neutrophils in normal and preeclamptic pregnancies. *Obstet Gynecol* 1993;81:536–540.

133. Walker JJ: Hypertension in pregnancy. *Br J Obstet Gynaecol* 1994;101:639–644.

134. Suhonen L, Teramo K: Hypertension and pre-eclampsia in women with gestational glucose intolerance. *Acta Obstet Gynecol Scand* 1993;72:269–272.

135. Sibai BM, Gordon T, Thom E, et al: Risk factors for preeclampsia in healthy nulliparous women: A prospective multicenter study. *Am J Obstet Gynecol* 1995;172:642–648.

136. Arbogast BW, Taylor RN: A unifying theory of preeclampsia. *Molecular Mechanisms of Preeclampsia.* Austin: RG Landes; 1996:175–187.

137. Arbogast BW, Leeper SC, Merrick RD, et al: Which plasma factors bring about disturbance of endothelial function in preeclampsia? *Lancet* 1994;343:340–341.

138. Herrera E, Lasuncion MA, Coronado DG, et al: Role of lipoprotein lipase activity on lipoprotein metabolism and the fate of circulating triglycerides in pregnancy. *Am J Obstet Gynecol* 1988;158:1575–1583.

139. Knopp RH, Bonet B, Lasuncion MA, et al: Lipoprotein metabolism in pregnancy. In: Herrera E, Knopp RH, eds. *Perinatal Biochemistry.* Boca Raton, FL: CRC Press, Inc.; 1992:20–51.

140. Potter JM, Nestel PJ: The hyperlipidemia of pregnancy in normal and complicated pregnancies. *Am J Obstet Gynecol* 1979;133:165–170.

141. Alvarez JJ, Montelongo A, Iglesias A, et al: Longitudinal study on lipoprotein profile, high density lipoprotein subclass, and postheparin lipases during gestation in women. *J Lipid Res* 1996;37:299–308.

142. Coleman RA: The role of the placenta in lipid metabolism and transport. *Semin Perinatol* 1989;13:180.

143. Boyd EM, Kingston CM: Blood lipids in preeclampsia. *Am J Obstet Gynecol* 1936;32: 937–944.
144. Gratacos E, Casals E, Sanllehy C, et al: Variation in lipid levels during pregnancy in women with different types of hypertension. *Acta Obstet Gynecol Scand* 1996;75:896–901.
145. Reaven GM: Syndrome X: 6 years later. *J Internat Med* 1994;236:13–22.
146. Haffner SM, Mykkanen L, Robbins D, et al: Preponderance of small dense LDL is associated with specific insulin, proinsulin and the components of the insulin resistance syndrome in non-diabetic subjects. *Diabetologia* 1995;38:1328–1336.
147. Bonora E, Targher G, Zenere MB, et al: Relationship of uric acid concentration to cardiovascular risk factors in young men. Role of obesity and central fat distribution. The Verona Young Men Atherosclerosis Risk Factors Study. *Int J Obesity* 1996;20:975–980.
148. Eskenazi B, Fenster L, Sidney S. A multivariate analysis of risk factors for preeclampsia. *JAMA* 1991;266:237–241.
149. Hubel CA, Lyall F, Gandley RE, Roberts JM: Small low-density lipoproteins and vascular cell adhesion molecule (VCAM-1) are increased in association with hyperlipidemia in preeclampsia. *Metabolism* 1998;47:1281–1288.
150. Sattar N, Bedomir A, Berry C, et al: Lipoprotein subfraction concentrations in preeclampsia: Pathogenic parallels to atherosclerosis. *Obstet Gynecol* 1997;89(3):403–408.
151. Sowers JR: Insulin resistance, hyperinsulinemia, dyslipidemia, hypertension, and accelerated atherosclerosis. *J Clin Pharmacol* 1992;32:529–535.
152. Knudsen P, Eriksson J, Lahdenpera S, et al: Changes of lipolytic enzymes cluster with insulin-resistance syndrome. *Diabetologia* 1995;38:344–350.
153. Biezenski JJ: Maternal lipid metabolism. *Obstet Gynecol Ann* 1974;3:203–233.
154. Hotamisligil GS, Arner P, Cro JF, et al: Increased adipose tissue expression of tumor necrosis factor-α in human obesity and insulin resistance. *J Clin Invest* 1995;95:2409–2415.
155. Kern PA, Saghizadeh M, Ong JM, et al: The expression of tumor necrosis factor in human adipose tissue: Regulation by obesity, weight loss, and relationship to lipoprotein lipase. *J Clin Invest* 1995;95:2111–2119.
156. Arbogast BW, Leeper SC, Merrick RD, et al: Plasma factors that determine endothelial cell lipid toxicity in vitro correctly identify women with preeclampsia in early and late pregnancy. *Hypertens Pregnancy* 1996;15(3):263–279.
157. Paolisso G, Gambardella A, Tagliamonte MR, et al: Does free fatty acid infusion impair insulin action also through an increase in oxidative stress? *J Clin Endocrinol Metab* 1996; 81:4244–4248.
158. Toborek M, Barger W, Mattson MP, et al: Linoleic acid and TNF-α cross-amplify oxidative inury and dysfunction of endothelial cells. *J Lipid Res* 1996;37:123–135.
159. Toborek M, Hennig B: Is endothelial cell autocrine production of tumor necrosis factor a mediator of lipid-induced endothelial dysfunction. *Med Hypoth* 1996;47:377–382.
160. Krauss RM: Genetic, metabolic, and dietary influences on the atherogenic lipoprotein phenotype. In: Simopoulos AP, ed. *World Review of Nutrition and Diet.* Basel: Karger; 1997:2–43.
161. Krauss RM: The tangled web of coronary risk factors. *Am J Med* 1991;90:2a–36a.
162. Lewis GF, Steiner G: Hypertriglyceridemia and its metabolic consequences as a risk factor for atherosclerotic cardiovascular disease in non-insulin-dependent diabetes mellitus. *Diabetes Metab Rev* 1996;12:37–56.
163. Hiramatsu K, Arimori S: Increased superoxide production by mononuclear cells of patients with hypertriglyceridemia and diabetes. *Diabetes* 1988;37:832–837.
164. Hoogerbrugge N, Verkerk A, Jacobs ML, et al: Hypertriglyceridemia enhances monocyte binding to endothelial cells in NIDDM. *Diabetes Care* 1996;19:1122–1125.
165. McNamara JR, Campos H, Ordovas JM, et al: Effect of gender, age, and lipid status on low density lipoprotein subfraction distribution. *Arteriosclerosis* 1987;7:483–490.
166. Griffin BA: Low-density lipoprotein heterogeneity. *Bailliére's Clin Endocrinol Metab* 1995;9: 687–703.
167. Krauss RM: Heterogeneity of plasma low-density lipoproteins and atherosclerosis risk. *Current Opin Lipidol* 1994;5:339–349.
168. Gardner CD, Fortmann SP, Krauss RM: Association of small low-density lipoprotein parti-

cles with the incidence of coronary artery disease in men and women. *JAMA* 1996;276: 875–881.

169. Stampfer MJ, Krauss RM, Ma J, et al: A prospective study of triglyceride level, low-density lipoprotein particle diameter, and risk of myocardial infarction. *JAMA* 1996;276:882–888.

170. Austin MA, Mykkanen L, Kuusisto J, et al: Prospective study of small LDLs as a risk factor for non-insulin dependent diabetes mellitus in elderly men and women. *Circulation* 1995; 92(7):1770–1778.

171. Selby JV, Austin MA, Newman B, et al: LDL subclass phenotypes and the insulin resistance syndrome in women. *Circulation* 1993;88:381–387.

172. Raal FJ, Areias AJ, Joffe BI: Low density lipoproteins and atherosclerosis—quantity or quality? *Redox Report* 1995;171–174.

173. Anber R, Griffin BA, McConnell M, et al: Influence of plasma lipid and LDL-subfraction profile on the interaction between low density lipoprotein with human arterial wall proteoglycans. *Atherosclerosis* 1996;124:261–271.

174. Nordestgaard BG, Nielsen LB: Atherosclerosis and arterial influx of lipoproteins. *Curr Opin Lipidol* 1994;5:252–257.

175. Tribble DL, Theil PM, vandenBerg JJM, Krauss RM: Differing α-tocopherol oxidative lability and ascorbic acid sparing effects in buoyant and dense LDL. *Arterioscler Thromb Vasc Biol* 1995;15:2025–2031.

176. Chait A, Brazg RL, Tribble DL, Krauss RM: Susceptibility of small, dense, low-density lipoproteins to oxidative modification in subjects with the atherogenic lipoprotein phenotype, pattern B. *Am J Med* 1993;94:350–356.

177. Austin MA: Genetic epidemiology of dyslipidaemia and atherosclerosis. *Ann Med* 1996; 28:459–464.

178. Dejager S, Bruckert E, Chapman MJ: Dense low density lipoprotein subspecies with diminished oxidative resistance predominate in combined hyperlipidemia. *J Lipid Res* 1993;34: 295–308.

179. Dimitriadis E, Griffin M, Owens D, et al: Oxidation of low-density lipoprotein in NIDDM: Its relationship to fatty acid composition. *Diabetologia* 1995;38:1300–1306.

180. Tribble DL, vandenBerg JJM, Motchnik PA, et al: Oxidative susceptibility of low density lipoprotein subfractions is related to their ubiquinol-10 and α-tocopherol content. *Proc Natl Acad Sci USA* 1994;91:1183–1187.

181. Weisser B, Locher R, deGraff J, et al: Low density lipoprotein subfractions increase thromboxane formation in endothelial cells. *Biochem Biophys Res Comm* 1993;192(3):1245–1250.

182. Weisser B, Locher R, Graaf J, Vetter W: Low density lipoprotein subfractions and $[Ca^{2+}]_i$ in vascular smooth muscle cells. *Circ Res* 1993;73:118–124.

183. Silliman K, Shore V, Forte TM: Hypertriglyceridemia during late pregnancy is associated with the formation of small dense low-density lipoproteins and the presence of large buoyant high-density lipoproteins. *Metabolism* 1994;43:1035–1041.

184. Hubel CA, Shakir Y, Gandley RE, et al: The hypertriglyceridemia of normal pregnancy is associated with increased formation of small low-density lipoproteins. *J Soc Gynecol Invest* 1997;4(1 suppl):141A(abstr).

185. Kulkarni KR, Garber DW, Jones MK, Segrest JP: Identification and cholesterol quantification of low density lipoprotein subclasses in young adults by VAP-II methodology. *J Lipid Res* 1995;36:2291–2302.

186. Williams PT, Krauss RM, Nichols AV, et al: Identifying the predominant peak diameter of high-density and low-density lipoproteins by electrophoresis. *J Lipid Res* 1990;31:1131–1139.

187. Pierucci F, Garnica JJP, Cosmi EV, Anceschi MM: Oxidability of low density lipoproteins in pregnancy-induced hypertension. *Br J Obstet Gynaecol* 1996;103:1159–1161.

188. Wang Y, Walsh SW, Guo J, Zhang J: The imbalance between thromboxane and prostacyclin in preeclampsia is associated with an imbalance between lipid peroxides and vitamin E in maternal blood. *Am J Obstet Gynecol* 1991;165:1695–1700.

189. Tabacova S, Little RE, Balabaeva L, et al: Complications of pregnancy in relation to maternal lipid peroxides, glutathione, and exposure to metals. *Reproduct Toxicol* 1994;8(3):217–224.

190. Uotila JT, Tuimala RJ, Aarnio TM, et al: Findings on lipid peroxidation and antioxidant function in hypertensive complications of pregnancy. *J Obstet Gynecol* 1993;100:270–276.

191. Kauppila A, Makila UM, Korpela H, et al: Relationship of serum selenium and lipid peroxidation in preeclampsia. In: Combs GF: *Selenium in Biology and Medicine*. New York: AVI Books; 1987:996–1001.

192. Jendryczko A, Drozdz M, Wojcik A: Serum 18:2 (9,11) linoleic acid in normal pregnancy and pregnancy complicated by pre-eclampsia. *Zent bl Gynakol* 1991;113:443–446.

193. Jain SK, Wise R: Relationship between elevated lipid peroxides, vitamin E deficiency and hypertension in preeclampsia. *Mol Cell Biochem* 1995;151:33–38.

194. Sane AS, Chokshi SA, Mishra VV, et al: Serum lipoperoxide levels in pregnancy-induced hypertension. *Panminerva Med* 1989;31:119–122.

195. Garzetti GG, Tranquilli AL, Cugini AM, et al: Altered lipid composition, increased lipid peroxidation, and altered fluidity of the membrane as evidence of platelet damage in preeclampsia. *Obstet Gynecol* 1993;81:337–340.

196. Sotnikova LG, Naumov AV, Kuznetsova VA: The value of some parameters of erythrocyte membrane lipid peroxidation in late gestosis. *Akush Ginekol* 1986;4:20–22.

197. Wang Y, Walsh SW, Guo J, Zhang J: Maternal levels of prostacyclin, thromboxane, vitamin E, and lipid peroxides throughout normal pregnancy. *Am J Obstet Gynecol* 1991,165: 1690–1694.

198. Minakami H, Kimura Z, Tamada T, et al: Hepatocellular lipofuscin in pre-eclampsia. *Asia-Oceania J Obstet Gynaecol* 1989;15:277–280.

199. Jansen H, Ghanem H, Kuypers JHSAM, Birkenhager JC: Autoantibodies against malondialdehyde-modified LDL are elevated in subjects with an LDL subclass pattern B. *Atherosclerosis* 1995;115:255–262.

200. Armstrong VW, Wieland E, Diedrich F, et al: Serum antibodies to oxidised low-density lipoprotein in pre-eclampsia and coronary heart disease. *Lancet* 1994;343:1570.

201. Branch DW, Mitchell MD, Miller E, et al: Pre-eclampsia and serum antibodies to oxidised low-density lipoprotein. *Lancet* 1994;343:645–646.

202. Kurki T, Ailus K, Palosuo T, Ylikorkala O: Oxidized low-density lipoprotein, cardiolipin, and phosphatidyl serine fail to predict the risk of preeclampsia. *Hypertens Pregnancy* 1996;15(2):251–256.

203. Retsky KL, Frei B: Vitamin C prevents metal ion-dependent initiation and propagation of lipid peroxidation in human low-density lipoprotein. *Biochim Biophys Acta* 1995;1257: 279–287.

204. Frei B: Ascorbic acid protects lipids in human plasma and low-density lipoprotein against oxidative damage. *Am J Clin Nutr* 1991;54:1113S–1118S.

205. Chappey B, Myara I, Benoit M-O, et al: Characteristics of ten charge-differing subfractions isolated from human native low-density lipoproteins (LDL). No evidence of peroxidative modifications. *Biochim Biophys Acta* 1995;1259:261–270.

206. Hodis HN, Kramsch DM, Avogaro P, et al: Biochemical and cytotoxic characteristics of an in vivo circulating oxidized low density lipoprotein (LDL). *J Lipid Res* 1994;35:669–677.

207. Zamburlini A, Maiorino M, Barbera P, et al: Measurement of lipid hydroperoxides in plasma lipoproteins by a new highly-sensitive 'single photon counting' luminometer. *Biochim Biophys Acta* 1995;1256:233–240.

208. Zamburlini A, Maiorino M, Barbera P, et al: Direct measurement by single photon counting of lipid hydroperoxides in human plasma and lipoproteins. *Anal Biochem* 1995;232: 107–113.

209. Halliwell B: Vitamin C: Antioxidant or pro-oxidant in vivo? *Free Rad Res* 1996;25:439–454.

210. Stocker R, Bowry VW: Tocopherol-mediated peroxidation of lipoprotein lipids and its inhibition by co-antioxidants. In: Cadenas E, Packer L, eds. *Handbook of Antioxidants*. New York: Marcel Dekker, Inc.; 1996:27–41.

211. Buettner GR, Jurkiewicz BA: Chemistry and biochemistry of ascorbic acid. In: Cadenas E, Packer L, eds. *Handbook of Antioxidants*. New York: Marcel Dekker, Inc.; 1996:91–115.

212. Basu TK, Schorah CJ: *Vitamin C in Health and Disease*. Westport, CT: AVI Publishing Co.; 1982:95–100.

213. Clemetson CAB, Andersen L: Ascorbic acid metabolism in preeclampsia. *Obstet Gynecol* 1964;24:774–782.

214. Roginsky VA, Stegmann HB: Ascorbyl radical as natural indicator of oxidative stress: Quantitative regularities. *Free Rad Biol Med* 1994;17(2):93–103.

215. Schiff E, Friedman SA, Stampfer M, et al: Dietary consumption and plasma concentrations of vitamin E in pregnancies complicated by preeclampsia. *Am J Obstet Gynecol* 1996; 175:1024–1028.

216. Traber MG: Determinants of plasma vitamin E concentrations. *Free Rad Biol Med* 1994;16(2): 229–239.

217. Bonet B, Chait A, Gown AM, Knopp RH: Metabolism of modified LDL by cultured human placental cells. *Atherosclerosis* 1995;112:125–136.

218. Mondon F, Alsat E, Berthelier M, et al: Presence of acetyl-like modified LDL in human placental blood. *Med Sci Res* 1987;15:385–386.

219. Alaiz M, Beppu M, Ohishi K, Kikugawa K: Modification of delipidated apoprotein B of low density lipoprotein by lipid oxidation products in relation to macrophage scavenger receptor binding. *Biol Pharm Bull* 1994;17(1):51–57.

220. Cester N, Staffolani R, Rabini RA, et al: Pregnancy induced hypertension: A role for peroxidation in microvillus plasma membranes. *Mol Cell Biochem* 1994;131:151–155.

221. Nelson GH, Zuspan FP, Mulligan LT: Defects of lipid metabolism in toxemia of pregnancy. *Am J Obstet Gynecol* 1966;94:310–315.

222. Morris J, Endresen MJR, Watts A, et al: Pre-eclamptic placental syncytiotrophoblast microvillous membranes have altered fluidity and inhibit endothelial cell proliferation. *Hypertens Pregnancy* 1996;16(1):78(abstr).

223. Murata M, Kodama H, Goto K, et al: Decreased very-low-density lipoprotein and low-density lipoprotein receptor messenger ribonucleic acid expression in placentas from preeclamptic pregnancies. *Am J Obstet Gynecol* 1996;175:1551–1556.

224. Uhlinger DJ, Burnham DN, Mullins RE, et al: Functional differences in human neutrophils isolated pre- and post-prandially. *FEBS Letter* 1991;286:28–32.

225. Bellinati-Pires R, Waitzberg DL, Salgado MM, Carneiro-Sampaio MM: Functional alterations of human neutrophils by medium-chain triglyceride emulsions: Evaluation of phagocytosis, bacterial killing, and oxidative activity. *J Leukoc Biol* 1993;53:404–410.

226. Herbert V, Shaw S, Jayatilleke E, Stopler-Kasdan T: Most free-radical injury is iron-related: It is promoted by iron, hemin, holoferritin and vitamin C, and inhibited by desferoxamine and apoferritin. *Stem Cells* 1994;12:189–303.

227. Gutteridge JMC: Antioxidant properties of the proteins caeruloplasmin, albumin and transferrin. A study of their activity in serum and synovial fluid from patients with rheumatoid arthritis. *Biochim Biophys Acta* 1986;869:119–127.

228. Gutteridge JMC, Quintan GJ: Antioxidant protection against organic and inorganic oxygen radicals by normal human plasma: The important primary role for iron-binding and iron-oxidising proteins. *Biochim Biophys Acta* 1993;1156:144–150.

229. Cranfield LM, Gollan JL, White AG, Dormandy TL: Serum antioxidant activity in normal and abnormal subjects. *Ann Clin Biochem* 1979;16:299–306.

230. Halliwell B, Gutteridge JM: Role of free radicals and catalytic metal ions in human disease: An overview. In: Packer L, Glazer AN, eds. *Oxygen Radicals in Biological Systems*. San Diego: Academic Press, Inc.; 1990:1–83.

231. Davidge ST, Hubel CA, Brayden RD, et al: Sera antioxidant activity in uncomplicated and preeclamptic pregnancies. *Obstet Gynecol* 1992;79(6):897–901.

232. Uotila JT, Kirkkola AL, Rorarius M, et al: The total peroxyl radical-trapping ability of plasma and cerebrospinal fluid in normal and preeclamptic parturients. *Free Rad Biol Med* 1994; 16:581–590.

233. Benzie IFF, Strain JJ: Uric acid: Friend or foe? *Redox Report* 1996;2:231–234.

234. Stratta P, Canavese C, Porcu M, et al: Vitamin E supplementation in preeclampsia. *Gynecol Obstet Invest* 1994;37:246–249.

235. Gulmezoglu AM, Oosthuizen MMJ, Hofmeyer GJ: Placental malondialdehyde and glu-

tathione levels in a controlled trial of antioxidant treatment in severe preeclampsia. *Hypertens Pregnancy* 1996;15:287–296.

236. Gulmezoglu AM, Hofmeyr GJ, Oosthuisen MMJ: Antioxidants in the treatment of severe preeclampsia: An explanatory randomized controlled trial. *Br J Obstet Gynecol* 1997;104: 689–696.

237. Cutler MG, Schneider R: Linoleate oxidation products and cardiovascular lesions. *Atherosclerosis* 1974;20:383–394.

238. Shunsaku H, Okamoto K, Morimatsu M: Lipid peroxide in the aging process. In: Yagi K, ed. *Lipid Peroxides in Biology and Medicine*. Orlando, FL: Academic Press; 1982:305–315.

239. Yoshioka T, Ichikawa L, Fogo A: Reactive oxygen metabolites cause massive, reversible proteinuria and glomecular sieving defect without apparent ultrastructural abnormality. *J Am Soc Nephrol* 1991;2:902–912.

240. Stamler FW: Fatal eclamptic disease of pregnant rats fed anti-vitamin E stress diet. 1959;35(6):1207–1231.

241. Nisell H, Hjemdahl P, Linde B: Cardiovascular responses to circulating catecholamines in normal pregnancy and pregnancy-induced hypertension. *Clin Physiol* 1985;5:479–493.

242. Gant NF, Daley GL, Chand S, et al: A study of angiotensin II pressor response throughout primigravid pregnancy. *J Clin Invest* 1973;52:2682–2689.

243. Auge N, Fitoussi G, Bascands JL, et al: Mildly oxidized LDL evokes a sustained Ca^{2+}-dependent retraction of vascular smooth muscle cells. *Circ Res* 1996;79:871–880.

244. Hubel CA, Davidge ST, McLaughlin MK: Lipid hydroperoxides potentiate mesenteric artery vasoconstrictor responses. *Free Rad Biol Med* 1993;14:397–407.

245. Watanabe K, Okatani Y, Sagara Y: Potentiating effect of hydrogen peroxide on the serotonin-induced vasocontraction in human umbilical artery. *Acta Obstet Gynecol Scand* 1996;75:783–789.

246. Knock GA, Poston L: Bradykinin-mediated relaxation of isolated maternal resistance arteries in normal pregnancy and preeclampsia. *Am J Obstet Gynecol* 1996;175:1668–1674.

247. Galle J, Ochslen M, Schollmeyer P, Wanner C: Oxidized lipoproteins inhibit endothelium-dependent vasodilation. *Hypertension* 1994;23:556–564.

248. Simon BC, Cunningham LD, Cohen RA: Oxidized low density lipoproteins cause contraction and inhibit endothelium-dependent relaxation in the pig coronary artery. *J Clin Invest* 1990;86:75 79.

249. Remuzzi G, Marchesi D, Zoja C, et al: Reduced umbilical and placental vascular prostacyclin in severe pre eclampsia. *Prostaglandins* 1980;20(1):105–110.

250. Falanga A, Doni MG, Delaini F: Unbalanced control of TxA2 and PGI_2 synthesis in vitamin E-deficient rats. *Am J Physiol* 1983;245(*Heart Circ Physiol*):H867–H870.

251. Taylor RN, Crombleholme WR, Friedman SA, et al: High plasma cellular fibronectin levels correlate with biochemical and clinical features of preeclampsia but cannot be attributed to hypertension alone. *Am J Obstet Gynecol* 1991;165:895–901.

252. Peters JH, Ginsberg MH, Bohl BP, et al: Intravascular release of intact cellular fibronectin during oxidant-induced injury of the in vitro perfused rabbit lung. *J Clin Invest* 1986; 78:1596–1603.

253. Baker PN, Davidge ST, Roberts JM: Plasma from patients with preeclampsia increases endothelial cell nitric oxide production. *Hypertension* 1995;26:244–248.

254. Davidge ST, Baker PN, Roberts JM: NOS expression is increased in endothelial cells exposed to plasma from women with preeclampsia. *Am J Physiol* 1995;269(*Heart Circ Physiol*): H1106–H1112.

255. Fries DM, Penha RG, D'Amico EA, et al: Oxidized low-density lipoprotein stimulates nitric oxide release by rabbit aortic endothelial cells. *Biochem Biophys Res Comm* 1995;207(1): 231–237.

256. Hirata K, Miki N, Kuroda Y, et al: Low concentration of oxidized low-density lipoprotein and lysophosphatidylcholine upregulate constitutive nitric oxide synthase mRNA expression in bovine aortic endothelial cells. *Circ Res* 1995;76:958–962.

257. Baker PN, Davidge ST, Barankiewicz J, Roberts JM: Plasma of preeclamptic women stimulates and then inhibits endothelial prostacyclin. *Hypertension* 1996;27:56–61.

258. Myers DE, Huang WN, Larkins RG: Lipoprotein-induced prostacyclin production in endothelial cells and effects of lipoprotein modification. *Am J Physiol* 1996;271:C1504–C1511.
259. Wang J, Zhen E, Guo Z, Lu Y: Effect of hyperlipidemic serum on lipid peroxidation, synthesis of prostacyclin and thromboxane by cultured endothelial cells: Protective effect of antioxidants. *Free Rad Biol Med* 1989;7:243–249.
260. Cunningham FG, Lowe T, Guss S, Mason R: Erythrocyte morphology in women with severe preeclampsia and eclampsia. *Am J Obstet Gynecol* 1985;153:358–363.
261. Samuels P, Main EK, Mennuti MT, Gabbe SG: The origin of increased serum iron in pregnancy-induced hypertension. *Am J Obstet Gynecol* 1987;157:721–725.
262. Chiu D, Lubin B, Sohet SB: Peroxidative reactions in red cell biology. In: Pryor WA, ed. *Free Radicals in Biology.* New York: Academic Press; 1982:115–120.
263. Nardulli G, Proverbio F, Limongi FG, et al: Preeclampsia and calcium adenosine triphosphate activity of red blood cell ghosts. *Am J Obstet Gynecol* 1994;171:1361–1365.
264. Kagan VE: *Lipid Peroxidation in Biomembranes.* Boca Raton, FL: CRC Press, Inc.; 1988:55–117.

15

Animal Models

Rocco C. Venuto and Marshall D. Lindheimer

In the first edition of this text, Chesley outlined some of the many hypotheses then proposed to explain the pathophysiology of de novo proteinuria and hypertension in pregnancy known as preeclampsia or toxemia.[1] In the chapter titled "Hypotheses," he discussed four broad categories of explanations:

1. Dietary
2. Renal
3. Placental
4. Immunologic

A generation later, the cause(s) of preeclampsia remains incompletely defined. There continues to be insufficient evidence to support the notions that either poor dietary intake or abnormalities of the kidney underlie the majority of episodes of preeclampsia. Immunologically mediated vascular injury as the initiating event in this disease process has not been excluded and remains as a possible cause of preeclampsia.[2] However, the last 20 years have witnessed increasing emphasis on the possible role of placental pathophysiology, specifically uteroplacental ischemia, as a crucial factor in the pathogenesis of many cases of this disease process.[3-5] Yet the role of uteroplacental hypoperfusion alone has not been confirmed as the primary and universal cause of preeclampsia.[6] Two decades ago, Chesley also suggested that alterations of the wall of the systemic arterioles might directly underlie the changes observed in the preeclamptic patient.[1] More recently, advances that describe how the endothelium controls systemic vascular tone have become a major focus for studies of the pathogenesis of preeclampsia.[7-10] The relevance of these developments to this chapter are clear. Evidence to support the leading hypothetical causes for this unique form of hypertension (i.e., uteroplacental ischemia and endothelial dysfunction) has resulted from studies in laboratory animals that elucidate and support clinical observations.

Although Chesley[1] and others[4] noted that the spontaneous development of preeclampsia is essentially limited to humans, research in laboratory mammals has proven to be a surprisingly fertile area to explore multiple hypotheses for human disease. Models have been developed in several species of laboratory animals that exhibit some or most of the findings observed in women. Manipulated to mimic preeclampsia, animal models could be used both to explore the pathophysiology of the human condition and to test theoretical treatment strategies. In most commonly employed laboratory animals, gestation is of shorter duration, can be accurately timed, and the subjects are usually homogenous. Human studies, on the other hand, raise profound ethical and legal problems, particularly since invasive techniques in acutely ill pregnant women could jeopardize the health or survival of both mother and fetus. This combination of factors has influenced the decision to focus research on animal models.

A compendium of every animal model utilized to study hemodynamics in either normal or abnormal gestations is beyond the scope of this chapter. Here we will review models used to explore the cardiovascular and renal hemodynamic changes in normal pregnancy and in particular studies which stress the role of prostaglandins and nitric oxide (NO), the potent endothelium-derived relaxing factor. The bulk of the chapter, however, is devoted to abnormal pregnancy and the animal models devised to explore the pathogenesis of preeclampsia.

PARALLELS BETWEEN HUMAN AND ANIMAL PREGNANCY

Overview

The changes in cardiovascular physiology experienced by women during pregnancy include dramatic increases in cardiac output and plasma volume. The potential for studies of laboratory animals to "vicariously" explore the physiology and pathophysiology of human pregnancy rests in part upon the similarities in gestational physiology shared by most mammalian species. Dogs, rabbits, rats, and sheep, as well as primates such as baboons and monkeys, have been used to investigate the cause of preeclampsia.[4,11-23] The use of these species in such research is predicated in part on the similarities in physiologic changes they experience during gestation and those observed in women (Table 15–1). Consequently, animal experimentation has also been beneficial to understanding the physiology of uncomplicated human pregnancy.

TABLE 15–1. PHYSIOLOGIC ADAPTATIONS OF THE CARDIOVASCULAR SYSTEM DURING PREGNANCY SHARED BY HUMAN AND COMMONLY EMPLOYED LABORATORY ANIMALS

1. Lowered systemic blood pressure
2. Increased cardiac output
3. Reduced renovascular resistance and ± enhanced renal function
4. Reduced response to hypertensive effect of pressor compounds

Kidney Function

The changes outlined in Table 15–1 are considered hallmarks of pregnancy. For example, improvement in renal function during human gestation is so consistent and dramatic that the esteemed Homer Smith stated in 1956, that "A pregnant woman is a very interesting phenomenon; I do not know any other way to increase glomerular filtration rate by 50% or better for prolonged periods."[24] Dr. Smith's comment clearly implied that unlocking this mystery would not only aid our understanding of the enhanced renal physiology during pregnancy, but might also profoundly influence the treatment of patients with reduced renal function. Despite the obvious importance of these physiologic adaptations and many years of clinical investigation, the factor(s) responsible remains as undefined as are those responsible for preeclampsia itself (see also Chap. 8).

Animal models have been employed extensively in the effort to further study the adaptation of the kidney to pregnancy. Data obtained from humans[25] were preceded by the results of studies performed in rabbits demonstrating that enhanced urinary excretion of vasodilator prostanoids, such as prostaglandin E_2 (PGE_2), were temporally correlated with the increase in renal hemodynamics during gestation.[26] Subsequently, tissue slices obtained from gravid and virgin rabbits were employed to more precisely define the intrarenal site and the pregnancy-induced differences in the rates of synthesis of several potentially vasoactive prostanoids.[27] Conrad and Colpoys administered a nonsteroidal antiinflammatory drug (NSAID) to extensively instrumented rats to explore whether enhanced synthesis of prostanoids via the cyclooxygenase cascade causally relates to the gestationally induced fall in systemic and renal vascular resistance and increase in renal function. They found that NSAID treatment failed to prevent the physiologic changes associated with pregnancy in these conscious rats.[28] Elegant micropuncture studies performed in rats by Baylis helped define glomerular hemodynamics during gestation.[29] Her data revealed that transglomerular hydrostatic pressure was not substantially increased despite the increase in glomerular flow and function. Clearly, experiments that required either renal tissue slices or chronic instrumentation could not be employed in the study of pregnant human subjects. The results of invasive studies in animals which sometimes employed potentially dangerous compounds may also broadly relate to humans. Such data emphasize the crucial role that animal research might play in enhancing our knowledge of pregnancy physiology.

Nonetheless, the very real limitations of observations in animals must be addressed. For example, neither rabbits nor rats experience a gestation-induced increase in renal blood flow or glomerular filtration rate similar in magnitude and/or duration to that observed in women experiencing uncomplicated pregnancy.[28,30,31] Further, investigations undertaken in rabbits chronically instrumented with renal artery flow probes and arterial catheters revealed that despite a substantial decline in renal vascular resistance, an absolute increase in renal blood flow was not detected during gestation in this species.[31] It cannot be overemphasized how these species differences influence any interpretation of experimental results from one to another.

Vascular Reactivity

Nearly 40 years ago, Abdul-Karim and Assali showed that the pressor response to infused angiotensin II was diminished in pregnant women.[32] This biologic phenomenon is another hallmark of human pregnancy shared by many mammals such as rats, rabbits, and sheep, which are often employed to explore gestational physiology.[33-35] The blunted pressor response to angiotensin II during mammalian pregnancy has been ascribed to a specific event, perhaps the high endogenous levels of plasma renin activity and angiotensin II which also characterize pregnancy.[36-38] These high blood levels may result in an attenuated response to exogenous angiotensin II by down-regulation of specialized receptors, as described in pregnant rabbits.[39] Although some evidence from animal studies suggested that the increased concentrations of angiotensin II are in turn the result of reduced metabolism of this peptide,[40] subsequent experimentation in women showed no difference in the metabolic clearance of angiotensin II between pregnant and nonpregnant individuals.[41] Furthermore, diminished sensitivity to pressor compounds during gestation has been demonstrated to be a more universal phenomenon and not limited only to angiotensin II. The report of Raab et al. in 1956, strongly suggested that pregnancy blunted the response of pregnant women to norepinephrine.[42] Subsequently, nonanesthetized pregnant rabbits were shown to be resistant to the hypertensive effect of norepinephrine,[43] while Paller reported that pregnant rats not only had a blunted pressor response to angiotensin II and norepinephrine, but to vasopressin as well.[35]

It seems likely that the reduced responsiveness to vasopressor peptides is a consequence of the generalized vasodilation permitting an increase in blood volume and a simultaneous decrease in systemic blood pressure during mammalian gestation. The decreased vascular tone, in turn, may be a function of increased local or circulating amounts of vasodilating prostaglandins such as prostocyclin or prostaglandin I_2 (PGI_2) and PGE_2. Support for this suggestion comes from data demonstrating increases in the concentrations of PGE_2 and PGI_2, both in the blood and vascular tissue of pregnant women[25,44] and pregnant mammals.[45-47]

Everett et al. pursued the possible causal relationship between increased synthesis of these prostanoids and the diminished pressor responsiveness.[48] They found that the quantity of angiotensin II required to raise mean arterial pressure by 20 mm Hg declined by 50% or more in 11 female subjects after the cyclooxygenase-inhibiting agent indomethacin was administered.[48,49] Drugs that inhibit prostaglandin synthesis may also decrease plasma renin activity and angiotensin II concentrations.[50] Gant et al. designed separate studies to exclude the possibility that the enhanced sensitivity to exogenous angiotensin II that developed following indomethacin administration resulted from lowered endogenous angiotensin II levels. They volume-expanded pregnant women in order to reduce endogenous angiotensin II.[51] This manipulation failed to alter the pressor response to infused angiotensin II. The authors concluded in a later report that gestationally induced increases in vasodilator prostaglandins may reduce the tone of vascular smooth muscle and thereby mediate the altered pressor responsiveness.[52] A review from other students of this specialized area of biology supports the hypothesis.[53]

Experiments that employ laboratory animals to expand and support observations made in human subjects are exemplified by rabbit studies designed to parallel the work in human subjects.[34] This work was done in animals remote from the effects of anesthesia and surgery, which itself can activate the renin–angiotensin system and heighten prostaglandin synthesis.[54-56] Conscious, chronically instrumented pregnant rabbits were resistant to the pressor effect of angiotensin II, however, following treatment with a cyclooxygenase inhibitor, pregnant rabbits required 50% or less angiotensin II to raise mean arterial pressure (MAP) by 20 mm Hg compared to nonpregnant control rabbits. Consistent with the observations made in pregnant women, experimental saline infusion in gravid rabbits did not alter the pressor response to exogenous angiotensin II, whereas the nonpregnant control rabbits required less angiotensin II to achieve the targeted 20 mm Hg increase in MAP.

These experiments also included measurements of plasma renin activity and serum PGE_2 concentrations. Plasma renin activity declined in both pregnant and nonpregnant animals following volume expansion. Administration of a cyclooxygenase inhibitor decreased plasma renin activity in gravid rabbits from the high levels that characterized pregnancy, but did not change renin levels in the control animals. Mean PGE_2 concentrations in pregnant rabbits were precipitously reduced from basal levels by the NSAID, meclofenamate. The pretreatment levels of PGE_2 were tenfold higher in pregnant than in the nonpregnant rabbits. Saline infusion did not influence the concentration of this prostanoid in either group. In a separate group of experiments, prostaglandin synthesis inhibition with meclofenamate restored the pressor effect of norepinephrine in pregnant rabbits.[43]

These experiments illustrate how animal research can allow for the selection of well-matched controls, frequent measurement of physiologic parameters, repeat blood and/or tissue sampling, as well as the use of potentially dangerous agents without the obvious ethical bars posed by this type of research in humans. Further, the species (rabbit) chosen is one characterized by high circulating PGE_2 levels (compared to humans), which rise during gestation and enhance the ability to detect changes in this parameter. Although it is tempting to generate hypotheses by combining the results obtained from animal studies and human-derived experimental data, the direct application of animal experiments to human physiologic events poses its own problems, as discussed.

Despite the apparent support provided by the results of studies in animals for the hypothesis of Gant et al.,[52] the explanation for the development of pressor resistance during gestation is not yet fully understood. An interplay between vasodilator (e.g., PGE_2, PGI_2) and vasoconstrictor (e.g., thromboxane A_2) prostanoids may help regulate the responses of the systemic vasculature in pregnancy,[5,44] but other data from experiments undertaken in conscious rats would appear to undermine the concept that vasorelaxing prostanoids play a primary role in the control of vascular tone during gestation.[28] Other prostanoids, cytokines, and hormones may contribute even more to this physiologic adaption. Indeed, the endothelium-derived relaxing factor, nitric oxide (NO),[7,57] has been postulated to be the primary factor responsible for the generalized flaccidity of the systemic vasculature during pregnancy.[58] This theory is based in part on animal-derived data that include the demonstration of increased NO biosynthesis in rats during gestation.[59] Nitric oxide must also be considered as one of the possible causes for the pregnancy-associated reduced responsiveness to vasopressors. Consistent with this notion, Molnar and Hertelendy recorded an increase in the blood pressure responses to both angiotensin II and norepinephrine, as well as arginine vasopressin in pregnant rats acutely infused with an inhibitor of NO synthesis.[60] The observation that the pressor responsiveness to vasopressors was restored in pregnant rats once NO production was blocked has been confirmed in other laboratories.[61,62] These recent results in pregnant rats may lead us to modify older concepts and eventually enhance our understanding of mechanisms of pressor hyporesponsiveness during human pregnancy.

ANIMAL STUDIES DESIGNED TO EXPLORE HYPOTHETICAL CAUSES OF PREECLAMPSIA

Selection of Models

The lack of a naturally occurring condition in animals that completely overlaps with human preeclampsia has been mentioned. However, edema and proteinuria have occasionally been observed in nonmanipulated pregnant subhuman primates.[63-65] Those findings are key features of the human condition and some are encouraged to believe that a disease identical to preeclampsia might occur spontaneously in animals. In their comprehensive review of the literature to 1988, Phippard and Horvath[4] found that if a similar disease existed in primates it must have a lower attack rate, and the reported biochemical changes were not identical to those seen in women. Additionally, since blood pressure measurements are difficult to attain in animals without sedation, documentation of the hypertension is problematic.[4]

Phippard and Horvath concluded that the syndrome which occasionally develops without intervention in some primates appears to parallel, rather than precisely imitate, human preeclampsia. Preeclampsia per se either does not appear to occur de novo in these animals most closely related to humans, or does so infrequently, that it cannot be studied in a systematic fashion. Consequently, the authors[4] suggested that either a great deal of good fortune and/or considerable manipulation of the subject animals would be required to use primates as surrogates to study the human condition. Indeed, pursuit of the pathophysiology of human preeclampsia using animal models typically involves inducing alterations that replicate a risk factor(s) like uteroplacental ischemia either theorized or documented to be linked to this disease process in women.[11-22]

The limitations of subhuman primates in the study of preeclampsia is not exclusively a consequence of the apparent, but subtle, differences between the disease process that sometimes complicates their pregnancy and the human condition. The ample overlap between the physiologic changes experienced by most mammals during pregnancy and those alterations which gravid women undergo have been defined. Perhaps appropriately manipulated mammals of many species would be more effective models for carefully selected aspects of preeclampsia than primates. This may be especially true when one considers duration of pregnancy, the expense of purchase and maintenance of primates, as well as the lack of docility that frequently characterizes those species phylogenetically closest to humans.

UTEROPLACENTAL HYPOPERFUSION

Uteroplacental hypoperfusion, as intimated, remains a key suspect in the pathogenesis of preeclampsia.[1,4] The initial basis for suspecting uteroplacental ischemia as a likely cause of toxemia arises from the repetitive clinical observations made in pregnant women. Some of these observations are listed in Table 15–2. A number of these clinical findings and their implications were first recognized many years ago.[66] It is not surprising, therefore, that experiments designed to induce acute uterine ischemia in pregnant animals were initiated not long after Goldblatt et al., in the mid-1930s, showed that an acute reduction of blood flow to another organ, the kidney, resulted in a rapid and sustained increase in systemic blood pressure.[67] Ogden et al. reported, in 1940, that partially occluding the infrarenal aorta of four pregnant, but not of four nonpregnant, dogs resulted in hypertension.[68] The blood pressure in these animals rose by a few mm Hg initially and then continued to rise further for up to 147 minutes, which was the duration of the longest experiment. The experiments of Ogden et al. were repeated by Bastiaanse and Mastboom several years later, with similar results.[69]

All of these animal studies were performed in an acute setting, and hemodynamic parameters were assessed relatively shortly after uteroplacental ischemia was induced in anesthetized animals. The problems with such determinations are manifold. They are limited by misinterpretations that can result from the afore-

TABLE 15–2. OBSERVATIONS SUPPORTING UTEROPLACENTAL ISCHEMIA AS A KEY FACTOR IN PREECLAMPSIA[1,3-6,70,93-99]

1. Occurs predominantly in primigravidas; ? "immature" uterine vasculature
2. Increased risk with more fetuses and placentae (twins)
3. Disease occurs late in gestation
4. Labor aggravates the clinical syndrome
5. High occurrence rate with large, rapidly growing hydatidiform moles
6. Increased incidence in patients with underlying microvascular disease, i.e., diabetes, hypertension, and systemic lupus erythematosus
7. Consistent abnormalities of the placenta and uteroplacental vascular interface

mentioned effects of anesthesia and surgery.[54-56] More important, these studies where uterine perfusion is precipitously lower bear only a faint resemblance to the clinical syndrome they were designed to imitate. Nonetheless, these data have been used as evidence to foster the concept that uteroplacental ischemia is a key factor in the induction of hypertension during pregnancy.[70] Berger and Cavanagh[13] attempted to show that placental, and not uterine, ischemia was the inciting element for the hypertension observed in pregnant animals subjected to acute reduction in uteroplacental blood flow. The investigators placed blood flow limiting "Z" sutures through the placentae of pregnant rabbits. This resulted in a transient decline in blood pressure, followed by a fairly rapid rise in systemic blood pressure about 5 minutes after the sutures were tightened. Blood pressure elevation peaked in about one hour and then gradually declined. Sera obtained from pregnant rabbits prepared with placental sutures caused blood pressure to rise when transfused into nonpregnant rabbits. Not only did the authors conclude that their results support the specificity of placental ischemia in this model of hypertension, but they also enhanced the conjecture made much earlier[71] that injured placentae released a pressor compound which could act systemically. In addition to the caveats that relate to acute anesthesia and surgery, this work lacked both statistical analysis of the data and quantification of the reduction in placental blood flow. Finally, the intriguing results of Berger and Cavanagh could not be reproduced by Smith and Taniguchi.[72]

Subsequently, animal experimentation employing uteroplacental ischemia began to focus on models designed to *chronically* limit circulation to the gravid uterus. Hodari described a series of experiments using dogs that had bilateral uteroovarian artery ligation and bands arranged around the uterine arteries which were nonconstrictive but fit snugly.[11] Dogs so treated did not develop hypertension until they became pregnant, which was several weeks after they had undergone the preparatory surgery. Once pregnant, the animals almost uniformly developed hypertension by about the third of their usual 7-week gestation and remained hypertensive into the postpartum period, at which time their blood pressures returned to normal. Proteinuria, assessed in a semiquantitative fashion occurred in virtually all banded dogs during gestation and cleared after delivery. This model was free of the criticism that it was an acute preparation, but suffered from several limitations: (1) many dogs were infertile following the initial surgery; (2) blood pressure was measured only after the animal had been again subjected to anesthesia, and then at infrequent intervals; and (3) quantitation of the reduction of the blood flow to the placenta was not possible.

Abitbol et al. undertook studies in rabbits,[15] and later in dogs,[12] which employed very precise constriction of the aorta below the renal arteries. Considerable care was also taken to limit the surgery. Unlike the experiments of Hodari, however, all studies were initiated during gestation. In rabbits, blood pressure increased progressively for up to 14 days postaortic banding, whereas about one-third of pregnant dogs failed to develop hypertension. The mean blood pressure was nonetheless higher in the group of dogs subjected to continuous reduction of distal aortic flow than in sham-operated or nonpregnant-banded animals. Proteinuria was detected in virtually all pregnant animals of both species following aortic constriction. Perhaps the most striking finding was the detection of changes in the kidneys which mimicked, in part, glomerular endotheliosis, one of the "hallmarks" of preeclampsia. These changes were much more prominent in the dog model and occurred in about 75% of the animals. There appeared to be a correlation with the length of time that the constriction was present and the severity of the histologic change. Criticism of these studies includes the potential nonphysiologic nature of aortic constriction, which can cause ischemia in all parts distal to the narrowing. Further, the validity of blood pressure measurements could be compromised, since in the dog model, the readings were obtained while the animals were anesthetized, whereas the blood pressure in rabbits was assessed using the indirect ear artery occlusion technique.

Cavanagh et al. studied pregnant baboons with reduced uteroplacental blood flow.[20,73] The surgical technique used to limit blood flow was virtually identical to that described by Hodari.[11] With few exceptions, subhuman primates bred after the surgery had higher blood pressure than nonpregnant or sham-operated control pregnant animals. In the 1977 report, animals were found to have glomerular endothelial cell swelling. These apparently promising studies suffered from similar methodologic problems that plagued the earlier investigation using this surgical approach. The measurement of blood pressure was undertaken during anesthesia and the reduction in uteroplacental blood flow was uncontrolled and unquantified. The authors could not exclude the possibility that collateral circulation had developed to supplement flow to the gravid uterus.

Despite the very enthusiastic comments by the investigators which suggested this would be "the future model" to study preeclampsia, this uterine artery constriction–ovarian artery plication technique was subsequently abandoned by Cavanagh et al. They found that the fertility rate of the animals was so low following surgery that the protocol took years to complete and resulted in nearly prohibitive expenses. Later experiments in baboons employed a constricting ligature placed around the infrarenal aorta just past the midpoint of gestation.[22] Once again, hypertension developed and a renal lesion somewhat similar to that seen in preeclamptic patients was visible by electron microscopy. Unfortunately, anesthesia was required to obtain the blood pressure readings, proteinuria was detected in only about 20% of the animals, and the flow beyond the narrowed section of the aorta increased as gestation progressed.

Experiments employing distal aortic constriction have evolved to become more refined and incorporated new technologies and techniques as they have been developed. For example, Losonczy et al. attempted to obviate the problems of acute anesthesia in surgery by studying conscious, chronically instrumented rabbits.[74] The animals had been trained to rest comfortably in metabolic cages while the physiologic assessments were performed.[34] Blood pressure and cardiac output could be determined repeatedly without additional invasion, anesthesia, or apparent discomfort to the animals at the time data were collected.[31] Because the entire study was of relatively short duration, the degree of aortic constriction in the experimental phase could be accurately quantified using a transit time ultrasonic flow probe.[31,75] The residual flow was sufficient to ensure adequate perfusion of the lower extremities of the rabbits, at least as reflected by the normal rear leg motion and strength.

The hypertension which followed the reduction in distal aortic flow was accompanied by an increase in total peripheral resistance, a feature commonly observed in women who are preeclamptic.[3] The rise in systemic blood pressure did not seem to be driven by endogenous angiotensin, since neither a specific angiotensin-receptor blocker nor an angiotensin-converting enzyme inhibitor caused the elevated blood pressure to decline. This possibility was explored because enhanced uteroplacental renin formation[76] has been noted in pregnancy and uterine ischemia stimulates the release of this potential pressor compound at least in rabbits.[77] The hypertension which results when uteroplacental perfusion pressure is reduced in conscious dogs likewise is not reversed by blocking the action of angiotension II.[78] Finally, the aortic-constricted pregnant rabbits exhibited increased sensitivity to the pressor effect of exogenous angiotensin II similar to those women who can be categorized as already being preeclamptic[32] or those who are likely to develop preeclampsia.[79] The rabbit model that employs conscious, instrumented aortic-constricted animals clearly has its own limitations in the study of pathophysiology of preeclampsia. These include the lack of progression of the hypertension, the short duration of the study period, and the larger percentage decline in blood pressure that rabbits develop during gestation when compared to women.[74,80]

Another example of the application of technical and methodologic improvements to the aortic-constriction model is provided by the work of Combs et al. in rhesus monkeys.[81] They undertook longitudinal studies from early pregnancy through delivery. These studies included at will, continuous measurement of blood pressure above and below the narrowed segment of the aorta, as well as use of the Doppler ultrasound probes to estimate the impact of constriction on distal aortic flow. A specially developed tethering device protected the arterial catheter but allowed the animals to be unrestricted in their movement within their cages and to live in a communal environment. Phippard and Horvath, years before, had espoused the value of maintaining in a communal environment those primates used in the study of pregnancy,[4] since the stress of isolation appears to affect the very physiologic parameters under scrutiny. Combs et al. were able to show, in their carefully designed monkey model, that if the degree of aortic constriction was precisely achieved, progressive hypertension, proteinuria, and glomerular endotheliosis uniformly developed. Despite the new technology, a very high rate of technical failure occurred related to the difficulty attaining and maintaining the precise degree of aortic constriction. The studies of Losonczy et al.[74] and Combs et al.[81] used animals free from the problems of anesthesia and surgery and employed protocols designed to answer relatively narrow questions. This appears to be a more reasoned and successful formula for the use of laboratory animals in this model of gestational hypertension.

In conclusion, the attempts to either acutely or chronically reduce uteroplacental perfusion have led to results that are sometimes difficult to interpret. An overview of the criticisms of this approach in the study of preeclampsia is synopsized in Table 15–3. Nonetheless, one cannot ignore the consistent rise in blood pressure observed in so many different species resulting from lowered blood flow to the gravid uterus. The hypothesis, eloquently expounded by Page,[70] that places inadequate delivery of blood to the pregnant uterus at the focal point in the pathophysiology of preeclampsia appears to be supported by research in a wide array of pregnant mammals. The strength of these observations in animal studies using uteroplacental ischemia is diffused when investigators overstate the importance of individual experiments. Despite obvious difference from the human condition, the phrase "model for preeclampsia" can usually be found somewhere in each new report of a technique used to limit uteroplacental flow in yet another mammal. Care needs to be taken by authors to recognize the potentially exciting new findings in each study but to temper the comments with realistic assessment of the methodologic difficulties posed by the particular models. The goal of subsequent investigations should be to further reduce the methodologic problems and pose questions in improved models so that animal research protocol can, in a stepwise manner, advance our knowledge of the pathophysiology of both animal pregnancy and human preeclampsia.

MODELS OF PREECLAMPSIA EMPLOYING DIETARY DEPRIVATION

Page's hypothesis placed uteroplacental hypoperfusion at the core of the etiopathogenesis of preeclampsia and reflected his belief that hypoxia could either initiate or aggravate placental injury.[70] He extended this hypothesis to include the notion that damage to the placenta could also result from inadequate delivery of key nutrients to this organ. A deficiency of essential food and/or elements at the maternal placental interface might result from inadequate diet. Ewes sometimes develop a syndrome late in pregnancy comprised of convulsions, proteinuria, and azotemia.[82-84]

TABLE 15–3. LIMITATIONS OF ISCHEMIA MODELS DESIGNED TO MIMIC PREECLAMPSIA

Acute Models[13,14,18,21,68,69,72]

1. Precipitous onset bears little resemblance to the human condition
2. Effects of anesthesia and surgery are unavoidable

Chronic Models[11,12,15,16,19,20-22,26,73,74,78,80,81]

1. Hypertension sometimes not attained or sustained[12,20,73,80]
2. Blood pressure frequently measured
   a. indirectly—tail cuff, earlobe[12,74]
   b. under anesthesia[11,20,22,73]
3. Reduction in blood flow to uteroplacental unit often not quantified[11,12,26,73]
4. Other features (reduced renal function,[22] proteinuria) are sometimes lacking

This disease process correlates with environmental stress, multiple fetuses, poor food intake, and starvation ketosis. Unlike human preeclampsia, the disorder in ewes includes a neurologic component of progressive motor weakness beginning in the hindlimbs. Although affected animals frequently convulse, the seizures have their onset late in the course and are not associated with papilledema or retinal hemorrhage.[84] These differences, including the lack of correlation of the severity of the syndrome with the inconsistently observed hypertension, markedly separate this disease from preeclampsia and eclampsia.[1,3,84] The clinical and pathologic finding of proteinuria, impaired renal function, and glomerular endothelial cell swelling do, however, bear a resemblance to the human condition.

Pregnant guinea pigs and rats also develop a highly fatal clinical syndrome if stressed or starved during gestation.[85,86] This metabolic disturbance has a high attack rate in obese guinea pigs, where documented abnormalities include markedly altered lipid metabolism, ketosis, and fatty degeneration of the liver as well as other solid organs.[85] Hypertension is not a feature of the guinea pig model, yet such animals develop proteinuria and histologic changes of the kidney which include glomerular endothelial swelling.[87] Results obtained in a few very ill animals subjected to aortography and distal aortic blood pressure monitoring suggested that the aorta becomes narrowed and perfusion pressure to the gravid uterus may decline in animals affected with this disease.[87]

In contrast, Thatcher and Keith found the blood pressure to be elevated in late pregnant ewes after a 3-day fast.[88] They suggested that the failure of Ferris et al.[84] to demonstrate hypertension reflected the technical limitations of the equipment available to assess these hemodynamic parameters in studies undertaken nearly a generation earlier, and the decision by the original investigators to study animals when they were in the terminal phase of this condition. Although a reduction in uterine blood flow and an increase in peripheral vascular resistance also occurred, no individual hemodynamic parameters were included and the data were derived from small numbers of animals studied by Thatcher and Keith.[88]

Prada et al. attempted to further define the metabolic disturbances in "sheep toxemia."[89] Since calcium has been speculated to play a role in blood pressure regulation,[90] perhaps especially during gestation,[91] they theorized that a deficiency of this cation may mediate this form of hypertension in sheep. Their data showed that hypertension developed inconsistently only in ewes deprived of food and calcium late in pregnancy. All ewes that developed hypertension had multiple fetuses. Those animals experiencing a rise in blood pressure had lower serum-ionized calcium levels than the remainder of the starved ewes also drinking calcium-free water. In affected sheep, a negative linear correlation was observed between the serum level of ionized calcium and the increase in blood pressure. Reciprocally, uterine blood flow correlated positively with blood calcium concentrations.

Several years earlier, dietary calcium deficiency has been correlated with a rise in blood pressure in pregnant rats by Belizan et al.[92] These studies, however, not only relied on indirect assessment of blood pressure, but calcium-depleted non-pregnant control rats became as hypertensive as did the pregnant animals. The metabolic demands of the tissues and bones of the rapidly maturing fetus during gestation are high. It is not surprising that dietary-deprived, late-pregnant animals, especially sheep with multiple fetuses, became calcium-depleted more rapidly than nonpregnant animals and pregnant animals nurturing a smaller burden of fetal and placental tissue. The simple fact that pregnant animals more readily develop hypocalcemia does not necessarily imply that the blood pressure elevating stimulus that results from low levels of this divalent cation is specific for the pregnant state alone.

The hypertension that is often induced in gravid animals by extreme dietary manipulation nonetheless remains a fascinating biologic phenomenon. One could argue that the disorders seen in sheep and rodents are consistent with Page's concept that inadequate delivery of essential nutrients to the fetal unit can result in preeclampsia.[70] However, with the exception of the renal pathology, the observed differences between starvation syndromes and human preeclampsia are substantial. Discussing the hypothetical causes of preeclampsia, Chesley addressed the inconsistencies between the appealing, albeit simplistic, concept that selected dietary deficiency will predispose to preeclampsia and the observations made in pregnant women which showed that dietary deficiencies are difficult to correlate with an increased risk of gestational hypertension.[1] The lack of correlation between the syndromes seen in animals and human preeclampsia, as well as the severity of the generalized illness that developed in affected animals suggest that models which rely upon severe restrictions of vital nutrients, at best, have only a narrow use in the study of preeclampsia. The data derived from experiments undertaken in calcium-depleted animals have, nonetheless, helped to stimulate the ongoing evaluation of the role of calcium supplementation in the prevention of hypertensive pregnancy.[93,94] So far the data derived from clinical research are conflicting, as the results of studies in women given supplementary calcium during pregnancy are nearly completely divergent; thus, although the negative results of the randomized, double-blind study[94] appear more powerful, these data continue to stimulate review and editorial comment.[95,96] The difficulty in understanding the variable effects of calcium on blood pressure during gestation may be reduced by recent evidence which positively links the level of extracellular calcium with the excretion of sodium and water.[97,98] Retained salt and water could have been a cause of the elevated blood pressure that was found by Prada et al.[89] in only those pregnant sheep that had become hypocalcemic.

Leffler et al. showed the crucial role that excess sodium may play in a model of preeclampsia when they observed that hypertension developed only in aortic-constricted pregnant ewes given supplemental sodium.[99] Perhaps low total body calcium may contribute to hypertension in gravid women as it appears to do in some animal models. Carefully undertaken metabolic balance studies, which are often best posed in the laboratory setting, might help answer this speculation.

A discussion concerning animal models of preeclampsia that employs techniques to limit the supply of oxygen or other essential nutrients to the uteroplacental unit and thereby mimic the effects of placental pathology requires mention of the species differences in uterine and placental anatomy and physiology. Ramsey and Donner have meticulously defined the wide variations between species in the placental vascular anatomy.[100] Despite vast other anatomic differences between species, rodents, like humans, have discoid placentae with hemochorial (maternal blood comes into direct contact with the fetal chorionic membranes) blood flow. This contrasts with dogs and sheep, where a cell layer separates the maternal blood from the fetal chorionic membrane. The placentae in the respective canine and ovine species are designated as zonary and cotyledonary. The gross structure of the placentae of women and those of species lower on the phylogenetic scale may have some remarkable overlap, but the resemblance between human placentation and that of primates is closer yet.[100] The baboon appears to be anatomically closest of all, but the invasion of the fetoplacental trophoblasts into the spinal arteries of uterine endothelium may not be as deep as in humans.[101,102]

Advancement of the invasion of trophoblastic cells into the spiral arteries appears to be a prerequisite for blood flow to the placenta to increase as human pregnancy progresses. Compromise of this process, along with other vascular changes including arteriolar hyalinosis and focal areas of infarction of the placenta, are the characteristic abnormalities of this organ in the preeclamptic patient.[103-105] The parallels between the anatomy and physiology of the placentae of primates and women ensures that primates will have a special role in studies designed to better understand human pregnancy physiology and pathophysiology. For example, a 1993 study in rhesus monkeys subjected to aortic constriction revealed that the depth of the trophoblast invasion into the spinal arteries was positively correlated with the development of uteroplacental ischemia.[23] This important finding emphasizes the value of using species that share similar physiology when studying selected aspects of preeclampsia-related research.

Measurement of Uteroplacental Blood Flow

The assumption that uteroplacental blood flow falls in preeclamptic patients appears solid, both from the aforementioned description of placental vascular pathology and the clinical settings which predispose to gestational hypertension (see Table 15–2). Unfortunately, precise quantitation of blood flow to the gravid human uterus has not been achieved. Current methodologies rely on extraction techniques such as washouts of radioactive inert gases[106,107] or use externally placed Doppler ultrasound probes.[108] Concerns about the possible effects of even minute quantities of ionizing radiation on the fetus limit the acceptance of techniques that employ isotopes, and any dilution methodology provides only an indirect estimate of flow. The Doppler ultrasound technique currently is quite widely used, and has the advantage of low risk of injury or discomfort to patient and fetus. Unfortunately, because the energy beam originates from an externally placed probe, the precise relationship with the artery is often variable and the results are highly dependent on the operator's approach.[108] Moreover, the multiple routes that blood can travel to the uterus during gestation make exact measurement of flow by Doppler ultrasound virtually impossible.

In contrast, uteroplacental blood flow can be fairly precisely quantitated in pregnant animals. Radiolabeled microspheres injected into the left ventricle can accurately and simultaneously define blood flow to multiple organs. Indeed, some of the first uses of this technique were in gravid animals.[109-110] Radiolabeled microspheres may be useful to determine cardiac output as well as organ blood flow, but well-recognized caveats, especially the possible escape of smaller size spheres through the uteroplacental unit, limit their use in gestational studies.[111] Another major restriction is that organs must be removed after the experiment and usually acid-digested to assess the number of spheres trapped in each organ. Despite these limitations, the ability to measure regional flow in animals provides a unique opportunity to answer selected questions which cannot be asked in humans. Implantable Doppler ultrasound probes should permit continuous measurement of uterine blood flow in animals. These probes are loosely placed around vessels and may avoid the problem inherent to electromagnetic flow probes, which must be fitted snugly around arteries and, therefore, might influence the pregnancy by preventing the expansion of the vessels during gestation. Doppler ultrasound probes are likely to be used even more in future animal studies of pregnancy.

ENDOTHELIAL DYSFUNCTION AND PREECLAMPSIA

Overview

Several approaches to explore the pathophysiology of preeclampsia have emerged from the widely discussed[6,9,10] but still unproven notion that dysfunction of endothelium is the cause of this disorder. The theoretical construct depicted in Figure 15–1 schematically shows two possible routes leading to impaired endothelial function. Placental ischemia could release substances which are potentially damaging to these blood vessel lining cells and to the adjacent underlying structures.[112,113] Alternatively, an undefined endothelial injury or insult may already exist in patients with underlying vascular or kidney disease, causing affected individuals to be vulnerable to progressive or new dysfunction of the endothelium, a tissue with many important regulatory roles.[6,114-116]

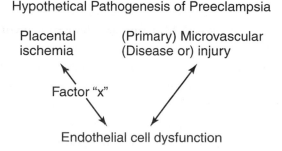

Figure 15–1. A possible explanation for the pathophysiology of preeclampsia that focuses on the endothelium.

Nitric Oxide

Exploration to define a role for the endothelium in the pathophysiology of preeclampsia has heavily focused on nitric oxide. The postulate that this endothelium-derived relaxing factor[57] may mediate the gestationally related reduction in systemic vascular tone has already been discussed. Extension of that theory would suggest that a deficiency in the synthesis of nitric oxide (NO) may result in hypertension during pregnancy.[58] L-arginine is the amino acid substrate for the vascular endothelial cell enzyme nitric oxide synthase (NOS) that generates NO.[117,118] Nitric oxide effects on the vasculature are mediated by the intracellular activation of soluble guanylate cyclase and the increased concentration of cyclic guanosine monophosphate (cGMP).[117]

Production of NO can be blocked in vivo by L-arginine analogs such as nitro-L-arginine methyl ester (L-NAME) which competitively inhibits NOS.[118] During pregnancy, rats have increased turnover of cGMP,[119] enhanced synthesis of NO,[57] and will develop hypertension if given L-NAME.[60,120-123] However, in most reports, the hypertensive response to L-NAME in gravid rats was not different from that observed in nonpregnant rats.[120-123]

The observations of Nathan et al., however, suggested that the hypertensive response of baroreceptor-blocked pregnant rats to acute NOS blockade was greater than in virgin controls.[61] Danielson and Conrad reported that constrictive response of the renal vasculature to the acute administration of L-arginine analogs was also greater in instrumented pregnant rats than in nonpregnant rats.[124] The results of these two studies imply that there may be a unique, pregnancy-enhanced response to the vasoconstrictor effect of NOS blockade. Indeed the constellation of symptoms, including hypertension, increased renal vascular tone, proteinuria, reduced plasma volume, and fetal growth retardation that have been reported when pregnant rats were chronically administered L-arginine analogs[122,123,125-128] has led to the suggestion that the NOS-blocked pregnant rat model for preeclampsia can be a useful one.[58,120,125-128] The importance of animal research in the study of pregnancy physiology and pathophysiology is further emphasized by the provocative results of studies that employed drugs and techniques unacceptable in human subjects. When coupled with the finding in sheep which showed the gestationally related increased expression of NOS was greater in uterine than systemic arteries[129] and the observation that systemic and/or local NO production may be decreased in some preeclamptic women,[130,131] altered NO synthesis has moved to the forefront of the potential causes of the endothelial dysfunction in preeclampsia.

Disturbing parallels exist, however, between recent speculation on altered NO synthesis in the pathophysiology of pregnancy hypertension and the roles proposed for other vasoactive compounds when discovered in greater quantities in pregnant mammals. History should temper the zeal to readily accept the latest hypothesis. We must consider that the enhanced synthesis of this vasoactive compound (NO) during gestation may be a reactive rather than an initiating event. Angiotensin II, for example, has already been considered as suspect in the etiopathogenesis of preeclampsia. It is now accepted that higher levels of the potent vasoconstrictor angiotensin II appear necessary to counteract the as yet undefined primary cause of systemic vasodilation during pregnancy and that levels of angiotensin II are decreased rather than increased in preeclampsia.[3,5]

Moreover, there are results obtained in laboratory animals that appear to conflict with the notion that pharmacologically induced NO deficiency preferentially results in greater vasoconstriction in pregnancy. Losonczy et al. found that nonpregnant rabbits showed a greater increase in total peripheral resistance when compared to pregnant rabbits given L-NAME.[132] Cardiac output declined substantially in both groups of animals after treatment with the NOS-blocking agent but the reduction was greater in the nonpregnant animals. These results cast doubt not only on the theory that enhanced NO synthesis may have a primary role in pregnancy-induced vasodilation but also question the usefulness of the L-arginine analogs in such studies because of the apparent cardiotoxic effects of these compounds.[132] Along these lines, Richer et al. found that a NO donor did not reverse the preeclamptic-like syndrome seen in rats given L-NAME chronically.[133] The latter results suggest that NO deficiency is not primarily responsible for this form of hypertension in rats.

The Role of the Prostanoids Prostacyclin and Thromboxane A_2

Nitric oxide is one of many compounds derived from and/or directly acting upon the endothelium, potentially affecting vascular tone and function during gestation. Two products of the arachidonic acid-cyclooxygenase cascade have also been of special interest. Prostacyclin is a vasodilator eicosanoid with potency similar to NO which is produced by the endothelium and other tissues. Prostacyclin can act locally in a paracrine manner and the endothelium is also capable of reacting to PGI_2 made at distant sites. Based in part on seminal work in animals, evidence accrues that vasodilator prostaglandins produced by the uteroplacental unit have a systemic action and may be the partial, or even the major, cause of the generalized vasorelaxation during gestation.[5,44,134] Prostacyclin has a role in assisting the endothelium to resist platelet aggregation on its surface and platelet aggregation, in turn, is associated with the local release of thromboxane A_2 (TXA_2), a very potent vasoconstrictor prostanoid.[44] Observations made in both humans and animals suggest that preeclampsia may result from an imbalance between the production of these two compounds in which the production of TXA_2 by platelets and perhaps the uteroplacental unit is favored relative to that of PGI_2.[135-139]

The notion that an imbalance of production between thromboxane and prostacyclin is linked to gestational hypertension has garnered considerable attention. This speculation has spurred studies in both animals[140,141] and human subjects[136,137] which employed low doses of aspirin. This treatment inhibits thromboxane synthesis by platelets while permitting continued synthesis of prostacyclin.[44] At present, the results of studies in humans suggest that the prophylactic use of aspirin appears to have limited value as prophylaxis in a large population of individuals with an increased risk to develop preeclampsia[142] and in several groups of patients classified to be at high risk to develop preeclampsia.[143]

Low-dose aspirin administered to both pregnant animals and humans has failed to clarify the role of TXA_2–PGI_2 imbalance in preeclampsia. Unfortunately, low-dose aspirin does not selectively reduce TXA_2 synthesis in all pregnant subjects.[144] Because the existing data are not definitive and since they possess such important actions on the endothelium, these eicosanoids remain the focus of intense study in preeclampsia pathogenesis. Free radical oxidation products are increased in the plasma of women with pregnancy-induced hypertension.[145] Such compounds, along with other circulating factors, all suspected to be of uteroplacental origin, may enhance TXA_2 production by the endothelium as well as by platelets,[44,112,146] and also reduce PGI_2 synthesis.[146,147]

We are unaware of any published animal study that has clearly defined the implications of this potential imbalance between the synthesis of these prostanoids during gestation. A series of investigations undertaken in pregnant rabbits, however, have indicated that thromboxane may be uniquely qualified to act as a systemic vasoconstrictor during pregnancy.[148-150] These findings suggest that the pressor effect of TXA_2 may be enhanced on the systemic vasculature and, seemingly paradoxically, reduced in the pulmonary circuit during gestation. Based on these results, the authors have suggested that altered sensitivity to TXA_2 during gestation may not only permit this prostanoid to play a key role in preeclampsia but also explain the short-term benefit that pregnancy affords those individuals who have primary pulmonary hypertension.[151]

Preliminary data in rats suggest that the systemic pressor action of TXA_2 is enhanced during gestation as it is in the pregnant rabbit.[152] Further, TXA_2 may mediate the action of endothelin, a potent vasoconstrictor derived from the endothelium.[153] Pregnancy does not blunt the pressor effect of endothelin in rats,[154] and endothelin levels are elevated in preeclamptic women.[155] Conscious pregnant sheep continuously infused with endothelin develop systemic hemodynamic and renal abnormalities which parallel those seen in preeclampsia.[156] Despite this growing body of evidence that may support a direct or indirect role for TXA_2 in gestational hypertension. These TXA_2 data combined with the recent discovery that in rabbits pregnancy increases the pressor action of a calcium channel enhancing agent suggests that mechanisms of blood pressure regulation during gestation are yet to be fully defined.[156a] The usual caveats must be applied against the extrapolation of these largely animal-derived data to the human condition.

Nonetheless, the previously mentioned findings of Conrad and Colpoys in rats strongly argue against vasodilator prostanoids as the primary mediators of the systemic vasodilation of pregnancy.[28] By contrast, recent studies, also in rats, from that same laboratory have shown that such prostaglandins may have a special role in protecting the renal vascular bed from excess constriction in response to inhibition of nitric oxide synthesis.[157]

Endotoxin Infusion

Pregnancy increases the sensitivity of animals to the so-called endotoxin-induced, generalized Schwartzman reaction.[158,159] Features of the Schwartzman reaction, including diffuse intravascular coagulation and thrombosis in the renal microvasculature, are seen in patients with severe preeclampsia.[160] Fass et al. injected rats with minute quantities of bacterial endotoxin intravenously on 14 consecutive days.[161] Pregnant animals given endotoxin beginning on day 1 of gestation developed hypertension, albuminuria, and fibrinogen deposition in the glomeruli while normally cycling female rats were unaffected by this dose. The triad of findings observed in the pregnant rats led these investigators to propose that administration of ultralow-dose endotoxin to pregnant rats could be a model of preeclampsia. Subsequently, Fass et al., using immunohistochemical techniques, showed that glomerular inflammation and production of adhesion molecules were much greater in pregnant rats than in nonpregnant rats given low-dose endotoxin.[162]

The action of endotoxin is thought to be mediated by a cascade of events which ultimately results in the release by monocytes of the cytokine tumor necrosis factor α (TNF-α).[163] Conrad and Benyo have hypothesized that TNF-α is likely to be the key cytokine overproduced by the placenta in response to local ischemia.[115] The review by Conrad and Benyo also details the multiple mechanisms through which TNF-α may damage the endothelium.[115] The potential relationship between endotoxin and endothelial injury would seem to support some role for the ultralow-dose endotoxin infusion model in the study of preeclampsia. There is evidence for an increase in TNF-α in preeclamptic patients; however, there is no direct evidence that endotoxin levels are increased in pregnant women.[115] An excess of cytokines appears to result from another cascade of changes initiated by uteroplacental ischemia, therefore, usefulness of this model to define the pathophysiology of toxemia may be limited.

OTHER MODELS OF PREECLAMPSIA

Two additional models of preeclampsia deserve comment. One relates to breakthroughs in molecular biology and genetic research, the other to the virtual lack of spontaneously developing preeclampsia in mammals other than humans.

Gene-Manipulated Animals

The interest in the activation of the renin–angiotensin system as a cause of preeclampsia has been recently rekindled by the observation that women who express a molecular variant of angiotensinogen have a much higher preeclampsia attack rate.[164,165] This gene abnormality has already been associated with an increased incidence of essential hypertension.[166] Moreover, expression of the molecular variant of angiotensinogen, angiotensinogen T235, was elevated in decidual spiral arteries of women.[167] This observation suggests that abnormal activation of the renin system may in turn be a cause of the atherotic changes in these vessels which are strongly linked to preeclampsia. These preliminary data are interesting because they bear on the uteroplacental unit which remains the focal point of the events tied to the pathogenesis of preeclampsia.

Animal models may be available to further explore this new approach. When female mice transgenic for human angiotensinogen[168] are mated with males transgenic for human renin,[169] hypertension develops beginning about day 14 of the usual 19- to 20-day gestation.[170] Control mice remained normotensive as did female mice transgenic for human renin when bred to males transgenic for human angiotensinogen.

This recent discovery is important in its own right and further hints at the potential of gene manipulation in the study of preeclampsia. Gene substitution could be used, for example, to either limit or enhance the enzymes that govern the synthesis of NO, PGI_2, or TXA_2. Such experiments in mice must be paralleled, however, by more extensive definition of the physiology of pregnancy in this species, since mice have, heretofore, only rarely been used in such studies. Enthusiasm for this approach must also be tempered by the complex and typically redundant mechanisms that characterize blood pressure regulatory physiology in mammals. Such adaptive responses may render futile attempts to isolate the effect of a particular vasoactive compound.

Ureteral Obstruction

Enhorning has proposed that preeclampsia is exclusively a disease of humans because of our upright posture and bipedal locomotion.[171] He hypothesizes that the pathogenesis of this unique form of hypertension is causally related to intermittent, but near complete, obstruction of ureters by the uterus at the pelvic brim. He further theorizes that the more muscular abdominal wall, which typifies the primigravid patient, would enhance the intraabdominal pressure that pushes the uterus back toward the ureters and thereby explain the increased susceptibility of this subgroup of individuals to preeclampsia. This theory is also compatible with the beneficial effect of rest in the left lateral recumbent position by patients with early manifestations of this condition. The results of preliminary experiments performed in a sheep subjected to intermittent ureteral occlusion are encouraging (G. Enhorning, personal communication). Although the data as yet are far from definitive, they are nonetheless intriguing.

ANIMALS WITH PREEXISTING DISEASES THAT MAY PREDISPOSE TO PREECLAMPSIA

Hypertension predisposes to preeclampsia. Various animals, especially rats, genetically disposed to develop hypertension,[172] have been used in an attempt to reproduce the clinical picture of hypertensive women who become pregnant.[29,173] The results of such studies have defined the effect of pregnancy on the kidney function and blood pressure of congenitally hypertensive animals. The gravid rats, however, rarely develop a syndrome that mimics preeclampsia and so differ from the situation in hypertensive women who become pregnant.

Likewise, the effect of pregnancy on several different models of kidney disease or injury has also been examined.[174,175] Baylis et al. found that rats with an antiglomerular basement membrane form of glomerulonephritis and reduced renal mass (five-sixths nephrectomy) experienced the expected beneficial effect of pregnancy on glomerular filtration rate. Further, during the study period, proteinuria did not increase and the animals appeared to fare well during gestation.

In contrast, Podjarny et al. studied rats treated with Adriamycin.[176] A dose of 4 mg/kg of this chemotherapeutic agent induces mild proteinuria in control rats with minimal histologic changes in the kidney. When Adriamycin-treated rats were mated, they developed hypertension and heavy proteinuria. Despite these findings there was no histologic abnormality detected in the kidney. The isolated glomeruli of the pregnant Adriamycin-treated rats, however, failed to increase the production of PGE_2 (as compared to untreated pregnant controls) and therefore the ratio of TXA_2 to PGE_2 was increased in the Adriamycin-treated pregnant rats. The glomerular pathology in this model does not mimic that seen in preeclampsia, and the altered ratio of vasoconstrictor to vasodilator prostaglandins in pregnant women with preeclampsia does not appear to be of renal origin[136,137] as it seems to be in these pregnant rats. Therefore, this model does not resemble the human condition and appears to be a circumscribed tool in preeclampsia research. More recently, Podjarny et al.[176a] have shown that exogenous insulin elevates systemic blood pressure and reduces NO excretion in pregnant rats. This model may provide an alternate route to study the role of NO in pregnancy.

An even more complex model has also been suggested to be used in pursuit of the study of preeclampsia. Wada et al. examined the effects of pregnancy on rats with genetic hypertension and neonatal streptozotocin-induced diabetes.[177] Pregnancy was associated with progressive albuminuria and hypertension in these rats. Unfortunately, these studies failed to include pathology of kidney and adequate control groups and must be considered preliminary at this time. Taken collectively, however, these results offer some promise for complex models to study the effects of pregnancy on the underlying hypertension and kidney disease. Whether rats with underlying renal and blood pressure abnormalities echo the physiology of women with similar afflictions remains unclear.

CONCLUSION

This discourse highlights some of the interrelationships between animal models devised to mimic preeclampsia and advancements made in the understanding of the pathophysiology of this condition. The scope of the work reviewed is outlined in Table 15–4. The results of experiments undertaken in animals have substantially strengthened the arguments for certain hypotheses regarding the pathophysiology

TABLE 15–4. ANIMAL MODELS DEVISED TO MIMIC PREECLAMPSIA

1. Uteroplacental ischemia
   a. Acute
      (1) Aortic constriction[14,18,21,68,69]
      (2) Placental vascular occlusion[13,72]
   b. Chronic
      (1) Aortic constriction[12,15,16,19,22,23,74,78,81,177]
      (2) Multiple vessel ligation[11,20,73]
2. Dietary manipulation
   a. Starvation[82-86]
   b. Calcium deficiency[89,92]
3. Alterations of vasodepressor–vasopressor balance? endothelial injury[6,9,10,12,112,113]
   a. NO inhibition of NO synthesis[57,58,60,61,120-133]
   b. Infusion of TXA_2[44,114,145,147-151]
   c. Endotoxin infusion[160,161]
4. Other models
   a. Gene-manipulated animals[167]
   b. Ureteral occlusion[170]
5. Animals with preexisting disease that predispose to preeclampsia
   a. Renal disease[173-175]
   b. Hypertension[29,172,176,176a]

of a condition that occurs spontaneously and frequently only in gravid women. Data derived from research in laboratory animals continue to support a key role for uteroplacental hypoperfusion in the pathogenesis of this condition. For example, the potential interaction between uteroplacental ischemia and endothelial injury has been strengthened by the results of recent experiments in subhuman primates.[178] The dangers inherent when attempting to directly extrapolate from the research in any species of animal to the human condition cannot be minimized. This perspective is useful when new information generated in either the research laboratory or the clinic purports to further define the pathophysiology of the still mysterious disease entity called preeclampsia.

REFERENCES

1. Chesley LC, ed: Hypothesis. In: *Hypertensive Disorders in Pregnancy*. New York: Appleton-Century Crofts; 1978:445–476.
2. El-Roeiy A, Gleicher N: The immunologic concept of pre-eclampsia. In: Rubin PC, ed. *Handbook of Hypertension*. Amsterdam: Elsevier Science Publishers B.V.; 1988:257–266.
3. Wallenburg HCS: Hemodynamics in hypertensive pregnancy. In: Rubin PC, ed.: *Handbook of Hypertension*. Amsterdam: Elsevier Science Publishers B.V.; 1988:66–101.
4. Phippard AF, Horvath JS: Animal Models of Pre-eclampsia. In: Rubin PC, ed. *Handbook of Hypertension*. Amsterdam: Elsevier Science Publishers B.V.; 1988:168–685.
5. Ferris TF: Hypertension and pre-eclampsia. In: Burrow GN, Ferris TF (eds.): *Medical Complications During Pregnancy*, ed 4. Philadelphia: WB Saunders; 1993:1–28.
6. Roberts JM, Redman CWG: Pre-eclampsia: More than pregnancy-induced hypertension. *Lancet* 1993;341:1447–1451.
7. Rubanyi GM: The role of endothelium in cardiovascular homeostasis and diseases. *J Cardiovasc Pharmacol* 1993;22(suppl 4):S1–S4.

8. De Meyer GRY, Herman AG: Vascular endothelial dysfunction. *Prog Cardiovasc Dis* 1997; 39:325–342.
9. Roberts JM, Taylor RN, Goldfein A: Clinical and biochemical evidence of endothelial cell dysfunction in the pregnancy syndrome of preeclampsia. *Am J Hypertens* 1991;4:700–708.
10. Roberts JM, Taylor RN, Goldfein A: Clinical and biochemical evidence of endothelial cell dysfunction in the pregnancy syndrome pre-eclampsia. *Am J Hypertens* 1991;4:700–708.
11. Hodari AA: Chronic uterine ischemia and reversible experimental "toxemia of pregnancy." *Am J Obstet Gynecol* 1967;97:597–607.
12. Abitbol MM, Pirani CL, Ober WB, et al: Production of experimental toxemia in the pregnant dog. *Obstet Gynecol* 1976;48:537–548.
13. Berger M, Cavanagh D: Toxemia of pregnancy. The hypertensive effect of acute experimental placental ischemia. *Am J Obstet Gynecol* 1963;87:293–305.
14. Berger M, Boucek RJ: Irreversible uterine and renal changes induced by placental ischemia (rabbit). *Am J Obstet Gynecol* 1964;89:230–240.
15. Abitbol MM, Gallo GR, Pirani CL, Ober WB: Production of experimental toxemia in the pregnant rabbit. *Am J Obstet Gynecol* 1976;124:460–470.
16. Abitbol MM: Simplified technique to produce toxemia in the rat: Considerations of cause of toxemia. *Clin Exp Hypertens* 1982;Part B:B1:93–103.
17. Fraser AHH, Godden W, Snook IC, Thomson W: Ketonanemia in pregnant ewes and its possible relation to pregnancy disease. *J Physiol* 1939;97:120–127.
18. Assali NS, Holm L, Hutchinson DL: Renal haemodynamics, electrolyte excretion and water metabolism in pregnant sheep before and after the induction of toxemia of pregnancy. *Circ Res* 1958;6:468–475.
19. Thatcher CD, Keith JC: Pregnancy-induced hypertension: Development of a model in the pregnant sheep. *Am J Obstet Gynecol* 1986;155:201–207.
20. Cavanagh D, Rao PS, Tung KSK, Lamat G: Eclamptogenic toxemia: The development of an experimental model in the subhuman primate. *Am J Obstet Gynecol* 1974;120:183–196.
21. Abitbol MM, Ober WB, Gallko GR, et al: Experimental toxemia of pregnancy in the monkey. *Am J Pathol* 1977;86:573–590.
22. Cavanagh D, Rao PS, Knuppel RA, et al: Pregnancy-induced hypertension: Development of a model in the pregnant primate (*Papio anubis*). *Am J Obstet Gynecol* 1985;151:987–999.
23. Zhou Y, Chiu K, Brescia RJ, et al: Increased depth of trophoblast invasion after chronic constriction of the lower aorta in rhesus monkeys. *Am J Obstet Gynecol* 1993;169:224–229.
24. Smith HG: Summary interpretation of observations of renal hemodynamics in pre-eclampsia. In: Fomon SJ, ed. *Report of First Ross Obstetric Research Conference.* Columbus, OH: Ross Laboratories; 1956:75.
25. Pedersen EB, Christensin NJ, Christensin P, et al: Preeclampsia—a state of prostaglandin deficiency? *Hypertension* 1983;5:105–111.
26. Venuto RC, Donker ABJM: Prostaglandin E2, plasma renal activity, and renal function throughout pregnancy. *J Lab Clin Med* 1982;99:239–246.
27. Brown G, Venuto R: In vitro renal eicosanoid production during pregnancy in rabbits. *Am J Physiol* 1988;254:E687–E693.
28. Conrad KP, Colpoys MC: Evidence against the hypothesis that prostaglandins are the vasodepressor agents of pregnancy. *J Clin Invest* 1986;77:236–245.
29. Baylis C, Reckelhoff JF: Renal hemodynamics in normal and hypertensive pregnancy: Lessons from micropuncture. *Am J Kidney Dis* 1991;27:98–104.
30. Conrad KP: Renal hemodynamics during pregnancy in chronically catheterized, conscious rats. *Kidney Int* 1984;26:24–29.
31. Brown G, Venuto RC: Renal blood flow response to angiotensin II infusions in conscious pregnant rabbits. *Am J Physiol* 1991;261:F51–F59.
32. Abdul-Karim R, Assali NS: Pressor response to angiotensin in pregnant and nonpregnant women. *Am J Obstet Gynecol* 1961;82:246–251.
33. Rosenfeld CR, Gant NF: The chronically instrumented ewe: A model for studying vascular reactivity to angiotensin II in pregnancy. *J Clin Invest* 1981;67:486–492.
34. Donker AJM, Min I, Venuto RC: The conscious instrumented rabbit: A model for the study of mechanisms of blood pressure regulation during pregnancy. *Hypertension* 1983;5:514–520.

35. Paller MS: Mechanism of decreased pressor responsiveness to Ang II, NE, and vasopressin in pregnant rats. *Am J Physiol* 1984;247:H100–H105.

36. August P, Levy T, Ales KL, et al: Longitudinal study of the renin-angiotensin aldosterone system in hypertensive pregnant women. *Am J Obstet Gynecol* 1990;163:1612–1621.

37. Weir RJ, Brown JJ, Fraser R, et al: Plasma renin, renin substrate, angiotensin II and aldosterone in hypertensive disease of pregnancy. *Lancet* 1973;1:291–294.

38. Hanssens M, Keirse MJ, Spitz B, Van Assche FA: Angiotensin II levels in hypertensive and normotensive pregnancies. *Br J Obstet Gynaecol* 1991;98:155–161.

39. Brown GP, Venuto RC: Angiotensin II receptor alterations during pregnancy in rabbits. *Am J Physiol* 1986;251:E58–E64.

40. Naden RP, Coutrup S, Arant BS, Rosenfeld CR: Metabolic clearance of angiotensin II in pregnant and non-pregnant sheep. *Am J Physiol* 1985;249:E49–E55.

41. Magness RR, Cox K, Rosenfeld CR, Gant NF: Angiotensin II metabolic clearance rate and pressor responses in non-pregnant and pregnant women. *Am J Obstet Gynecol* 1994;171: 668–679.

42. Raab W, Schroeder G, Wagner R, Gigse W: Vascular reactivity and electrolytes in normal and toxemic pregnancy. *J Clin Endocrinol* 1956;16:1196–1216.

43. Venuto R, Min I, Barone P, et al: Blood pressure control in pregnant rabbits: Norepinephrine and prostaglandin interactions. *Am J Physiol* 1984;247:R786–R791.

44. Fitzgerald DJ, Fitzgerald GA: Eicosanoids in the pathogenesis of preeclampsia. In: Laragh JH, Brenner BM, eds. *Hypertension Pathophysiology, Diagnosis and Management*. New York: Raven Press; 1990:1789–1807.

45. Chaudhuri GP, Barone P, Lianos E, et al: Uterine and peripheral blood concentrations of vasodilator prostaglandins in conscious pregnant rabbits. *Am J Obstet Gynecol* 1982;144: 760–767.

46. Gerber JG, Payne NA, Murphy RC, Nies AS: Prostacyclin produced by the pregnant uterus in the dog may act as a circulating vasodepressor substance. *J Clin Invest* 1981;67:632–636.

47. Magness RR, Osei-Boaten K, Mitchell MD, Rosenfeld CR: In vitro prostacyclin production by ovine uterine and systemic arteries. *J Clin Invest* 1985;76:2206–2212.

48. Everett RB, Worley RJ, MacDonald PC, Gant NF: Effect of prostaglandin synthetase inhibitors on pressor response to angiotensin II in human pregnancy. *J Clin Endocrinol Metab* 1978;46:1007–1010.

49. Flower RJ: Drugs which inhibit prostaglandin biosynthesis. *Pharmacol Rev* 1974;26:33–67.

50. Romero JC, Dunlap CL, Strong C: The effect of indomethacin and other anti-inflammatory drugs on the renin angiotensin system. *J Clin Invest* 1976;58:282–288.

51. Gant NF, Chand S, Whalley PJ, MacDonald PC: The nature of pressor responsiveness to angiotensin II in human pregnancy. *Obstet Gynecol* 1974;43:854–860.

52. Gant NF, Worley RJ, Everett RB, MacDonald PC: Control of vascular responsiveness during human pregnancy. *Kidney Int* 1986;18:253–258.

53. Paller MS, Ferris TF: The kidney and hypertension in pregnancy. In: Brenner BM, ed. *The Kidney*, ed 5. Philadelphia: WB Saunders; 1996:1731–1763.

54. Zins GR: Renal prostaglandins. *Am J Med* 1975;58:14–24.

55. Terragno N, Terragno D, McGiff J: Contribution of prostaglandins to the renal circulation in the conscious anesthetized and laparotomized dogs. *Circ Res* 1977;40:590–593.

56. Burger BM, Hopkins T, Tulloch A, Hollenberg NK: The role of angiotensin in the canine renal vascular response to anesthesia. *Circ Res* 1976;38:196–202.

57. Palmer RMJ, Ashton DS, Moncada S: Nitric oxide release accounts for the biologic activity of endothelium derived relaxing factor. *Nature* 1987;327:524–526.

58. Sladek SM, Magness RR, Conrad CP: Nitric oxide and pregnancy. *Am J Physiol* 1997; 272:R441–R463.

59. Conrad KP, Joffed GM, Kruszyna R, et al: Identification of increased nitric oxide biosynthesis during pregnancy in rats. *FASEB J* 1993;7:566–571.

60. Molnar M, Hertelendy F: N^{ω}-nitro L-arginine, an inhibitor of nitric oxide synthesis, increases blood pressure in rats and reverses the pregnancy-induced refractoriness to vasopressor agents. *Am J Obstet Gynecol* 1992;166:1560–1567.

61. Nathan L, Cuevas J, Chaudhuri G: The role of nitric oxide in the altered vascular reactivity of pregnancy in the rat. *Br J Pharmacol* 1995;114:955–960.
62. Allen R, Castro L, Arora C, et al: Endothelium-derived relaxing factor inhibition and the pressor response to norepinephrine in the pregnant rat. *Obstet Gynecol* 1994;83:92–96.
63. Stout C, Lemmon WB: Glomerular capillary endothelial swelling in a pregnant chimpanzee. *Am J Obstet Gynecol* 1969;105:212–215.
64. Baird J: Eclampsia in a lowland gorilla. *Am J Obstet Gynecol* 1981;141:345–346.
65. Palmer AE, London WT, Sly DL, Rice JM: Spontaneous pre-eclamptic toxemia of pregnancy in the Patas monkey (*Erythrocebus patas*). *Lab Anim Sci* 1979;29:102–106.
66. Page EW: The relation between hydatid moles, relative ischemia of the uterus and the placental origin of eclampsia. *Am J Obstet Gynecol* 1939;37:291–293.
67. Goldblatt H, Lynch J, Hanzel R, Summerville W: Studies on experimental hypertension: Production of persistent elevation of systolic blood pressure by means of renal ischemia. *J Exp Med* 1934;59:347–379.
68. Ogden E, Hildebrand GJ, Page EW: Rise in blood pressure during ischemia of the gravid uterus. *Proc Soc Exper Biol & Med* 1940;43:49–51.
69. Bastiaanse MA, Mastboom JL: Kidney and pregnancy. *Gynecologia* 1949;127:1–22.
70. Page EW: On the pathogenesis of preeclampsia and eclampsia. *J Obstet Gynaecol B Commonw* 1972;79:883–894.
71. Young J: Recurrent pregnancy toxemia and its relation to placental damage. *Trans Edinburgh Obstet Soc* 1927;47:61–76; *Edinburgh Med J* 1927;34.
72. Smith RW, Taniguchi AG: Angiotensin sensitivity in experimental uteroplacental ischemia. *Am J Obstet Gynecol* 1960;94:303–307.
73. Cavanagh D, Rao P, Stai C, O'Connor T: Experimental toxemia in the pregnant primate. *Am J Obstet Gynecol* 1977;128:75–88.
74. Losonczy G, Brown G, Venuto R: Increased peripheral resistance during reduced uterine perfusion pressure hypertension in pregnant rabbits. *Am J Med Sci* 1992;303:233–240.
75. Drost CJ, Dobson A, Sellers AF, et al: An implantable transit time ultrasonic flowmeter for long term measurement of blood volume flow. *Fed Proc* 1984;43:538–543.
76. Dzau FJ, Gonzales D, Ellison DK, et al: Characterization of purified rabbit uterine renin: Influence of pregnancy on uterine inactive renin. *Endocrinology* 1987;120:358–364.
77. Ferris TF, Stein JH, Kauffman J: Uterine blood flow and uterine renin secretion. *J Clin Invest* 1972;51:2827–2833.
78. Woods LL, Brooks VL: Role of the renin angiotensin system in hypertension during reduced uteroplacental perfusion pressure. *Am J Physiol* 1989;257:R204–R209.
79. Gant NF, Daley GL, Chand S, et al: A study of angiotensin II pressor response throughout primigravida pregnancy. *J Clin Invest* 1973;52:2682–2689.
80. Losonczy GY, Todd H, Palmer DC, Hertelendy F: Prostaglandins, norepinephrine, angiotensin II and blood pressure changes induced by uteroplacental ischemia in rabbits. *Clin Exp Hyper* 1986;B5:271–294.
81. Combs CA, Katz MA, Kitzmiller JL, Brescia RJ: Experimental preeclampsia produced by chronic constriction of the lower aorta: Validation with longitudinal blood pressure measurements in conscious rhesus monkeys. *Am J Obstet Gynecol* 1993;169:215–223.
82. Fraser AHH, Godden W, Snook IC, Thomson W: Ketonaemia in pregnant ewes and its possible relation to pregnancy disease. *J Physiol* 1939;97:120–127.
83. Reid RL: Pregnancy toxaemia in sheep. *Agriculture* (London) 1952;4:20–26.
84. Ferris TF, Herdson PB, Dunnill MS, Radcliffe LM: Toxemia of pregnancy in sheep: A clinical, physiological and pathological study. *J Clin Invest* 1969;48:1643–1655.
85. Ganaway JR, Sr, Allen AM: Obesity predisposes to pregnancy toxemia (ketosis) of guinea pigs. *Lab Anim Sci* 1971;2:40–44.
86. Stamler FW: Fatal eclamptic disease of pregnant rats fed anti-vitamin E stress diet. *Am J Path* 1967;35:1207–1211.
87. Seidl DC, Hughes HC, Bertolet R, Lang CM: True pregnancy toxemia (preeclampsia) in the guinea pig (*Cania porcellus*). *Lab Anim Sci* 1979;29:472–478.
88. Thatcher CD, Keith JC: Pregnancy-induced hypertension: Development of a model in the pregnant sheep. *Am J Obstet Gynecol* 1986;155:201–207.

89. Prada JA, Ross R, Clark JKE: Hypocalcemia and pregnancy induced hypertension produced by maternal fasting. *Hypertension* 1992;20:620–626.
90. Karanja N, McCarron DA: Calcium and hypertension. *Ann Rev Nutri* 1986;6:475–494.
91. Belizan JM, Villar J, Repke J: The relationship between calcium intake and edema, proteinuria, and hypertension-gestosis. An hypothesis. *Am J Clin Nutr* 1980;33:2202–2210.
92. Belizan JM, Pineda O, Sainz E, et al: Rise of blood pressure in calcium-deprived pregnant rats. *Am J Obstet Gynecol* 1981;141:163–169.
93. Bucher HC, Guyatt GH, Cook, RJ, et al: Effect of calcium supplementation on pregnancy-induced hypertension and preeclampsia. *JAMA* 1996;275:113–117.
94. Levine RJ, Hauth JC, Curet LB, et al: Trial of calcium to prevent preeclampsia. *N Engl J Med* 1997;337:69–76.
95. Sibai BM: Hypertension in pregnancy. In: Gabbe SG, Niebyl JR, Simpsin JL, eds. *Obstetrics—Normal and Problem Pregnancies*. New York: Churchill Livingstone, Inc.; 1996:935–996.
96. Roberts JM: Prevention or early treatment of preeclampsia (editorial). *N Engl J Med* 1997;337:124–125.
97. Brown E, Hebert S: A cloned Ca^{2+} sensing receptor. A mediator of direct effects of extracellular Ca^{2+} on renal function? *J Am Soc Nephrol* 1995;6:1530–1540.
98. Hebert SC, Brown EM: The scent of an ion: Calcium sensing and its roles in health and disease. *Curr Opin Nephrol & Hypertens* 1996;5:45–53.
99. Leffler CW, Hessler JR, Green RS, Fletcher AM: Effects of sodium chloride on pregnant sheep with reduced uteroplacental perfusion pressure. *Hypertension* 1986;8:62–65.
100. Ramsey EM, Donner MW: *Placental Vasculature and Circulation*. Philadelphia: WB Saunders; 1980.
101. Ramsey EM, Houston ML, Harris JWS: Interactions of the trophoblast and maternal tissues in three closely related primate species. *Am J Obstet Gynecol* 1976;124:647–652.
102. Lee MM, Yeh M: Fetal circulation of the placenta: A comparative study of human and baboon placenta by scanning electron microscopy of vascular casts. *Placenta* 1983;4:515–526.
103. Zeek-Minning P, Assali NS: Vascular changes in the decidua associated with eclamptogenic toxemia of pregnancy. *Am J Clin Pathol* 1950;20:1099–1109.
104. Brosens IM, Robertson NB, Dixon HG: The physiological response of the vessels of the placental bed to normal pregnancy. *J Path Bacteriol* 1967;93:569–579.
105. Zuspan FP: Abnormal placentation in hypertensive disorders of pregnancy. In: Laragh JH, Brenner BM, eds. *Hypertension. Pathophysiology, Diagnosis and Management*. New York: Raven Press, Ltd; 1990:1778–1779.
106. Clavero-Nunez JA: Uteroplacental blood flow in pregnant women: Its measurement by radioisotope techniques. In: Moawad AH, Lindheimer MD, eds. *Uterine and Placental Blood Flow*. New York: Masson Publishing; 1982:53–59.
107. Lunell NO, Joelsson I, Lewander R, et al: Clinical determination of uteroplacental blood flow: Methodology and application. In: Moawad AH, Lindheimer MD, eds. *Uterine and Placental Blood Flow*. New York: Masson Publishing; 1982:61–66.
108. Cunningham FG, MacDonald PC, Gant NF, et al, eds: Doppler and ultrasound. In: *Williams' Obstetrics*. Stamford, CT: Appleton & Lange; 1997:1023–1044.
109. Rosenfeld CR: Distribution of cardiac output in ovine pregnancy. *Am J Physiol* 1977;232:H231–H235.
110. Assali NS, Numayhid B, Zugaib M: Control of the uteroplacental circulation in health and disease. *Eur J Obstet Gynecol Reprod Biol* 1978;8:43–48.
111. Venuto RC: The use of radiolabelled microspheres to measure uteroplacental blood flow. In: Moawad AH, Lindheimer MD, eds. *Uterine and Placental Blood Flow*. New York: Masson Publishing; 1982:39–44.
112. Walsh SW, Wang Y: Trophoblast and placental villus core production of lipid peroxide thromboxane, and prostacyclin in preeclampsia. *J Clin Endocriol Metab* 1995;80:1888–1893.
113. Warso MA, Lands WEM: Lipid peroxidation in relation to prostacyclin and thromboxane physiology and pathophysiology. *Br Med Bull* 1983;39:277–280.
114. Roberts JN, Taylor RN, Musci TJ, et al: Preeclampsia: An endothelial cell disorder. *Am J Obstet Gynecol* 1989;161:1200–1204.

115. Conrad KP, Benyo DF: Placental cytokines and the pathogenesis of preeclampsia. *Am J Reprod Immunol* 1997;37:240–249.
116. Ness RB, Roberts JM: Heterogeneous causes constituting the single syndrome of preeclampsia: A hypothesis and its implications. *Am J Obstet Gynecol* 1996;175:1365–1370.
117. Moncada S, Higgs A: The L-arginine-nitric oxide pathway. *N Engl J Med* 1993;329:2002–2012.
118. Palmer RJF, Ashton DS, Moncada S: Vascular endothelial cells synthesize nitric oxide from L-arginine. *Nature* 1988;333:664–666.
119. Conrad KP, Vernier KA: Plasma level, urinary excretion and metabolic production of cGMP during gestation in rats. *Am J Physiol* 1989;257:R847–R853.
120. Umans JB, Lindheimer MD, Barron WM: Pressor effect of endothelium derived relaxing factor inhibition in conscious virgin and gravid rats. *Am J Physiol* 1990;28:F293–F296.
121. Ahokas RA, Mercer BM, Sibai BM: Enhanced endothelium-derived relaxing factor activity in pregnant spontaneously hypertensive rats. *Am J Obstet Gynecol* 1991;165:801–807.
122. Baylis C, Engels K: Adverse interactions between pregnancy and a new model of systemic hypertension produced by chronic blockade of endothelial derived relaxing factor (EDRF) in the rat. *Clin Exp Hypertens Pregnancy* 1992;B11:117–129.
123. Edwards DL, Arora CP, Brui DT, Castro LC: Long-term nitric oxide blockade in the pregnant rat: Effects on blood pressure and plasma levels of endothelin-1. *Am J Obstet Gynecol* 1996;175:484–488.
124. Danielson LA, Conrad CP: Acute blockade of nitric oxide synthase inhibits renal vasodilation and hyperfiltration during pregnancy in chronically instrumented conscious rats. *J Clin Invest* 1995;96:482–490.
125. Yallampalli C, Garfield RE: Inhibition of nitric oxide synthesis in rats during pregnancy produces signs similar to those of preeclampsia. *Am J Obstet Gynecol* 1993;169:1316–1320.
126. Molnar M, Suto T, Toth T, Hertelendy F: Prolonged blockade of nitric oxide synthesis in gravid rats produces sustained hypertension, proteinuria, thrombocytopenia and intrauterine growth retardation. *Am J Obstet Gynecol* 1994;170:1458–1466.
127. Diket AL, Pierce MR, Munshi UK, et al: Nitric oxide inhibition causes intrauterine growth retardation and hind limb disruptions in rats. *Am J Obstet Gynecol* 1994;171:1248–1250.
128. Salas SP, Altermatt AF, Campos M, et al: Effects of long term nitric oxide synthesis inhibitors on plasma volume expansion and fetal growth in pregnant rats. *Hypertens Dallas* 1995;26:1019–1023.
129. Magness RR, Shaw CE, Phernetton IM, et al: Endothelial vasodilation production by uterine and systemic arteries. II. Pregnancy effects on NO synthase expression. *Am J Physiol* 1997;272:H1730–H1740.
130. Pinto A, Sorrentino R, Sorrentino P: Endothelial-derived relaxing factor release by endothelial cells of human umbilical vessels and its impairment in pregnancy induced hypertension. *Am J Obstet Gynecol* 1991;164:507–513.
131. Davidge ST, Stranko CP, Roberts JM: Urine but not plasma nitric oxide metabolites are decreased in women with preeclampsia. *Am J Obstet Gynecol* 1996;174:1008–1013.
132. Losonczy GY, Mucha I, Muller V, et al: The vasoconstrictor effects of L-NAME, a nitric oxide synthase inhibitor, in pregnant rabbits. *Br J Pharmacol* 1996;118:1012–1018.
133. Richer C, Boulanger H, Es-Slami S, Giudicelli J: Lack of beneficial effects of the NO-donor, molsidomine in the L-NAME-induced pre-eclamptic syndrome in pregnant rats. *Br J Pharmacol* 1996;119:1642–1648.
134. Gerber JG, Payne NA, Murphy RC, Nies AS: Prostacyclin produced by the pregnant uterus in the dog may act as a circulating vasodepressor substance. *J Clin Invest* 1981;67:632–636.
135. Walsh SW: Preeclampsia: An imbalance in placental prostacyclin and thromboxane production. *Am J Obstet Gynecol* 1985;152:335–340.
136. Schiff E, Peleg E, Goldenberg M, et al: The use of aspirin to prevent pregnancy-induced hypertension and lower the ratio of thromboxane A_2 to prostacyclin in relatively high risk pregnancies. *N Engl J Med* 1989;321:351–356.
137. Benigni A, Gregorini G, Fusca T, et al: Effect of low dose aspirin on fetal and maternal generation of thromboxane by platelets in women at risk for pregnancy-induced hypertension. *N Engl J Med* 1989;321:357–362.
138. Keith JC, Jr, Miller K, Eggleston MK, et al: Effects of thromboxane synthetase inhibition on

maternal–fetal homeostasis in gravid ewes with ovine pregnancy-induced hypertension. *Am J Obstet Gynecol* 1989;161:1305–1313.

139. Keith JC Jr, Thatcher CD, Schaub RG: Beneficial effects of U-63,557A, a thromboxane synthetase inhibitor, in an ovine model of pregnancy-induced hypertension. *Am J Obstet Gynecol* 1987;157:199–203.

140. Woods LL: Importance of prostaglandins in hypertension during reduced uteroplacental perfusion pressure. *Am J Physiol* 1989;257:R1558–R1561.

141. Schafer W, Tielsch J, Casper FW, et al: Urinary excretion of 6-keto-PGF$_{1\alpha}$ TXB$_2$ and PGE$_2$ in a rat animal model for preeclampsia-like syndrome. *Prostaglandins* 1993;46:167–175.

142. CLASP: A randomized trial of low-dose aspirin for the prevention and treatment of preeclampsia among 9364 pregnant women. *Lancet* 1994;343:629–632.

143. Caritis S, Sibai B, Hauth J, et al: Low-dose aspirin to prevent preeclampsia in women at high risk. *N Engl J Med* 1998;338:701–705.

144. Brown CEL, Gant NF, Cox K, et al: Low-dose aspirin II. Relationship of angiotensin II pressor responses, circulating eicosanoids, and pregnancy outcome. *Am J Obstet Gynecol* 1990;163:1853–1861.

145. Wickens D, Wilkins M, Lunec J, et al: Free radical oxidation (peroxidation) products in plasma in normal and abnormal pregnancy. *Ann Clin Biochem* 1981;18:158–162.

146. Wang Y, Walsh SW, Kay W: Placental lipid peroxides and thromboxane are increased and prostacyclin is decreased in women with preeclampsia. *Am J Obstet Gynecol* 1992;167:946–949.

147. Baker PN, Davidge ST, Barankiewicz J, Roberts JM: Plasma of preeclamptic women stimulates then inhibits endothelial prostacyclin. *Hypertension* 1996;27:56–61.

148. Losonczy G, Mucha I, DiPirro J, et al: The effect of pregnancy on the response to the TXA$_2$/PGH$_2$ analogue U-46619 in rabbits. *Am J Physiol* 1993;265:R772–R780.

149. Losonczy G, Singh JP, Schoenl M, et al: Pregnancy enhances the pressor response to thromboxane analogues in rabbits. *Am J Physiol* 1995;262:R720–R725.

150. Losonczy G, Brown G, Mucha I, et al: Gestational resistance to the pulmonary vasoconstrictor effect of the TXA$_2$ mimetic U-46619: Possible mechanism. *Am J Physiol* 1997;272:R1734–R1739.

151. Losonczy G, Brown G, Venuto R: Pregnant or nonpregnant—Systemic or pulmonary hypertension induced by thromboxane A$_2$ and deficiency of prostaglandins: A hypothesis. *Hypertens Pregnancy* 1996;15:281–285.

152. Losonczy G, Kriston T, Engels K, et al: Pregnancy enhances the pressor response to the TXA$_2$ agonist U46619 in rats. *J Am Soc Nephrol* 1996;7:1537(abstr).

153. Howarth SR, Vallance P, Wison CA: Role of thromboxane A$_2$ in the vasoconstrictor response to endothelin-1, angiotensin II and 5-hydroxytryptamine in human placental vessels. *Placenta* 1995;16:679–689.

154. Molnar M, Hertelendy F: Pressor responsiveness to endothelin is not attenuated in gravid rats. *Life Sci* 1990;47:1463–1468.

155. Taylor RN, Varma M, Teng NNH, Roberts JM: Women with preeclampsia have higher plasma endothelin levels than women with normal pregnancies. *J Clin Endocrinol Metab* 1990;71:1675–1677.

156. Greenberg SG, Baker RS, Yang D, Clark KE: Effects of continuous infusion of endothelin-1 in pregnant sheep. *Hypertension* 1997;30:1585–1590.

156a. Venuto R, Losonczy G, Brown G, et al: Pregnancy enhances the pressor response to the calcium channel activator BAY-K 8644. *J Am Soc Neph* 1988;9:318A.

157. Danielson LA, Conrad K: Prostaglandins maintain renal vasodilation and hyperfiltration during chronic nitric oxide synthase blockade in conscious pregnant rats. *Circ Res* 1996;79:1161–1166.

158. Wong TC: A study on the generalized Schwartzman reaction in pregnant rats induced by bacterial endotoxin. *Am J Obstet Gynecol* 1982;84:786–799.

159. Beller FK, Schmidt EH, Holzgreve W, Hauss J: Septicemia during pregnancy: A study in different species of experimental animals. *Am J Obstet Gynecol* 1985;151:967–975.

160. Brozna JP: Schwartzman reaction. *Semin Thromb Hemost* 1990;16:326–332.

161. Fass MM, Schuiling GA, Baller AS, et al: A new animal model for human preeclampsia: Ultra low-dose endotoxin infusion in pregnant rats. *Am J Obstet Gynecol* 1994;171:158–164.

162. Fass MM, Schuiling GA, Baller JFW, Bakker WW: Glomerular inflammation in pregnant rats after infusion of low dose endotoxin. *Am J Pathol* 1995;147:1510–1518.

163. Cybulsky MI, Chan MKW, Movat HZ: Biology of disease, acute inflammation and microthrombosis induced by endotoxin, interleukin-1 and tumor necrosis factor and their implications in gram negative infections. *Lab Invest* 1988;58:365–378.

164. Ward K, Hata A, Jeunemaitre X, et al: A molecular variant of angiotensinogen associated with preeclampsia. *Nature Genet* 1993;4:59–61.

165. Armgrimisson R, Purandare S, Connor M, et al: Angiotensinogen: A candidate gene involved in preeclampsia. *Nature Genet* 1993;4:114–115.

166. Jeunemaitre X, Soubrier F, Koteleutsev YV, et al: Molecular basis of human hypertension: Role of angiotensinogen. *Cell* 1992;71:169–180.

167. Morgan T, Craven C, Nelson L, et al: Angiotensin T235 expression is elevated in decidual spiral arteries. *J Clin Invest* 1997;100:1406–1415.

168. Takahashi S, Fukamizu A, Hasegawa T, et al: Expression of the human angiotensin gene in transgenic mice and transfected cells. *Biochem Biophys Res Comm* 1991;180;1103–1109.

169. Fukamizu A, Seo MS, Hatae T, et al: Tissue specific expression of the human renin gene in transgenic mice. *Biochem Biophy Res Comm* 1989;165:826–832.

170. Takimoto E, Ishida J, Sugiyama F, et al: Hypertension induced in pregnant mice by placental renin and maternal angiotensinogen. *Science* 1996;274:995–998.

171. Enhorning G: Pre-eclampsia. A hypothesis for its pathogenesis. *Acta Obstet Gynecol Scand Suppl* 1984;118:7–11.

172. Yamori Y, Okamotu K: The Japanese spontaneously hypertensive rat (SHR). *Clin Experi Pharmacol & Physiol Suppl* 1976;3:1–4.

173. Lindheimer MD, Katz AT, Koeppen BM, et al: Kidney function and sodium handling in the pregnant spontaneously hypertensive rat. *Hypertension* 1983;5:498–506.

174. Baylis C, Reese K, Wilson CB: Glomerular effects of pregnancy in a model of glomerulonephritis in the rat. *Am J Kidney Dis* 1989;14:456–460.

175. Deng A, Baylis C: Glomerular hemodynamic response to pregnancy in rats with severe reduction of renal mass. *Kidney Internat* 1995;48:39–44.

176. Podjarny E, Bernheim J, Rathaus M, et al: Adriamycin nephropathy: A model to study effects of pregnancy on renal disease in rats. *Am J Physiol* 1992;263:F711–F715.

176a. Podjarny E, Bernheim J, Katz B, et al: Chronic exogenous hyperinsulinemia in pregnancy: A rat model of pregnancy-induced hypertension. *J Am Soc Nephrol* 1998,9:9–13.

177. Wada M, Iwase M, Wakisaka M, et al: A new model of diabetic pregnancy with genetic hypertension: Pregnancy in spontaneously hypertensive rats with neonatal streptozotocin-induced diabetes. *Am J Obstet Gynecol* 1995;172:626–630.

178. De Groot CJM, Merrill DC, Taylor RN, et al: Increased von Willebrand factor expression in an experimental model of preeclampsia produced by reduction of uteroplacental perfusion pressure in conscious rhesus monkeys. *Hypertens Pregnancy* 1997,16.177–186.

VI

Prevention and Management of Preeclampsia

16

Prevention of Preeclampsia

Baha M. Sibai and F. Gary Cunningham

The incidence of hypertensive disorders as discussed in Chapter 2, varies among institutions, regions, and countries, and it complicates from 6 to 8% of pregnancies in the United States.[1,2] These disorders are a major cause of maternal and perinatal mortalities and morbidities worldwide, especially in developing countries.[3] Because most of the mortality and morbidity is related to proteinuric hypertension—either primary or superimposed preeclampsia and eclampsia—prevention of these disorders would have worldwide clinical implications.

PREVENTION OF PREECLAMPSIA

Prevention of disease usually requires knowledge of its etiology and pathophysiology, as well as methods to predict patients at high risk. However, as discussed in Chapters 11 and 12, the etiology of preeclampsia is largely unknown. Thus, it is not surprising that most studies designed to reduce the incidence of preeclampsia in either low- or high-risk women have had negative results.[4]

Coincidentally, a number of clinical, biophysical, or biochemical tests have been proposed for the prediction or early detection of preeclampsia.[5] Unfortunately, most suffer from poor sensitivity and positive predictive value and the majority are not suitable for routine use in clinical practice. As a result, prevention studies have enrolled women with demographic, clinical, or medical factors that increase their risk for preeclampsia (Table 16–1).

During the past two decades, numerous clinical reports and randomized trials have described the use of various methods to prevent or reduce the incidence and/or severity of preeclampsia. Because the etiology is unknown, these were necessarily empirical and attempted to correct a pathophysiologic abnormality, biochemical imbalance, or dietary excess or deficiency (Table 16–2).

TABLE 16–1. CHARACTERISTICS OF WOMEN ENROLLED IN RANDOMIZED TRIALS TO PREVENT PREECLAMPSIA

- Nulliparous
- Poor outcome in previous pregnancies
  - preeclampsia–hypertension
  - fetal growth restriction
  - abruptio placentae
  - perinatal death
- Abnormal uterine Doppler studies at 18 to 24 weeks
  - resistance index > 0.58
  - presence of diastolic notch
- Angiotensin-II sensitivity at 28 weeks
- Positive "roll-over test" at 28 weeks
- Chronic hypertension or renal disease
- Insulin-dependent diabetes
- Multifetal gestation

Low-Salt Diet

In the past, widespread use of salt restriction during pregnancy was recommended for the prevention of various hypertensive disorders, including preeclampsia. In their 1990 review, Steegers et al.[6] found no convincing evidence that salt restriction during pregnancy reduces the incidence of preeclampsia. This group,[7] as well as Knuist et al.[8] performed randomized trials on this subject and again found no benefit.

Diuretics and Other Antihypertensive Drugs

According to most studies, women with preexisting chronic hypertension are at significantly higher risk for preeclampsia compared with normotensive women.[9] As shown in Table 16–3, there have been several randomized trials—only one was placebo-controlled—that evaluated the use of various antihypertensive drugs to re-

TABLE 16–2. METHODS USED IN TRIALS TO PREVENT PREECLAMPSIA

- Low-salt diet
- Diuretics
- Antihypertensive drugs
- Nutritional supplementation
  - magnesium
  - zinc
  - fish oil
  - antioxidants–vitamins C, E
  - calcium
- Antithrombotic agents
  - low-dose aspirin
  - aspirin/dipyridamole
  - aspirin plus heparin
  - aspirin plus ketanserin

TABLE 16–3. RANDOMIZED TRIALS OF THERAPY TO PREVENT PREECLAMPSIA IN WOMEN WITH MILD CHRONIC HYPERTENSION

Study	Gestation at Entry (wk) (weeks ± SEM)	Preeclampsia[a] (%)
Redman et al.[10]		
Control (N = 107)	20.6 ± 0.5	4.7
Treated (N = 101)	21.9 ± 0.5	6.7
Arias & Zamora[11]		
Control (N = 29)	16.4 ± 1.1	10.3
Treated (N = 29)	14.7 ± 1.0	3.4
Weitz et al.[12]		
Control (N = 12)	< 34	33.3
Treated (N = 13)	< 34	38.4
Sibai et al.[14]		
Control (N = 90)	11.3 ± 0.2	15.6
Treated (N = 173)	11.2 ± 0.2	17.3

[a] Preeclampsia = increased blood pressure plus proteinuria

duce the incidence of superimposed preeclampsia in women with chronic hypertension. A critical analysis of these trials failed to demonstrate such a reduction.[13,15] Because none had an adequate sample size to evaluate this, potential benefits of such therapy are unclear.

Because of the presumed efficacy of low-salt diets that were, in the past, given to treat edema and hypertension or (?) preeclampsia, it is not surprising that diuretic therapy became popular in the 1960s. However, a meta-analysis of nine randomized trials totaling more than 7000 women given diuretics during pregnancy showed only a decreased incidence of edema and hypertension, but not of preeclampsia.[16]

Magnesium Supplementation

Probably because of the efficacy of magnesium sulfate in prevention and treatment of eclampsia, the relationship between dietary magnesium deficiency and hypertension has been the subject of experimental and observational studies. In some of these, prenatal dietary magnesium deficiency has been implicated in the pathogenesis of preeclampsia and fetal growth retardation.[17-19] In the two randomized studies done to evaluate the use of elemental magnesium in pregnancy, no such benefits were found.

Spatling and Spatling[18] studied 568 women who were randomized to receive either magnesium aspartate hydrochloride or aspartic acid as a placebo. Supplementation was given daily starting at less than 16 weeks' gestation and continued throughout pregnancy. The incidence of preeclampsia was similar in both groups (0.7%). This single-blinded study had limited sample size for that purpose. Sibai et al.[19] conducted a double-blind randomized trial in 400 nulliparas who were randomized at 13 to 24 weeks to receive either 365 mg of elemental magnesium or a

TABLE 16–4. PREVENTION OF PREECLAMPSIA BY DIETARY MAGNESIUM SUPPLEMENTATION

| Study | Entry | Preeclampsia (No./%) | |
		Magnesium	Placebo
Spatling & Spatling[18]	≤ 16 wks	2/278 (0.7)	2/290 (0.7)
Sibai et al.[19]	13–24 wks	32/187 (17.3)[a]	35/190 (18.5)[a]

[a] Includes hypertension ± proteinuria

matching placebo. The authors found no differences between the two groups regarding the incidence of preeclampsia. Both trials are described further in Table 16–4.

Zinc Supplementation

Plasma and leukocyte zinc concentrations, as well as placental zinc levels, are reduced in women with pregnancy hypertension or preeclampsia–eclampsia compared with levels in normotensive pregnant women.[20,21] There have been two small randomized trials done to assess zinc supplementation to prevent preeclampsia. Hunt et al.[22] found a reduced incidence of pregnancy-induced hypertension and preeclampsia among low-income Mexican-American women living in Los Angeles who received zinc supplementation during pregnancy. In contrast, Mahomed et al.[23] found no reduction in preeclampsia among British women who received such supplementation (Table 16–5). These differences are possibly related to baseline zinc status between the two study populations and/or to differences in definitions of preeclampsia. Neither study had adequate sample size to evaluate a potential benefit, thus, more data are needed to establish any benefits from zinc supplementation.

Fish Oil

Interest in beneficial effects of fish oil on lowering the incidence of preeclampsia arose from observational studies and one uncontrolled trial.[24-26] Beneficial effects of N-3 fatty acids may be related to inhibition of platelet thromboxane A_2 production

TABLE 16–5. PREVENTION OF PREECLAMPSIA BY ZINC SUPPLEMENTATION

| Study | Entry | Preeclampsia (No./%) | |
		Zinc	Placebo
Hunt et al.[22]	19.6 wks ± 4.6[a]	2/87 (2.3)[b]	14/90 (15.6)[b]
Mahomed et al.[23]	< 20 wks	11/241 (4.6)	3/238 (1.3)

[a] Mean ± SD
[b] Includes women with hypertension ± proteinuria

with simultaneous production of only small amounts of a physiologically inactive thromboxane A_3. In endothelial cells, the production of prostacyclin (PGI_2) is not inhibited, thus shifting the balance toward reduced platelet aggregation and increased vasodilation.[27] Beneficial effects may also be related to altered angiotensin II (AII) sensitivity. Adair et al.[28] evaluated the effects of N-3 fatty acid supplementation on vascular reactivity measured by angiotensin II sensitivity in 10 normotensive pregnant women between 24 and 34 weeks. Infusions were performed before, and 28 days after, supplementation with capsules containing 3.6 g per day of eicosapentaenoic acid. The effective pressor dose of angiotensin II was significantly increased after N-3 fatty acid supplementation (35.8 ± 15.9 vs. 13.6 ± 6.3 ng/kg/min, $P = 0.001$).

One uncontrolled study[26] involving over 5000 pregnant women suggested that supplementation with several nutrients and vitamins including fish oil resulted in lowered incidence of preeclampsia in 1530 nulliparous women. Women given supplementation had different prenatal care than the other group and diagnoses of hypertension and preeclampsia were not well defined. More recently, three randomized trials were reported that described effects of fish oil supplementation in women at high risk for preeclampsia.[29-31] These studies, summarized in Table 16–6, show no reduction in the incidence of preeclampsia in the treated group. Moreover, the results of a large European multicenter trial comparing fish oil to olive oil in women with previous preeclampsia and twin gestation have just become available. The results indicate no difference in the incidence of preeclampsia (JJ Walker, Leeds, England, personal communication).

Calcium Supplementation

The relationship between dietary calcium intake and hypertension has been the subject of several experimental and observational studies as reviewed by Hatton

TABLE 16–6. FISH OIL FOR PREVENTION OF HYPERTENSION OR PREECLAMPSIA

Study	Hypertension Only (No./%)	Preeclampsia (No./%)
Bulstra-Ramakers et al.[29,a]		
Fish oil (N = 32)	7 (22.0)	5 (16.0)
Placebo (N = 31)	4 (13.0)	3 (10.0)
Onwude et al.[30,a]		
Fish oil (N = 113)	38 (34.0)	15 (13.0)
Placebo (N = 119)	35 (30.0)	18 (15.0)
Salvig et al.[31,b]		
Fish oil (N = 266)	8 (3.0)	0
No oil (N = 131)	2 (1.5)	1 (0.7)

[a] Women at risk for hypertension or fetal growth retardation
[b] Healthy women

and McCarron.[32] Reduced calcium excretion has been observed at the time of diagnosis of preeclampsia as well as several weeks prior to clinical hypertension.[33,34] Belizan et al.[35] reported an inverse association between calcium intake and maternal blood pressure as well as the incidences of preeclampsia–eclampsia. Possible mechanisms of action of calcium in preventing preeclampsia are unknown. Belizan et al.[35] suggested that calcium supplementation reduces maternal blood pressure by influencing parathyroid hormone release and intracellular calcium availability. Also, calcium supplementation during pregnancy was shown to reduce angiotensin II vascular sensitivity.[36]

Numerous clinical studies have compared the use of calcium supplementation with no treatment or a placebo in pregnancy. The studies differed regarding the population studied (low risk or high risk for developing hypertension or preeclampsia), study design (randomization, placebo use, or double-blind), gestational age at start of supplementation (13–32 weeks), sample size (22–2295 subjects), and the dose of elemental calcium used (156–2000 mg/d). In addition, these studies differed regarding the definition of hypertension and preeclampsia, and several did not differentiate between the two. A critical analysis of the design of these studies was reported by Levine et al.[37] and the results of these studies were included in two meta-analyses.[38,39]

Only eight of the calcium-supplementation randomized trials were placebo-controlled, but one did not report the incidence of preeclampsia.[40] The results of the remaining seven trials are described in Table 16–7. Four trials[41-43,46] conducted in women at very high risk for preeclampsia (16–44% in the placebo groups) demonstrated significant reductions in the incidence of preeclampsia in the calcium group. However, the results of two of these trials[41,42] are suspect considering the high incidence of preeclampsia (24%) in nulliparous women and the fact that all women who developed hypertension were considered to have preeclampsia. Of importance, the two trials with the largest sample size conducted in healthy nulliparous women demonstrated no significant reduction in the incidence of preeclampsia with calcium supplementation.[45,47] One Argentinian study demonstrated a beneficial effect on maternal hypertension overall and on preeclampsia in a subgroup of women with probable calcium deficiency early in pregnancy.[45] Another recent study by Herrera et al.[48] suggested that a combination of linoleic acid and calcium supplementation lowers preeclampsia incidence in high-risk women. In contrast, the large NICHD study showed no effects on maternal hypertension or preeclampsia in any of the subgroups analyzed based on calcium intake.[47]

Antithrombotic Agents

Preeclampsia is characterized by vasospasm, endothelial cell dysfunction, and activation of the coagulation–hemostasis systems. Enhanced platelet activation with

TABLE 16–7. RANDOMIZED DOUBLE-BLIND PLACEBO TRIALS OF CALCIUM SUPPLEMENTATION TO PREVENT PREECLAMPSIA

Study	Risk Factors	Enrollment (wks)	Intervention (No.)		Preeclampsia (%)	
			Calcium	*Placebo*	*Calcium*	*Placebo*
Lopez-Jaramillo et al.[41]	Nulliparous	24	55	51	3.6	24[b]
Lopez-Jaramillo et al.[42]	Positive ROT[a]	24–32	22	34	0	24[b]
Villar & Repke[44]	Nulliparous (85%)	24	90	88	0	3.4
Belizan et al.[45]	Nulliparous	20	579	588	2.6	3.9
Sanchez-Ramos et al.[43]	Positive ROT & Ang II[a]	24–28	29	34	14	44[b]
Levine et al.[47]	Nulliparas	13–21	2295	2294	6.9	7.3
Lopez-Jaramillo et al.[46]	Nulliparas	20	125	135	3.2	16

[a] ROT = roll-over test; Ang II = angiotensin sensitivity test
[b] P < 0.05

resultant increased platelet thromboxane production appears to play an important role in some of these pathophysiologic abnormalities (see Chap. 10). Results of biochemical studies suggest that these abnormalities are caused partly by an imbalance in the production of vasoconstricting prostaglandins (thromboxane A_2) and vasodilating prostaglandins (prostacyclin). This imbalance may lead to pathologic vascular lesions within multiple organ systems including the uteroplacental and fetoplacental vascular systems. Indeed, there is evidence to suggest that thromboxane A_2 production is markedly increased while prostacyclin is reduced in women with well-established preeclampsia and prior to the onset of clinical preeclampsia. In addition, placental infarcts and thrombosis of spiral arteries have been demonstrated in pregnancies complicated by preeclampsia, particularly in those with severe fetal growth restriction and/or fetal death.[49,50] Consequently, there have been numerous studies of antithrombotic agents given in an attempt to reduce the incidence of preeclampsia.

The majority of randomized trials for the prevention of preeclampsia have used low-dose aspirin. When given in doses of 50 to 150 mg/d, aspirin in pregnancy effectively inhibits platelet thromboxane A_2 biosynthesis with minimal effects on vascular prostacyclin production, thus altering the balance in favor of prostacyclin.[51] In addition, low-dose aspirin was shown to affect angiotensin II sensitivity during pregnancy. Findings from these studies suggested that enhanced vascular responsiveness to angiotensin II infusions may be corrected in some women by the use of low-dose aspirin.[52-54]

Several early prospective studies suggested that aspirin administration reduces the incidence of preeclampsia. The first prospective randomized trial was an open study that compared a combination of 150 mg/d of aspirin plus 300 mg/d of dipyridamole with no treatment in pregnant women at very high risk for preeclampsia among 48 treated women.[55] This study had several methodologic problems. The first randomized placebo-controlled double-blind study to assess prevention of preeclampsia in nulliparous women with low-dose aspirin was reported in 1986 by Wallenburg et al.[56] This study included 46 women who were found to have a positive angiotensin II sensitivity test at 28 weeks. There was a significant reduction in the incidence of preeclampsia in 21 women given low-dose aspirin.

These studies were followed by five trials that included a limited number of subjects who were identified to be at high risk for preeclampsia on the basis of a poor obstetric history,[57,58] chronic hypertension,[59] positive roll-over test,[60] or abnormal Doppler studies of the uterine vessels.[61] The findings of these studies were the subject of a review[48] and a meta-analysis[62] that concluded that low-dose aspirin was highly effective to prevent preeclampsia and fetal growth restriction in women judged at high risk for these complications.

The encouraging results of the above trials led to the design and completion of eight large trials in different populations worldwide. Six of these trials were multicenter[63-68] and seven were double-blind and placebo-controlled. The results of these trials are summarized in Table 16–8. Only one of these trials included women

TABLE 16–8. RANDOMIZED TRIALS OF LOW-DOSE ASPIRIN TO PREVENT PREECLAMPSIA

Study	Risk Factors	Enrollment (wks)	No. of Women Developing Preeclampsia		
			Aspirin (No./%)		Placebo (No./%)
Hauth et al.[69]	Nulliparas	24	302	1.7	302	5.6[a]
Sibai et al.[64]	Nulliparas	13–26	1485	4.6	1500	6.3
Italian study[63,b]	Obstetric[c]	16–32	565	2.9	477[a]	2.7
CLASP[65]	Obstetric	12–32	4659	6.7	4650	7.6
ECPPA[66]	Obstetric	12–32	476	6.7	494	6.1
Golding[70]	Nulliparas	12–32	3022	7.1	3024	6.3
Caritis et al.[67]	High risk	13–26	1254	18.4	1249	20.3
Rotchell et al.[68]	None	12–32	1819	2.2	1822	2.5

[a] P = 0.009
[b] No treatment
[c] History of poor obstetric outcomes

at high risk for preeclampsia (20% in the placebo group),[67] whereas the others included women at mild-to-moderate risk (2.7–7.6% in the placebo group). In addition, only one of these trials demonstrated a significant reduction in preeclampsia in the aspirin group.[69] Overall, the results of these trials that included over 27,000 women demonstrated minimal to no reduction in the incidence of preeclampsia with low-dose aspirin.

Despite these overall findings, the debate continues regarding the efficacy of low-dose aspirin given prophylactically. Grant[71] suggested that the failure of large trials to demonstrate major benefits may be related to dilution of the trial population with women at low risk for preeclampsia, and that future trials should focus only on women who are at very high risk. There is, however, inconsistency regarding results of trials conducted in women at very high risk. For example, of three randomized trials evaluating low-dose aspirin in women with abnormal Doppler studies in uterine vessels, the sample size is limited, and the results are inconsistent (Table 16–9). Nevertheless, the data suggest that low-dose aspirin may be beneficial in some of these women.

Women who are sensitive to infused angiotensin II are considered at very high risk for preeclampsia. Three randomized studies were conducted to evaluate low-dose aspirin in such women (Table 16–10). Results of these studies are inconsistent and cast doubts about the benefits of low-dose aspirin in the these women.

The highest incidence of preeclampsia is usually reported in women with previous preeclampsia, those with multifetal gestation, women with chronic hypertension, and those with insulin-dependent diabetes. Subsequent incidence is particularly increased in those who had hypertension and proteinuria prior to 20 weeks. The recent NICHD randomized trial reported by Caritis et al.[67] evaluated the effects of low-dose aspirin in these subgroups of women (Table 16–11). They found that low-dose aspirin does not reduce the incidence of preeclampsia in these high-risk women.

TABLE 16–9. LOW-DOSE ASPIRIN IN WOMEN WITH ABNORMAL UTERINE ARTERY DOPPLER FLOW STUDIES

	Gestational Hypertension (No./%)	Preeclampsia (No./%)
McParland et al.[61]		
Aspirin (N = 48)	5 (10.2)	1 (2.1)[a]
Placebo (N = 52)	3 (5.8)	10 (19.2)[a]
Morris et al.[72]		
Aspirin (N = 52)	8 (17.2)	4 (7.7)
Placebo (N = 50)	7 (14.0)	7 (14.0)
Bower et al.[73]		
Aspirin (N = 31)	—	9 (29.0)[b]
Placebo (N = 29)	—	12 (41.4)[b]

[a] $P \le 0.023$
[b] $P = 0.03$ for severe preeclampsia

TABLE 16–10. LOW-DOSE ASPIRIN IN WOMEN WHO ARE ANGIOTENSIN-II SENSITIVE

	Gestational Hypertension (No./%)	Preeclampsia (No./%)
Wallenburg et al.[56]		
Aspirin (N = 21)	2 (9.5)	0
Placebo (N = 23)	4 (17.0)	8 (35.0)[a]
Kyle et al.[74]		
Aspirin (N = 44)	6 (13.6)	7 (11.5)
Placebo (N = 36)	4 (11.1)	0
Brown et al.[75]		
Aspirin (N = 31)	11 (50.0)	4 (18.2)

[a] P < 0.01

Other criticisms of large randomized trials included poor compliance, gestational age at randomization (before and after 20 weeks), and the aspirin dose used. The issue of compliance is irrelevant since randomized trials are designed to discover whether an intervention works under real clinical conditions rather than investigational conditions. In addition, the lack of benefit from aspirin cannot be attributed to either the aspirin dose or time of enrollment because most randomized trials with positive results used a 60-mg dose in women randomized up to 28 weeks. Moreover, most trials showed no difference in the incidence of preeclampsia between those enrolled before or after 20 weeks.

Low-dose aspirin has also been studied in combination with heparin as well as ketanserin, a selective serotonin-2 receptor antagonist. Stein and Odendaal[76] reported a randomized trial of ketanserin and aspirin to prevent preeclampsia in 138 pregnant women who had diastolic blood pressure persistently above 80 mm Hg before 20 weeks. Each group included 69 women; one group received aspirin

TABLE 16–11. NICHD TRIAL OF LOW-DOSE ASPIRIN IN WOMEN AT HIGH RISK FOR PREECLAMPSIA

Entry Criteria	No.	Preeclampsia (%)[a]	
		Aspirin	Placebo
Normotensive, no proteinuria	1613	14.5	17.7
Proteinuria and hypertension	119	31.7	22.0
Proteinuria only	48	25.0	33.3
Hypertension only	723	24.8	25.0
Insulin-dependent diabetes	462	18.3	21.6
Chronic hypertension	763	26.0	24.6
Multifetal gestation	678	11.5	15.9
Previous preeclampsia	600	16.7	19.0

[a] No difference for any of the aspirin vs. placebo groups
Data from Caritis SN, Sibai BM, Hauth J, et al: Low-dose aspirin to prevent preeclampsia in women at high risk. N Engl J Med 1998;338:701–705.

plus ketanserin and the other was given aspirin plus placebo. The incidence of preeclampsia was significantly lower in the ketanserin group (3 vs. 19%, P = 0.006). The authors concluded that further studies were indicated to confirm their preliminary data.

Currently, there are trials exploring the benefits of dietary supplementation with L-arginine, antioxidants, and other unknown agents in preventing preeclampsia. Rather than conducting such trials aimed at prevention, it would seem reasonable that efforts should be directed at finding the etiology of preeclampsia as well as finding methods to predict women at high risk for its development.

PREVENTION OF ECLAMPSIA

Eclampsia is defined as the development of convulsions or coma during pregnancy or postpartum in women with signs and symptoms of preeclampsia. The precise pathogenesis of eclamptic convulsions remains an enigma. At present, the two most common etiologic factors considered are cerebral vasospasm[77] and hypertensive encephalopathy.[78]

Prevention of eclampsia can be primary by preventing the development of preeclampsia or secondary by using agents that prevent convulsions in women with established preeclampsia. Prevention can also be tertiary by preventing subsequent convulsions in women with eclampsia.

The incidence of eclampsia in hypertensive women not receiving anticonvulsive prophylaxis is unknown. A few observational studies describing the frequency of eclampsia in such patients are shown in Table 16–12. The incidence of eclampsia ranges from 0.13% for women with gestational hypertension only to 2.8% for women with severe preeclampsia. The heterogeneity of women studied in these reports warrants cautious interpretation of data. Nonetheless, the data from these studies were used by several authorities outside the United States as an argument against the use of any prophylactic anticonvulsants in women with gestational hypertension or preeclampsia.[79,81,82]

In the United States, parenteral magnesium sulfate is the drug of choice for the prevention and treatment of eclamptic convulsions. Witlin and Sibai[84] recently reviewed this subject. Alternative drugs that have been recommended for this purpose include antihypertensive drugs for aggressive control of maternal blood pressure and "traditional" anticonvulsants such as phenytoin, diazepam, and lytic cocktail. It is important to emphasize that seizure prophylaxis is recommended only during labor and for 24 hours postpartum. Therefore, it will prevent only about half of all eclampsia cases because half develop antepartum.[85]

Five randomized trials have been conducted that compare magnesium sulfate with either phenytoin or placebo for women with hypertensive disorders of pregnancy (Table 16–13). Only the trial of Lucas et al.[89] had an adequate sample size to

TABLE 16–12. OBSERVATIONAL STUDIES OF THE INCIDENCE OF ECLAMPSIA IN HYPERTENSIVE WOMEN NOT GIVEN SEIZURE PROPHYLAXIS

Study	Classification of Disease	Patients	Eclampsia	
			No.	(%)
Nelson (1951–1953)[80]	Gestational hypertension	527	2	0.38
	Preeclampsia[a]	216	6	2.8
Walker (1981–1989)[81]	Hypertensive disorders	3885	7	0.18
Odendaal & Hall (1983–1993)[83]	Severe preeclampsia	491	3	0.6
Burrows & Burrows (1986–1993)[82]	Gestational hypertension	745	1	0.13
	Preeclampsia[a]	457	9[b]	1.9
Chua & Redman (1987–1990)[79]	Preeclampsia[a]	78	1	1.3

[a] Includes mild and severe preeclampsia
[b] Includes only intrapartum and postpartum convulsions

TABLE 16–13. RANDOMIZED TRIALS OF MAGNESIUM SULFATE VS. PHENYTOIN OR PLACEBO TO PREVENT ECLAMPSIA IN WOMEN WITH HYPERTENSIVE DISORDERS OF PREGNANCY

		Eclamptic Convulsions	
Study	Control Drug	MgSO$_4$	Control
Appleton et al.[86]	Phenytoin	0/24	0/23
Friedman et al.[87]	Phenytoin	0/60	0/43
Atkinson et al.[88]	Phenytoin	0/28	0/26
Lucas et al.[89]	Phenytoin	0/1049	10/1089[a]
Witlin et al.[90]	Placebo	0/67	0/68
Total		0/1228[a]	10/1249 (0.8%)[a]

[a] $P < 0.001$

evaluate the effects of seizure prophylaxis in these women, the remainder evaluated mostly side effects of magnesium therapy. In this trial, over 2000 women with various hypertensive disorders of pregnancy were randomized to either an intramuscular magnesium regimen or to an intravenous/oral phenytoin regimen administered peripartum. The authors observed no seizures among 1049 women given magnesium sulfate and 10 cases of eclampsia (1%) among 1089 women given phenytoin. This trial indicates that magnesium sulfate is superior to phenytoin for seizure prophylaxis in such women. It is important to note that there are no placebo-controlled trials with adequate sample sizes to address the efficacy of magnesium sulfate for this purpose.

Four randomized trials compared the use of antihypertensive drugs alone vs. antihypertensive drugs plus magnesium sulfate to prevent seizures with severe preeclampsia (Table 16–14). Only two of these had an adequate sample size. The trial by Belfort et al.[93] compared the use of magnesium sulfate with nimodipine, a calcium-channel blocker with cerebral vasodilatory effects. The authors found a lower but nonsignificant incidence of eclampsia in the magnesium sulfate group (1.5% vs. 3.6%). Coetzee et al.[94] reported a double-blind study which compared intravenous magnesium sulfate to saline placebo in 685 women with severe preeclampsia. They found a significant tenfold reduction in development of eclampsia in the magnesium-treated group (Table 16–14). From these data, it is apparent that magnesium sulfate prophylaxis should be used in all women with severe preeclampsia during labor and postpartum.

Anticonvulsant Agents in Eclampsia

It is of general agreement that anticonvulsant agents are necessary for the prevention of recurrent seizures in patients with eclampsia. In the United States, magnesium sulfate has been used for this purpose for over 60 years. Until recently, its use

TABLE 16–14. RANDOMIZED TRIALS OF ANTIHYPERTENSIVE THERAPY WITH AND WITHOUT MAGNESIUM SULFATE TO PREVENT CONVULSIONS IN WOMEN WITH SEVERE PREECLAMPSIA

Study	Antihypertensive Drugs	Eclamptic Convulsions		Relative Risk (95% Confidence Intervals)
		MgSO$_4$ (%)	Control (%)	
Moodley & Moodley[91]	Dihydralazine, nifedipine	1/112 (0.9)	0/116 (0)	N/A
Chen et al.[92]	Hydralazine, methyldopa, nifedipine	0/34	0/34	N/A
Belfort et al.[93]	Nimodipine, hydralazine	5/324 (1.5)	11/303 (3.6)	0.43 (0.15–1.21)
Coetzee et al.[94]	Hydralazine, labetalol	1/345 (0.3)	11/340 (3.2)[a]	0.09 (0.01–0.69)
Total		7/815 (0.86)	22/793 (2.8)	0.31 (0.13–0.72)

[a] Placebo-controlled

for this purpose was criticized as empirical and dogmatic because it had never been tested in a randomized trial.[95]

Magnesium sulfate does not always prevent recurrent seizures in eclamptic women. Six observational studies describe the rate of subsequent seizures in eclamptic women given magnesium sulfate for anticonvulsant therapy (Table 16–15). The overall rate of recurrent seizures among these studies is 10%. This failure rate was also used as a reason to conduct randomized trials comparing magnesium sulfate with other traditional anticonvulsants.

During recent years, several randomized trials were reported that compared the efficacy of magnesium sulfate with other anticonvulsants in eclamptic women (Table 16–16). Only one multicenter trial had an adequate sample size to compute a significant difference. The Collaborative Eclampsia Trial[105] was conducted in several centers in South Africa and South America. The trial included 1680 eclamptic women who were randomized to either magnesium sulfate, phenytoin, or diazepam in two different randomization schemes. The trial demonstrated that magnesium sulfate was superior to both phenytoin and diazepam for the prevention of recurrent seizures in eclamptic women (Table 16–16). In addition, the data by Bhalla et al.[103] indicate that magnesium sulfate is superior to lytic cocktail in preventing recurrent eclamptic seizures.

These randomized trials also had adequate information to compare maternal death rates between women given magnesium sulfate with those given other agents (Table 16–17). The overall results of these studies demonstrate that magnesium sulfate therapy was associated with significantly lower maternal mortality in eclampsia than that observed with other anticonvulsants (3.0% vs. 4.8%, $P < 0.05$).

In summary, a review of randomized trials indicates that magnesium sulfate is the ideal agent to use as a prophylaxis in women with severe preeclampsia and for treatment of eclamptic convulsions. There is limited information regarding the need of magnesium sulfate for prophylaxis in women with mild hypertension or preeclampsia, but there is a need for double-blind placebo controlled studies to address this.

TABLE 16–15. OBSERVATIONAL STUDIES OF SUBSEQUENT CONVULSIONS IN ECLAMPTIC WOMEN GIVEN MAGNESIUM SULFATE

Study	Eclampsia	Recurrent Convulsion(s)	
		No.	*(%)*
Pritchard et al.[96]	85	3	3.5
Gedekoh et al.[97]	52	1	1.9
Pritchard et al.[98]	83	10	12.0
Dunn et al.[99]	13	5	38.5
Sibai & Ramanathan[100]	315	41	13.0
Dommisse[101]	100	3	3.0
Total	648	63	9.7

TABLE 16–16. RANDOMIZED TRIALS COMPARING MAGNESIUM SULFATE WITH OTHER ANTICONVULSANTS IN WOMEN WITH ECLAMPSIA

Study	Antihypertensive Drugs	Recurrent Seizures		Relative Risk (95% Confidence Interval)
		$MgSO_4$ (%)	Other (%)	
Dommisse[101]	Dihydralazine	0/11 (0)	4/11 (37)[a]	
Crowther[102]	Dihydralazine	5/24 (21)	7/27 (26)[b]	0.80 (0.29–2.2)
Bhalla et al.[103]	Nifedipine	1/45 (2.2)	11/45 (24)[c]	0.09 (0.1–0.68)
Friedman et al.[104]	Nifedipine, labetalol	0/11 (0)	2/13 (15)[a]	
Collaborative Eclampsia Trial[105]	Not reported	60/453 (13.2)	126/452 (28)[b]	0.48 (0.36–0.63)
		22/388 (5.7)	66/387 (17)[c]	0.33 (0.21–0.53)
Total		88/922 (9.4)	216/935 (23)	0.41 (0.32–0.51)

[a] Phenytoin
[b] Diazepam
[c] Lytic cocktail

TABLE 16–17. MATERNAL DEATHS IN TRIALS COMPARING MAGNESIUM SULFATE WITH OTHER ANTICONVULSANTS IN WOMEN WITH ECLAMPSIA

Study	Comparison Group	Maternal Deaths		Relative Risk (95% Confidence Interval)
		$MgSO_4$ (%)	Other (%)	
Dommisse[101]	Phenytoin	0/11	0/11	
Crowther[102]	Diazepam	1/24 (4.2)	0/27	
Bhalla et al.[103]	Lytic cocktail	0/45	2/45 (4.4)	
Friedman et al.[104]	Phenytoin	0/11	0/13	
Collaborative Eclampsia Trial[105]	Phenytoin	10/388 (2.5)	20/387 (5.2)	0.50 (0.24–1.00)
	Diazepam	17/453 (3.8)	23/452 (5.1)	0.74 (0.40–1.36)
Total		28/932 (3.0)	45/935 (4.8)	0.62 (0.39–0.99)

REFERENCES

1. Sibai BM: Hypertension in pregnancy. *Obstet Gynecol Clin North Am* 1992;19(4):615–632.
2. American College of Obstetricians and Gynecologists: Hypertension in pregnancy. Technical Bulletin 219; January 1996.
3. National High Blood Pressure Education Program Working Group: Report on High Blood Pressure in Pregnancy. *Am J Obstet Gynecol* 1990;163:1689–1712.
4. Sibai BM: Prevention of preeclampsia: A major disappointment. *Am J Obstet Gynecol* 1998 (in press).
5. Dekker GA, Sibai BM: Early detection of preeclampsia. *Am J Obstet Gynecol* 1991;165:160–172.
6. Steegers EAP, Eskes TKAB, Jongsma HW, Hein PR: Dietary sodium restriction during pregnancy: A historical review. *Eur J Obstet Gynecol Reprod Biol* 1991;40:83–90.
7. Steegers EAP, VanLakwijk HPJM, Jongsma HW, et al: Pathophysiological implications of chronic dietary sodium restriction during pregnancy: A longitudinal prospective randomized study. *Br J Obstet Gynaecol* 1991;98:980–987.
8. Knuist M, Bonsel GJ, Zondervan HA, Treffers PE: Low sodium diet and pregnancy-induced hypertension: A multi-centre randomized trial. *Br J Obstet Gynaecol* 1998;105:430–434.
9. Sibai BM, Lindheimer M, Hauth J, et al, and the National Institute of Child Health and Human Development Network of Maternal–Fetal Medicine Units: Risk factors for preeclampsia, abruptio, and adverse neonatal outcome in women with chronic hypertension. *N Engl J Med* 1998;339:667–671.
10. Redman CWG, Beilin LJ, Bonner J, et al: Fetal outcome in trial of antihypertensive treatment in pregnancy. *Lancet* 1976;2:753–756.
11. Arias F, Zamora J: Antihypertensive treatment and pregnancy outcome in patients with mild chronic hypertension. *Obstet Gynecol* 1979;53:489–494.
12. Weitz C, Khouzami V, Maxwell K, Johnson JWC: Treatment of hypertension in pregnancy with methyldopa, randomized double-blind study. *Int J Gynaecol Obstet* 1987;25:35–40.
13. Sanchez-Ramos L, Mora CS: Effect of antihypertensive therapy on the development of superimposed preeclampsia in patients with chronic hypertension: A meta-analysis. *Am J Obstet Gynecol* 1999 (in press).
14. Sibai BM, Mabie WC, Shamsa F, et al: A comparison of no medication versus methyldopa or labetalol in chronic hypertension during pregnancy. *Am J Obstet Gynecol* 1990;162:960–967.
15. Sibai BM: Treatment of hypertension in pregnant women. *N Engl J Med* 1996;335:257–265.
16. Collins R, Yusuf S, Peto R. Overview of randomized trials of diuretics in pregnancy. *Br Med J* 1985;29:17–23.
17. Altura BM, Altura BT, Carella A: Magnesium deficiency induced spasm of umbilical vessels: Relation to preeclampsia, hypertension, growth retardation. *Science* 1983;221:376–378.
18. Spatling L, Spatling G: Magnesium supplementation in pregnancy: A double-blind study. *Br J Obstet Gynaecol* 1988;950:120–125.
19. Sibai BM, Villar MA, Bray E: Magnesium supplementation during pregnancy: A double-blind randomized controlled clinical trial. *Am J Obstet Gynecol* 1989;161:115–119.
20. Lazebrik N, Kuhnert BR, Kuhnert PM: Zinc, cadmium and hypertension in parturient women. *Am J Obstet Gynecol* 1989;161:437–440.
21. Adeniyi AAF: The implications of hypozincemia in pregnancy. *Acta Obstet Gynaecol Scand* 1987;66:579–585.
22. Hunt IF, Murphy NJ, Cleaver AE, et al: Zinc supplementation during pregnancy: Effects on selected blood constituents and on progress and outcome of pregnancy in low-income women of Mexican descent. *Am J Clin Nutr* 1984;40:508–521.
23. Mahomed K, James DK, Golding J, McCabe R: Zinc supplementation during pregnancy: A double-blind randomised controlled trial. *Br Med J* 1989;299:826–829.
24. Andersen HJ, Andersen LF: Diet, pre-eclampsia, and intrauterine growth retardation. *Lancet* 1989;i:1146.
25. Olsen SF, Secher NJ: A possible preventive effect of low-dose fish oil on early delivery and preeclampsia: Indications from a 50-year-old controlled trial. *Br J Nutr* 1990;64:599–609.

26. Secher NJ, Olsen SF: Fish oil and pre-eclampsia. *Br J Obstet Gynaecol* 1990;97:1077–1079.

27. Sorensen JD, Olsen SF, Pedersen AK, Boris J, et al: Effects of fish oil supplementation in the third trimester of pregnancy on prostacyclin and thromboxane production. *Am J Obstet Gynecol* 1993;168:915–922.

28. Adair CD, Sanchez-Ramos L, Briones DL, Ogburn P: The effect of high dietary N-3 fatty acid supplementation on angiontensin II pressor response in human pregnancy. *Am J Obstet Gynecol* 1996;75:688–691.

29. Bulstra-Ramakers MTEW, Huisjes HJ, Visser GHA: The effects of 3 g eicosapentaenoic acid daily on recurrence of intrauterine growth retardation and pregnancy induced hypertension. *Br J Obstet Gynaecol* 1994;102:123–126.

30. Onwude JL, Lilford RJ, Hjartardottier H, et al: A randomised double blind placebo controlled trial of fish oil in high risk pregnancy. *Br J Obstet Gynaecol* 1995;109:95–100.

31. Salvig JD, Olsen SF, Secher NJ: Effects of fish oil supplementation in late pregnancy on blood pressure: A randomised controlled trial. *Br J Obstet Gynaecol* 1996;103:529–533.

32. Hatton DC, McCarron DA: Dietary calcium and blood pressure in experimental models of hypertension: A review. *Hypertension* 1994;23:513–530.

33. Taufield PA, Ales KL, Resnick LM, et al: Hypocalciuria in preeclampsia. *N Engl J Med* 1987;316:715–718.

34. Sanchez-Ramos L, Jones DC, Cullen MT: Urinary calcium as an early marker for preeclampsia. *Obstet Gynecol* 1991;77:685–689.

35. Belizan JM, Villar J, Repke J: The relationship between calcium intake and pregnancy induced hypertension: Up-to-date evidence. *Am J Obstet Gynecol* 1988;158:898–902.

36. Kawasaki N, Matsui K, Ito M, et al: Effect of calcium supplementation on the vascular sensitivity to angiotensin II in pregnant women. *Am J Obstet Gynecol* 1985;153:576–582.

37. Levine RJ, Esterlitz JR, Raymond EG, et al: Trial of calcium for preeclampsia prevention (CPEP): Rationale, design, and methods. *Control Clin Trials* 1996;17:442–469.

38. Carrolli G, Duley L, Belizan JM, Villar J: Calcium supplementation during pregnancy: A systemic review of randomised controlled trials. *Br J Obstet Gynaecol* 1994;101:753–758.

39. Bucher HC, Guyatt GH, Cook RJ, et al: Effect of calcium supplementation on pregnancy-induced hypertension and preeclampsia: A metaanalysis of randomized controlled trials. *JAMA* 1996;275:1113–1117.

40. Villar J, Repke J, Belizan JM, Pareja G: Calcium supplementation reduces blood pressure during pregnancy: Results from a randomized clinical trial. *Obstet Gynecol* 1987;70:317–322.

41. Lopez-Jaramillo P, Narvaez M, Weigel RM, Yepez R: Calcium supplementation reduces the risk of pregnancy-induced hypertension in an Andes population. *Br J Obstet Gynaecol* 1989;96:648–655.

42. Lopez-Jaramillo P, Narvaez M, Felix C, Lopez A: Dietary calcium supplementation and prevention of pregnancy hypertension (letter). *Lancet* 1990;335:293.

43. Sanchez-Ramos L, Briones DK, Kaunitz AM, et al: Prevention of pregnancy-induced hypertension by calcium supplementation in angiotensin II-sensitive patients. *Obstet Gynecol* 1994;84:349–353.

44. Villar J, Repke J: Calcium supplementation during pregnancy may reduce preterm delivery in high-risk populations. *Am J Obstet Gynecol* 1990;163:1124–1131.

45. Belizan JM, Villar J, Gonzalez L, et al: Calcium supplementation to prevent hypertensive disorders of pregnancy. *N Engl J Med* 1991;325:1399–1405.

46. Lopez-Jaramillo P, Delgado F, Jacome P, et al: Calcium supplementation and the risk of preeclampsia in Ecuadorian pregnant teenagers. *Obstet Gynecol* 1997;90(2):162–167.

47. Levine RJ, Hauth JC, Curet LB, et al, and the Maternal–Fetal Medicine Units Network. Trial of calcium to prevent preeclampsia. *N Engl J Med* 1997;337:69–76.

48. Herrera JA, Arevalo-Herrera M, Herrera S: Prevention of preeclampsia by linoleic acid and calcium supplementation: A randomized controlled trial. *Obstet Gynecol* 1998;91:585–590.

49. Frusca T, Morassi L, Pecorelli S, et al: Histological features of uteroplacental vessels in normal and hypertensive patients in relation to birthweight. *Br J Obstet Gynaecol* 1989;96:835–839.

50. Pijnenborg R, Anthony J, Davey DA, et al: Placental bed spiral arteries in the hypertensive disorders of pregnancy. *Br J Obstet Gynaecol* 1991;98:648–655.

51. Thorp JA, Walsh SW, Brath PC: Low-dose aspirin inhibits thromboxane, but not prostacyclin production by human placental arteries. *Am J Obstet Gynecol* 1988;159:1381–1384.
52. Sanchez-Ramos L, O'Sullivan MJ, Garrido-Calderon J: Effect of low-dose aspirin on angiotensin pressor response in human pregnancy. *Am J Obstet Gynecol* 1987;156:193–194.
53. Spitz B, Magness RR, Cox SM, et al: Low-dose aspirin. Effect on angiotensin II pressor responses and blood prostaglandin concentrations in pregnant women sensitive to angiotensin II. *Am J Obstet Gynecol* 1988;159:1035–1043.
54. Wallenburg HCS, Dekker GA, Makovitz JW, Rotmans N: Effect of low-dose aspirin on vascular refractoriness in angiotensin-sensitive primigravid women. *Am J Obstet Gynecol* 1991;164:1169–1173.
55. Beaufils M, Donsimoni R, Uzan S, Colau JC: Prevention of pre-eclampsia by early antiplatelet therapy. *Lancet* 1985;1:840–842.
56. Wallenburg HCS, Dekker A, Makovitz JW, Rotmans P: Low dose aspirin prevents pregnancy-induced hypertension and preeclampsia in angiotensin-sensitive primigravidae. *Lancet* 1986;1:1–3.
57. Azar R, Turpin D: Effect of antiplatelet therapy in women at high-risk for pregnancy-induced hypertension. Proceedings of the VII World Congress of Hypertension in Pregnancy. Perugia, Italy; October 1990:257(abstr 74).
58. Uzan S, Beaufils M, Breart G, et al: Prevention of fetal growth retardation with low-dose aspirin: Findings of the EPREDA trial. *Lancet* 1991;337(8775):1427–1431.
59. Viinikka L, Hartikainen-Sorri AL, Lumme R, et al: Low dose aspirin in hypertensive pregnant women: Effect on pregnancy outcome and prostacyclin-thromboxane balance in mother and newborn. *Br J Obstet Gynaecol* 1993;100:809–812.
60. Schiff E, Peleg E, Goldenberg M, et al: The use of aspirin to prevent pregnancy-induced hypertension and lower the ratio of thromboxane A_2 to prostacyclin in relatively high risk pregnancies. *N Engl J Med* 1989;321:351–356.
61. McParland P, Pearce JM, Chamberlain GVP: Doppler ultrasound and aspirin in recognition and prevention of pregnancy-induced hypertension. *Lancet* 1990;335:1552–1555.
62. Imperiale TF, Petrulis AS: A meta-analysis of low-dose aspirin for the prevention of pregnancy-induced hypertensive disease. *JAMA* 1991;266:260–264.
63. Italian Study of Aspirin in Pregnancy Group: Low-dose aspirin in prevention and treatment of intrauterine growth retardation and pregnancy-induced hypertension. *Lancet* 1993;341:396–400.
64. Sibai BM, Caritis SN, Thom E, et al: Prevention of preeclampsia with low-dose aspirin in healthy, nulliparous, pregnant women. The National Institute of Child Health and Human Development Network of MFM Units. *N Engl J Med* 1993;329:1213–1218.
65. CLASP: A randomized trial of low-dose aspirin for the prevention and treatment of preeclampsia among 9,364 pregnant women. *Lancet* 1994;343:619–629.
66. ECPPA: Randomised trial of low-dose aspirin for the prevention of maternal and fetal complications in high risk pregnant women. *Br J Obstet Gynaecol* 1996;103:39–47.
67. Caritis SN, Sibai BM, Hauth J, et al: Low-dose aspirin to prevent preeclampsia in women at high risk. *N Engl J Med* 1998;338:701–705.
68. Rotchell YE, Cruickshank JK, Phillips GM, et al: Barbados low-dose aspirin study in pregnancy (BLASP): A randomized trial for the prevention of pre-eclampsia and its complications. *Br J Obstet Gynaecol* 1998;105:286–292.
69. Hauth JC, Goldenberg RL, Parker CR Jr, et al: Low-dose aspirin therapy to prevent preeclampsia. *Am J Obstet Gynecol* 1993;168:1083–1093.
70. Golding J: A randomized trial of low-dose aspirin for primiparae in pregnancy. *Br J Obstet Gynaecol* 1998;105:293–299.
71. Grant JM: Multicentre trials in obstetrics and gynecology. Smaller explanatory trials are required. *Br J Obstet Gynaecol* 1996;103:599–602.
72. Morris JM, Fay RF, Ellwood DA, et al: A randomized controlled trial of aspirin in patients with abnormal uterine artery blood flow. *Obstet Gynecol* 1996;87:74–78.
73. Bower SJ, Harrington KF, Schuchter K, et al: Prediction of pre-eclampsia by abnormal uterine Doppler ultrasound and modification by aspirin. *Br J Obstet Gynaecol* 1996;103:625–629.

74. Kyle PM, Buckley D, Kissane J, et al: The angiotensin sensitivity test and low-dose aspirin are ineffective methods to predict and prevent hypertensive disorders in nulliparous pregnancy. *Am J Obstet Gynecol* 1995;173:865–872.

75. Brown CEL, Gant NF, Cox K, et al: Low-dose aspirin. II. Relationship of angiotensin II pressor responses, circulating eicosanoids, and pregnancy outcome. *Am J Obstet Gynecol* 1990;163:1853–1861.

76. Steyn W, Odendaal HJ: Randomised controlled trial of ketanserin and aspirin in prevention of pre-eclampsia. *Lancet* 1997;350:1267–1271.

77. Naidu K, Moodley J, Corr P, Hoffmann M: Single photon emission and cerebral computerised tomographic scan and transcranial Doppler sonographic findings in eclampsia. *Br J Obstet Gynaecol* 1997;104:1165–1172.

78. Morriss MC, Twickler DM, Hatab MR, et al: Cerebral blood flow and cranial magnetic resonance imaging in eclampsia and severe preeclampsia. *Obstet Gynecol* 1997;89:561–568.

79. Chua S, Redman CWG: Are prophylactic anticonvulsants required in severe preeclampsia? *Lancet* 1991;337:250–251.

80. Nelson TR: A clinical study of preeclampsia. Part II. *J Obstet Gynaecol Br Empire* 1955;62:58–66.

81. Walker JJ: Hypertensive drugs in pregnancy. *Hypertens Pregnancy* 1991;18:845–872.

82. Burrows RF, Burrows EA: The feasibility of a control population for a randomized controlled trial of seizure prophylaxis in the hypertensive disorders of pregnancy. *Am J Obstet Gynecol* 1995;173:929–935.

83. Odendaal HJ, Hall DR: Is magnesium sulfate prophylaxis really necessary in patients with severe preeclampsia? *J Maternal Fetal Invest* 1996;6:14–18.

84. Witlin AG, Sibai BM: Magnesium sulfate in preeclampsia and eclampsia. *Obstet Gynecol* 1998;92:883–889.

85. Sibai BM: Eclampsia VI. Maternal–perinatal outcome in 254 consecutive cases. *Am J Obstet Gynecol* 1990;163:1049–1055.

86. Appleton MP, Kuehl TJ, Raebel MA, et al: Magnesium sulfate versus phenytoin for seizure prophylaxis in pregnancy-induced hypertension. *Am J Obstet Gynecol* 1991;165:907–913.

87. Friedman SA, Lim KH, Baker CA, Repke JT: Phenytoin versus magnesium sulfate in preeclampsia: A pilot study. *Am J Perinatol* 1993;10:233–238.

88. Atkinson MW, Guinn D, Owen J, Hauth JC: Does magnesium sulfate affect the length of labor induction in women with pregnancy-associated hypertension? *Am J Obstet Gynecol* 1995;173:1219–1222.

89. Lucas MJ, Leveno KJ, Cunningham FG: A comparison of magnesium sulfate with phenytoin for the prevention of eclampsia. *N Engl J Med* 1995;333:201–205.

90. Witlin AG, Friedman SA, Sibai BM: The effect of magnesium sulfate therapy on the duration of labor in women with mild preeclampsia at term: A randomized, double-blind, placebo-controlled trial. *Am J Obstet Gynecol* 1997;176:623–627.

91. Moodley J, Moodley VV: Prophylactic anticonvulsant therapy in hypertensive crises of pregnancy—the need for a large randomized trial. *Hypertens Pregnancy* 1994;13(3):245–252.

92. Chen F, Chang S, Chu K: Expectant management in severe preeclampsia: Does magnesium sulfate prevent the development of eclampsia? *Acta Obstet Gynecol Scand* 1995;74:181–185.

93. Belfort M, Anthony J, Saade G, and the Nimodipine Study Group: Interim report of the nimodipine vs. magnesium sulfate for seizure prophylaxis in severe preeclampsia study: An international, randomized, controlled trial. *Am J Obstet Gynecol* 1998 (in press).

94. Coetzee EJ, Dommisse J, Anthony J: A randomized controlled trial of intravenous magnesium sulfate versus placebo in the management of women with severe pre-eclampsia. *Br J Obstet Gynecol* 1998;105:300–303.

95. Donaldson JO: Does magnesium sulfate treat eclamptic convulsions? *Clin Neuropharmacol* 1986;9:37–45.

96. Pritchard JA, Pritchard SA: Standardized treatment of 154 consecutive cases of eclampsia. *Am J Obstet Gynecol* 1975;123:543–552.

97. Gedekoh RH, Hayashi TT, MacDonald HM: Eclampsia at Magee-Women's Hospital 1970 to 1980. *Am J Obstet Gynecol* 1981;140:860–866.

98. Pritchard JA, Cunningham FG, Pritchard SA: The Parkland Memorial Hospital protocol for treatment of eclampsia: Evaluation of 245 cases. *Am J Obstet Gynecol* 1984;148:951–963.

99. Dunn R, Lee W, Cotton DB: Evaluation of computerized axial tomography of eclamptic women with seizures refractory to magnesium sulfate therapy. *Am J Obstet Gynecol* 1986; 155:267–268.

100. Sibai BM, Ramanathan J: The case for magnesium sulfate in preeclampsia–eclampsia. *Int J Obstet Anesth* 1992;1:167–175.

101. Dommisse J: Phenytoin sodium and magnesium sulfate in the management of eclampsia. *Br J Obstet Gynaecol* 1990;97:104–109.

102. Crowther C: Magnesium sulfate versus diazepam in the management of eclampsia: A randomized controlled trial. *Br J Obstet Gynaecol* 1990;97:110–117.

103. Bhalla AK, Dhall GI, Dhall K: A safer and more effective treatment regimen for eclampsia. *Aust NZ J Obstet Gynecol* 1994;34:144–148.

104. Friedman SA, Schiff E, Kao L, Sibai BM: Phenytoin versus magnesium sulfate in patients with eclampsia: Preliminary results from a randomized trial. Poster presented at 15th Annual Meeting of the Society of Perinatal Obstetricians. Atlanta; January 23–28, 1995 (abstr 452). *Am J Obstet Gynecol* 1995;172(1):384, pt 2.

105. Which anticonvulsant for women with eclampsia: Evidence from the Collaborative Eclampsia Trial. *Lancet* 1995;345(8963):1455–1463.

17

Management of Preeclampsia

Kenneth J. Leveno and F. Gary Cunningham

Leon Chesley was a PhD, and although he associated most of his career with hospitals and academic clinical departments, he did not practice obstetrics. Still, he devoted two chapters—"A Survey of Management and Case Mortality" and "Management of Preeclampsia and Eclampsia"—to the treatment of the hypertensive disorders in the single-authored first edition of this text. These chapters bear rereading, for they display Chesley's critical assessment of the literature with an acumen that surpassed that of most obstetricians and hypertension experts of his time. The Survey chapter contains a historical compilation of treatment approaches through the ages, complementing the introductory chapter of this edition. The Management chapter contains Chesley's pioneering clinical studies on the fate of infused magnesium sulfate in preeclampsia, as well prescient analyses of published treatment regimens used in the 1960s and 1970s.

The goal of this chapter is somewhat different. Its primary aim is to aid physicians in the day-to-day management of preeclampsia–eclampsia, stressing the regimens used at Parkland Hospital in Dallas, an obstetric tertiary care center where the authors have practiced during a period when over 250,000 women were delivered and tens of thousands of preeclamptics, many quite severe, were managed. Thus, our approach will stress the practical aspects of treatment, emphasizing those references that have had the most influence on our practice.

Management of preeclampsia depends upon its severity as well as the gestational age that it becomes clinically apparent. Although in the majority of cases diagnosis is made by the appearance of new-onset pregnancy hypertension and de novo proteinuria, observations over the last decade—which are discussed in detail in other chapters in this edition of the text—have emphasized the importance of endothelial cell injury and multi-organ dysfunction in preeclampsia.

As discussed in Chapter 1, there are many extant classification schemata proposed for hypertension identified in pregnancy. In this chapter, the management of women with *new-onset* hypertensive diseases is according to the classification of the National High Blood Pressure Education Program's (NHBPEP) Working Group.[1]

This is summarized in Table 17–1; Korotkoff phase 5 is used for diastolic pressure. As of 1998, however, updates of several national working groups, including NHBPEP and the Australasian Hypertension Society were in progress. While 140/90 mm Hg has been designated as the value definitively considered normal, *increases in systolic and diastolic blood pressure after midpregnancy can either be normal physiologic changes or signs of developing pathology.* The separation of normal but profound pregnancy-induced physiologic changes from those of disease is often difficult during prenatal care. The prudent physician can only increase surveillance and be aware of further changes in blood pressure, as well as the development of signs and symptoms discussed below.

Preeclampsia

The diagnosis of preeclampsia has traditionally required the identification of de novo hypertension plus new-onset proteinuria *or* generalized edema. Today, most authorities believe that edema, even of the hands and face, is such a common finding in pregnant women that its presence should not validate the diagnosis of preeclampsia any more than its absence should preclude it.[1] The clinical spectrum of preeclampsia is detailed in Chapter 5. Some of this will be summarized below as background for management.

Proteinuria is an important sign of preeclampsia and Chesley[2] rightfully concluded that the diagnosis is questionable in its absence (see Chap. 8). Proteinuria is defined as 300 mg or more of urinary protein per 24 hours or 30 mg/dL or more in at least two random urine specimens collected 6 or more hours apart. This often correlates with "1+ dipstick" or greater in a random urine determination. The de-

**TABLE 17–1. CLASSIFICATION OF HYPERTENSIVE DISORDERS
COMPLICATING PREGNANCY**

Preeclampsia–eclampsia: Hypertension that develo̶p̶s̶   ̶sequenc̶
regresses postpartum.

1. Hypertension is accompanied by protein̶
2. Hypertension includes: (a) systolic BP
   increase of 15 mm Hg or more compa̶
   prior BPs are not known, then 140/90
3. Proteinuria is defined as excretion of 3(
4. Eclampsia is diagnosed when otherwise
   preeclampsia.

Chronic hypertension: Chronic underlying hypert̶
persists postpartum.

Preeclampsia superimposed on chronic hypertensio̶.   ̶ed
by pregnancy and accompanied by proteinuria.

Transient hypertension: Hypertension which develops after th̶   ̶ancy or
first day postpartum. This form of hypertension regresses after deliv̶   *̶n in*
subsequent gestations.

Modified from National High Blood Pressure Education Program Working Group Report on High Blood Pressure in Pregnancy. *Am J Obstet Gynecol* 1990;163:1691–1712. (See also Chapter 1 for full discussion.)

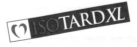

gree of proteinuria may fluctuate widely over any 24-hour period, even in severe cases. Therefore, a single random sample may fail to demonstrate significant proteinuria.[3] While proteinuria is *defined* as > 300 mg/24 h, it should be appreciated that the upper limit of normal protein excretion varies from institution to institution dependent on the analytic procedure utilized. A better approach may be to consider twice the upper limit of normal for nonpregnant subjects at an individual institution as abnormal for pregnancy.

When blood pressure rises appreciably during the latter half of pregnancy, it is dangerous—especially to the fetus—not to take action simply because proteinuria has not yet developed. As Chesley[2] emphasized, 10% of eclamptic seizures develop before overt proteinuria. Thus, from pathophysiologic and epidemiologic perspectives, it is clear that hypertension is the sine qua non of preeclampsia. Once blood pressure reaches 140/90 mm Hg or more, then pregnancy hypertension is diagnosed and the woman treated accordingly. Proteinuria is a sign of worsening hypertensive disease, specifically preeclampsia; and when it is overt and persistent, maternal and fetal risks are increased.

Severity of Hypertension in Pregnancy

The severity of hypertension complicating pregnancy is assessed by the frequency and intensity of the abnormalities listed in Chapter 5, Table 5–2. The more profound the frequency and intensity of these aberrations, the more likely is the need for pregnancy termination. *It is important to note that apparently mild disease may progress rapidly to severe disease.*

Blood pressure alone is not always a dependable indicator of severity. Indeed, 20% of women have eclamptic seizures with blood pressures less than 140/90 mm Hg. For example, a thin adolescent female may have 3+ proteinuria (300 mg/dL) and convulsions while her blood pressure is 140/85 mm Hg, whereas most women with blood pressures as high as 180/120 mm Hg do not have seizures. Convulsions are usually preceded by an unrelenting severe headache or visual disturbances; thus, these symptoms are considered ominous.

Proteinuria is an important indicator of severity because it usually develops late in the course of the disease. Certainly, persistent proteinuria of 2+ (100 mg/dL) or more, or 24-hour urinary excretion in the nephrotic range, suggests severe preeclampsia. With severe renal involvement, glomerular filtration may be impaired, as evidenced by increased plasma creatinine and oliguria.

Epigastric or *right upper quadrant pain* likely results from hepatocellular necrosis, edema, and ischemia that stretches the Glisson capsule. The characteristic pain is frequently accompanied by elevated serum liver enzymes, and *usually* is a sign to terminate the pregnancy. Such pain can presage hepatic infarction and hemorrhage as well as catastrophic rupture of a subcapsular hematoma. Fortunately, hepatic rupture is rare and most often associated with hypertension in older and parous women.

Thrombocytopenia is characteristic of worsening preeclampsia, and is often caused by microangiopathic hemolysis which some believe is induced by severe vasospasm. Whatever the cause, evidence of gross hemolysis such as hemoglobinemia, hemoglobinuria, or hyperbilirubinemia is indicative of severe disease.

Finally, there are other complications usually associated with severe hypertension, and that are more common when preeclampsia is superimposed on chronic underlying hypertension. These include cardiac dysfunction with pulmonary edema as well as fetal growth restriction.

Eclampsia

Neglected or fulminant cases of preeclampsia may progress to a convulsive phase called eclampsia. The grand mal seizures may appear before, during, or after labor. Seizures that develop more than 48 hours postpartum, however, especially in primiparas, may be encountered up to 10 days postpartum.[4,5]

Chronic Hypertension and Superimposed Preeclampsia

All *chronic hypertensive disorders*, regardless of their cause, predispose to development of superimposed preeclampsia or eclampsia.[6] This is discussed in detail in Chapter 19. Primary or essential hypertension is the cause of underlying vascular disease in more than 90% of pregnant women. This diagnosis is suggested by: (1) hypertension (140/90 mm Hg or greater) antecedent to pregnancy; (2) hypertension (140/90 mm Hg or greater) detected before 20 weeks (unless there is gestational trophoblastic disease); or (3) persistent hypertension long after delivery. Additional historical factors that help support the diagnosis are multiparity and hypertension complicating a previous pregnancy other than the first one. A strong family history is also usually evident.

Chronic hypertension causes morbidity whether or not a woman is pregnant. Specifically, it may lead to premature cardiovascular deterioration resulting in cardiac decompensation and/or cerebrovascular accidents. Intrinsic renal damage may also result. Dangers specific to pregnancy complicated by chronic hypertension include the risk of superimposed preeclampsia, which may develop in as many as 20% of women.[6] The risk of abruptio placentae also is increased substantively. Finally, the fetus of the woman with chronic hypertension is at increased risk for growth restriction and death.

Preexisting chronic hypertension worsens in some women, typically after 24 weeks. This should not be confused with *superimposed preeclampsia* in which hypertension accompanied by proteinuria or pathologic edema develops in a chronically hypertensive woman. Often, the onset of superimposed preeclampsia develops earlier in pregnancy than pure preeclampsia, and it tends to be quite severe and accompanied in many cases by fetal growth restriction.

The diagnosis requires documentation of chronic underlying hypertension. Pregnancy-induced changes in chronic hypertension are characterized by worsening hypertension, although one must keep in mind that both systolic and diastolic pressures normally rise as gestation increases. Preeclampsia is accompanied by proteinuria, pathologic edema, or both. Indicators of severity shown in Table 5–1 (Chap. 5, p. 171) are also used to further characterize these disorders.

Transient Hypertension

This condition is diagnosed retrospectively. *An attempt to make the diagnosis of transient hypertension in an antepartum woman with hypertension, especially a nullipara, is unwise because hypertension may worsen rapidly and progress to preeclampsia or eclampsia.* This classification likely includes a mixture of hypertensive etiologies including hypertension that has not yet progressed to overt preeclampsia, chronic hypertension of many different etiologies, and the provocation of hypertension in women destined to develop chronic hypertension later in life.

MANAGEMENT OF PREECLAMPSIA

Basic management objectives for any pregnancy complicated by preeclampsia are (1) termination of pregnancy with the least possible trauma to mother and fetus; (2) birth of an infant who subsequently thrives; and (3) complete restoration of health to the mother. In certain cases of preeclampsia, especially in women at or near term, all three objectives are served equally well by induction of labor. *Therefore, the most important information that the obstetrician has for successful management of pregnancy, and especially a pregnancy that becomes complicated by hypertension, is precise knowledge of the age of the fetus.*

Early Prenatal Detection

Traditionally, the timing of prenatal examinations has been scheduled at intervals of 4 weeks until 28 weeks, and then every 2 weeks until 36 weeks, and weekly thereafter. Increased prenatal visits during the third trimester facilitates early detection of preeclampsia. Women with overt hypertension ($\geq$ 140/90 mm Hg) are frequently admitted to the hospital for 2 to 3 days to evaluate the severity of new-onset pregnancy hypertension. Those with persistent severe disease are observed closely and many are delivered. Conversely, women with mild disease are often managed as outpatients.

Management of women without overt hypertension but in whom early preeclampsia is suspected during routine prenatal visits is primarily based upon increased surveillance. The protocol used successfully for many years at Parkland Hospital in women during the third trimester and with new-onset diastolic blood pressure readings between 81 and 89 mm Hg or sudden abnormal weight gain includes return visits at 3- to 4-day intervals. Such outpatient surveillance is continued unless overt hypertension, proteinuria, visual disturbances, or epigastric discomfort supervene.

Hospital Management

Hospitalization is considered at least initially for women with new-onset hypertension if there is persistent or worsening hypertension or development of proteinuria. A systematic evaluation is instituted to include the following:

1. Detailed medical examination followed by daily scrutiny for clinical findings such as headache, visual disturbances, epigastric pain, and rapid weight gain.
2. Admittance weight and every day thereafter.
3. Admittance analysis for proteinuria and at least every 2 days thereafter.
4. Blood pressure readings in sitting position with an appropriate-size cuff every 4 hours, except between midnight and morning.
5. Measurements of plasma or serum creatinine, hematocrit, platelets, and serum liver enzymes, the frequency to be determined by the severity of hypertension.
6. Frequent evaluation of fetal size and amnionic fluid volume either clinically or with sonography.

If these observations lead to a diagnosis of severe preeclampsia, further management is the same as described subsequently for eclampsia.

Although not proven in rigorous studies, reduced physical activity throughout much of the day seems beneficial. Absolute bed rest is not necessary, and sedatives and tranquilizers are not prescribed. Ample, but not excessive, protein and calories should be included in the diet. Sodium and fluid intakes should not be limited or forced. Further management depends upon (1) severity of preeclampsia, determined by presence or absence of conditions cited in Table 5–1, (2) duration of gestation, and (3) condition of the cervix. Fortunately, many cases prove to be sufficiently mild and near enough to term that they can be managed conservatively until labor commences spontaneously or until the cervix becomes favorable for labor induction. Complete abatement of all signs and symptoms, however, is uncommon until after delivery. *Almost certainly, the underlying disease persists until after delivery.*

Termination of Pregnancy

Delivery is the only cure for preeclampsia. Headache, visual disturbances, or epigastric pain likely indicate that convulsions are imminent, and oliguria is another ominous sign. Severe preeclampsia demands anticonvulsant and usually antihypertensive therapy followed by delivery. Treatment is identical to that described subsequently for eclampsia. The prime objectives are to forestall convulsions, to prevent intracranial hemorrhage and serious damage to other vital organs, and to deliver a healthy infant.

When the fetus is known or suspected to be preterm, however, the tendency is to temporize in the hope that a few more weeks in utero will reduce the risk of neonatal death or serious morbidity. As discussed, such a policy certainly is justified in milder cases. Assessments of fetal well being and placental function have been attempted, especially when there is hesitation to deliver the fetus because of prematurity. Most recommend frequent performance of various tests currently used to assess fetal well being and amnionic fluid volume, such as the nonstress test or the *biophysical profile*. Measurement of the lecithin–sphingomyelin ratio in amnionic fluid may provide evidence of lung maturity. Even when this ratio is less than 2.0, however, respiratory distress may not develop; and if it does, it is usually not fatal.

With moderate or severe preeclampsia that does not improve after hospitalization, delivery is usually advisable for the welfare of both mother and fetus. Labor should be induced by intravenous oxytocin. Many clinicians favor preinduction cervical ripening with a prostaglandin or osmotic dilator. Whenever it appears that labor induction almost certainly will not succeed, or attempts at induction of labor have failed, cesarean delivery is indicated for more severe cases of preeclampsia.

For a woman near term, with a soft, partially effaced cervix, even milder degrees of preeclampsia probably carry more risk to the mother and her fetus-infant than does induction of labor by carefully monitored oxytocin induction. This is not likely to be the case, however, if the preeclampsia is mild but the cervix is firm and closed, indicating that abdominal delivery might be necessary if pregnancy is to be terminated. The hazard of cesarean delivery may be greater than that of allowing the pregnancy to continue *under close observation* until the cervix is more suitable for induction.

Antihypertensive Drug Therapy

The use of antihypertensive drugs in attempts to prolong pregnancy or modify perinatal outcomes in pregnancies complicated by various types and severities of hypertensive disorders has been of considerable interest. These are discussed in detail in Chapter 18.

Mild Hypertension

Drug treatment for early mild preeclampsia has been disappointing (Table 17–2). Sibai et al.[7] performed a well-designed randomized study to evaluate the effectiveness of labetalol and hospitalization compared with hospitalization alone. They evaluated 200 nulliparous women with proteinuric hypertension diagnosed between 26 and 35 weeks. Although women given labetalol had significantly lower mean blood pressures, there were no differences between the groups for mean pregnancy prolongation, gestational age at delivery, or birth weight (see Table 17–2). The cesarean delivery rates were similar, as were the number of infants admitted to special-care nurseries. *Growth-restricted infants were twice as frequent in women given labetalol compared with those treated by hospitalization alone (19% vs. 9%).* Since that time, at least three other studies have been done to compare either the beta-blocking agent, labetalol, or calcium-channel blockers (nifedipine and isradi-

TABLE 17–2. SUMMARY OF RANDOMIZED PLACEBO-CONTROLLED CLINICAL TRIALS OF ANTIHYPERTENSIVE THERAPY FOR EARLY, MILD DE NOVO HYPERTENSION IN LATE PREGNANCY

Study	Study Drug (N)	Prolongation Pregnancy (days)	Severe Hypertension[a] (%)	Cesarean Delivery (%)	Abruptio Placentae	Mean Birthweight (g)	Growth Restriction (g)	Neonatal Deaths
Sibai et al. (1987)[7] 200 inpatients	Labetalol (100)	21.3	15[b]	32	0	2260	9[b]	0
	Placebo (100)	20.1	5	36	2	2205	19	1
Sibai et al. (1992)[8] 200 outpatients	Nifedipine (100)	22.3	18[b]	35	2	2510	4	0
	Placebo (100)	22.5	9	43	3	2405	8	0
Pickles et al. (1992)[9] 144 outpatients	Labetalol (70)	26.6	9	24	NS[c]	NS	NS	NS
	Placebo (74)	23.1	10	26	NS	NS	NS	NS
Wide-Swensson et al. (1995)[10] 111 outpatients	Isradipine (54)	23.1	22	26	NS	NS	NS	0
	Placebo (57)	29.8	29	19	NS	NS	NS	0

[a] Includes intrapartum hypertension
[b] Significant (P < 0.05) when study drug compared with placebo
[c] NS = not stated

Reprinted, with permission, from Cunningham FG, et al *Williams Obstetrics*, ed 20. Stamford, CT: Appleton & Lange; 1997.

pine) with placebo. Results are shown in Table 17–2, and in none of these studies were benefits of antihypertensive treatment shown.

Severe Preeclampsia

Theoretically, antihypertensive therapy has potential usefulness when preeclampsia severe enough to warrant termination of pregnancy develops before neonatal survival is likely. Such management currently is controversial, and it may be catastrophic. Sibai et al.[11] attempted to prolong pregnancy because of fetal immaturity in 60 women with severe preeclampsia diagnosed between 18 and 27 weeks. *The total perinatal mortality rate was 87%, and although no mothers died, 13 suffered placental abruption, 10 developed eclampsia, 5 had consumptive coagulopathy, 3 experienced renal failure, 2 had hypertensive encephalopathy, 1 suffered an intracerebral hemorrhage, and 1 had a ruptured hepatic hematoma.*

Closer scrutiny of this study also reveals that the authors' appeal for "conservative" management was more apparent than real. They temporized as long as blood pressure could reasonably be controlled, and in the absence of ominous signs and symptoms such as headache, blurred vision, epigastric pain, evidence of coagulation or liver abnormalities, or indications of fetal jeopardy. This is essentially what authorities have recommended for decades, in essence, this "randomized trial" was a cogent demonstration that when managing women with hypertension in pregnancy, we do not treat the diagnosis per se, but rather the evolving disease.

Sibai et al.[12] subsequently performed a randomized controlled trial of expectant vs. aggressive management of severe preeclampsia in 95 women at more advanced gestations of 28 to 32 weeks. Aggressive management included glucocorticoid administration followed by delivery in 48 hours. Expectantly managed patients were treated with bed rest and either labetalol or nifedipine given orally. Pregnancy was prolonged for a mean of 15.4 days in the expectant management group with an improvement in neonatal outcome and decreased intensive-care hospitalization. Of note, 4% in each group sustained placental abruption.

Visser and Wallenburg[13] compared clinical outcomes of expectant management in 256 women with severe preeclampsia prior to 34 weeks. Half of these women had *HELLP syndrome* (Hemolysis, ELevated liver enzymes, and Low Platelets), and the other half had only severe preeclampsia. The authors were able to prolong pregnancy in both groups for 10 to 14 days, but 13 (5%) had a placental abruption and 3 (1.2%) women developed eclampsia. The cesarean delivery rate was 83% and perinatal mortality was 144 per 1000.

Finally, Banias et al.[14] found that temporization of delivery was not possible in 60 of 67 women with severe preeclampsia at 26 to 32 weeks. Similarly, Oláh et al.[15] reviewed outcomes in 56 severely preeclamptic women between 24 and 36 weeks. While neonatal outcome was improved in women managed expectantly, maternal morbidity was increased.

We find temporizing delivery with evidence of HELLP syndrome to be quite risky. We live in an epoch when maternal deaths are rare in industrial nations, and even a small increase in the number of maternal deaths is unacceptable. Therefore, we hope that clinicians will continue to be aggressive in terminating pregnancies complicated by severe preeclampsia using the criteria for severity noted by us and Sibai et al.,[12] which they paradoxically label "conservative" management. Also because of concerns for maternal safety, we further agree with Sibai and colleagues[12] that if such management is attempted, it should be done in a tertiary-care center.

Glucocorticoids

In attempts to enhance fetal lung maturation, glucocorticoids have been administered to severely hypertensive pregnant women remote from term. Treatment does not seem to worsen maternal hypertension, and a decrease in the incidence of respiratory distress and improved fetal survival has been accepted. Martin et al.[16] provided preliminary data that such treatment might enhance maternal outcome in women with preeclampsia and HELLP syndrome. This remains to be substantiated.

High-Risk Pregnancy Unit

An inpatient high-risk pregnancy unit was established at Parkland Hospital in 1973 to provide care as just described; initial results were reported by Hauth[17] and Gilstrap[18] and their colleagues. The majority of women hospitalized have a salutary response characterized by disappearance or improvement of hypertension. *It is important to note that these women are not "cured," because nearly 90% have recurrent hypertension before or during labor.* Through 1997, more than 7000 nulliparous women with mild to moderate early-onset hypertension during pregnancy have been successfully managed in the High-Risk Pregnancy Unit. The costs of providing the relatively simple physical facility, modest nursing care, no drugs other than iron supplement, and the very few laboratory tests that are essential are slight compared with the cost of neonatal intensive care for a preterm infant.

Home Health Care

Many clinicians feel that further hospitalization is not warranted if hypertension abates within a few days. Most third-party payors in the United States refuse hospital reimbursement; thus many women with mild to moderate hypertension, and without heavy proteinuria, are consequently managed at home. Such management may continue as long as the disease does not worsen and fetal jeopardy is not suspected. Sedentary activity throughout the greater part of the day is recommended. Home blood pressure and urine protein monitoring or frequent evaluations by a visiting nurse are acceptable. These women should be instructed in detail about reporting symptoms.

Barton et al.[19] managed 592 predominately nulliparous women with mild hypertension in such a manner. All were 24 to 36 weeks at enrollment and one-fourth had proteinuria. Gestation was prolonged for a mean of 4 weeks and 60% were delivered after 37 weeks. However, half of the women developed severe hypertension and 10% had fetal jeopardy. These investigators concluded that in highly motivated women such management produced results similar to inpatient care. Helewa et al.[20] reached similar conclusions with a home-care program.

In a preliminary study from Parkland Hospital, Horsager et al.[21] randomly assigned 72 nulliparas with new-onset hypertension from 27 to 37 weeks to continued hospitalization or outpatient care. In all of these women, proteinuria had receded to less than 500 mg/day. Outpatient management included daily blood pressure monitoring by the patient or her family and weight and urine protein were determined three times weekly. A home health nurse visited twice weekly and the women were seen weekly in the clinic. Although perinatal outcomes were similar, recurrence of severe preeclampsia was more common in the home group than the hospitalized women (40% vs. 25%).

Another approach that has been evaluated on a limited basis is day care. Tuffnell et al.[22] randomly studied 54 women with nonproteinuric hypertension after 26 weeks to either day care or routine management by their individual physicians. Hospitalizations, proteinuric hypertension, and labor inductions were significantly increased in the control group.

Whichever option is chosen, careful surveillance for worsening of preeclampsia is mandatory. The women must have immediate access to the health-care team if symptoms of severe preeclampsia develop. Measures must be taken to monitor blood pressure and urine protein excretion either at home or in a clinic setting.

CLINICAL ASPECTS OF ECLAMPSIA

Eclampsia is characterized by generalized tonic–clonic convulsions that develop in some women with hypertension induced or aggravated by pregnancy. Fatal coma without convulsions has also been called eclampsia; however, it is better to limit the diagnosis to women with convulsions and to regard deaths in nonconvulsive cases as due to severe preeclampsia. There appears to be little advantage, as claimed by López-Llera,[23] to subclassify eclampsia into clinical types and subtypes. Once eclampsia has ensued, the risk to both mother and fetus is appreciable.

Clinical Course

Depending on whether convulsions appear before, during, or after labor, eclampsia is designated as antepartum, intrapartum, or postpartum. Eclampsia is most common in the last trimester and becomes increasingly more frequent as term approaches. In 254 eclamptic women cared for at the University of Mississippi Medical Center, about 3% first developed seizures more than 48 hours postpartum.[24] *Other diagnoses should be considered in women with the onset of convulsions more than 48 hours postpartum.*

Almost without exception, preeclampsia precedes the onset of eclamptic convulsions. Isolated cases are occasionally cited of an eclamptic convulsion developing without warning in women who were apparently in good health. Usually such women had not been examined by their physician for some days or—more likely—weeks previously.

The convulsive movements usually begin about the mouth in the form of facial twitchings. After a few seconds, the entire body becomes rigid in a generalized muscular contraction. This phase may persist for 15 to 20 seconds. During this phase, unless protected, the woman's tongue is bitten by the violent action of the jaws (Fig. 17–1). This phase, in which the muscles alternately contract and relax, may last about a minute. Throughout the seizure the diaphragm has been fixed, with respiration halted. After seizure activity terminates, the woman takes a long, deep, stertorous inhalation, and breathing is resumed. Coma then ensues. She will not remember the convulsion or, in all probability, events immediately before and afterward.

The first convulsion is usually the forerunner of others, which may vary in number from one or two in mild cases to 100 or more in severe, untreated cases. In rare instances, convulsions follow one another so rapidly that the woman appears to be in a prolonged, almost continuous convulsion.

The duration of coma after a convulsion is variable. When the convulsions are

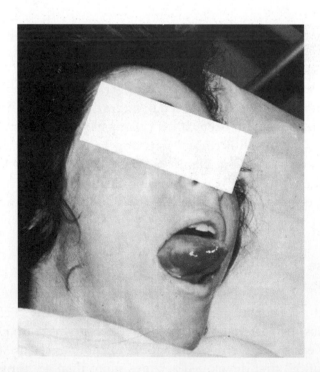

Figure 17–1. Hematoma of tongue from laceration during eclamptic convulsion. Thrombocytopenia may have contributed to the bleeding. (*Reprinted, with permission, from Cunningham FG, MacDonald PC, et al:* Williams Obstetrics, *ed 20. Stamford, CT: Appleton & Lange; 1997.*)

infrequent, the woman usually recovers some degree of consciousness after each attack. As the woman arouses, a semiconscious combative state may ensue. In very severe cases, the coma persists from one convulsion to another, and death may result before she awakens. In rare instances, a single convulsion may be followed by coma from which the woman may never emerge, although, as a rule, death does not occur until after frequent repetitive convulsions.

Respirations after an eclamptic convulsion are usually increased in rate and may reach 50 or more per minute in response presumably to hypercarbia from lactic acidemia, as well as to varying intensities of hypoxia. Cyanosis may be observed in severe cases. Fever of 39°C or more is a very grave sign, because it is probably the consequence of a central nervous system hemorrhage.

Proteinuria is almost always present and frequently pronounced. Urine output is likely diminished appreciably, and occasionally anuria develops. Hemoglobinuria is common, but hemoglobinemia is observed only rarely. Some degree of edema is probably present in all women with eclampsia. Often, as shown in Figure 17–2, the edema is pronounced—at times, massive—but it may also be occult.[25]

As with severe preeclampsia, after delivery an increase in urinary output is usually an early sign of improvement. Proteinuria and edema ordinarily disappear

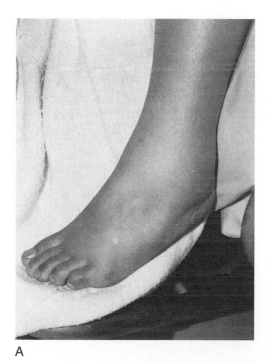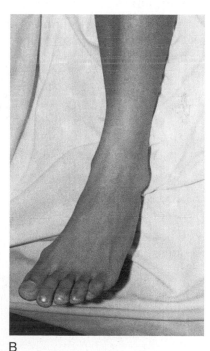

A   B

Figure 17–2. A. Severe edema in a young primigravida with antepartum eclampsia and a markedly reduced blood volume compared with normal pregnancy. **B.** The same woman 3 days after delivery. The remarkable clearance of pedal edema, accompanied by diuresis and a 28-lb weight loss, was spontaneous and unprovoked by any diuretic therapy. (*Reprinted, with permission, from Cunningham FG, Pritchard JA: How should hypertension during pregnancy be managed? Experience at Parkland Memorial Hospital.* Med Clin North Am *1984;68:505–526.*)

within a week (see Fig. 17–2). In most cases, blood pressure returns to normal within 2 weeks after delivery. The longer hypertension persists postpartum, the more likely that it is the consequence of chronic vascular or renal disease.

In antepartum eclampsia labor may begin spontaneously, shortly after convulsions ensue and progress rapidly to completion, sometimes before the attendants are aware that the unconscious or stuporous woman is having effective uterine contractions. If the attack occurs during labor, contractions may increase in frequency and intensity, and the duration of labor may be shortened. Because of maternal hypoxemia and lactic acidosis caused by convulsions, it is not unusual for fetal bradycardia to follow a seizure (Fig. 17–3). This usually recovers within 3 to 5 minutes; if it persists more than 10 minutes, however, another cause must be considered, such as placental abruption or imminent delivery.[26]

Pulmonary edema, may follow eclamptic convulsions. There are at least two sources: (1) aspiration pneumonitis may follow inhalation of gastric contents if simultaneous vomiting accompanies convulsions; and (2) cardiac failure may be the result of a combination of severe hypertension and vigorous IV fluid administration.

In some women with eclampsia, sudden death occurs synchronously with a convulsion or follows shortly thereafter as the result of a massive cerebral hemorrhage (see Chap. 5, Fig. 5–10). Hemiplegia may result from sublethal hemorrhage. Cerebral hemorrhages are more likely in older women with underlying chronic hypertension; they may rarely be due to a ruptured berry aneurysm or arteriovenous malformation. Occasionally, persistent coma or substantively altered consciousness follows a seizure. In our experiences,[27] at least in some cases, this is due to extensive cerebral edema (see Chap. 5, Fig. 5–13). If this occurs, uncal herniation may cause death.

Blindness may follow a seizure, or it may arise spontaneously with preeclamp-

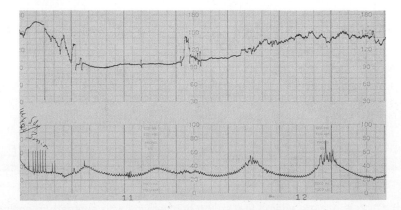

Figure 17–3. Fetal bradycardia developing in a woman with an intrapartum eclamptic convulsion. Bradycardia resolved and beat-to-beat variability returned after about 5 minutes following the seizure. (*Reprinted, with permission, from Cantrell DC, Cunningham FG: Epilepsy complicating pregnancy. In:* Williams' Obstetrics, *ed 19 (suppl #8). Norwalk, CT: Appleton & Lange; 1994.*)

sia. There are at least two causes: (1) varying degrees of retinal detachment and (2) occipital lobe ischemia or infarction. Whether due to cerebral or retinal pathology, the prognosis for return of normal vision is good and usually complete within a week.[28] Rarely, eclampsia is followed by psychosis, and the woman becomes violent. This usually lasts for several days to 2 weeks, but the prognosis for return to normal is good, provided there was no preexisting mental illness. Chlorpromazine or haloperidol in carefully titrated doses has proved effective in the few cases of posteclampsia psychosis treated at Parkland Hospital.

Differential Diagnosis

Generally, eclampsia is more likely to be diagnosed too frequently rather than overlooked because epilepsy, encephalitis, meningitis, cerebral tumor, cysticercosis, and ruptured cerebral aneurysm during late pregnancy and the puerperium may simulate eclampsia. *Until other such causes are excluded, however, all pregnant women with convulsions should be considered to have eclampsia.*

Prognosis

The prognosis for eclampsia is always serious; this is one of the most dangerous conditions that can afflict a pregnant woman and her fetus. Fortunately, maternal mortality due to eclampsia has decreased in the past three decades from 5 to 10% to less than 3% of cases.[23,29-31] These experiences clearly underscore that eclampsia, as well as severe preeclampsia, are to be considered overt threats to maternal life. Indeed, 25% of maternal deaths recorded in the United States during 1994 were related to pregnancy hypertension and accounted for at least 66 deaths.[32]

TREATMENT OF ECLAMPSIA

In 1955, Pritchard initiated a standardized treatment regimen at Parkland Hospital, and this has been used since that time to manage women with eclampsia. The carefully analyzed results of treatment of 245 cases of eclampsia, typically the severest form of pregnancy-induced or pregnancy-aggravated hypertension, were reported by Pritchard et al.[29] Most eclampsia regimens used in the United States adhere to a similar philosophy.[33] The tenets of such treatment include:

1. Control of convulsions with magnesium sulfate, using an intravenously administered loading dose along with an intramuscular loading dose if this route is chosen. This is followed by either a continuous infusion or by periodic IM injections.
2. Intermittent IV administration of an antihypertensive medication to lower blood pressure whenever the diastolic pressure is considered dangerously high. Some clinicians treat at 100 mm Hg, some at 105 mm Hg, and some at 110 mm Hg.

3. Avoidance of diuretics and limitation of IV fluid administration unless fluid loss is excessive. "Volume expansion" with albumin, starch polymers, or crystalloid solutions is avoided.
4. Delivery.

Magnesium Sulfate to Control Convulsions

In more severe cases of preeclampsia, as well as eclampsia, magnesium sulfate administered parenterally is an effective anti-eclamptic agent that does not produce central nervous system depression in either the mother or the infant. It may be given intravenously by continuous infusion or intramuscularly by intermittent injection (Table 17–3). The dosage schedule for severe preeclampsia is the same as for eclampsia. Because the period of labor and delivery is a more likely time for convulsions to develop, women with preeclampsia–eclampsia usually are given magnesium sulfate during labor and for 24 hours postpartum. *Magnesium sulfate is not given to treat hypertension.* Based on a number of studies cited below, as well as extensive clinical observations, magnesium most likely exerts a specific anticonvulsant action on the cerebral cortex. Typically, the mother stops convulsing after the initial administration of magnesium sulfate, and within an hour or two regains consciousness sufficiently to be oriented as to place and time.

TABLE 17–3. MAGNESIUM SULFATE DOSAGE SCHEDULE FOR SEVERE PREECLAMPSIA AND ECLAMPSIA

Continuous Intravenous Infusion[a]

1. Give 6-g loading dose of magnesium sulfate diluted in 100 mL of IV fluid administered over 15–20 min.
2. Begin 2 g/h in 100 mL of IV maintenance infusion.
3. Measure serum magnesium level at 4–6 h and adjust infusion to maintain levels between 4–6 mEq/L (4.8–9.6 mg/dL).
4. Magnesium sulfate is discontinued 24 h after delivery.

Pritchard Regimen—Intermittent Intramuscular Injection[b]

1. Give 4 g of magnesium sulfate ($MgSO_4 \cdot 7H_2O$, USP) as a 20% solution intravenously at a rate not to exceed 1 g/min.
2. Follow promptly with 10 g of 50% magnesium sulfate solution, one-half (5 g) injected deeply in the upper outer quadrant of both buttocks through a 3-inch-long 20-gauge needle. (Addition of 1.0 mL of 2% lidocaine minimizes discomfort.) If convulsions persist after 15 min, give up to 2 g more intravenously as a 20% solution at a rate not to exceed 1 g/min. If the woman is large, up to 4 g may be given slowly.
3. Every 4h thereafter give 5 g of a 50% solution of magnesium sulfate injected deeply in the upper outer quadrant of alternate buttocks, but only after assuring that
   a. the patellar reflex is present
   b. respirations are not depressed
   c. urine output the previous 4 h exceeded 100 mL
4. Magnesium sulfate is discontinued 24 h after delivery.

[a] From Sibai BM: Hypertension in pregnancy. In: Gabbe SG, Niebyl JR, Simpson, JL, eds. *Obstetrics: Normal and Problem Pregnancies,* ed 3. New York: Churchill Livingstone, Inc; 1996:961.
[b] From Pritchard JA, Cunningham FG, Pritchard SA: The Parkland Memorial Hospital protocol for treatment of eclampsia: Evaluation of 245 cases. *Am J Obstet Gynecol* 1984;148:951–963.

Magnesium sulfate may be given intramuscularly or intravenously by continuous infusion. The dosage schedules presented in Table 17–3 usually result in plasma magnesium levels illustrated in Figure 17–4. If given intravenously, serum magnesium levels need to be monitored at 4- to 6-hour intervals after a steady-state concentration is achieved. When given to arrest and prevent recurrent eclamptic seizures, about 10 to 15% of women will have a subsequent convulsion. An addi-

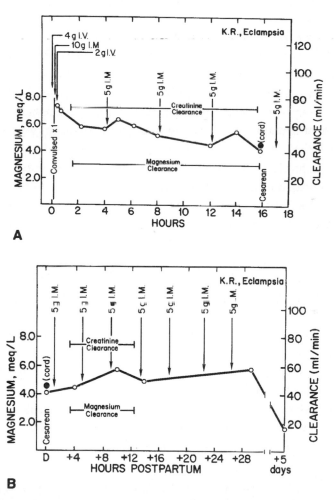

Figure 17–4. A. Plasma magnesium levels are plotted for a woman with antepartum eclampsia in whom 4 g of magnesium sulfate intravenously and 10 g intramuscularly were administered at the outset. When she soon convulsed again, 2 g more were injected slowly followed by 5 g intramuscularly every 4 hours, as described in Table 17–3 (Pritchard Regimen). She did not convulse again. **B.** The same woman as in (A). Maternal magnesium levels during the first 28 hours postpartum and 4 days after magnesium sulfate was discontinued are plotted. Before and the day after delivery the renal clearance of magnesium sulfate remained relatively constant at about 35% of the somewhat depressed creatinine clearance. (*Reprinted, with permission, from Pritchard JA, Cunningham FG, Pritchard SA: The Parkland Memorial Hospital protocol for treatment of eclampsia: Evaluation of 245 cases. Am J Obstet Gynecol 1984;148:951–963.*)

tional 2-g dose of magnesium sulfate in a 20% solution is administered slowly intravenously. In a small woman, an additional 2-g dose may be used once, and twice if needed in a larger woman. It was only necessary to use supplementary medication to control convulsions in 5 of 245 women with eclampsia at Parkland Hospital.[29] Sodium amobarbital is given slowly intravenously in doses up to 250 mg. Thiopental is also suitable. Maintenance magnesium sulfate therapy for eclampsia is continued for 24 hours after delivery. For eclampsia that develops postpartum, magnesium sulfate is administered for 24 hours after the onset of convulsions.

Pharmacology and Toxicology of Magnesium Sulfate

Magnesium sulfate United States Pharmacopeia is $MgSO_4 \cdot 7H_2O$ and not $MgSO_4$. Parenterally administered magnesium is cleared almost totally by renal excretion, and magnesium intoxication is avoided by ensuring that urine output is adequate, the patellar reflex is present, and there is no respiratory depression. Eclamptic convulsions are almost always prevented by plasma magnesium levels maintained at 4 to 7 mEq/L.

When administered as described in Table 17–3, the drug will almost always arrest eclamptic convulsions and prevent their recurrence. The initial IV infusion of 4 to 6 g is used to establish a prompt therapeutic level that is maintained by the nearly simultaneous IM injection of 10 g of the compound, followed by 5 g intramuscularly every 4 hours, or by continuous infusion at 2 g/hour. With these dosage schedules, therapeutically effective plasma levels of 4 to 7 mEq/L are achieved compared with pretreatment plasma levels of less than 2.0 mEq/L.[34,35] Magnesium sulfate injected deeply into the upper outer quadrant of the buttocks, as described above, has not resulted in erratic absorption and consequent erratic plasma levels.

Sibai et al.[36] performed a prospective study in which they compared continuous IV magnesium sulfate and IM magnesium sulfate. There was no significant difference between mean magnesium levels observed after IM magnesium sulfate and those observed following a maintenance IV infusion of 2 g/hour (Fig. 17–5).

Patellar reflexes disappear when the plasma magnesium level reaches 10 mEq/L, presumably because of a curariform action. This sign serves to warn of impending magnesium toxicity because a further increase will lead to respiratory depression.

When plasma levels rise above 10 mEq/L, respiratory depression develops, and at 12 mEq/L or more, respiratory paralysis and arrest follow. Somjen et al.[37] induced in themselves, by IV infusion, marked hypermagnesemia, achieving plasma levels up to 15 mEq/L. *Predictably, at such high plasma levels, respiratory depression developed that necessitated mechanical ventilation, but depression of the sensorium was not dramatic as long as hypoxia was prevented.* Treatment with calcium gluconate, 1 g intravenously, along with the withholding of magnesium sulfate usually reverses mild to moderate respiratory depression. Unfortunately, the effects of intravenously administered calcium may be short-lived. For severe respiratory depression and arrest, prompt tracheal intubation and mechanical ventilation are lifesaving. Direct toxic effects on the myocardium from high levels of magnesium are

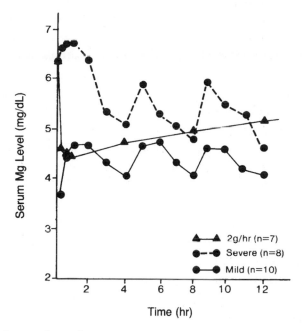

Time (hr)

Figure 17–5. Comparison of serum magnesium levels following use of the Pritchard Regimen: mild preeclampsia—10-g IM loading dose of magnesium sulfate and a 5-g maintenance dose every 4 hours (•-•) and severe preeclampsia—4-g IV loading dose followed by the same maintenance regimen (•—•). The IV method described in Table 17–3 (a 4-g loading dose was given instead of 6-g dose): 4-g IV loading dose followed by a continuous infusion of 2g/h (▲-▲). (*Reprinted, with permission, from Sibai BM, Graham JM, McCubbin JH: A comparison of intravenous and intramuscular magnesium sulfate regimens in preeclampsia. Am J Obstet Gynecol 1984;150:728–733.*)

uncommon. In humans, it appears that the cardiac dysfunction is associated with magnesium due to respiratory arrest and hypoxia. With appropriate ventilation, cardiac action is satisfactory even when plasma levels are exceedingly high.[38]

Because magnesium is cleared almost exclusively by renal excretion, plasma magnesium concentration, using the doses described above, will be excessive if glomerular filtration is decreased substantively. It is emphasized that renal insufficiency does not alter the loading doses shown in Table 17–3. Renal function is estimated by measuring plasma creatinine, and whenever it is 1.3 mg/dL or higher, we administer only half of the maintenance IM magnesium sulfate dose outlined in Table 17–3. With this renal impairment dosage, plasma magnesium levels are usually within the desired range of 4 to 7 mEq/L. If magnesium sulfate is being given intravenously by continuous infusion, serum magnesium levels are used to adjust the infusion rate. *With either method, when there is renal insufficiency, plasma magnesium levels must be checked periodically.*

Acute cardiovascular effects of parenteral magnesium ion in women with severe preeclampsia have been studied by Cotton et al.,[39] who obtained data using pulmonary and radial artery catheterization. Following a 4-g IV dose administered over 15 minutes, mean arterial blood pressure decreased slightly, accompanied by a 13% increase in cardiac index. Thus, magnesium decreased systemic vascular resistance and mean arterial pressure, and at the same time increased cardiac output, without evidence of myocardial depression. These findings were coincidental with transient nausea and flushing, and the cardiovascular effects persisted for only 15 minutes despite continued infusion of magnesium sulfate at 1.5 g/h.

As discussed in Chapter 10, presumably mediated by prostacyclin, magnesium inhibits platelet aggregation.[40] Recently, Leaphart et al.[41] reported an independent, direct magnesium-blocking effect on platelet activation mediated via adenosine diphosphate-induced stimulation. Others have questioned the findings of magnesium stimulation of prostacyclin.[42,43]

Thurnau et al.[44] have demonstrated a small but significant increase in cerebrospinal fluid magnesium concentration after magnesium therapy for preeclampsia. The magnitude of the increase was directly proportional to the corresponding serum concentration. This increase cannot be due to the disease itself because cerebrospinal fluid magnesium levels are unchanged in untreated severely preeclamptic women when compared with normotensive controls.[45]

Lipton and Rosenberg[46] attribute anticonvulsant effects to blocked neuronal calcium influx through the glutamate channel. Cotton et al.[47] induced seizure activity in the hippocampus region of rats because it is a region with a low seizure threshold and a high density of N-methyl-D-aspartate receptors. These receptors are linked to various models of epilepsy. Because hippocampal seizures can be blocked by magnesium, it is believed that this implicated the N-methyl-D-aspartate receptor in eclamptic convulsions.[48] It should be noted that results such as these suggest magnesium has a central nervous system effect in blocking seizures.

Uterine Effects

Magnesium ions in relatively high concentration will depress myometrial contractility both in vivo and in vitro. With the regimen described above and the plasma levels that have resulted, no evidence of myometrial depression has been observed beyond a transient decrease in activity during and immediately after the initial IV loading dose. Indeed, Leveno et al.[49] compared labor and delivery outcomes in 480 nulliparous women given phenytoin for preeclampsia with outcomes in 425 similar women given magnesium sulfate. Magnesium sulfate did not significantly alter oxytocin stimulation of labor, admission-to-delivery intervals, or route of delivery. Similar results have been reported by others.[50,51]

The cellular mechanisms by which magnesium might inhibit uterine contractility is not established but is generally assumed to depend on its effect on intracellular calcium.[52] The regulatory pathway leading to uterine contraction begins with an increase in the intracellular free Ca^{++} concentration which activates myosin light chain kinase.[53] High concentrations of extracellular magnesium have been reported not only to inhibit calcium entry into myometrial cells but to also lead to high intracellular magnesium levels.

This latter effect has been reported to inhibit calcium entry into the cell—

presumably by blocking calcium channels.[53] These mechanisms for inhibition of uterine contractility appear to be dose-dependent because serum magnesium levels of at least 8 mEq/L are necessary to inhibit uterine contractions.[52] This dose dependence likely explains why there is no uterine effect clinically when magnesium sulfate is given for eclampsia treatment or prophylaxis. Specifically, magnesium sulfate when given either intravenously or intramuscularly for preeclampsia or eclampsia, consistently results in serum magnesium levels less than the 8 mEq/L necessary to inhibit uterine contractility (see Fig. 17–4).

Fetal Effects

Magnesium administered parenterally to the mother promptly crosses the placenta to achieve equilibrium in fetal serum and less so in amnionic fluid.[54] Atkinson et al.[50] reported a statistically significant, but clinically insignificant, decrease in short-term fetal heart rate variability. They observed no changes in long-term variability or accelerations. Others, however, have reported reductions both in short- and long-term variability.[55] Gray et al.[56] reported that magnesium sulfate for tocolysis did not alter the biophysical profile in 25 fetuses studied. The neonate may be depressed only if there is *severe* hypermagnesemia at delivery. We have not observed neonatal compromise after IM therapy with magnesium sulfate,[25] nor have Green et al.[57]

There is a suggestion of a possible protective effect of magnesium against cerebral palsy in very low birth weight infants.[58,59] Murphy et al.[60] found that preeclampsia, rather than magnesium sulfate, was protective against cerebral palsy in these very small infants. Kimberlin et al.[61] found no advantage of maternal magnesium sulfate tocolysis in infants born weighing less than 1000 g.

Clinical Efficacy of Magnesium Sulfate Therapy

In 1995, results were reported from the multinational controlled clinical trial of eclampsia therapy. The Eclampsia Trial Collaborative Group[31] study was funded in part by the World Health Organization and coordination was provided by the National Perinatal Epidemiology Unit in Oxford, England. This study included 1687 women with eclampsia who were randomly allocated to different anticonvulsant regimens. The primary outcome measures were recurrence of convulsions and maternal deaths. In one study, 453 women were randomized to magnesium sulfate compared with 452 given diazepam. Another 388 eclamptic women were randomized to magnesium sulfate and compared with 387 women given phenytoin.

As shown in Figure 17–6, women allocated to magnesium sulfate therapy had a 50% reduction in incidence of recurrent seizures compared with those given diazepam. As shown in Table 17–4, it is important to note that maternal deaths were reduced in women given magnesium sulfate, and although these differences are clinically impressive, they are not statistically significant. Specifically, there were 3.8% deaths among 453 women randomized to magnesium sulfate compared with

Magnesium sulphate versus diazepam

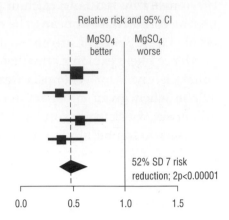

| Entry characteristic | Recurrent convulsion/women | | Relative risk and 95% CI |
	MgSO$_4$	Diazepam	
Before delivery	46/325	83/308	
After delivery	14/128	43/144	
No prior anticonvulsant[1]	33/198	64/218	
Prior anticonvulsant[1]	25/244	60/227	
All women	60/453 (13.2%)	126/452 (27.9%)	52% SD 7 risk reduction; 2p<0.00001

Magnesium sulphate versus phenytoin

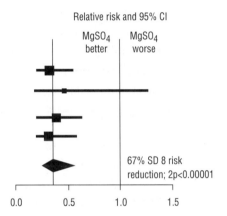

| Entry characteristic | Recurrent convulsion/women | | Relative risk and 95% CI |
	MgSO$_4$	Phenytoin	
Before delivery	17/309	56/319	
After delivery	5/79	10/68	
No prior anticonvulsant[2]	10/91	23/73	
Prior anticonvulsant[2]	12/294	43/308	
All women	22/388 (5.7%)	66/387 (17.1%)	67% SD 8 risk reduction; 2p<0.00001

Figure 17–6. Effects of magnesium sulfate vs. diazepam and phenytoin on recurrent convulsions. (*Reprinted, with permission, from Eclampsia Trial Collaborative Group: Which anticonvulsant for women with eclampsia? Evidence from the collaborative eclampsia trial.* Lancet *1995;345:1455–1463 © by The Lancet Ltd. 1995.*)

5.1% among 452 given diazepam. Maternal and perinatal morbidity were not different between these two groups, and there was no difference in the number of labor inductions or cesarean deliveries.

In a second comparison, also shown in Figure 17–6, women randomized to receive magnesium sulfate compared with phenytoin had a 67% reduction in recurrent convulsions. As shown in Table 17–4, maternal mortality was lower in the magnesium group compared with the phenytoin group (2.6% vs. 5.2%). This clinically impressive decreased maternal mortality of 50% again was not significant statistically.

In other comparisons, women allocated to magnesium sulfate therapy were less likely to be artificially ventilated, to develop pneumonia, or to be admitted to intensive-care units than those given phenytoin. Neonates of women given magnesium sulfate were significantly less likely to require intubation at delivery and to

TABLE 17–4. MATERNAL MORTALITY IN ECLAMPSIA TRIAL COLLABORATIVE GROUP

Regimen	No.	Mortality	
		Maternal (%)	Perinatal
Magnesium sulfate	453	3.8	25/1000
Diazepam	452	5.1	22/1000
Magnesium sulfate	388	2.6	22/1000
Phenytoin	387	5.2	31/1000

From Eclampsia Trial Collaborative Group: Which anticonvulsant for women with eclampsia? Evidence from the collaborative eclampsia trial. *Lancet* 1995;345:1455–1463.

be admitted to the neonatal intensive care unit compared with infants whose mothers received phenytoin.

The Eclampsia Trial Collaborative Group concluded: "There is now compelling evidence in favour of magnesium sulphate, rather than diazepam or phenytoin, for the treatment of eclampsia."[31] *These results are even more impressive when it is emphasized that women in this study who received IV magnesium sulfate received only 1 g/h.*

Antihypertensive Treatment Alone to Control Seizures

A question of whether antihypertensive medications alone can be used to prevent seizures remains unanswered.[62,63] It is difficult and unwise to recommend withholding magnesium sulfate because even with the excellent results reported using both anticonvulsants and antihypertensive agents in the Eclampsia Trial Collaborative Group,[31] maternal mortality was still 4.1% of 1690 women, or almost 1 death per 25 women.

Prevention of Eclampsia

Magnesium sulfate therapy also is superior to phenytoin in preventing eclamptic seizures. Lucas et al.[64] reported results of a prospective study from Parkland Hospital in which pregnant women with hypertension were randomized to receive magnesium sulfate or phenytoin during labor. These were women with sustained blood pressures that exceeded 140/90 mm Hg and no regard was given to presence or absence of proteinuria. The magnesium sulfate therapy consisted of the Pritchard Regimen presented in Table 17–3. The phenytoin regimen consisted of a 1000-mg loading dose infused over a 1-hour period, followed by a 500-mg oral dose 10 hours later. Anticonvulsant therapy in both groups was continued for 24 hours postpartum. Ten of the 1089 women randomly assigned to the phenytoin regimen had eclamptic convulsions. There were no convulsions in the 1049 women randomly assigned to magnesium sulfate (P = 0.004). There were no significant differences in any risk factors for eclampsia between the two groups of women studied. Maternal and neonatal outcomes were similar in the two study groups. As shown in Figure 17–7, women given phenytoin who developed eclampsia did so despite "therapeutic" serum levels (10–25 μg/mL).

Debate still ensues—mostly outside the United States—over whether magnesium sulfate prophylaxis should be given routinely to all women in labor who have hypertension.[65,66] Burrows and Burrows[67] described 467 women with preeclampsia (proteinuric hypertension) in whom seizure prophylaxis was not given. A total of 3.9% developed eclamptic seizures. This is in contrast to a failure rate of prophylaxis of 1 in 750 women treated with the regimen shown in Table 17–3 reported by Cunningham and Leveno.[68] Because of the risk of maternal death with eclampsia (see Table 17–4), we continue to use magnesium sulfate seizure prophylaxis for all women with preeclampsia. After a recent review, Lindheimer[69] as well as Sibai[70] also continue to recommend such prophylaxis.

The next section of this chapter is concerned with the treatment of acute and severe hypertension, often during labor. The specific agents are detailed in Chapter 18. Here we focus more selectively on management issues.

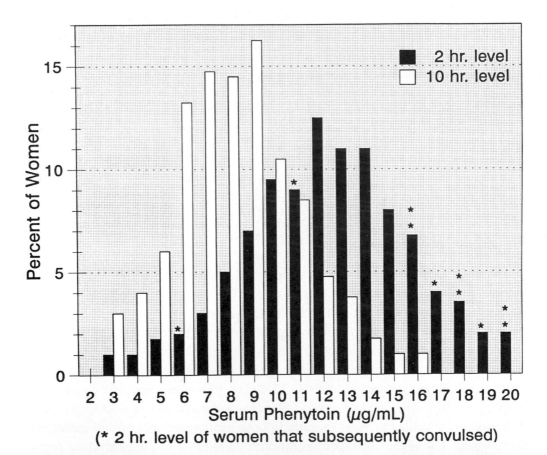

Figure 17–7. Distribution of serum phenytoin levels 2 and 10 hours after initiation of therapy. Women given phenytoin and who developed eclampsia (indicated by asterisks) did so despite "therapeutic" serum levels (10–25 μg/mL). (*Reprinted, with permission, from Lucas MJ, Leveno KJ, Cunningham FG: A comparison of magnesium sulfate with phenytoin for the prevention of eclampsia.* N Engl J Med *1995;333: 201–205. Copyright © 1995 Massachusetts Medical Society. All rights reserved.*)

Hydralazine to Control Severe Hypertension

Following $MgSO_4$ treatment, about 60% of severe preeclamptics need additional medications to lower blood pressure.[70a] We administer hydralazine intravenously whenever the diastolic blood pressure is 110 mm Hg or higher. Some recommend treatment of diastolic pressures over 100 mm Hg and some use 105 mm Hg as a cut-off.[70,71] Hydralazine is administered in 5- to 10-mg doses at 15- to 20-minute intervals until a satisfactory response is achieved. A satisfactory response antepartum or intrapartum is defined as a decrease in diastolic blood pressure to 90 to 100 mm Hg, but not lower lest placental perfusion be compromised.

Hydralazine administered in this manner has proven remarkably effective in the prevention of cerebral hemorrhage. At Parkland Hospital, approximately 8% of all women with pregnancy-induced hypertension are given hydralazine as described, and we estimate that more than 3500 women have been treated with this compound. Other antihypertensive agents were seldom needed because of poor response to hydralazine. In most European hospitals, hydralazine is also favored.[72,73] In recent years, injectable hydralazine was at times difficult to obtain because its primary manufacturer ceased production; however, these shortages are no longer a problem.

The tendency to give a larger initial dose of hydralazine when the blood pressure is higher must be avoided. Figure 17–8 shows mean arterial blood pressure responses to 5-mg hydralazine bolus doses.[74] The response to even 5- to 10-mg doses cannot be predicted by the level of hypertension; thus we always give 5 mg as the initial dose. An example of very severe hypertension in a woman with chronic hy-

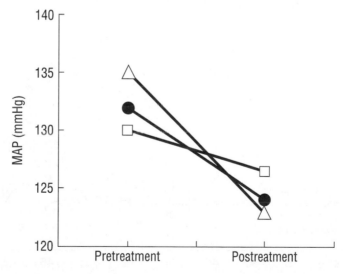

Figure 17–8. Effect of successive treatments with bolus hydralazine on mean arterial pressure (MAP). Δ = first bolus (N = 109), change in MAP −12.0 mm Hg (95% CI −14 to −10); ● = second bolus (N = 41), change in MAP −9.0 mm Hg (95% CI −12 to −6 × 5); □ = third bolus (N = 14), change in MAP −5.0 mm Hg (95% CI −10 to −1). (*Reprinted, with permission, from Paterson-Brown S, Robson SC, Redfern N, De Swiet M: Hydralazine boluses for the treatment of severe hypertension in preeclampsia.* Br J Obstet Gynaecol *1994;101:409–413.*)

pertension complicated by superimposed eclampsia that responded to repeated IV injections of hydralazine is shown in Figure 17–9. Hydralazine was injected more frequently than recommended in the protocol, and blood pressure decreased in less than 1 hour from 240–270/130–150 mm Hg to 110/80 mm Hg. Uteroplacental insufficiency-type fetal heart rate decelerations were evident when the pressure fell to 110/80 mm Hg, and persisted until maternal blood pressure increased.

Labetalol

Intravenous labetalol is also used to treat acute hypertension of pregnancy. In 1994, hydralazine was not always available in the United States and more experience was gained with this alpha-1 and nonselective beta-blocker. It lowers blood pressure by decreasing heart rate and contractility, and it is not a vasodilator. Mabie et al.[75] compared IV hydralazine with labetalol for blood pressure control in 60 peripartum women. Labetalol lowered blood pressure more rapidly and associated tachycardia was minimal, but hydralazine lowered mean arterial pressure to safe levels more effectively. We have evaluated labetalol given intravenously for women with severe preeclampsia and our results are very similar. Our protocol initially calls for 10 mg intravenously. If the blood pressure has not decreased to the desirable level in 10 minutes, then a 20-mg dose is given. The next 10-minute incremental doses are 40 mg followed by another 40 mg, and then 80 mg if a salutary response is not yet achieved.

Other Antihypertensive Agents

Belfort et al.[76] administered the calcium antagonist, *verapamil*, by IV infusion at 5 to 10 mg/h. Mean arterial pressure was lowered by 20%. Scardo et al.[77] gave 10 mg

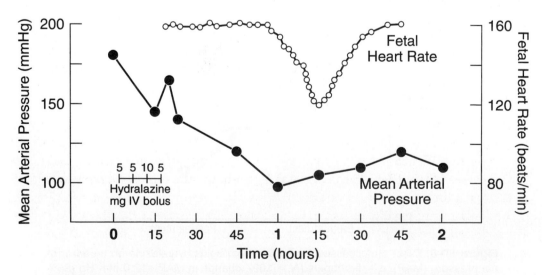

Figure 17–9. Effects of acute blood pressure decrease on fetal status. Hydralazine was given at 5-min intervals instead of 15-min intervals and mean arterial pressure decreased from 180 to 90 mm Hg within 1 h. This was associated with fetal bradycardia.

nifedipine orally to 10 women with preeclamptic hypertensive emergencies and reported no hypotension or fetal compromise. Mabie et al.[78] administered nifedipine sublingually to 34 women with peripartum hypertension, and because its antihypertensive effects were potent and rapid, two women developed worrisome hypotension. Similar effects in nonpregnant patients have caused cerebrovascular ischemia, myocardial infarction, conduction disturbances, and death, leading Grossman et al.[79] to call for a moratorium for its use in hypertensive emergencies. Belfort et al.[80] found that *nimodipine* given by continuous infusion as well as orally[81] was effective to lower blood pressure in women with severe preeclampsia. Bolte et al.[82] reported good results in 169 preeclamptic women treated with IV *ketanserin,* a selective serotonin-2 receptor blocker.

Intravenously administered *diazoxide* has been championed by some for use in preeclampsia–eclampsia because of its very potent antihypertensive action. Unfortunately, IV diazoxide therapy is accompanied by many adverse side effects. For example, it likely is to arrest labor. It causes retention of sodium, water, and uric acid, as well as serious hyperglycemia in mother and neonate. It should also be noted that it may produce irreversible, and therefore lethal, hypotension when administered with or after other antihypertensive agents. Undoubtedly, many of the serious adverse reactions reported were associated with the standard 300-mg bolus dose recommended for nonpregnant patients; titration using intermittent small boluses of 30 to 60 mg is apparently safer.[1] Diazoxide is seldom used in the United States, although some nonobstetricians continue to recommend it.

Nitroglycerin given intravenously has been used for acute hypertension control.[39] It is not recommended by the Working Group of the National High Blood Pressure Education Program[1] because of fetal cyanide toxicity in animal models.

Persistent Postpartum Hypertension

The potential problem of serious compromise of placental perfusion and fetal well being is obviated by delivery. If there is a problem after delivery in controlling severe hypertension and IV hydralazine is being used repeatedly early in the puerperium to control persistent severe hypertension, then other regimens can be used. Ascarelli et al.[82a] randomized 266 postpartum preeclamptics to no treatment versus furosemide, 20 mg orally for 5 days. Blood pressure was significantly lower by the second day in women given furosemide and only 5.7% (vs. 26% given no furosemide) required antihypertensive therapy at discharge. We have had success with *intramuscular* hydralazine, usually in 10- to 25-mg doses at 4- to 6-hour intervals. Once repeated blood pressure readings remain near normal, hydralazine is stopped. If hypertension of appreciable intensity persists or recurs *in these postpartum women,* oral labetalol or a thiazide diuretic are given for as long as necessary. A variety of other antihypertensive agents have been utilized for this purpose, including other beta-blockers and calcium-channel antagonists. The persistence or refractoriness of hypertension is likely due to at least two mechanisms: (1) underlying chronic hypertension and/or (2) mobilization of edema fluid with redistribution into the intravenous compartment. Labetalol and a diuretic are effective treatment for both mechanisms.

Persistent HELLP Syndrome

Over the years, the group at the University of Mississippi Medical Center has described an atypical syndrome in which preeclampsia–eclampsia persists despite delivery. They described 18 such women over a 10-year period during which time they delivered nearly 43,000 patients.[83] They advocate single or multiple plasma exchange for these women and in some cases, 3 L of plasma (representing 12–15 donors), was exchanged three times before a response was forthcoming. In our experiences of over 40,000 hypertensive women in nearly 300,000 pregnancies, we have not encountered this syndrome. It also has not been encountered by investigators at the University of Tennessee.[84] In a very few women, persistent hypertension, thrombocytopenia, and renal dysfunction were found to be due to thrombotic microangiopathy.[84,85]

Diuretics and Hyperosmotic Agents

Potent diuretics further compromise placental perfusion because their immediate effects include intravascular volume depletion which most often is already reduced compared with normal pregnancy. Therefore, diuretics are not used to lower blood pressure lest they enhance the intensity of the maternal hemoconcentration and its adverse effects on the mother and the fetus.

Once delivery is accomplished, in almost all cases of severe preeclampsia and eclampsia there is a spontaneous diuresis that usually begins within 24 hours and results in the disappearance of excessive extravascular extracellular fluid over the next 3 to 4 days, as demonstrated in Figure 17–2.

With infusion of hyperosmotic agents, such as albumin or starch polymers, the potential exists for an appreciable intravascular influx of fluid and, in turn, subsequent escape of intravascular fluid in the form of edema into vital organs, especially the lungs and brain. Moreover, an oncotically active agent that leaks through capillaries into lungs and brain promotes accumulation of edema at these sites. Most important, a sustained beneficial effect from their use has not been demonstrated. For all of these reasons, hyperosmotic agents have not been administered, and use of furosemide or similar drugs has been limited to the rare instances in which pulmonary edema was identified or strongly suspected.

Fluid Therapy

Lactated Ringer solution is administered routinely at the rate of 60 mL to no more than 125 mL per hour unless there was unusual fluid loss from vomiting, diarrhea, or diaphoresis, or more likely, excessive blood loss at delivery. Even at these relatively low infusion rates, a substantive sodium load accrues at 24 to 48 hours. Oliguria, common in cases of severe preeclampsia and eclampsia, coupled with the knowledge that maternal blood volume is very likely constricted compared with normal pregnancy, makes it tempting to administer IV fluids more vigorously. The rationale for controlled, conservative fluid administration is that the typical eclamptic woman already has excessive extracellular fluid that is inappropriately distributed between the intravascular and extravascular spaces. Infusion of large fluid volumes could, and does, enhance the maldistribution of extravascular fluid and, thereby appreciably increases the risk of pulmonary and cerebral edema.[86-88]

Pulmonary Edema

Women with severe preeclampsia–eclampsia who develop pulmonary edema most often do so postpartum.[88-90] Aspiration of gastric contents, the result of convulsions or perhaps from anesthesia, or oversedation, should be excluded; however, the majority of these women have cardiac failure if IV fluids have been limited. Some normal pregnancy changes, magnified by preeclampsia, predispose to pulmonary edema (see also Chap. 5). It is important to note that plasma oncotic pressure decreases appreciably in normal term pregnancy because of decreases in serum albumin, and oncotic pressure falls even more with preeclampsia.[91,92] Moreover, Øian et al.[93] described increased extravascular fluid oncotic pressure in preeclamptic women, and this favors capillary fluid extravasation. Brown et al.[94] verified increased capillary permeability in preeclamptic women. Bhatia et al.[95] reported a correlation between plasma colloid osmotic pressure and fibronectin concentration; this suggested to them that vascular protein loss was the result of increased vascular permeability caused by vessel injury.

The frequent findings of hemoconcentration, and more recently findings by some of reduced central venous and pulmonary capillary wedge pressures in women with severe preeclampsia, have tempted some to infuse various fluids, starch polymers, or albumin concentrates, or all three, in attempts to expand blood volume and, thereby, somehow to relieve vasospasm and reverse organ deterioration. Thus far, clearcut evidence of benefits from this approach is lacking, however, serious complications, especially pulmonary edema, have been reported (see Chap. 5 for a more detailed discussion). López-Llera[23] reported that vigorous volume expansion was associated with the highest incidence of pulmonary edema in his series of more than 700 eclamptic women. Benedetti et al.[89] described pulmonary edema in seven of ten severely preeclamptic women who were given colloid therapy. Sibai et al.[88] cited excessive colloid and crystalloid infusions as causing most of 37 cases of pulmonary edema associated with severe preeclampsia–eclampsia. Pulmonary edema is a common cause of maternal morbidity as well as mortality in women with HELLP syndrome.[95a,95b] Finally, Lehmann et al.[96] reported that pulmonary edema caused nearly one-third of maternal deaths due to pregnancy-associated hypertension.

For these reasons, until it is understood how to contain more fluid within the intravascular compartment and, at the same time, less fluid outside the intravascular compartment, we remain convinced that, in the absence of marked fluid loss, fluids can be administered safely only in moderation. To date, no serious adverse effects have been observed from such a policy. It should be mentioned that dialysis for renal failure was not required for any of the more than 450 cases of eclampsia managed in this manner.

Invasive Hemodynamic Monitoring

Much of what has been learned within the past decade about cardiovascular and hemodynamic pathophysiologic alterations associated with severe preeclampsia–eclampsia has been made possible by invasive hemodynamic monitoring using a flow-directed pulmonary artery catheter. The need for clinical implementation of such technology for the woman with preeclampsia–eclampsia, however, has not been established. The subject has been reviewed by Nolan et al.,[97] Hankins and Cunningham,[98] and Clark and Cotton.[99] Two conditions frequently cited as indications for such monitoring are preeclampsia associated with oliguria and preeclampsia associated with pulmonary edema. *Perhaps somewhat paradoxically, it is usually vigorous treatment of the former that results in most cases of the latter.* In addition, urine volume, per se, does not relate to renal function, and oliguria should always be analyzed in relation to the trend in serum creatinine levels. *Otherwise uncomplicated severe preeclampsia–eclampsia is not an indication for pulmonary artery catheterization.*[100,101]

Because vigorous IV hydration or other attempts at volume expansion are avoided at Parkland Hospital in women with severe preeclampsia and eclampsia, hemodynamic monitoring has not been used for the vast majority of these women. Such measures are usually reserved for women with accompanying severe cardiac disease and/or renal disease or in cases of refractory hypertension, oliguria, and pulmonary edema. Similar indications are used by Clark and Cotton,[99] Cowles et al.,[102] and Easterling et al.,[103] and have been reported in Technical Bulletins published by the American College of Obstetricians and Gynecologists.[100,101] The routine use of such monitoring, even if pulmonary edema develops, is questionable. Most of these women respond quickly to furosemide given intravenously. Afterload reduction with intermittent doses of IV hydralazine to lower blood pressure, as described above, may also be necessary because women with chronic hypertension and severe superimposed preeclampsia are more likely to develop heart failure.[90] Obese women in these circumstances are even more likely to develop heart failure.[104]

Invasive monitoring should be considered for those women with multiple clinical factors such as intrinsic heart disease and/or advanced renal disease that might cause pulmonary edema by more than one mechanism. This is particularly relevant if pulmonary edema is inexplicable or refractory to treatment. Still, in most of these cases it is not necessary to perform pulmonary artery catheterization for clinical management.

Delivery

To avoid maternal risks from cesarean delivery, steps to effect vaginal delivery are initially employed. After an eclamptic seizure, labor often ensues spontaneously or can be induced successfully even in women remote from term. An immediate cure does not immediately follow delivery by any route, but serious morbidity is less common during the puerperium in women delivered vaginally.

Blood Loss at Delivery

Hemoconcentration, or lack of normal pregnancy-induced hypervolemia, is an almost predictable feature of severe preeclampsia. *The woman with severe preeclampsia or eclampsia, who consequently lacks normal pregnancy hypervolemia, is much less tolerant of blood loss than is the normotensive pregnant woman.* It is of great importance to recognize that an appreciable fall in blood pressure very soon after delivery most often means excessive blood loss and not sudden dissolution of vasospasm. When oliguria follows delivery, the hematocrit should be evaluated frequently to help detect excessive blood loss that, if identified, should be treated appropriately by careful blood transfusion.

Analgesia and Anesthesia

In the past, both spinal and epidural anesthesia were avoided in women with severe preeclampsia and eclampsia.[29] Physiologic changes leading to these concerns centered on the hypotension induced by sympathetic blockade and, in turn, on dangers from pressor agents or large volumes of IV fluid used to correct iatrogenically induced hypotension. For example, rapid infusion of large volumes of crystalloid or colloid, given to counteract maternal hypovolemia caused by a variety of situations, including epidural analgesia, has been implicated as a cause of pulmonary edema.[88] There have also been concerns about fetal safety because sympathetic blockade-induced hypotension can dangerously lower uteroplacental perfusion.[105] Another concern is that attempts to restore blood pressure pharmacologically with vasopressors may be hazardous because women with preeclampsia are extremely sensitive to such agents.

As regional analgesic techniques were improved during the past decade, epidural analgesia was promoted by some proponents for women with severe preeclampsia to ameliorate vasospasm and lower hypertension.[106] Moreover, many who favored epidural blockade believed that general anesthesia was inadvisable because stimulation caused by tracheal intubation may result in sudden hypertension, which may cause pulmonary edema, cerebral edema, or intracranial hemorrhage.[23,107-109] Others have also cited that tracheal intubation may be particularly hazardous in women with airway edema due to preeclampsia.[110-112]

These differing perspectives on the advantages, disadvantages, and safety of the anesthetic method used in the cesarean delivery of women with severe preeclampsia have evolved so that some authorities believe that epidural analgesia is the preferred method, whereas others are more circumspect. Wallace et al.[113] evaluated these important issues by conducting a randomized investigation in women with severe preeclampsia cared for at Parkland Hospital. There were 80 women with severe preeclampsia who were to be delivered by cesarean and who were randomized to general anesthesia or epidural or combined spinal–epidural analgesia. Their mean preoperative blood pressure was approximately 170/110 mm Hg, and all had proteinuria. Anesthetic and obstetric management included antihypertensive drug therapy and limited IV fluids and other drug therapy. The infants, whose mean gestational age at delivery was 34.8 weeks, were all born in good condition as assessed by Apgar scores and umbilical arterial blood gas determinations. Maternal hypotension resulting from regional analgesia was managed without excessive IV fluid administration. Similarly, maternal blood pressure was managed without severe hypertensive effects in women undergoing general anesthesia (Figure 17–10). There were no serious maternal or fetal complications attributable to any of the three anesthetic methods. We concluded that both general and regional anesthetic methods are equally acceptable for cesarean delivery in pregnancies complicated by severe preeclampsia if steps are taken to ensure a careful approach to either method.

The immense popularity and increasing availability of epidural analgesia for labor has led many anesthesiologists as well as obstetricians to develop the viewpoint that epidural analgesia is an important factor in the treatment of women with preeclampsia.[111,114] Although epidural analgesia is widely used during labor in women with preeclampsia, the effects of such analgesia on the mother and fetus have not been extensively investigated. In an ongoing study at Parkland Hospital, a total of 738 women with singleton cephalic pregnancies at 36 weeks or more, and preeclampsia of various severity, have been randomized to epidural analgesia (372) or patient-controlled IV meperidine analgesia (366) during labor.[115] Ephedrine for hypotension was given intravenously to 11% of women with epidural analgesia and none of those

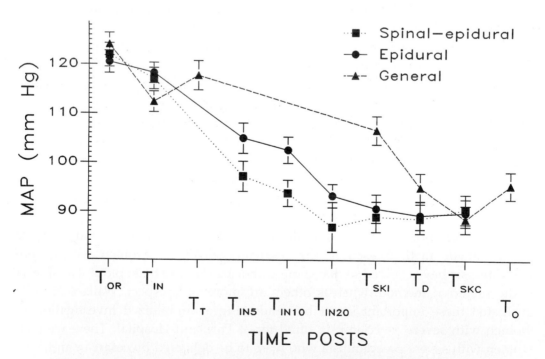

Figure 17–10. Blood pressure effects of general anesthesia vs. epidural or spinal–epidural analgesia for cesarean delivery in 80 women with severe preeclampsia. (*Reprinted from Wallace DH, Leveno KJ, Cunningham FG, et al: Randomized comparison of general and regional anesthesia for cesarean delivery in pregnancies complicated by severe preeclampsia. Obstet Gynecol 1995;86:193–199. Reprinted with permission from the American College of Obstetricians and Gynecologists.*)

given IV meperidine. Importantly, there were no differences in maternal and neonatal outcomes, and there were no adverse effects related to either method of analgesia.

Potential Side Effects of Regional Anesthesia/Analgesia

Newsome et al.[116] demonstrated that lowered mean arterial pressure followed epidural blockade in women with severe preeclampsia. Despite this, the cardiac index did not fall, but as shown in Figure 17–11, IV fluid loading caused elevation of pulmonary capillary wedge pressures as compared with women in whom fluids were restricted. Although the intravascular volume of women with severe preeclampsia is not expanded as for normal pregnancy, total body water is increased. It is also generally recognized that there is a capillary leak with severe preeclampsia, and that this is manifested as pathologic peripheral edema, proteinuria, and ascites. Aggressive volume replacement in these women increases their risk for pulmonary edema, especially in the first 72 hours postpartum.[118,119] When pulmonary edema develops there is also concern for development of cerebral edema. Finally, Heller et al.[120] demonstrated that the majority of cases of pharyngolaryngeal edema were related to aggressive volume therapy.

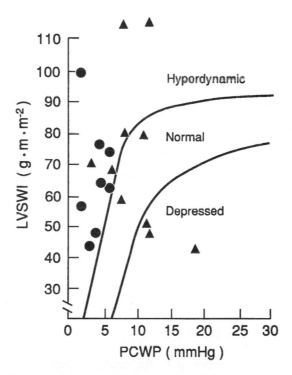

Figure 17–11. Comparison of ventricular function curves in women with severe preeclampsia. The solid circles represent values from women with eclampsia managed with fluid restriction.[117] The triangles represent women with epidural analgesia given intravenous fluid preloading. (LVSWI = left ventricular stroke work index; PCWP = pulmonary capillary wedge pressure. (*Modified, with permission, from Newsome LR, Bramwell RS, Curling PE: Severe preeclampsia: Hemodynamic effects of lumbar epidural anesthesia.* Anesth Analg *1986;65:31–36.*)

REFERENCES

1. National High Blood Pressure Education Program Working Group Report on High Blood Pressure in Pregnancy. *Am J Obstet Gynecol* 1990;163:1691–1712.
2. Chesley LC: Diagnosis of preeclampsia. *Obstet Gynecol* 1985;65:423–425.
3. Meyer NL, Mercer BM, Friedman SA, Sibai BM: Urinary dipstick protein: A poor predictor of absent or severe proteinuria. *Am J Obstet Gynecol* 1994;170:137–141.
4. Brown CEL, Cunningham FG, Pritchard JA: Convulsions in hypertensive, proteinuric primiparas more than 24 hours after delivery: Eclampsia or some other cause? *J Reprod Med* 1987;32:499–503.
5. Lubarsky SL, Barton JR, Friedman SA, et al: Late postpartum eclampsia revisited. *Obstet Gynecol* 1994;83:502–505.
6. Sibai BM, Lindheimer M, Hauth J, et al, and the National Institute of Child Health and Human Development Network of Maternal–Fetal Medicine Units: Risk factors for preeclampsia, abruptio, and adverse neonatal outcome in women with chronic hypertension. *N Engl J Med* 1998;339:667–671.
7. Sibai BM, Gonzalez AR, Mabie WC, Moretti M: A comparison of labetalol plus hospitalization versus hospitalization alone in the management of preeclampsia remote from term. *Obstet Gynecol* 1987;70:323–327.
8. Sibai BM, Barton JR, Akl S, et al: A randomized prospective comparison of nifedipine and bed rest versus bed rest alone in the management of preeclampsia remote from term. *Am J Obstet Gynecol* 1992;167:879–884.
9. Pickles CJ, Broughton Pipkin F, Symonds EM: A randomized placebo controlled trial of labetalol in the treatment of mild to moderate pregnancy induced hypertension. *Br J Obstet Gynaecol* 1992;99:964–968.
10. Wide-Swensson DH, Ingemarsson I, Lunnell N-O, et al: Calcium channel blockade (isradipine) in treatment of hypertension in pregnancy: A randomized placebo-controlled study. *Am J Obstet Gynecol* 1995;173:872–878.
11. Sibai BM, Taslimi M, Abdella TN, et al: Maternal and perinatal outcome of conservative management of severe preeclampsia in midtrimester. *Am J Obstet Gynecol* 1985;152:32–37.
12. Sibai BM, Mercer BM, Schiff E, Friedman SA: Aggressive versus expectant management of severe preeclampsia at 28 to 32 weeks' gestation: A randomized controlled trial. *Am J Obstet Gynecol* 1994;171:818–822.
13. Visser W, Wallenberg HCS: Temporizing management of severe pre-eclampsia with and without the HELLP syndrome. *Br J Obstet Gynaecol* 1995;102:111–117.
14. Banias BB, Devoe LD, Nolan TE: Severe preeclampsia in preterm pregnancy between 26 and 32 weeks' gestation. *Am J Perinatol* 1992;9:357–360.
15. Oláh KS, Redman CWG, Gee H: Management of severe, early preeclampsia: Is conservative management justified? *Eur J Obstet Gynaecol Reprod Biol* 1993;51:175–180.
16. Martin JN Jr, Perry KG Jr, Blake PG, et al: Better maternal outcomes are achieved with dexamethasone therapy for postpartum HELLP (hemolysis, elevated liver enzymes, and thrombocytopenia) syndrome. *Am J Obstet Gynecol* 1997;177:1011–1017.
17. Hauth JC, Cunningham FG, Whalley PJ: Management of pregnancy-induced hypertension in the nullipara. *Obstet Gynecol* 1976;48:253–259.
18. Gilstrap LC, Cunningham FG, Whalley PJ: Management of pregnancy-induced hypertension in the nulliparous patient remote from term. *Semin Perinatol* 1978;2:73–81.
19. Barton JR, Stanziano G, Sibai BM: Monitored outpatient management of mild gestational hypertension remote from term. *Am J Obstet Gynecol* 1994;170:765–769.
20. Helewa M, Heaman M, Robinson M-A, Thompson L: Community-based home-care program for the management of pre-eclampsia: An alternative. *Can Med Assoc J* 1993;149:829–834.
21. Horsager R, Adams M, Richey S, et al: Outpatient management of mild pregnancy-induced hypertension. *Am J Obstet Gynecol* 1995;172:383.
22. Tuffnell DJ, Lilford RJ, Buchan PC, et al: Randomized controlled trial of day care for hypertension in pregnancy. *Lancet* 1992;339:224–227.

23. López-Llera M: Complicated eclampsia: Fifteen years' experience in a referral medical center. *Am J Obstet Gynecol* 1982;142:28–35.
24. Miles JF, Martin JN Jr, Blake PG, et al: Postpartum eclampsia: A recurring perinatal dilemma. *Obstet Gynecol* 1990;76:328–331.
25. Cunningham FG, Pritchard JA: How should hypertension during pregnancy be managed? Experience at Parkland Memorial Hospital. *Med Clin North Am* 1984;68:505–526.
26. Cantrell DC, Cunningham FG: Epilepsy complicating pregnancy. In: *Williams' Obstetrics,* ed 19 (suppl #8). Norwalk, CT: Appleton & Lange; 1994.
27. Brown CEL, Purdy PD, Cunningham FG: Head computed tomographic scans in women with eclampsia. *Am J Obstet Gynecol* 1988;159:915–920.
28. Cunningham FG, Fernandez CO, Hernandez C: Blindness associated with preeclampsia and eclampsia. *Am J Obstet Gynecol* 1995;172:1291–1298.
29. Pritchard JA, Cunningham FG, Pritchard SA: The Parkland Memorial Hospital protocol for treatment of eclampsia: Evaluation of 245 cases. *Am J Obstet Gynecol* 1984;148:951–963.
30. Bhalla AK, Dhall GI, Dhall K: A safer and more effective treatment regimen for eclampsia. *Aust NZ J Obstet Gynaecol* 1994;34:144–148.
31. Eclampsia Trial Collaborative Group: Which anticonvulsant for women with eclampsia? Evidence from the collaborative eclampsia trial. *Lancet* 1995;345:1455–1463.
32. Singh GK, Kochaneb KD, MacDorman MF: Advance report of the final mortality statistics, 1994. Monthly vital statistics report. Hyattsville, MD: National Center for Health Statistics; 1996:vol 45, no 3(suppl).
33. Sibai BM: Hypertension in pregnancy. In: Gabbe SG, Niebyl JR, Simpson JL, eds. *Obstetrics, Normal and Problem Pregnancies,* ed 3. New York: Churchill Livingstone; 1996:961 (chap 28).
34. Chesley LC, Tepper I: Plasma levels of magnesium attained in magnesium sulfate therapy for preeclampsia and eclampsia. *Surg Clin North Am* 1957 (April);353–360.
35. Stone SR, Pritchard JA: Effect of maternally administered magnesium sulfate on the neonate. *Obstet Gynecol* 1970;35:574–578.
36. Sibai BM, Graham JM, McCubbin JH: A comparison of intravenous and intramuscular magnesium sulfate regimens in preeclampsia. *Am J Obstet Gynecol* 1984;150:728–733.
37. Somjen G, Hilmy M, Stephen CR: Failure to anesthetize human subjects by intravenous administration of magnesium sulfate. *J Pharmacol Exp Ther* 1966;154:652–659.
38. McCubbin JH, Sibai BM, Abdella TN, Anderson GD: Cardiopulmonary arrest due to acute maternal hypermagnesemia. *Lancet* 1981;1:1058–1059.
39. Cotton DB, Longmire S, Jones MM, et al: Cardiovascular alterations in severe pregnancy-induced hypertension: Effects of intravenous nitroglycerin coupled with blood volume expansion. *Am J Obstet Gynecol* 1986;154:1053–1059.
40. Watson KV, Moldow CF, Ogburn PL, Jacob JS: Magnesium sulfate: Rationale for its use in preeclampsia. *Proc Natl Acad Sci USA* 1986;83:1075–1078.
41. Leaphart WL, Meyer MC, Capeless EL, Tracy PB: Adenosine diphosphate-induced platelet activation inhibited by magnesium in a dose-dependent manner. *Obstet Gynecol* 1998;91:421–425.
42. O'Brien WF, Williams MC, Benoit R, et al: The effect of magnesium sulfate infusion on systemic and renal prostacyclin production. *Prostaglandins* 1990;40:529–538.
43. Hsu CD, Hong SF, Chung YK, Copel JA: Effect of magnesium sulfate on nitric oxide levels in preeclamptic pregnancy. *Am J Obstet Gynecol* 1996;174:450–456.
44. Thurnau GR, Kemp DB, Jarvis A: Cerebrospinal fluid levels of magnesium in patients with preeclampsia after treatment with intravenous magnesium sulfate: A preliminary report. *Am J Obstet Gynecol* 1987;157:1435–1438.
45. Fong J, Gurewitsch ED, Vlpe L, et al: Baseline serum and cerebrospinal fluid magnesium levels in normal pregnancy and preeclampsia. *Obstet Gynecol* 1995;85:444–448.
46. Lipton SA, Rosenberg PA: Excitatory amino acids as a final common pathway for neurologic disorders. *N Engl J Med* 1994;330:613–622.
47. Cotton DB, Janusz CA, Berman RF: Anticonvulsant effects of magnesium sulfate on hippocampal seizures: Therapeutic implications in preeclampsia-eclampsia. *Am J Obstet Gynecol* 1992;166:1127–1134.

48. Hallak M, Hotca JW, Evans JB: Magnesium sulfate affects the n-methyl-D-aspartate receptor binding in maternal rat brain. *Am J Obstet Gynecol* 1998;178:S112.

49. Leveno KJ, Alexander JM, McIntire DD, Lucas MJ: Does magnesium sulfate given for prevention of eclampsia affect the outcome of labor? *Am J Obstet Gynecol* 1998;178:707–711.

50. Atkinson MW, Guinn D, Owen J, Hauth JC: Does magnesium sulfate affect the length of labor induction in women with pregnancy-associated hypertension. *Am J Obstet Gynecol* 1995;173:1219–1222.

51. Witlin AG, Friedman SA, Sibai BM: The effect of magnesium sulfate therapy on the duration of labor in women with mild preeclampsia at term: A randomized, double-blind, placebo-controlled trial. *Am J Obstet Gynecol* 1997;176:623–627.

52. Watt-Morse ML, Caritis SN, Kridgen PL: Magnesium sulfate is a poor inhibitor of oxytocin-induced contractility in pregnant sheep. *J Maternal Fetal Med* 1995;4:139–143.

53. Mizuki J, Tasaka K, Masumoio N, et al: Magnesium sulfate inhibits oxytocin induced calcium mobilization in human puerperal myometrial cells: Possible involvement of intracellular free magnesium concentration. *Am J Obstet Gynecol* 1993;109:134–139.

54. Hallak M, Berry SM, Madincea F, et al: Fetal serum and amniotic fluid magnesium concentrations with maternal treatment. *Obstet Gynecol* 1993;81:185–188.

55. Guzman ER, Conley M, Steward R, et al: Phenytoin and magnesium sulfate effects on fetal heart rate tracings assessed by computer analysis. *Obstet Gynecol* 1993;82:375–379.

56. Gray SE, Rodis JF, Lettieri L, et al: Effect of intravenous magnesium sulfate on the biophysical profile of the healthy preterm fetus. *Am J Obstet Gynecol* 1994;170:1131–1136.

57. Green KW, Key TC, Coen R, Resnik R: The effects of maternally administered magnesium sulfate on the neonate. *Am J Obstet Gynecol* 1983;146:29–33.

58. Nelson KB, Grether JK: Can magnesium sulfate reduce the risk of cerebral palsy in very low birthweight infants? *Pediatrics* 1995;95:263–269.

59. Schendel DE, Berg CJ, Yeargin-Allsopp M, et al: Prenatal magnesium sulfate exposure and the risk for cerebral palsy or mental retardation among very low birthweight children aged 3 to 5 years. *JAMA* 1996;276:1805–1810.

60. Murphy DJ, Sellers S, Mackenzie IZ, et al: Case-control study of antenatal and intrapartum risk factors for cerebral palsy in very preterm singleton babies. *Lancet* 1995;346:449–454.

61. Kimberlin DF, Hauth JC, Goldenberg RL, et al: The effect of maternal $MgSO_4$ treatment on neonatal morbidity in $\leq$ 1000g neonates. *Am J Obstet Gynecol* 1996;174:469–472.

62. Duley L, Johanson R: Magnesium sulphate for preeclampsia and eclampsia: The evidence so far. *Br J Obstet Gynaecol* 1994;101:565–568.

63. Ramsay MM, Rimoy GH, Rubin PC: Are anticonvulsants necessary to prevent eclampsia? *Lancet* 1994;343:540–541.

64. Lucas MJ, Leveno KJ, Cunningham FG: A comparison of magnesium sulfate with phenytoin for the prevention of eclampsia. *N Engl J Med* 1995;333:201–205.

65. Neilson JP: Magnesium sulphate: The drug of choice in eclampsia. *Br Med J* 1995;311:702–703.

66. Robson SC: Magnesium sulphate: The timing of reckoning. *Br J Obstet Gynaecol* 1996;103:99–102.

67. Burrows RF, Burrows EA: The feasibility of a control population for a randomized control trial of seizure prophylaxis in the hypertensive disorders of pregnancy. *Am J Obstet Gynecol* 1995;173:929–935.

68. Cunningham FG, Leveno KJ: Management of pregnancy-induced hypertension. In: Rubin PC, ed. *Handbook of Hypertension. Vol X. Hypertension in Pregnancy.* Amsterdam: Elsevier Science; 1988:290–298.

69. Lindheimer MD: Preeclampsia-eclampsia 1996: Preventable? Have disputes on its treatment been resolved? *Curr Opin Nephrol Hypertens* 1996;5:452–458.

70. Sibai BM: Treatment of hypertension in pregnant women. *N Engl J Med* 1996;335:257–265.

70a. Belfort MA, Anthony J, Carrillo JF, et al: $MgSO_4$ is an effective antihypertensive agent in preeclampsia. *Am J Obstet Gynecol* 1999 (in press).

71. Cunningham FG, Lindheimer MD: Hypertension in pregnancy. Current concepts. *N Engl J Med* 1992;326:927–932.

72. Hutton JD, James DK, Stirrat GM, et al: Management of severe pre-eclampsia and eclampsia by UK consultants. *Br J Obstet Gynaecol* 1992;99:554–556.

73. Redman CWG, Roberts JM: Management of pre-eclampsia. *Lancet* 1993;341:1451–1454.
74. Paterson-Brown S, Robson SC, Redfern N, De Swiet M: Hydralazine boluses for the treatment of severe hypertension in pre-eclampsia. *Br J Obstet Gynaecol* 1994;101:409–413.
75. Mabie WC, Gonzalez AR, Sibai BM, Amon E: A comparative trial of labetalol and hydralazine in the acute management of severe hypertension complicating pregnancy. *Obstet Gynecol* 1987;70:328–333.
76. Belfort MA, Anthony J, Buccimazza A, Davey DA: Hemodynamic changes associated with intravenous infusion of the calcium antagonist verapamil in the treatment of severe gestational proteinuric hypertension. *Obstet Gynecol* 1990;75:970–974.
77. Scardo JA, Vermillion ST, Hogg BB, Newman RB: Hemodynamic effects of oral nifedipine in preeclamptic hypertensive emergencies. *Am J Obstet Gynecol* 1996;175:336–338.
78. Mabie WC, Sibai BM, Anderson GD, et al: Nifedipine in the treatment of severe peripartum hypertension. Presented at the Eighth Annual Meeting of the Society of Perinatal Obstetricians. Las Vegas, February 1988; abstract 87.
79. Grossman E, Messerli FH, Grodzicki T, Kowey P: Should a moratorium be placed on sublingual nifedipine capsules given for hypertensive emergencies and pseudoemergencies? *JAMA* 1996;276:1328–1331.
80. Belfort MA, Taskin O, Buhur A, et al: Intravenous nimodipine in the management of severe preeclampsia: Double blind, randomized, controlled clinical trial. *Am J Obstet Gynecol* 1996;174:451–457.
81. Belfort M, Anthony J, Saade G and the Nimodipine Study Group: Interim report of the nimodipine vs. magnesium sulfate for seizure prophylaxis in severe preeclampsia study: An international, randomized, controlled trial. *Am J Obstet Gynecol* 1998;178:S7.
82. Bolte AC, Gafar S, van Eyck J, et al: Ketanserin, a better option in the treatment of preeclampsia? *Am J Obstet Gynecol* 1998;178:S118.
82a. Ascarelli MH, Johnson V, McCreary H, et al: Adjunctive postpartive treatment of preeclampsia with furosemide. *Am J Obstet Gynecol* 1999 (in press).
83. Martin JN Jr, Files JC, Blake PG, et al: Postpartum plasma exchange for atypical preeclampsia–eclampsia as HELLP (hemolysis, elevated liver enzymes, and low platelets) syndrome. *Am J Obstet Gynecol* 1995;172:1107–1125.
84. Egerman R, Sibai BM (letter). *Am J Obstet Gynecol* 1997;176:1397.
85. Dashe JS, Ramin SM, Cunningham FG: The long-term consequences of thrombotic microangiopathy (thrombotic thrombocytopenic purpura and hemolytic uremic syndrome) in pregnancy. *Obstet Gynecol* 1998;91:662–668.
86. Benedetti TJ, Quilligan EJ: Cerebral edema in severe pregnancy-induced hypertension. *Am J Obstet Gynecol* 1980;137:860–862.
87. Gedekoh RH, Hayashi TT, MacDonald HM: Eclampsia at Magee–Women's Hospital, 1970–1980. *Am J Obstet Gynecol* 1981;140:860–866.
88. Sibai BM, Mabie BC, Harvey CJ, Gonzalez AR: Pulmonary edema in severe preeclampsia–eclampsia: Analysis of thirty-seven consecutive cases. *Am J Obstet Gynecol* 1987;156:1174–1179.
89. Benedetti TJ, Kates R, Williams V: Hemodynamic observations in severe preeclampsia complicated by pulmonary edema. *Am J Obstet Gynecol* 1985;152:330–334.
90. Cunningham FG, Pritchard JA, Hankins GDV, et al: Peripartum heart failure: Idiopathic cardiomyopathy or compounding cardiovascular events? *Obstet Gynecol* 1986;67:157–168.
91. Benedetti TJ, Carlson RW: Studies of colloid osmotic pressure in pregnancy-induced hypertension. *Am J Obstet Gynecol* 1979;135:308–311.
92. Zinaman M, Rubin J, Lindheimer MD: Serial plasma oncotic pressure levels and echoencephalography during and after delivery in severe preeclampsia. *Lancet* 1985;1:1245–1247.
93. Øian P, Maltau JM, Noddleland H, Fadnes HO: Transcapillary fluid balance in preeclampsia. *Br J Obstet Gynaecol* 1986;93:235–239.
94. Brown MA, Zammit VC, Lowe SA: Capillary permeability and extracellular fluid volumes in pregnancy-induced hypertension. *Clin Sci* 1989;77:599–604.
95. Bhatia RK, Bottoms SF, Saleh AA, et al: Mechanisms for reduced colloid osmotic pressure in preeclampsia. *Am J Obstet Gynecol* 1987;157:106–108.
95a. Terrone DA, Isler CM, May WL, et al: Cardiopulmonary morbidity as a complication of severe preeclampsia HELLP syndrome. *Am J Obstet Gynecol* (in press).

95b. Mattar FM, Usta I, Sibai BM: Eclampsia risk factors for maternal mortality and morbidity. *Am J Obstet Gynecol* 1999 (in press).

96. Lehmann DK, Mabie WC, Miller JM Jr, Pernoll ML: The epidemiology and pathology of maternal mortality: Charity Hospital of Louisiana in New Orleans, 1965–1984. *Obstet Gynecol* 1987;69:833–840.

97. Nolan TE, Wakefield ML, Devoe LD: Invasive hemodynamic monitoring in obstetrics. A critical review of its indications, benefits, complications, and alternatives. *Chest* 1992;101:1429–1433.

98. Hankins GDV, Cunningham FG: Severe preeclampsia and eclampsia: Controversies in management. In: *Williams' Obstetrics*, ed 18 (suppl #12). Norwalk, CT: Appleton & Lange; 1991.

99. Clark SL, Cotton DB: Clinical indications for pulmonary artery catheterization in the patient with severe preeclampsia. *Am J Obstet Gynecol* 1988;158:453–458.

100. American College of Obstetricians and Gynecologists: *Invasive Hemodynamic Monitoring in Obstetrics and Gynecology.* October 1988; Tech Bull No. 121.

101. American College of Obstetricians and Gynecologists: *Hypertension in Pregnancy.* January 1996; Tech Bull No. 219.

102. Cowles T, Saleh A, Cotton DB: Hypertensive disorders in pregnancy. In: James DK, Steer PJ, Weiner CP, Gonik B, eds. *High Risk Pregnancy. Management Options.* London; Saunders; 1994; 253 (chap 18).

103. Easterling TR, Benedetti TJ, Schmucker BC, Carlson KL: Antihypertensive therapy in pregnancy directed by noninvasive hemodynamic monitoring. *Am J Perinatol* 1989;6:86–89.

104. Mabie WC, Ratts TE, Ramanathan KB, Sibai BM: Circulatory congestion in obese hypertensive women: A subset of pulmonary edema in pregnancy. *Obstet Gynecol* 1988;72:553–558.

105. Montan S, Ingemarsson I: Intrapartum fetal heart rate patterns in pregnancies complicated by hypertension. *Am J Obstet Gynecol* 1989;160:283–288.

106. Gutsche BB, Cheek TG: Anesthesia considerations in preeclampsia–eclampsia. In: Shnider SM, Levinson G, eds. *Anesthesia for Obstetrics*, ed 3. Baltimore: Williams & Wilkins; 1993:321.

107. Fox EJ, Sklar GS, Hill CH, et al: Complications related to the pressor response to endotracheal intubation. *Anesthesiology* 1977;47:524–525.

108. Lavies NG, Meiklejohn BH, May AE, et al: Hypertensive and catecholamine response to tracheal intubation in patients with pregnancy-induced hypertension. *Br J Anaesth* 1989;63: 429–434.

109. Hodgkinson R, Husain FJ, Hayashi RH: Systemic and pulmonary blood pressure during caesarean section in parturients with gestational hypertension. *Can Anaesth Soc J* 1980;27: 389–394.

110. Morgan M: Anaesthetic contribution to maternal mortality. *Br J Anaesth* 1987;59:842–855.

111. Chadwick HS, Easterling T: Anesthetic concerns in the patient with preeclampsia. *Semin Perinatol* 1991;15:397–409.

112. Turnbull A, Tindall VR, Beard RW: *Report on Confidential Enquiries into Maternal Deaths in England and Wales.* 1982–84. London: Her Majesty's Stationary Office, 1989.

113. Wallace DH, Leveno KJ, Cunningham FG, et al: Randomized comparison of general and regional anesthesia for cesarean delivery in pregnancies complicated by severe preeclampsia. *Obstet Gynecol* 1995;86:193–199.

114. Ramanathan J: Anesthetic considerations in preeclampsia. *Clin Perinatol* 1991;18:875–889.

115. Lucas MJ, Sharma S, McIntire D, et al: A randomized trial of epidural analgesia on pregnancy-induced hypertension. *Am J Obstet Gynecol* 1999 (in press).

116. Newsome LR, Bramwell RS, Curling PE: Severe preeclampsia: Hemodynamic effects of lumbar epidural anesthesia. *Anesth Analg* 1986;65:31–36.

117. Hankins GDV, Wendel GD, Cunningham FG, Leveno KJ: Longitudinal evaluation of hemodynamic changes in eclampsia. *Am J Obstet Gynecol* 1984:150:506–512.

118. Clark SL, Divon MY, Phelan JP: Preeclampsia/eclampsia: Hemodynamic and neurologic correlations. *Obstet Gynecol* 1985;66:337–340.

119. Cotton DB, Jones MM, Longmire S, et al: Role of intravenous nitroglycerine in the treatment of severe pregnancy-induced hypertension complicated by pulmonary edema. *Am J Obstet Gynecol* 1986;154:91–93.

120. Heller PJ, Scheider EP, Marx GF: Pharyngo-laryngeal edema as a presenting symptom in preeclampsia. *Obstet Gynecol* 1983;62:523–525.

18

Antihypertensive Treatment

Jason G. Umans and Marshall D. Lindheimer

In the first edition of this text, discussion of antihypertensive therapy in pregnancy was mainly historical; the drugs noted included veratrum alkaloids, opium and its derivatives, a host of sedatives, and even spinal anesthesia (it was often unclear in this old literature whether drugs had been prescribed for hypertension per se or to treat an eclamptic convulsion). More emphasis, however, was given to diuretics (which were vehemently opposed by Chesley), and to the recurring theme that hypertension in preeclampsia might paradoxically be treated by volume expansion. Space prohibits republishing these historical vignettes, which bear rereading. It is of interest though, that use of veratrum viride was incorporated into the treatment of eclampsia even before physicians were aware that a rise of blood pressure accompanied the "puerperal convulsion." Also, for many years, use of veratrum was called the "Brooklyn treatment," which is noted here for two minor reasons: Chesley spent most of his career on the faculty of the State University of New York in Brooklyn, and both authors of this chapter were born there.

There are several reasons for the paucity of information on antihypertensive treatment during pregnancy in this text's first edition. Effective and tolerable drugs to lower blood pressure are a phenomenon of the last three decades. Before then, many considered hypertension as "protective," the increased pressure needed to perfuse vital organs such as the kidney in the setting of arteriosclerosis. This view persisted longer in the pregnancy literature, where it was feared that lowering of blood pressure would lead to decreased placental perfusion, and that blood flow bringing nutrients to the fetus was already compromised. This topic will be addressed further below. More important, was the absence of multicenter randomized trials of a scale large enough to assess the safety and efficacy of specific antihypertensive medications during pregnancy, including risks of congenital anomalies and follow-up data on neonates. This, too, will be revisited below. Of interest, though, a landmark study by Redman et al. reporting their randomized trial of methyldopa to treat chronic hypertension in pregnant women,[1] appeared in 1976, and was noted by Chesley. This report, followed later by periodic evaluation of the offspring for an additional 7.5 years, focused attention on the need for appropriate trials in pregnant women, heralding a rash of literature during the 1980s and continuing through the present. Many of these studies will be reviewed below.

GOALS OF ANTIHYPERTENSIVE DRUG THERAPY

The availability of safe and effective antihypertensive drugs permits an operational definition of hypertension, independent of those derived from evaluation of the normal distribution of blood pressures within the population or from associations with morbid sequelae at different levels of pressure. Now, hypertension could be defined as a level of arterial pressure whose pharmacologic control would improve outcome for the population at risk. In nonpregnant adults, blood pressure control can decrease the *long-term* incidence of stroke, coronary heart disease, congestive heart failure, and cardiovascular mortality.[2] Each of these morbid outcomes (and others, such as hypertensive nephrosclerosis) is due only in part to hypertension per se; risk is also attributable to smoking, dyslipidemia, diabetes mellitus, race, age, sex, and familial predisposition. In addition to these comorbidities, the ability to detect improved outcome due to blood pressure control also depends on the severity of hypertension (and the presence of target organ damage),[3] the completeness of blood pressure control,[4] and perhaps the pathophysiology leading to hypertension and the drugs used to treat it.[2] For example, treatment trials have been most easily designed to show decreases in stroke incidence in patients with severe hypertension; much larger, longer, or more restrictively designed trials were required to show benefits for coronary disease or in patients with only mild or moderate hypertension.

Hypertension in pregnant women is different. Here, the major goals of treatment are to safeguard the mother from *acute* dangers or irreversible insults during or immediately after the pregnancy while delivering a healthy infant. In this respect, one balances *short-term* maternal outcome against possible *long-term* consequences of intrauterine drug exposure on fetal and childhood growth and development. While comorbidities such as diabetes mellitus, target organ dysfunction at baseline, and (uncommon) secondary causes of hypertension may certainly interact with maternal hypertension and alter strategies for its control, these concerns will not apply to most hypertensive gravidas. The majority of women with blood pressures high enough to warrant treatment during pregnancy will either have chronic essential hypertension or preeclampsia leading to threatening levels of pressure which occur when there are compelling reasons to extend the length of the pregnancy. It should be noted that the balance of risks and benefits for antihypertensive therapy will differ for women with chronic hypertension present from early in gestation, whose fetuses may have greater drug exposure during early stages of development, compared with women who develop hypertension (either transient hypertension or preeclampsia) closer to term. Well-designed and adequately powered trials, of which there are *shamefully few,* need to account for this clinical heterogeneity. Maternal risks which may justify pharmacotherapy include that of super-imposed preeclampsia which, with its morbid outcomes, appears to account for most complications ascribed to chronic hypertension.[5] Additional risks are those of placental abruption, accelerated hypertension leading to hospitalization or to target organ damage, and cerebrovascular catastrophe. Risks to the fetus include death, growth restriction, and early delivery, the latter occurring in many cases due to concerns regarding maternal safety.

GENERAL PRINCIPLES IN THE CHOICE OF ANTIHYPERTENSIVE AGENTS

Blood pressure, in its simplest conceptualization, is determined as the product of cardiac output and systemic vascular resistance. The latter is sensitive to the structure of small arterial and arteriolar resistance vessels, activity of local vasodilator and vasoconstrictor systems, humoral influences such as the renin–angiotensin system, and the activity of the autonomic nervous system. The former is most sensitive to changes in volume status and autonomic tone; other influences on intrinsic myocardial contractility are usually minor in healthy women. These physiologic targets, sometimes obscured in the chronic state by vascular autoregulation or our limited ability to measure relevant volumes or pressures with precision,[6] provide the rationale for each of the available pharmacologic strategies for control of hypertension. Further, due to the homeostatic nature of blood pressure control, even when pathologically elevated, this simple physiologic construct suggests likely mechanisms of apparent resistance to antihypertensive drugs, especially when used as single agents. In nonpregnant hypertensives, choice of a specific antihypertensive drug is usually rationalized by the severity of hypertension and immediate risk of end-organ damage, the desired time–action characteristics of the drug, specific comorbidities, spectrum of possible adverse drug effects, cost, and known secondary causes of the hypertension. As well, therapy can be based on outcomes of well-conducted, large clinical trials or on broad, population-based assumptions regarding the likely physiologic mechanisms leading to hypertension in a given patient. Following is a brief review of the above considerations, which should be tempered by the knowledge that, in mild-to-moderate hypertension, most available agents appear effective in a similar proportion of patients when used as monotherapy, and most hypertension can be adequately controlled by a combination of two rationally paired drugs.

In nonpregnant adults with hypertensive emergencies (systolic BP ≥ 200 mm Hg or diastolic BP ≥ 120 mm Hg, or lower values with evolving target organ damage), blood pressure is usually controlled acutely, albeit only to a target of ~160 mm Hg systolic so as not to compromise organ perfusion, by use of rapidly and short-acting, easily titrated parenteral agents. These include sodium nitroprusside (a nitric oxide donor), enalaprilat (an ACE inhibitor), hydralazine (a direct vasodilator), diazoxide (a potassium channel-activating hyperpolarizing vasodilator), labetalol (a combined α- and β-adrenergic antagonist), nicardipine (a dihydropyridine calcium entry blocker), and fenoldopam (a specific dopamine-receptor antagonist). Short-acting (i.e., immediate-release) oral or sublingual nifedipine, used until recently for acute blood pressure control, is often avoided due to concerns by many regarding unpredictable hypotensive responses, excessive autonomic activation, and precipitation of acute myocardial ischemia. Results of large randomized controlled trials provide compelling evidence that angiotensin-converting enzyme (ACE) inhibitors should be the cornerstone of antihypertensive therapy in nonpregnant patients with established diabetic nephropathy because they significantly slow the progression of renal failure.[7] Extrapolation from these findings and the results of other studies support the use of these drugs in diabetic patients with less evident nephropathy or in patients with proteinuric nondiabetic renal insufficiency;[8] similar reasoning supports use of angiotensin-receptor antagonists in such patients who are intolerant of ACE inhibitors. Similarly strong evidence supports the use of β-blockers (lacking intrinsic sympathomimetic activity) to prevent death in patients who have suffered a myocardial infarction[9] and the use of ACE inhibitors in postmyocardial infarction patients with systolic dysfunction.[10] ACE inhibitors prolong survival and improve functional status in patients with (systolic) congestive heart failure irrespective of hypertension;[11] angiotensin antagonists may act similarly.[12] Finally, diuretics appear especially efficacious in avoiding a variety of morbid complications in patients with isolated systolic hypertension, especially in the elderly;[13] in at least one large prospective trial[14] this benefit was not shared by β-blockers.

In the absence of compelling data from controlled trials, drug choice may be influenced by reasoned extrapolation of the impact of known pharmacology of specific antihypertensive agents on medical comorbidities in individual patients. For example, β-blockers, even those with claims of β_1 selectivity, are routinely avoided in asthmatic patients due to their ability to provoke bronchospasm. Similarly, these agents are avoided in some patients due to exacerbation of systolic heart failure (except carvedilol), their ability to mask autonomic symptoms of hypoglycemia in diabetics, and their capacity to worsen atrial–ventricular conduction defects. Conversely, β-blockers are rational agents in hypertensive patients also suffering from angina, supraventricular tachyarrythmias, benign essential tremor, or migraine, as they are often useful in these conditions when hypertension is absent. Likewise, thiazide diuretics are reasonably avoided in some patients due to their capacity to exacerbate hyperuricemia and gout, to impair glucose tolerance, or to worsen hypercalcemia in patients with primary hyperparathyroidism. Potassium-sparing diuretics, ACE inhibtors, or angiotensin antagonists are all reasonably avoided in patients with a potassium excretory defect, most commonly due to hyperkalemic distal renal tubular acidosis and associated with diabetes mellitus, sickle-cell nephropathy, or obstructive uropathy.

In general, hypertension in young men is more often associated with increased cardiac output and is responsive to monotherapy with β-blockers.[15] Likewise, in spite of a striking lack of conformity in the clinical assessment of salt sensitivity,[16] African Americans and elderly women more often manifest low-renin hypertension, relative defects in the renal excretion of a salt load, or enhanced blood pressure increments with volume expansion. It is not surprising that these groups demonstrate a greater tendency to effective blood pressure control with diuretic or calcium entry blocker monotherapy, with lesser rates of response to β-blockers or ACE inhibitors.[17] In spite of these population differences, careful titration of even haphazardly selected antihypertensive drugs usually leads to acceptable blood pressure control in individual patients, casting some doubt on the importance of such "physiologically based" drug choice strategies in the absence of outcome data from well-designed prospective treatment trials.

FETAL SAFETY AND DRUG USE IN PREGNANT WOMEN

While new regulations are beginning to encourage testing of some drugs in pregnant women,[18] such clinical information is generally unavailable for most currently prescribed agents. Indeed, rigorous evaluation of pharmacokinetics, biotransformation, maternal efficacy, fetal exposure, and long-term fetal effects of drugs used during pregnancy are generally lacking. Available information, save for assessment of teratogenicity in laboratory animals, is limited and selective. The US Food and Drug Administration (FDA) encourages use of its classification scheme to categorize potential fetal risks (Table 18–1), though there are plans to modify this scheme within the next few years.

TABLE 18–1. US FOOD AND DRUG ADMINISTRATION CLASSIFICATION OF DRUG RISK IN PREGNANCY[a]

Category A	Controlled studies in women fail to demonstrate risk to the fetus in the first trimester, and there is no evidence of risk in later trimesters. The possibility of fetal harm appears remote.
Category B	Either animal reproduction studies have not demonstrated a fetal risk but no controlled studies have been performed in pregnant women, or animal reproduction studies have shown an adverse effect (other than a decrease in fertility) that was not confirmed in controlled studies in women in the first trimester. There is no evidence of risk in later trimesters.
Category C	Either studies in animals have revealed adverse effects on the fetus (teratogenic or embryocidal effects or other) and there are no controlled studies in women, or studies in women and animals are not available. Drugs should only be given if the potential benefit justifies the potential risk to the fetus.
Category D	There is positive evidence of human fetal risk, but the benefits of use in pregnant women may be acceptable despite the risk (e.g., if the drug is needed in a life-threatening situation or for a serious disease for which safer drugs cannot be used or are ineffective). There is an appropriate statement in the "warnings" section of the labeling.
Category X	Studies in animals or humans have demonstrated fetal abnormalities, or there is evidence of fetal risk based on human experience, or both, and the risk of the use of the drug in pregnant women clearly outweighs any possible benefit. The drug is contraindicated in women who are or may become pregnant. There is an appropriate statement in the "contraindications" section of the labeling.

[a] Plans have been made to modify this classification within the next 2 years.

Unfortunately, because data from human and animal studies are so limited, most drugs are listed in FDA category C, with the caveat that they should be used only if potential benefit justifies the potential risk to the fetus. This category is so broad as to be considered useless; it includes those antihypertensive drugs with the greatest history of safe use in pregnant women but, until only 6 years ago also included the ACE inhibitors, which are contraindicated in pregnancy. Indeed, we would classify these latter agents as category X (rather than D). Even when drugs are placed in category B, their presumed safety may be a function of the insensitivity of animal tests to predict subtle clinical effects, such as fetal ability to withstand hypoxic stress, changes in functional physiologic development, and altered postnatal neurocognitive development. Limited evidence of clinical safety is often extended injudiciously, such that drugs that lack teratogenic potential in early pregnancy may exert devastating effects on fetal organ function nearer to term; conversely, drugs that are safe in the third trimester may have irreversible effects on fetal growth or development when used earlier. By contrast, one can easily err too strongly against drug use in pregnancy, as when discontinuation of required category D drugs might jeopardize both mother and fetus. Examples of this latter scenario would include the mistake of discontinuing immunosuppressives in a pregnant renal transplant recipient or of prophylactic agents in a pregnant woman with a seizure disorder. Therefore, we include FDA classifications for each of the drugs discussed below, stressing however the need to take all clinical information into account when making a prescribing decision in a particular patient.

CHOICE OF AN ANTIHYPERTENSIVE DRUG FOR USE IN PREGNANCY

Following this background on the rationale for choosing an antihypertensive drug, we now turn to consideration of each of the classes of agents available in common practice. *Below, we consider each of these drug classes, their apparent mechanisms of action, and in terms of this chapter's primary goals, their suitability for use during pregnancy.*

Sympathetic Nervous System Inhibition

The modern era of effective antihypertensive therapy was heralded by introduction of agents to decrease peripheral activity of the sympathetic nervous system. Strategies for sympathoinhibition have included ganglionic blockade (using drugs such as guanethidine), depletion of norepinephrine from sympathetic nerve terminals (with agents such as reserpine, the first antihypertensive to have proven benefit in a prospective clinical trial[19]), use of α_2-adrenergic agonists to decrease sympathetic outflow from the central nervous system (e.g., α-methlydopa, clonidine), and use of specific antagonists of α- or β-adrenergic receptors (e.g., α-antagonists: prazosin, terazosin, doxazosin; β-blockers: propranolol, atenolol, metoprolol; combined α/β-antagonists: labetalol, carvedilol). Figure 18–1 shows a physiologic scheme for sym-

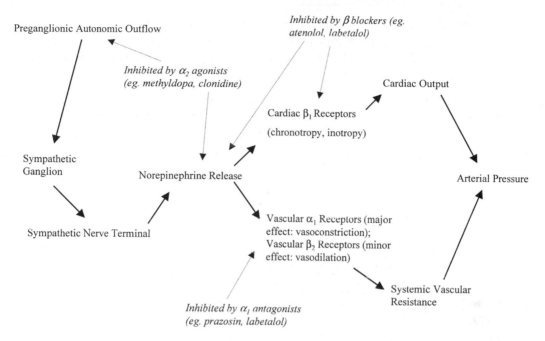

Figure 18–1. Scheme showing major influences of sympathetic nervous system on physiologic determinants of arterial pressure. Bold arrows denote endogenous mechanisms leading from central nervous system to maintenance of blood pressure. Dotted arrows show sites at which sympatholytic antihypertensive drugs used in pregnancy might exert their effects.

pathetic nervous system influences on arterial pressure, along with sites of action for drugs such as α_2-adrenergic agonists and peripheral adrenergic antagonists, which remain widely used in pregnancy.

Centrally Acting α_2-Adrenergic Agonists

Methyldopa (the prototypical agent of this class) is a prodrug metabolized to α-methylnorepinephrine, which then replaces norepinephrine in the neurosecretory vesicles of adrenergic nerve terminals. Since its efficacy is equivalent to that of norepinephrine at peripheral alpha-1 receptors, vasoconstriction is unimpaired. Centrally, however, it is resistant to degradation by monoamine oxidase, resulting in enhanced effect at the alpha-2 sites which govern sympathetic outflow. Decreased sympathetic tone reduces systemic vascular resistance, accompanied by only minor decrements in cardiac output, at least in young, otherwise healthy hypertensive patients. Blood pressure control is gradual, over 6 to 8 hours, due to the indirect mechanism of action. There do not appear to be significant decreases in renin and, while the hypotensive effect is greater in the upright than supine posture, orthostatic hypotension is usually minor. Clonidine, a selective α_2-agonist acts similarly.

Adverse effects are mostly predictable consequences of central α_2-agonism or decreased peripheral sympathetic tone. These drugs act at sites in the brainstem to decrease mental alertness, impair sleep, lead to a sense of fatigue or depression in some patients, and decrease salivation, resulting in xerostomia. Peripheral sympatho-inhibition may impair cardiac conduction in susceptible patients. Methyldopa can induce hyperprolactinemia and Parkinsonian signs in some patients. In addition, it can cause some potentially serious dose-independent adverse effects. Approximately 5% of patients receiving methyldopa will have elevated liver enzymes, with some manifesting frank hepatitis and, rarely, hepatic necrosis. Likewise, many patients will develop a positive antiglobulin (Coombs') test with chronic use, a small fraction of these progressing to hemolytic anemia.

Pregnancy

Methyldopa, which has been assessed in a number of prospective trials in pregnant women, compared with placebo[1,20,21] or with alternative hypotensive agents,[20,22-25] is unique in that careful studies have also assessed remote development of children exposed to this drug in utero.[26] Methyldopa remains the agent of choice for nonemergent blood pressure control during pregnancy since no "modern" antihypertensive has proven more efficacious or better tolerated, and no other drug possesses a comparable history of clinical safety, bolstered by prospective long-term follow-up. Indeed, observations of increased sympathetic nerve activity to the skeletal muscle vasculature in preeclamptic women, reverting to normal along with blood pressure after delivery,[27] now lends a compelling physiologic rationale to control of preeclamptic hypertension with agents that decrease sympathetic outflow.

Treatment with methyldopa decreases the subsequent incidence of severe hypertension[28] and is well tolerated by the mother without any apparent adverse effects on uteroplacental or fetal hemodynamics[29] or on fetal well being.[20] One placebo-controlled trial (> 200 women with diastolic BP > 90 mm Hg at entry) noted fewer midpregnancy losses in patients randomized to methyldopa;[1] this observation was not confirmed in a more recent trial of similar size.[20] It is important to note that birth weight, neonatal complications, and development during the first year were similar in children exposed to methlydopa compared with those in the placebo group.[30,31] While Cockburn et al.[26] noted somewhat smaller head circumference at 7 years of age in the subset of male offspring exposed to methyldopa at 16 to 20 weeks' gestation, these children exhibited intelligence and neurocognitive development similar to controls.

Studies of clonidine have been more limited; one third-trimester comparative trial vs. methyldopa showed similar efficacy and tolerability,[24] while a small, controlled follow-up study of 22 neonates reported an excess of sleep disturbance in clonidine-exposed infants.[32] Clonidine should be avoided in early pregnancy due to suspected embryopathy; there appears to be little justification for its later use in preference to methlydopa given their similar mechanisms of action and the proven safety of the latter agent.

Peripherally Acting Adrenergic-Receptor Antagonists

Cardiac β-1 receptors mediate the chronotropic and inotropic effects of sympathetic stimulation while receptors in the kidney modulate renin synthesis in response to renal sympathetic input; activation of β_2 receptors leads to relaxation of airway smooth muscle and to peripheral vasodilation. Acutely, nonselective β-blockade decreases cardiac output; there is little change in arterial pressure, however, due to increased systemic vascular resistance. Over time, vascular resistance falls to predrug levels, resulting in a persisting hypotensive response that parallels decreased cardiac output. Moderate decrements in renin, and thus in angiotensin II and aldosterone, may contribute to the chronic antihypertensive efficacy of β-blockers in some patients, likely accounting for their greater efficacy in patient groups not believed to have salt-sensitive hypertension.[15,17] Some agents, like pindolol or oxprenolol, are partial β-receptor agonists (i.e., they possess some limited degree of "intrinsic sympathomimetic activity"); these drugs lead to lesser decrements in cardiac output and β_2 stimulation may even result in significant decrements of vascular resistance. Individual drugs may also possess selective potency at $\beta_1 > \beta_2$ receptors (e.g., atenolol and metoprolol), the additional capacity to block vascular α_1 receptors (e.g., labetalol), and may differ in their lipid solubility, such that hydrophilic agents gain less access to the central nervous system.

β-receptor antagonists are first-line agents for hypertension in nonpregnant adults because of their demonstrated benefit, second only to diuretics in multiple randomized clinical trials.[2] They are the preferred agents in patients who have experienced myocardial infarction,[2,9] but appear to provide less benefit than diuretics in elderly patients with isolated systolic hypertension.[14] Unlike other agents, long-term use of β-blockers is not associated with remodeling of small resistance arteries which have been hypertrophied due to hypertension;[33] the clinical consequences of this observation are unknown.

Adverse effects can mostly be predicted as consequences of β-receptor blockade. They may include fatigue and lethargy, exercise intolerance due mostly to (nonselective) β_2 effects in skeletal muscle vasculature, peripheral vasoconstriction secondary to decreased cardiac output, sleep disturbance with use of more lipid-soluble drugs, and bronchoconstriction. Predictably, cardiac effects could worsen congestive heart failure or lead to heart block in susceptible patients (although carvedilol is beneficial in patients with congestive failure[34]).

Pregnancy

β-blockers have been used extensively in pregnancy and subjected to several randomized trials;[22,23,35-41] their utility and fetal safety, however, remain unclear. Animal studies and anecdotal clinical observations led to concerns that these agents could cause intrauterine growth restriction, impair uteroplacental blood flow, and exert detrimental cardiovascular and metabolic effects in the fetus. However, most prospective studies, which focused on drug administration in the third trimester and included a mix of hypertensive disorders, have demonstrated effective control of maternal hypertension without significant adverse effects to the fetus. Further reassurance is derived from a one-year follow-up study which showed normal development of infants exposed to atenolol in utero.[42] By contrast, when atenolol therapy for chronic hypertension was started between 12 and 24 weeks' gestation, it resulted in clinically significant growth restriction, along with decreased placental weight;[38] this observation was supported in a subsequent retrospective review comparing atenolol with alternative therapies.[43] Similarly, several more intensively monitored studies have demonstrated fetal and neonatal bradycardia, adverse influences on uteroplacental and fetal circulations, or evidence of other fetal insults following nonselective β-blockade; these effects may be mitigated with the partial agonist, pindolol.[41,44]

Labetalol, which is also an antagonist at vascular α_1 receptors, appears to be the β-blocking drug most widely prescribed in pregnancy. Parenterally, it is used to treat severe hypertension, apparently with efficacy and tolerability equivalent to parenteral hydralazine; individual small studies favoring one agent over the other.[45-47] When administered orally in chronic hypertension, it appeared safe[20,25,48-51] and equi-effective with methyldopa, though high doses may result in neonatal hypoglycemia.[52] Of further concern, its use was associated with fetal growth restriction or neonatal difficulties in one placebo-controlled study.[51]

Peripherally acting α-adrenergic antagonists are second-line antihypertensive drugs in nonpregnant adults, which have their clearest indication during pregnancy in the management of hypertension due to suspected pheochromocytoma. Both prazosin and phenoxybenzamine have been used, along with β-blockers as adjunctive agents, in the management of this life-threatening diagnosis.[53] Since there is but limited and primarily anecdotal additional experience with these agents in pregnancy, their more routine use cannot be advocated.

Diuretics

Diuretics represent the most commonly used antihypertensive agents, and are among the drugs most clearly associated with beneficial outcome in randomized, controlled trials relating to hypertension in nonpregnant adults. They lower blood pressure by promoting natriuresis and subtle decrements of intravascular volume. Evidence for this mechanism includes observations that the acute hypotensive effect of thiazide diuretics parallels net sodium loss (usually 100–300 mEq, equivalent to 1–2 L of extracellular fluid) over the first few days of therapy, that the hypotensive effect is absent in animals or patients with renal failure, that a high-salt diet blocks the fall in blood pressure, that salt restriction perpetuates the hypotensive response even following diuretic withdrawal, and that infusion of salt or colloid solutions reverses the hypotensive effect.[54-56] This early phase of volume depletion decreases cardiac preload and thus cardiac output. Decrements in blood pressure reflect the failure of counterregulatory mechanisms, including activation of the renin–angiotensin and sympathetic nervous systems, to raise peripheral resistance enough to defend elevated arterial pressure. Curiously, the chronic antihypertensive effect of diuretics is maintained in spite of partial restoration of plasma volume and normalization of cardiac output, due to persisting *decrements* in systemic vascular resistance. Numerous studies have failed to reveal neurohumoral mechanisms, mediators, or direct actions on the vasculature which lead to this prolonged secondary vasodilator response; at present it is best ascribed to the phenomenon of total body autoregulation.[6] Those patients most apt to have maintained responses to diuretics are those who most effectively achieve this secondary vasodilated state without persisting decrements in cardiac output leading to vasoconstrictor responses (i.e., salt-sensitve, low-renin hypertensives). For diuretic-refractory hypertensives, addition of a β-blocker or ACE inhibitor may be especially efficacious.

The adverse effects of diuretics are mainly due to their precipitation of fluid, electrolyte, and solute disturbances; complications that could be predicted from their known effects on renal salt handling. By blocking renal tubular sodium reabsorption, thiazides enhance sodium delivery to distal sites in the nephron. These are sites at which sodium may be exchanged for potassium or protons; modest volume contraction resulting from diuretic use may thus be accompanied by hypokalemia and metabolic alkalosis. If volume depletion is more marked, it may evoke both thirst and nonosmotic secretion of vasopressin, favoring hyponatremia in some patients. Similarly, decreased renal perfusion may lead to azotemia if severe, but will normally lead to increased proximal reclamation of salt, fluid, and solutes, resulting in hyperuricemia.

Pregnancy

There have been many prospective trials of diuretics or dietary salt restriction in pregnancy, primarily focused on prevention of preeclampsia rather than on treatment of hypertension. A meta-analysis published in 1985[57] suggested that diuretics did indeed prevent preeclampsia, noting, however, no decrease in the incidence of proteinuric hypertension; thus the claim of efficacy could be ascribed to use of an improper definition of clinical outcome. In addition, only limited data support the value of salt restriction, which some consider deleterious. Thus, neither of the above interventions appear successful, though diuretics prevent most of the physiologic volume expansion which normally accompanies pregnancy.[58] While volume contraction might be expected to limit fetal growth,[59] outcome data have not supported these concerns.[57] However, the enhanced proximal renal tubular reabsorption which results from this volume contraction can lead to hyperuricemia; this may complicate the already difficult clinical diagnosis of superimposed preeclampsia. Also, observations of volume depletion and primary systemic vasoconstriction in preeclampsia[60] make diuretics physiologically irrational agents in this disorder.

By contrast, diuretics are commonly prescribed in essential hypertension prior to conception and, given their apparent safety, there is general agreement, articulated by the National High Blood Pressure Education Program (NHBPEP) Working Group on High Blood Pressure in Pregnancy, that they may be continued through gestation or used in combination with other agents, especially for women deemed likely to have salt-sensitive hypertension.[61] In this sense, their greatest utility may be as second or third agents which might act synergistically with other antihypertensives in drug-resistant patients. By contrast, we note that gestational vasodilation itself often normalizes the modestly elevated blood pressures most often controlled by diuretics, leading many to suggest that these agents be discontinued in most hypertensive patients lacking another indication for their continued use. Indeed, one of several small trials of diuretics in chronically hypertensive gravidas found no greater need for addition of antihypertensive medications in patients withdrawn from thiazides than in those who continued to receive diuretics through pregnancy.[58] Finally, there is an old literature, albeit anecdotal, reviewed in the first edition of this text, which called attention to cases of severe hyponatremia, hypokalemia, volume depletion, or thrombocytopenia in pregnant women treated with diuretics. Given that most of these are predictable consequences of diuretic pharmacology in susceptible patients, caution is still advised.

Calcium Channel Antagonists

All available agents in this class inhibit influx of Ca^{+2} via (voltage-dependent, slow) L-type calcium channels. Principal cardiovascular sites of action include smooth muscle cells of arterial resistance vessels, cardiac myocytes, and cells of the cardiac-conducting system. These drugs appear to have little effect on the venous circulation, do not act via the endothelium and, despite the presence of target channels in the central nervous system, appear to exert their hemodynamic effects peripherally. Since contraction of vascular myocytes is a direct function of free cytosolic Ca^{+2}, which depends in part on influx via voltage-gated channels, these drugs act as direct vasodilators, antagonizing vasoconstriction, regardless of the original neural or humoral stimulus. Of the prototypical agents, verapamil is most selectively a negative chronotrope and negative inotrope, with significant, but lesser effects as a direct vasodilator. Dihydropyridines, by contrast, of which nifedipine is the prototype, are vasoselective agents with lesser effects on the heart; diltiazem is intermediate in its tissue selectivity.

Following calcium antagonist administration, blood pressure falls acutely due to decreased peripheral resistance; the response is blunted by reflex activation of the sympathetic nervous and renin–angiotensin systems. While these drugs often lead to dependent edema, likely due to local microvascular effects, they do not usually result in compensatory renal volume retention. This observation points to likely important contributions of drug-induced natriuresis, mediated primarily by effects on intrarenal hemodynamics including prominent afferent arteriolar vasodilation, but also perhaps at tubular sites, to the sustained antihypertensive effect of these agents. Indeed, increments in sodium excretion have paralleled decrements in blood pressure following isradapine[62] and other dihydropyridines, an effect opposite that seen with other classes of direct vasodilators. This secondary na-triuretic effect likely explains results from population studies which demonstrate that calcium antagonist monotherapy is most likely to prove efficacious in those groups that respond preferentially to diuretics rather than to β-blockers (i.e., salt-sensitive hypertensives).[17] Likewise, it is consistent with some observations of lim-ited benefit to combined therapy with calcium antagonists and diuretics while these agents are effectively combined with ACE inhibitors.[63]

A controversial emerging literature calls attention to an apparent excess inci-dence of myocardial infarction and death in hypetensive patients with concomitant coronary artery disease who mostly received higher doses of short-acting dihy-dropyridine calcium antagonists.[64] The possibility that a precipitous fall in blood pressure, coupled with excessive sympathetic nervous system response could lead to myocardial ischemia in patients with underlying coronary disease appears rea-sonable. Similarly convincing data currently fail to suggest such a risk for long-acting or sustained-release preparations of dihydropyridine calcium antagonists. While individual trials might be interpreted by some to suggest such risks, others appear to support the safety of these agents, even in high-risk populations.[65]

Pregnancy

Calcium entry blockers have been used both to treat chronic hypertension and mild preeclampsia presenting late in gestation and urgent hypertension in preeclampsia. There are no adequate studies of their use early in pregnancy, save for a small ret-rospective analysis arguing against significant teratogenic effect.[66] Most investiga-tors have focused on use of nifedipine,[67,68] though there are sporadic reports on nicardipine,[40] isradipine,[69] felodipine,[70] and verapamil.[71] Some have advocated oral or sublingual (immediate-release) nifedipine as a preferred agent in severely hypertensive preeclamptics;[72] there being no difference in nifedipine pharmacoki-netics or time–effect curves by these two routes of administration.[73] Indeed, the re-sults of small comparative studies suggest that this drug controls blood pressure in such patients with efficacy similar to that of parenteral hydralazine, with a similar spectrum of maternal adverse effects (mostly ascribed to vasodilation).[74-76a]

When treating severe hypertension, the data appear to conflict regarding the influence of calcium channel blockers on uteroplacental blood flow and fetal well being, especially in comparison with other agents. In two studies,[74,77] one which in-volved maternal hemodynamic monitoring via a pulmonary artery catheter,[77] the authors claimed less fetal distress with nifedipine than with hydralazine. However, in one of these very limited trials, this observation may have been due to a greater hypotensive effect of the hydralazine doses used; several other studies have failed to discern such differences, finding no significant fetal benefit to nifedipine or al-ternative agents. Of interest too, is an animal study where chronically instrumented pregnant sheep demonstrated fetal hypoxia and acidosis following high-dose ma-ternal nifedipine infusion, unexplained by changes in maternal or uteroplacental hemodynamics ;[78] we know of no corroborative clinical data for this worrisome ob-servation.

Calcium channel antagonists also relax uterine smooth muscle and are effective tocolytics in preterm labor, but there appear to be no data to suggest that their use as antihypertensives compromises the progression of labor or leads to ineffective hemostasis following delivery. The major concern with use of calcium antagonists for urgent blood pressure control in preeclampsia relates to the widespread use of magnesium sulfate to prevent eclamptic seizures. Magnesium itself can interfere with calcium-dependent contractile signaling in excitable tissue and in muscle; combined use with calcium antagonists might result in increased risk of neuromuscular blockade or circulatory collapse. Indeed, there are isolated reports of such complications,[79,80] while others argue against such adverse outcomes with routine therapy.[81]

In summary, these agents are unstudied other than in late pregnancy; numerous, albeit limited, studies suggest that they are relatively safe and effective antihypertensive agents in chronically hypertensive or preeclamptic pregnant women. In spite of these reassuring reports, however, the potential for precipitous decrements in blood pressure, nonhemodynamic effects on the fetus, and untoward interactions with magnesium therapy make them alternative second-line agents in pregnancy.

Direct Vasodilators

Commonly prescribed direct vasodilators exert their antihypertensive effects by one of three pharmacologic mechanisms. Diazoxide, like the active metabolite of minoxidil, opens ATP-sensitive K^+ channels, hyperpolarizing and relaxing arteriolar smooth muscle, with little effect on capacitance vessels. Sodium nitroprusside is a direct nitric oxide (NO)-donor; the spontaneously released NO nonselectively relaxes both arteriolar and venular vascular smooth muscle, principally due to activation of soluble guanylyl cyclase and cyclic guanosine 3',5'-monophosphate (cGMP) accumulation. By contrast, hydralazine and related phthalazine vasodilators selectively relax arteriolar smooth muscle by an as yet unknown mechanism. These agents all have their greatest utility in the urgent control of severe hypertension, or as third-line agents for multidrug control of refractory hypertension.

Hydralazine-induced vasodilation leads to striking reflex activation of the sympathetic nervous system, increments in plasma renin, and compensatory fluid retention. The sympathetic activation, combined with hydralazine's lack of effect on epicardial coronary arteries, can precipitate myocardial ischemia or infarction in hypertensive patients with coronary atherosclerosis. These same compensatory mechanisms rapidly attenuate the hypotensive effect, requiring combination therapy with sympatholytic agents and diuretics for long-term blood pressure control. It is effective orally or intramuscularly; parenteral administration is useful for rapid control of severe hypertension. Adverse effects are mostly those due to excessive vasodilation or sympathetic activation, such as headache, nausea, flushing, or palpitations; chronic use can lead to a pyridoxine-responsive polyneuropathy or to a variety of immunologic reactions including a drug-induced lupus syndrome.

Nitroprusside, administered only by continuous intravenous infusion, is easily titrated because it has a nearly immediate onset of action with a duration of effect of only about 3 minutes. Cardiac output tends to fall during nitroprusside administration in patients with normal myocardial function due to decreased preload, while it increases in those with systolic heart failure due to afterload reduction. Reflex sympathetic activation is the rule. Nitroprusside metabolism releases cyanide, which can reach toxic levels with high-infusion rates; cyanide is metabolized to thiocyanate, whose own toxicity usually occurs after 24 to 48 hours of nitroprusside infusion, unless its excretion is delayed due to renal insufficiency.

Use of diazoxide is limited to urgent parenteral control of severe hypertension; minoxidil is the alternative agent for prolonged use due to intolerable adverse effects when diazoxide was used chronically. Since diazoxide leads to profound activation of the sympathetic and renin–angiotensin systems, its hypotensive effect is enhanced by use of sympatholytic agents and diuretics. An intravenous bolus of diazoxide lowers blood pressure within 30 seconds, with maximum effect in 5 minutes, allowing easy titration by repeated administration. Most side effects are due to excessive vasodilation, as with hydralazine, though stimulation of ATP-sensitive K^+ channels in the pancreas can inhibit insulin secretion, leading to striking hyperglycemia.

Pregnancy

Of these agents, hydralazine is most often used in pregnant women, either as a second agent for hypertension uncontrolled following methyldopa (or a β blocker) or, more commonly, as a parenteral agent for control of severe hypertension. Its use is justified not by pharmacologic selectivity but by long clinical experience with tolerable side effects. Several studies of hydralazine (or related compounds) in preeclamptic women monitored with pulmonary artery catheters have highlighted concerns regarding its safety, including precipitous falls in cardiac output and blood pressure with oliguria; though these might have been predicted from its known pharmacology along with the primary vasoconstriction and relative volume contraction characteristic in these patients.[76a,77,82] Effects on uteroplacental blood flow are unclear, likely due to variation in the degree of reflex sympathetic activation, though fetal distress may result with precipitous control of maternal pressure.[45,74,83] There is a report of neonatal thrombocytopenia following intrauterine hydralazine exposure.[84] Many investigators have suggested that urgent blood pressure control might be better achieved with less fetal risk by use of other agents such as labetalol or nifedipine; objective outcome data currently fail to support significant differences between hydralazine (or dihydralazine) and these alternative therapies.

Diazoxide, even when dosed carefully, can lead to excessive hypotension,[85] and animal studies suggest that this may compromise uterine blood flow.[86] It is possible, however, that slow infusion may avoid these complications. Additionally, relaxation of uterine smooth muscle can arrest labor and both maternal and neonatal hyperglycemia are reported. Finally, there are concerns from animal studies that repeated administration could result in pancreatic islet cell degeneration;[87] this has not been addressed by follow-up studies in humans. Presently, this class of drugs seems to have fallen into disuse in both pregnant and nonpregnant populations. While in 1990, the working group of the NHBPEP had listed diazoxide as a major second-line alternative for use when parenteral hydralazine fails, it would not be surprising if they were to downgrade this view the next time their report is updated.

Nitroprusside has only been used sporadically in pregnancy, usually in life-threatening refractory hypertension.[88] Adverse effects include those due to excessive vasodilation, apparently including cardioneurogenic (i.e., paradoxically bradycardic) syncope in volume-depleted preeclamptic women.[89] The risk of fetal cyanide intoxication remains unknown. Given the long experience with hydralazine and alternative utility of calcium channel blockers or parenteral labetalol, these two drugs must be considered agents of last resort.

Angiotensin-Converting Enzyme Inhibitors and Angiotensin Receptor Antagonists

Angiotensin-converting enzyme inhibitors block ACE (kininase II), the enzyme responsible for conversion of angiotensin I (itself cleaved from angiotensinogen by renin) to angiotensin II (AII). Inhibition of this enzyme, localized to the endothelium and most abundant in the pulmonary microvasculature, predictably leads to decrements in AII and also in levels of aldosterone, whose synthesis in the zona glomerulosa of the adrenal cortex is AII-dependent. These agents lower blood pressure primarily by blocking AII-induced vasoconstriction; their efficacy in patients with low circulating renin and AII may reveal contributions of a parallel "tissue" renin–angiotensin axis distributed in the arterial wall.[90] In some hypertensive patients, accumulation of bradykinin, an endothelium-dependent vasodilator, and also an endogenous substrate for ACE, may contribute to the antihypertensive effect. Indeed, adverse effects, including the common ACE inhibitor-induced dry cough, appear to be due, at least in part, to bradykinin.[91] Long-term blood pressure control may be favored by an apparent natriuretic effect of these drugs, partially due to decrements in aldosterone synthesis, but mainly to a resetting of the normal relationship between salt excretion and renal perfusion pressure.[6] It is unclear what long-term benefits may be derived from nonhemodynamic effects of ACE inhibition, as AII is a potent growth factor for a variety of cardiovascular cells.

As predicted, these drugs are most efficacious in patients with renin-dependent hypertension, such as those with unilateral renal artery stenosis. Their benefit in diabetic nephropathy, their ability to decrease proteinuria in patients with glomerular diseases, and their possible "renal protective" effect in other (principally proteinuric) diseases leading to progressive renal insufficiency derives from their effects in the renal microvasculature. Since AII acts selectively to constrict the efferent arteriole (its effect in the afferent arteriole being antagonized by locally synthesized NO[92]), its absence, or antagonism, lowers intraglomerular pressure out of proportion to any effect on systemic arterial pressure. It is important to note that in those cases where preservation of glomerular filtration rate in the face of decreased renal perfusion depends on selective efferent arteriolar vasoconstriction by AII (e.g., renal artery stenosis, volume depletion, congestive heart failure), ACE inhibition may lead not only to exaggerated hypotension, but also to acute renal failure.

The recent introduction of antagonists for the AT1 subtype of AII receptors provides alternative agents with a pharmacology virtually identical to that of ACE inhibitors, save for hypersensitivity reactions and those effects due to bradykinin accumulation. Indeed, the fidelity with which these agents recapitulate the beneficial effects of ACE inhibition casts doubt on the contributions of bradykinin accumulation to the blood pressure-lowering effect in most patients. It also raises important questions regarding any hemodynamic effects of AT2 receptors, which are presumably activated by the elevated levels of AII which follow use of AT1 blockers.

Pregnancy

The renin–angiotensin system is activated in normal human pregnancy;[93] even in preeclampsia, where AII levels are lower than in normal gestation, there may be simultaneous up-regulation of AT1 receptors.[94] Thus, ACE inhibitors might have seemed attractive antihypertensive agents in pregnant women. Concerns regarding use of these drugs might have been anticipated, however, from excess fetal wastage in animal studies. Indeed, their use in human pregnancy has been associated with frequent reports of a specific fetopathy (including renal dysgenesis and calvarial hypoplasia), oligohydramnios (likely a result of fetal oliguria), intrauterine growth restriction, and neonatal anuric renal failure leading to death.[95,96] Thus, these agents are contraindicated in pregnancy. ACE inhibitors do not appear to be teratogens; drug use seems to have started during the second or third trimester in most reported cases of malformations. Whether these adverse outcomes are due to a hemodynamic effect in the fetus or to specific (nonhemodynamic) requirements for AII as a fetal growth factor remain unknown. While clinical experience is virtually nil, and adverse effects are yet to be reported, observation that the AT1 antagonist losartan also causes fetal and neonatal renal failure in the rat leads us to similarly reject the use of any AII receptor antagonists in pregnancy.[97] Of note, many women at risk for hypertension during pregnancy, particularly those with underlying diabetes mellitus, may benefit from use of ACE inhibitors prior to conception. Since all cases of ACE inhibitor-associated fetopathy or renal failure occurred with drug use in the latter two trimesters, it seems reasonable to use these drugs when appropriate, counseling women that they should either change to alternate agents when attempting to conceive or discontinue them early in pregnancy.

DRUG USE WHILE BREASTFEEDING

No well-designed studies are available that assess neonatal effects of maternally administered antihypertensive drugs delivered via breast milk. The pharmacokinetic principles which govern drug distribution to milk and subsequently infant exposure are well established.[98,99] Milk, secreted by alveolar cells, is a suspension of fat globules in a protein-containing aqueous solution whose pH is lower than that of maternal plasma. Factors that favor drug passage into milk are a small maternal volume of distribution, low plasma protein binding, high lipid solubility, and lack of charge at physiologic pH. Even when drugs are ingested by nursing infants, exposure depends on volume ingested, intervals between drug administration and nursing, oral bioavailability, and the capacity of the infant to clear the drug.

Neonatal exposure to methyldopa via nursing is likely low and it is generally considered safe. Atenolol and metoprolol are concentrated in breast milk, possibly to levels that could affect the infant; by contrast, exposure to labetalol and propranolol appears low.[100] While milk concentrations of diuretics are limited, these agents can decrease milk production significantly.[101] There are brief reports of calcium channel blocker transfer into breast milk,[102] apparently without adverse effects. Given concerns regarding effects of ACE inhibitors and AT1 receptor antagonists on neonatal renal function, these drugs should be avoided, even though levels of captopril in milk appear to be low.

CONCLUSION

Use of antihypertensive agents in pregnancy is either for the urgent control of severe hypertension (Table 18–2) or for control of chronic hypertension (Table 18–3),

TABLE 18–2. DRUGS FOR URGENT CONTROL OF SEVERE HYPERTENSION IN PREGNANCY[a,b]

Drug (FDA Risk)[c]	Dose and Route	Concerns or Comments[d]
Hydralazine (C)	5 mg IV or IM, then 5–10 mg every 20–40 min; or constant infusion of 0.5–10 mg/h	Drug of choice according to NHBPEP Working Group; long experience of safety and efficacy.
Labetalol (C)	20 mg IV, then 20–80 mg every 20–30 min, up to maximum of 300 mg; or constant infusion of 1–2 mg/min	Experience in pregnancy less than with hydralazine. Probably less risk of tachycardia and arrhythmia than with other vasodilators.
Nifedipine (C)	5–10 mg p.o., repeat in 30 min if needed, then 10–20 mg every 2–6 h	Possible interference with labor; may interact synergistically with magnesium sulfate.
Diazoxide (C)	30–50 mg IV every 5–15 min	Use is waning; may arrest labor; causes hyperglycemia.
Relatively Contraindicated		
Nitroprusside (C)[e]	Constant infusion of 0.5–10 εg/kg/min	Possible cyanide toxicity; agent of last resort.

[a] Indicated for acute elevation of diastolic BP ≥ 105 mm Hg; goal is gradual reduction to 90–100 mm Hg.
[b] There are periodic reports of serotonin receptor antagonists (e.g., ketanserin). Data are too fragmentary to analyze.
[c] US Food and Drug Administration classification, see Table 18–1.
[d] Adverse effects for all agents, except as noted, may include headache, flushing, nausea, and tachycardia (primarily due to precipitous hypotension and reflex sympathetic activation).
[e] We would classify in category D.

TABLE 18–3. DRUGS FOR CHRONIC HYPERTENSION IN PREGNANCY[a,b]

Drug (FDA Risk)[c]	Dose	Concerns or Comments
Preferred Agent		
Methyldopa (C)	0.5–3.0 g/d in 2–3 divided doses	Drug of choice according to NHBPEP Working Group; safety after 1st trimester well documented, including 7-yr follow-up of offspring.
Second-Line Agents[d]		
Hydralazine (C)	50–300 mg/d in 2–4 divided doses	Few controlled trials, long experience with few adverse events documented; useful only in combination with sympatholytic agent. May cause neonatal thrombocytopenia.
Labetalol (C)	200–1200 mg/d in 2–3 divided doses	May be associated with fetal growth restriction and neonatal difficulties.
β-receptor blockers (C)	Depends on specific agent	May cause fetal bradycardia and decrease uteroplacental blood flow, this effect may be less for agents with partial agonist activity. May impair fetal response to hypoxic stress; risk of growth restriction when started in 1st or 2nd trimester.
Nifedipine (C)	30–120 mg/d of a slow-release preparation	May inhibit labor and have synergistic interaction with magnesium sulfate. Limited experience other calcium entry blockers.
Thiazide diuretics (C)[e]	Depends on specific agent	Majority of controlled studies in normotensive pregnant women rather than hypertensive patients; can cause volume depletion and electrolyte disorders. May be useful in combination with methyldopa and vasodilator to mitigate compensatory fluid retention.
Contraindicated		
ACE inhibitors and AT1 receptor antagonists (D)[f]	Depends on specific agent	Leads to fetal loss in animals; human use associated with fetopathy, oligohydramnios, growth restriction, and neonatal anuric renal failure which may be fatal.

[a] No antihypertensive has been proven safe for use during 1st trimester.
[b] Drug therapy indicated for uncomplicated chronic hypertension when diastolic BP ≥ 100 mm Hg (Korotkoff 5). Treatment at lower levels may be indicated for patients with diabetes mellitus, renal disease, or target organ damage.
[c] US Food and Drug Administration classification, see Table 18–1.
[d] We omit some agents (e.g., clonidine, alpha-blockers) due to limited data on use for chronic hypertension in pregnancy.
[e] Classified as category D by Briggs et al.[103]
[f] We would classify in category X.

realizing that this latter indication may include patients with a variety of hypertensive disorders including early preeclampsia. Tables 18–2 and 18–3 summarize clinical data on the use of drugs discussed above, including FDA risk classification, usual doses, and special concerns.

Currently, there is little evidence to support the notion that blood pressure control in gravidas with chronic hypertension will prevent the subsequent occurrence of preeclampsia,[104,105a] itself the cause for most adverse outcomes in these patients. Indeed, given the pathophysiologic hypotheses which ascribe this disorder to events in early pregnancy,[106] it would seem unreasonable to expect such a benefit. As well, there are no data to suggest that antihypertensive therapy will lessen the incidence of placental abruption. There have been few studies that have rigorously assessed the prevention of severe or accelerated hypertension, focusing on avoidance of the perceived need for hospitalization or urgent early delivery. What is clear is that effective agents can control hypertension during pregnancy with acceptable risks to mother and fetus. Desperately needed, however, are adequately powered prospective clinical trials that distinguish between women with essential hypertension, transient hypertension, or preeclampsia, and stratify treatment both by severity of hypertension and by gestational age. Such trials should include systematic assessment of uteroplacental hemodynamics and fetal well being as well as long-term functional and developmental assessment of postnatal outcome. Only through such research will we ever gain the confidence to rationally select from a broader armamentarium of antihypertensive agents to benefit pregnant women.

REFERENCES

1. Redman CWG, Beilin LJ, Bonnar J, Ounsted MK: Fetal outcome in trial of antihypertensive treatment in pregnancy. *Lancet* 1976;2:753–756.
2. The Sixth Report of the Joint National Committee on Prevention, Detection, Evaluation, and Treatment of High Blood Pressure. *Arch Intern Med* 1997;157:2413–2446. (Also reprinted as NIH Publication No. 98-4080 and available via the world wide web at www.nhlbi.nih.gov/nhlbi/cardio/hbp/prof/jnc6.pdf
3. Black HR, Yi JY: A new classification scheme for hypertension based on relative and absolute risk with implications for treatment and reimbursement. *Hypertension* 1996;28:719–724.
4. Hansson L, Zanchetti A, Carruthers SG, et al: Effects of intensive blood-pressure lowering and low-dose aspirin in patients with hypertension: Principal results of the hypertension Optimal Treatment (HOT) randomised trial. HOT Study Group. *Lancet* 1998;351:1755–1762.
5. Sibai BM, Abdella TN, Anderson GD: Pregnancy outcome in 211 patients with mild chronic hypertension. *Obstet Gynecol* 1983;61:571–576.
6. Guyton AC: Blood pressure control—special role of the kidneys and body fluids. *Science* 1991;252:1813–1816.
7. Lewis EJ, Hunsicker LG, Bain RP, Rohde RD (for the Collaborative Study Group): The effect of angiotensin converting enzyme inhibition on diabetic nephropathy. *N Engl J Med* 1993;329:1456–1462.
8. Giatras I, Lau J, Levey AS (for the Angiotensin Converting Enzyme Inhibition and Progresssive Renal Insufficiency Study Group): Effect of angiotensin converting enzyme inhibition on the progression of nondiabetic renal disease; a meta-analysis of randomized trials. *Ann Intern Med* 1997;127:337–345.
9. Yusuf S, Peto R, Lewis J, et al: Beta blockade during and after myocardial infarction: An overview of the randomized trials. *Prog Cardiovasc Dis* 1985;27:335–371.
10. Pfeffer MA, Braunwald E, Moyé LA (for the SAVE Investigators): Effect of captopril on mortality and morbidity in patients with left ventricular dysfunction after myocardial infarction: Results of the Survival and Ventricular Enlargement Trials. *N Engl J Med* 1992;327:669–677.
11. Garg R, Yusuf S (for the Collaborative Group on ACE Inhibitor Trials): Oveview of randomized trials of angiotensin converting enzyme inhibitors on mortality and morbidity in patients with heart failure. *JAMA* 1995;273:1450–1456.
12. Pitt B, Segal R, Martinez FA (for the ELITE Study Investigators): Randomised trial of losar-

tan versus captopril in patients over 65 with heart failure (Evaluation of Losartan in the Elderly Study, ELITE). *Lancet* 1997;349:375–380.

13. SHEP Cooperative Research Group: Prevention of stroke by antihypertensive drug treatment in older persons with isolated systolic hypertension: Final results of the Systolic Hypertension in the Elderly Program (SHEP). *JAMA* 1991;265:3255–3264.

14. MRC Working Party: Medical Research Council trial of treatment of hypertension in older adults: Principal results. *Br Med J* 1992;304:405–412.

15. Materson BJ, Reda DJ, Cushman WC (for the Department of Veterans Affairs Cooperative Study Group on Antihypertensive Agents): Single drug therapy for hypertension in men: A comparison of six antihypertensive agents with placebo. *N Engl J Med* 1993;328:914–921.

16. Weinberger MH, Stegner JE, Fineberg NS: A comparison of two tests for the assessment of blood pressure responses to sodium. *Am J Hypertens* 1993;6:179–184.

17. Kiowski W, Bühler FR, Fadayomi MO, et al: Age, race, blood pressure and renin; predictors for antihypertensive treatment with calcium antagonists. *Am J Cardiol* 1985;56:81H–85H.

18. Merkatz RB, Temple R, Subel S, et al: Women in clinical trials of new drugs. A change in Food and Drug Administration policy. The Working Group on Women in Clinical Trials. *N Engl J Med* 1993;329:292–296.

19. Veterans Administration Cooperative Study Group on Antihypertensive Agents: Effects of treatment on morbidity in hypertension: Results in patients with diastolic blood pressures averaging 115 through 129 mm Hg. *JAMA* 1967;202:1028–1034.

20. Sibai BM, Mabie WC, Shamsa F, et al: A comparison of no medication versus methyldopa or labetalol in chronic hypertension during pregnancy. *Am J Obstet Gynecol* 1990;162:960–967.

21. Leather HM, Humphreys DM, Paker PB, Chadd MA: A controlled trial of hypotensive agents in hypertension in pregnancy. *Lancet* 1968;2:488–490.

22. Fidler J, Smith V, Fayers P, de Swiet M: Randomized controlled comparative study of methyldopa and oxprenolol in treatment of hypertension in pregnancy. *Br Med J* 1983;286:1927–1930.

23. Gallery EDM, Ross MR, Gyory AZ: Antihypertensive treatment in pregnancy: Analysis of different responses to oxprenolol and methyldopa. *Br Med J* 1985;291:563–566.

24. Horvath JS, Phippard A, Korda A, et al: Clonidine hydrochloride—a safe and effective antihypertensive agent in pregnancy. *Obstet Gynecol* 1985;66:634–638.

25. Plouin PF, Breart G, Maillard F, et al: Comparison of antihypertensive efficacy and perinatal safety of labetalol and methyldopa in the treatment of hypertension in pregnancy: A randomized controlled trial. *Br J Obstet Gynaecol* 1988;95:868–876.

26. Cockburn J, Moar VA, Ounsted M, Redman CW: Final report of study on hypertension during pregnancy: The effects of specific treatment on the growth and development of the children. *Lancet* 1982;1:647–649.

27. Schobel HP, Fischer T, Heuszer K, et al: Preeclampsia—a state of sympathetic overactivity. *N Engl J Med* 1996;335:1480–1485.

28. Redman CW, Beilin LJ, Bonnar J: Treatment of hypertension in pregnancy with methyldopa: Blood pressure control and side effects. *Br J Obstet Gynaecol* 1977;84:419–426.

29. Montan S, Anandakumar C, Arulkumaran S, et al: Effects of methyldopa on uteroplacental and fetal hemodynamics in pregnancy-induced hypertension. *Am J Obstet Gynecol* 1993;168:152–156.

30. Mutch LM, Moar VA, Ounsted MK, Redman CW: Hypertension during pregnancy, with and without specific hypotensive treatment. I. Perinatal factors and neonatal morbidity. *Early Human Develop* 1977;1:47–57.

31. Mutch LM, Moar VA, Ounsted MK, Redman CW: Hypertension during pregnancy, with and without specific hypotensive treatment. II. The growth and development of the infant in the first year of life. *Early Human Develop* 1977;1:59–67.

32. Huisjes HJ, Hadders-Algra M, Touwen BC: Is clonidine a behavioural teratogen in the human? *Early Human Develop* 1986;14:43–48.

33. Schiffrin EL: Vascular remodeling and endothelial function in hypertensive patients: Effects of antihypertensive therapy. *Scand Cardiovasc J* 1998;47:15–21S.

34. Bristow MR, Gilbert EM, Abraham WT, et al: Carvedilol produces dose-related improvements in left ventricular function and survival in subjects with chronic heart failure. MOCHA Investigators. *Circulation* 1996;94:2807–2816.

35. Rubin PC, Butters L, Clark DM, et al: Placebo-controlled trial of atenolol in treatment of pregnancy-associated hypertension. *Lancet* 1983;1:431–434.

36. Wichman K, Ryden G, Karlberg BE: A placebo controlled trial of metoprolol in the treatment of hypertension in pregnancy. *Scand J Clin Lab Med Invest* 1984;44(suppl 169):90–94.

37. Hogstedt S, Lindeberg S, Axelsson O, et al: A prospective controlled trial of metoprolol-hydralazine treatment in hypertension during pregnancy. *Acta Obstet Gynecol Scand* 1985;64:505–510.

38. Butters L, Kennedy S, Rubin PC: Atenolol in essential hypertension during pregnancy. *Br Med J* 1990;301:587–589.

39. Plouin PF, Breart G, Llado J, et al: A randomized comparison of early with conservative use of antihypertensive drugs in the management of pregnancy-induced hypertension. *Br J Obstet Gynaecol* 1990;97:134–141.

40. Jannet D, Carbonne B, Sebban E, Milliez J: Nicardipine versus metoprolol in the treatment of hypertension during pregnancy: A randomized comparative trial. *Obstet Gynecol* 1994;84:354–359.

41. Paran E, Holzberg G, Mazor M, et al: Beta-adrenergic blocking agents in the treatment of pregnancy-induced hypertension. *Int J Clin Pharmacol Ther* 1995;33:119–123.

42. Reynolds B, Butters L, Evans J, et al: First year of life after the use of atenolol in pregnancy associated hypertension. *Arch Dis Child* 1984;59:1061–1063.

43. Lip GY, Beevers M, Churchill D, et al: Effect of atenolol on birthweight. *Am J Cardiol* 1997;79:1436–1438.

44. Montan S, Ingemarsson I, Marsal K, Sjoberg NO: Randomised controlled trial of atenolol and pindolol in human pregnancy: Effects on fetal haemodynamics. *Br Med J* 1992;304:946–949.

45. Mabie WC, Gonzalez AR, Sibai BM, Amon E: A comparative trial of labetalol and hydralazine in the acute management of severe hypertension complicating pregnancy. *Obstet Gynecol* 1987;70:328–333.

46. Michael CA: Intravenous labetalol and intravenous diazoxide in severe hypertension complicating pregnancy. *Aust NZ J Obstet Gynaecol* 1986;26:26–29.

47. Ashe RG, Moodley J, Richards AM, Philpott RH: Comparison of labetalol and dihydralazine in hypertensive emergencies in pregnancy. *S Afr Med J* 1987;71:354–356.

48. Pickles CJ, Symonds EM, Pipkin FB: The fetal outcome in a randomized double-blind controlled trial of labetalol versus placebo in pregnancy-induced hypertension. *Br J Obstet Gynaecol* 1989;96:38–43.

49. Redman CWG: A controlled trial of the treatment of hypertension in pregnancy: Labetalol compared with methyldopa. In: Riley A, Symonds EM, eds. *The Investigation and Management of Hypertension in Pregnancy.* Amsterdam: Exerpta Medica; 1982:111–122.

50. el-Qarmalawi AM, Morsy AH, al-Fadly A, et al: Labetalol vs. methyldopa in the treatment of pregnancy-induced hypertension. *Int J Gynaecol Obstet* 1995;49:125–130.

51. Sibai BM, Gonzalez AR, Mabie WC, Moretti M: A comparison of labetalol plus hospitalization versus hospitalization alone in the management of preeclampsia remote from term. *Obstet Gynecol* 1987;70:323–327.

52. Munshi UK, Deorari AK, Paul VK, Singh M: Effects of maternal labetalol on the newborn infant. *Indian Pediatr* 1992;29:1507–1512.

53. Freier DT, Thompson NW: Pheochromocytoma and pregnancy: The epitome of high risk. *Surgery* 1993;114:1148–1152.

54. Wilson IM, Freis IM: Relationship between plasma and extracellular fluid volume depletion and the antihypertensive effect of chlorothiazide. *Circulation* 1959;20:1028–1036.

55. Roos JC, Boer P, Koomaans HA, et al: Haemodynamic and hormonal changes during acute and chronic diuretic treatment in essential hypertension. *Eur J Clin Pharmacol* 1981;19:107–112.

56. Bennett WM, McDonald WJ, Kuehnel E, et al: Do diuretics have antihypertensive properties independent of natriuresis? *Clin Pharmacol Ther* 1977;22:499–504.

57. Collins R, Yusuf S, Peto R: Overview of randomised trials of diuretics in pregnancy. *Br Med J* 1985;290:17–23.

58. Sibai BM, Grossman RA, Grossman HG: Effects of diuretics on plasma volume in pregnancies with long-term hypertension. *Am J Obstet Gynecol* 1984;150:831–835.

59. Gallery EDM, Hunyor SN, Gyory AZ: Plasma volume contraction: A significant factor in

both pregnancy-associated hypertension (preeclampsia) and chronic hypertension in pregnancy. *Q J Med* 1979;192:593–602.

60. Visser W, Wallenburg HCS: Central hemodynamic observations in untreated preeclamptic patients. *Hypertension* 1991;17:1072–1077.

61. National High Blood Pressure Education Program Working Group report on high blood pressure in pregnancy. *Am J Obstet Gynecol* 1990;163:1689–1712. (Also reprinted as NIH Publication No. 91-3029 and available via the world wide web at gopher://fido.nhlbi.nih.gov:70/11/nhlbi/health/cardio/hbp/prof/hbp)

62. Krusell LR, Jespersen LT, Schmitz A, et al: Repetitive natriuresis and blood pressure. Long-term calcium entry blockade with isradipine. *Hypertension* 1987;10:577–581.

63. Brouwer RM, Bolli P, Erne P, et al: Antihypertensive treatment using calcium antagonists in combination with captopril rather than diuretics. *Cardiovasc Pharmacol* 1985;7:S88–S91.

64. Furberg CD, Psaty BM, Meyer JV: Nifedipine: Dose-related increase in mortality in patients with coronary heart disease. *Circulation* 1995;92:1326–1331.

65. Chobanian AV: Calcium channel blockers. Lessons learned from MIDAS and other clinical trials. *JAMA* 1996;276:829–830.

66. Magee LA, Schick B, Donnenfeld AE, et al: The safety of calcium channel blockers in human pregnancy: A prospective, multicenter cohort study. *Am J Obstet Gynecol* 1996;174:823–828.

67. Sibai BM, Barton JR, Akl S, et al: A randomized prospective comparison of nifedipine and bed rest versus bed rest alone in the management of preeclampsia remote from term. *Am J Obstet Gynecol* 1992;167:879–884.

68. Ismail AA, Medhat I, Tawfic TA, Kholeif A: Evaluation of calcium-antagonist (Nifedipine) in the treatment of pre-eclampsia. *Int J Gynaecol Obstet* 1993;40:39–43.

69. Wide-Swensson DH, Ingemarsson I, Lunell NO, et al: Calcium channel blockade (isradipine) in treatment of hypertension in pregnancy: A randomized placebo-controlled study. *Am J Obstet Gynecol* 1995;173:872–878.

70. Casele HL, Windley KC, Prieto JA, et al: Felodipine use in pregnancy. Report of three cases. *J Reprod Med* 1997;42:378–381.

71. Belfort MA, Anthony J, Buccimazza A, Davey DA: Hemodynamic changes associated with intravenous infusion of the calcium antagonist verapamil in the treatment of severe gestational proteinuric hypertension. *Obstet Gynecol* 1990;75:970–974.

72. Gallery ED, Györy AZ: Sublingual nifedipine in human pregnancy. *Aust NZ J Med* 1997;27:538–542.

73. van Harten J, Burggraaf K, Danhof M, et al: Negligible sublingual absorption of nifedipine. *Lancet* 1987;2:1363–1365.

74. Fenakel K, Fenakel G, Appelman Z, et al: Nifedipine in the treatment of severe preeclampsia. *Obstet Gynecol* 1991;77:331–337.

75. Seabe SJ, Moodley J, Becker P: Nifedipine in acute hypertensive emergencies in pregnancy. *S Afr Med J* 1989;76:248–250.

76. Martins-Costa S, Ramos JG, Barros E, et al: Randomized, controlled trial of hydralazine versus nifedipine in preeclamptic women with acute hypertension. *Clin Exp Hypertens* [B] 1992;11:25–44.

76a. Von Dadelszen P, Ornstein MP, Magee LA: Hydralazine is not the drug of choice for the control of severe pregnancy hypertension: A review of the randomized controlled trials. *Am J Obstet Gynecol* 1999 (abstract in press).

77. Visser W, Wallenburg HC: A comparison between the hemodynamic effects of oral nifedipine and intravenous dihydralazine in patients with severe preeclampsia. *J Hypertens* 1995; 13:791–795.

78. Blea CW, Barnard JM, Magness RR, et al: Effect of nifedipine on fetal and maternal hemodynamics and blood gases in the pregnant ewe. *Am J Obstet Gynecol* 1997;176:922–930.

79. Waisman GD, Mayorga LM, Camera MI, et al: Magnesium plus nifedipine: Potentiation of hypotensive effect in preeclampsia? *Am J Obstet Gynecol* 1988;159:308–309.

80. BenAmi M, Giladi Y, Shalev E: The combination of magnesium sulphate and nifedipine: A cause of neuromuscular blockade. *Br J Obstet Gynaecol* 1994;101:262–263.

81. Scardo JA, Vermillion ST, Hogg BB, Newman RB: Hemodynamic effects of oral nifedipine in preeclamptic hypertensive emergencies. *Am J Obstet Gynecol* 1996;175:336–338.

82. Wallenburg HCS: Hemodynamics in hypertensive pregnancy. In: Rubin PC, ed. *Hypertension in Pregnancy.* New York: Elsevier; 1988:66–101. (second edition in press 1999 or 2000)

83. Vink GJ, Moodley J, Philpott RH: Effect of dihydralazine on the fetus in the treatment of maternal hypertension. *Obstet Gynecol* 1980;55:519–522.

84. Widerlov E, Karlman I, Storsater J: Hydralazine-induced neonatal thrombocytopenia. *N Engl J Med* 1980;303:1235.

85. Dudley DKL: Minibolus diazoxide in the management of severe hypertension in pregnancy. *Am J Obstet Gynecol* 1985;151:196–200.

86. Nuwayhid B, Brinkman CR, Katchen B, et al: Maternal and fetal hemodynamic effects of diazoxide. *Obstet Gynecol* 1975;46:197–203.

87. Boulos BM, Davis LE, Almond CH, Jackson RL: Placental transfer of diazoxide and its hazardous effect on the newborn. *J Clin Pharmacol New Drugs* 1971;11:206–210.

88. Shoemaker CT, Meyers M: Sodium nitroprusside for control of severe hypertensive disease of pregnancy: A case report and discussion of potential toxicity. *Am J Obstet Gynecol* 1984;149:171–173.

89. Wasserstrum N: Nitroprusside in preeclampsia. Circulatory distress and paradoxical bradycardia. *Hypertension* 1991;18:79–84.

90. Rosenthal J: Role of renal and extrarenal renin-angiotensin system in the mechanism of arterial hypertension and its sequelae. *Steroids* 1993;58:566–572.

91. Takahama K, Araki T, Fuchikami J, et al: Studies on the magnitude and the mechanism of cough potentiation by angiotensin-converting enzyme inhibitors in guinea pigs: Involvement of bradykinin in the potentiation. *J Pharm Pharmacol* 1996;48:1027–1033.

92. Ito S, Arima S, Ren YL, et al: Endothelium-derived relaxing factor/nitric oxide modulates angiotensin II action in the isolated microperfused rabbit afferent but not efferent arteriole. *J Clin Invest* 1993;91:2012–2019.

93. August P, Mueller FB, Sealey JE, Edersheim TG: Role of renin-angiotensin system in blood pressure regulation in pregnancy. *Lancet* 1995;345:896–897.

94. Baker PN, Pipkin FB, Symonds EM: Comparative study of platelet angiotensin II binding and the angiotensin II sensitivity test as predictors of pregnancy-induced hypertension. *Clin Sci* (Colch) 1992;83:89–95.

95. Pryde PG, Sedman AB, Nugent CE, Barr M Jr: Angiotensin-converting enzyme inhibitor fetopathy. *J Am Soc Nephrol* 1993;3:1575–1582.

96. Buttar HS: An overview of the influence of ACE inhibitors on fetal-placental circulation and perinatal development. *Mol Cell Biochem* 1997;176:61–71.

97. Spence SG, Zacchei AG, Lee LL, et al: Toxicokinetic analysis of losartan during gestation and lactation in the rat. Teratology 1996;53:245–252.

98. Atkinson HC, Begg EJ, Darlow BA: Drugs in human milk: Clinical pharmacokinetic considerations. *Clin Pharmacokinet* 1988;14:217–240.

99. Breitzka RL, Sandritter TL, Hatzopoulos FK: Principles of drug transfer into breast milk and drug disposition in the nursing infant. *J Human Lact* 1997;13:155–158.

100. Atkinson H, Begg EJ: Concentrations of beta-blocking drugs in human milk. *J Pediatr* 1989;114:478–480.

101. White WB: Management of hypertension during lactation. *Hypertension* 1984;6:297–300.

102. Ehrenkranz RA, Ackerman BA, Hulse JD: Nifedipine transfer into human milk. *J Pediatr* 1989;114:478–480.

103. Briggs GG, Freeman RK, Yaffe SJ: *A Reference Guide to Fetal and Neonatal Risk: Drugs in Pregnancy and Lactation,* ed 4. Baltimore: Williams & Wilkins; 1994.

104. Redman CWG: Controlled trials of antihypertensive drugs in pregnancy. *Am J Kidney Dis* 1991;17:149–153.

105. Sibai BM: Treatment of hypertension in pregnant women. *N Engl J Med* 1996;335:257–265.

105a. Sanchez-Ramos L, Mora CS: Effect of antihypertensive therapy on the development of superimposed preeclampsia in patients with chronic hypertension: A meta-analysis. *Am J Obstet Gynecol* 1999 (abstract in press).

106. Conrad KP, Benyo DF: Placental cytokines and the pathogenesis of preeclampsia. *Am J Reprod Immunol* 1997;37:240–249.

19

Chronic Hypertension and Pregnancy

Phyllis August and Marshall D. Lindheimer

Chronic hypertension in pregnancy received but modest attention in the first edition of this text. It was discussed with renal diseases in the final chapter, where Chesley noted briefly that most patients had the "essential variety," 85% of whom did well, and that many of these women had an exaggerated decrease in blood pressure in early gestation. He cited personal experience to support his view that "accelerated (malignant)" hypertension was an unusual pregnancy complication. He also discussed the difficulty in diagnosing "superimposed preeclampsia" in these women, and by applying his own stringent criteria, suggested an incidence lower than most studies. There were also short discussions of renovascular hypertension, aldosteronism, and pheochromocytoma. Chesley's summary reflected the paucity of contemporary data, not only in relation to chronic hypertension in pregnancy, but knowledge of the disease in nonpregnant populations as well. Research in both areas has progressed substantially in the last 25 years.

In this chapter, the natural history, diagnosis, and treatment of chronic hypertension complicating pregnancy are reviewed, followed by an overview of specific diagnostic categories including essential, renal, renovascular, and adrenal hypertension. Evaluation and treatment of hypertension postpartum is also discussed.

BACKGROUND

The prevalence of hypertension in premenopausal women may be as high as 25% in whites, and 30% in blacks, and increases with age.[1] High blood pressure, therefore, is an important cardiovascular risk factor in this population which has significant implications for pregnancy outcome. The incidence of preexisting or chronic hypertension in pregnant women has not been exactly quantified. Based on current estimates of the prevalence of hypertensive disorders during gestation, chronic hypertension likely complicates about 2 to 5% of pregnancies.[2] Also, because preeclampsia in multiparous women is often misdiagnosed and is really unrecognized chronic hypertension,[3,4] the incidence may be higher. Finally, in certain parts of the world, particularly industrialized urban areas, many women postpone childbearing, and thus, the incidence of preexisting hypertension complicating pregnancy is more common.

Definition

Chronic hypertension complicating pregnancy is diagnosed by high blood pressure known to predate conception.[2] One problem with this is that criteria for diagnosing hypertension in premenopausal women are not well established. In late 1997, the Joint National Committee for the Detection and Treatment of High Blood Pressure sponsored by the National Institutes of Health recommended that for the adult population *stage 1* hypertension (previously called "mild") be defined as a blood pressure of 140 to 159/90 to 99 mm Hg[1] (Table 19–1). Most women with chronic hypertension will have essential (also called primary) hypertension, but as many as 10% may have underlying renal or endocrine disorders, i.e., secondary hypertension.

Diagnosis

When hypertension has been clearly documented prior to conception, the diagnosis of chronic hypertension in pregnancy is straightforward. It is also the most likely diagnosis when hypertension is present prior to 20 weeks' gestation, although isolated, rare cases of preeclampsia before this time have been reported, particularly in the presence of hydatidiform mole.[5]

Difficulties arise when pregnant women with stage 1, and even stage 2 hypertension, present initially in the second trimester, after having experienced the pregnancy-associated "physiologic" decrease in blood pressure. These women will have been presumed to be normotensive, and later erroneously diagnosed with preeclampsia if blood pressure rises in the third trimester. In such cases, a diagnosis of either transient (late) hypertension of pregnancy or of chronic hypertension is most likely when the increased blood pressure is not accompanied by proteinuria

TABLE 19–1. CLASSIFICATION OF BLOOD PRESSURE FOR ADULTS AGE 18 AND OLDER

Category	Systolic (mm Hg)		Diastolic (mm Hg)
Normal	< 130	and	< 85
High normal	130–139	or	85–89
Hypertension			
Stage 1 (mild)	140–159	or	90–99
Stage 2 (moderate)	160–179	or	100–109
Stage 3 (severe)	≥ 180	or	≥ 110

Reprinted from The Sixth Report of the Joint National Committee on Prevention, Detection, Evaluation, and Treatment of High Blood Pressure. *Arch Intern Med* 1997;157:2413–2446.

and other classic laboratory abnormalities consistent with preeclampsia (see Chap. 5) are absent. Because 15 to 25% of women with chronic hypertension develop *superimposed* preeclampsia, it may be impossible to diagnose chronic hypertension in this setting until well after delivery. In other instances, women with well-documented hypertension prior to conception will demonstrate normal blood pressures throughout their entire pregnancy, only to return to prepregnancy hypertensive levels postpartum. Thus, an understanding of the normal pregnancy-induced physiologic changes, as well as an appreciation of the clinical and laboratory features of preeclampsia, are essential for correct diagnosis and management of women with chronic hypertension. These principles, reviewed here briefly, are more extensively discussed in Chapters 3 and 4.

Cardiac and Hemodynamic Alterations

Normal pregnancy is characterized by generalized vasodilation, so marked that despite increases in cardiac output and blood volume of 40 to 50%, mean arterial pressure decreases approximately 10 mm Hg[6-8] (see Chaps. 3 and 4). The decrement apparent in the first trimester, reaches a nadir by midpregnancy. Blood pressure then increases gradually, approaching prepregnancy values at term, but may transiently increase to values slightly above the women's nonpregnant level during the puerperium. Women with preexisting or chronic hypertension also manifest such decrements that may be as great as 15 to 20 mm Hg[9] (Fig. 19–1).

Blood pressure control in normal pregnancy, including the influence of pressor systems (autonomic nerves and catecholamines, renin–angiotensin, and vasopressin), baroreceptor function, endothelial cell function, and volume-mediated changes (detailed elsewhere in this text), has not been well evaluated in pregnant women. Animal studies are frequently contradictory, in part because of species differences. Thus, there is a critical need to explain normal vascular physiology in gestation in order to understand the blood pressure alterations in chronically hypertensive women.

Conflicting data regarding whether the autonomic nervous system is more active in the control of blood pressure during pregnancy is another issue to be addressed. In one well-designed study there were no differences in sympathetic nerve activity in normotensive gravidas compared with nonpregnant controls.[10] On the other hand, the renin–angiotensin system is markedly stimulated,[8] and normotensive pregnant women have an exaggerated hypotensive response to angiotensin-converting enzyme inhibition, compared with nonpregnant women.[11] These data suggest that this system is stimulated to help maintain normal blood pressure.

Some evidence exists, mainly from animal models, that basal and stimulated nitric oxide production increase in pregnancy, and may account for the marked vasodilation and lower blood pressure.[12] There are conflicting data on endothelial cell function in human pregnancy as discussed in Chapter 12. The link between markedly increased placental hormones, particularly estrogen and progesterone, and alterations in vascular endothelial function is another area of active investigation. Fi-

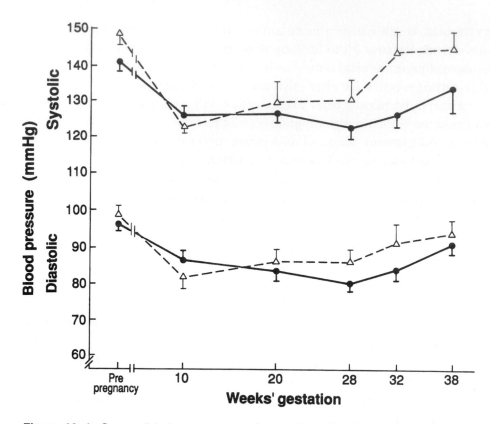

Figure 19–1. Sequential changes in systolic and diastolic blood pressure throughout pregnancy in women with uncomplicated chronic hypertension (N = 17, •-•), and women with chronic hypertension with superimposed preeclampsia (N = 13, Δ---Δ) (mean ± SEM). In cases of uncomplicated chronic hypertension blood pressure decreases in the first and second trimesters, rising to early pregnancy or pregnancy levels in the third trimester. In contrast, blood pressure did not decrease after 10 weeks in women who developed superimposed preeclampsia, but remained constant or increased until the third trimester when preeclampsia was diagnosed. (*Reprinted, with permission, from August P, Lenz T, Ales KL, et al: Longitudinal study of the renin–angiotensin–aldosterone system in hypertensive pregnant women: Deviations related to development of superimposed preeclampsia. Am J Obstet Gynecol 1990;163:1612–1621.*)

nally, preliminary studies of a vasoactive peptide produced by neural tissue, calcitonin gene-related peptide (CGRP),[13] further suggest that the vasculature in pregnant women is modulated by multiple factors.

Other pregnancy-associated cardiovascular alterations that impact on blood pressure are increased cardiac output and blood volume.[6-8] The relationship between these changes in women with chronic hypertension seems not to have been studied, though such data are important for optimal management.

The profound alterations in renal hemodynamics in normal pregnancy which include increases in glomerular filtration rate and renal blood flow of ~50% are also detailed elsewhere[14] (see Chap. 8). The impact of these changes on blood pressure control and on responsiveness to antihypertensive agents in women with chronic hypertension is not known. It does seem probable, though, that these hemodynamic alterations contribute to the greater ease of blood pressure control during pregnancy, that is, in the absence of superimposed preeclampsia.

Finally, the extent to which excessive weight gain during gestation compromises therapeutic blood pressure control is also poorly understood. Some dietary habits, such as increased consumption of dairy products high in sodium, may also impact blood pressure control in the chronically hypertensive pregnant woman. Credible investigations of dietary modification have not been performed.

Effects of Chronic Hypertension on the Mother

There is considerable confusion regarding the maternal and fetal risks associated with preexisting hypertension. This is largely due to a failure to distinguish outcomes in women with superimposed preeclampsia from those with uncomplicated chronic hypertension. While there is little doubt that women with chronic hypertension who develop *superimposed preeclampsia* have increased perinatal morbidity as well as mortality compared with hypertensive pregnant women with uncomplicated preexisting essential hypertension,[4,15] the maternal and fetal risks of pregnancies in this latter group, are less clear.

Some women will experience accelerated hypertension during pregnancy, with resultant target organ damage, e.g., to the heart, brain, and kidneys, although in the absence of preeclampsia, this is extremely uncommon. One exception may be the rare women with severe hypertension (stage 3 or 4) prior to conception, many of whom have underlying renal disease or secondary hypertension. In the well-designed study by Rey and Couturier of women with chronic hypertension complicating pregnancy, there was an increased incidence of gestational diabetes.[16] This may reflect similar risk factors for both conditions (obesity) as well as similar pathogenetic mechanisms (insulin resistance).

Placental abruption is associated with life-threatening maternal hemorrhage, and its risk is increased threefold in women with chronic hypertension.[17] Some women with secondary forms of hypertension, such as from chronic renal disease and collagen disorders, may suffer from irreversible deterioration in renal function. In the case of systemic lupus erythematosus, there may be multiorgan system morbidity, regardless of the development of superimposed preeclampsia. Finally, although the expectation is that pregnancies in women with uncomplicated chronic hypertension will be successful, these women are more likely to be hospitalized for hypertension and to undergo cesarean delivery.[16]

Chronic Hypertension with Superimposed Preeclampsia

As discussed, underlying hypertension is a recognized risk factor for preeclampsia. Depending on diagnostic criteria, etiology (essential vs. secondary), duration, and the severity of hypertension, the incidence of superimposed preeclampsia ranges between 4 to 40%.[18-21a] A major reason for this wide range in incidence is that the definition of superimposed preeclampsia was used too liberally in some studies. Criteria proposed by the National Institutes of Health Working Group Report (and most appealing to us) include a significant increase in blood pressure (30 mm Hg systolic, 15 mm Hg diastolic) in association with new onset proteinuria ($\geq$ 300 mg/day), and hyperuricemia or features of "HELLP" syndrome (*h*emolysis, *e*levated *l*iver enzymes, *l*ow *p*latelet counts) occurring after midpregnancy. In one series in which these criteria were applied there was an incidence of superimposed preeclampsia of 21% in consecutively enrolled patients.[16] These investigators also observed that the risk increased with higher first trimester diastolic blood pressure.[16] Sibai et al.[20] prospectively studied 300 women with "mild" chronic hypertension, defined as baseline blood pressure between 140/90 to 160/110 mm Hg, and reported similar incidences of superimposed preeclampsia; 15.6% in untreated women compared with 18.4% and 16.3% in women treated with either methyldopa or labetalol, respectively. Experiences at the primary author's institution (Cornell University) are similar, and using the NIH Working Group's criteria for diagnosis,[2] the incidence of superimposed preeclampsia is 15% in mild essential hypertensives, and as high as 30% in women with severe or secondary hypertension (P. August, unpublished data).

The above noted results were recently verified, in a multicenter, randomized blind trial to assess low-dose aspirin therapy for preeclampsia prevention in high-risk women. In chronic hypertensives, (N = 774), the incidence of superimposed preeclampsia was similar in the treatment and placebo groups, averaging 26% and 25%, respectively.[22] An even higher incidence was noted in women whose hypertension had been present for 4 or more years.[21a] An intriguing question is why women with preexisting hypertension are at greater risk for the development of superimposed preeclampsia. There are few studies addressing this, but it has been suggested that women at risk for preeclampsia have genetic, biochemical, and metabolic abnormalities similar to women with essential hypertension.[23] This list includes a higher incidence of polymorphisms in the angiotensinogen gene, obesity, hypertriglyceridemia, and insulin resistance. Such observations raise the possibility that the genesis of "superimposed" preeclampsia in hypertensive pregnant women may be related to the underlying genetic and metabolic disturbances that led to hypertension, rather than the elevated blood pressure itself. This is clearly an exciting area worthy of further investigation.

Effects of Chronic Hypertension on Fetal Outcome

Perinatal mortality is higher in pregnancies associated with chronic hypertension. Moreover, these excess losses are primarily due to superimposed preeclampsia. Rey and Couturier[16] reported a relative risk of perinatal death of 3.6 in women with "superimposed preeclampsia" in comparison to those with uncomplicated chronic hypertension. It should be noted that the incidence of perinatal death was also significantly higher in the latter group compared with outcomes in normotensive controls (relative risk 2.3). Preterm delivery was more common only if there was superimposed preeclampsia. Fetal growth restriction is also more common with chronic hypertension, especially when superimposed preeclampsia develops. Rey and Couturier[16] reported the incidence of fetal growth restriction as 35% in women with superimposed preeclampsia vs. 11% in women with uncomplicated chronic hypertension. Sibai et al.[19] reported a similar incidence of small-for-gestational-age infants in their large clinical trial of women with mild chronic hypertension.

An unquantified risk to fetal well being is exposure in utero to antihypertensive medications. Careful clinical trials evaluating maternal outcomes as well as long-term outcomes of exposed offspring have been conducted with a limited number of agents, primarily methyldopa (see Chap. 18). Because of its proven safety, this drug remains the drug of choice for hypertension during pregnancy.

SPECIFIC HYPERTENSIVE DISORDERS

Essential Hypertension

Approximately 50 million adult Americans have hypertension.[1] In the majority, no identifiable cause is apparent and such individuals are considered to have "essential" hypertension. The disorder is more prevalent in African Americans, in whom it is associated with greater morbidity, particularly renal damage.[24] Its prevalence in women of childbearing age is estimated to be 20 to 25%, with blood pressure rising to abnormal levels ($\geq$ 140/90 mm Hg) usually during the third and fourth decades. In all likelihood essential hypertension is a heterogeneous disorder, with variable pathogenetic features. While a detailed discussion of the pathophysiology of essential hypertension is beyond the scope of this chapter, there are several important biochemical, hormonal, metabolic, and genetic abnormalities that have been described that are intriguing from the viewpoint of pregnancy interaction. For example, there is emerging evidence that previously normotensive women with preeclampsia demonstrate similar abnormalities to women with chronic hypertension. The brief overview of important pathophysiologic features relating to essential hypertension which follows focuses on their impact during pregnancy.

Genetic Basis for Essential Hypertension

Primary hypertension is a polygenic disorder which does not follow classic Mendelian rules of inheritance. Thus, the likelihood of identifying one or a few genes that have a major impact on the development of hypertension is small. Nevertheless, it is also likely that within the spectrum of individuals currently characterized as essential hypertensives that some cases of monogenic hypertension will be discovered. Polymorphisms in several genes have been linked to the development of essential hypertension in humans, including the angiotensinogen gene, the angiotensin-converting enzyme gene, and the α adducin gene.[25-27] Interestingly, the same polymorphism in the angiotensinogen gene that has been associated with essential hypertension has also been associated with preeclampsia[28,29] (see also Chap. 13).

Renal Basis for Essential Hypertension

Abundant evidence shows that renal mechanisms, either directly or indirectly, play an important role in subpopulations of hypertensive individuals. Subclinical renal abnormalities observed in some individuals with essential hypertension include focal renal ischemia leading to chronic nonsuppressible renin secretion, renal sodium retention, reduced renal mass, decreased glomerular filtration rate, and a compromised sodium excretory capacity.[30-32]

Therapeutically, the role for renal sodium retention in the pathogenesis of hypertension is supported by the efficacy in many hypertensive individuals of diuretic therapy. Similarly, a role for nonsuppressible renin secretion is supported by the efficacy of agents that interrupt the renin–angiotensin system. The relationship between subtle abnormalities in renal function, and pregnancy outcome has not been investigated in detail. Given the significant impact of reduced renal function on the risk of preeclampsia, this is an area of investigation of potential importance.

Hormonal Basis for Essential Hypertension

Alterations in the renin–angiotensin system are important aspects of the pathophysiology of primary aldosteronism and renovascular hypertension. Conversely, in essential hypertension there is considerable heterogeneity in renin and aldosterone levels.[33] Some patients have normal or high plasma renin activity, whereas about one-third of hypertensive individuals have low or suppressed plasma renin activity. The latter values are those expected if volume overload is present, and indeed, low-renin hypertension is often associated with increased sensitivity to salt restriction or diuretic therapy. Because pregnancy is characterized by activation of the renin–angiotensin system, adverse perinatal outcomes in women with essential hypertension who have alterations in the renin system is a real possibility.

Sympathetic Nervous System and Essential Hypertension

The role of the sympathetic nervous system in the pathogenesis of primary hypertension is supported by a large number of indirect experimental and clinical observations. These include increased heart rate and plasma catecholamine levels in response to a variety of stimuli in hypertensive individuals and in animals.[34] While sympathetic nervous system activity and function are difficult to measure accurately in humans, there are a few studies that link preeclampsia to its activation.[10]

Vascular Structure and Function and Hypertension

It is beyond the scope of this chapter to review the expanding field of vascular biology and the role of abnormalities of vascular structure and function that are important in the genesis and the maintenance of elevated blood pressure. However, several key areas of investigation are worth mentioning, particularly those with relevance to the pathophysiology of preeclampsia. Mechanisms for vascular hypertrophy blood vessel remodeling, as well as alterations in ion transport and signal transduction in vascular smooth muscle and endothelial cells are the focus of active investigation. The resultant functional consequences with respect to the ability of vascular endothelial cells to generate vasodilatory (e.g., nitric oxide and prostacyclin), as well as vasoconstrictor substances (e.g., endothelin) are also relevant to the pathophysiology of essential hypertension because these substances are important mediators of vascular muscle tone and function. Additionally, interactions between nitric oxide and prostacyclin with platelets and lipids are important in relation to the development of atherosclerotic lesions. Current evidence supports a role for dysregulation of these processes in the pathogenesis of preeclampsia.[35] The role of these processes in the increased tendency of women with preexisting hypertension to develop preeclampsia deserves study.

Metabolic Disturbances and Hypertension

The common occurrence of obesity, type II diabetes, and hypertension, as well as the observation that a significant number of nonobese hypertensives will have insulin resistance and hyperinsulinemia has led to the concept of insulin resistance in the genesis of primary hypertension.[36] This has relevance to pregnancy hypertension because insulin resistance is claimed to be more prevalent in preeclamptic women, and women with overt and gestational diabetes are reported to be at greater risk for preeclampsia.[4,21a,22,37]

Dietary Factors

The role of sodium in the pathogenesis of some if not most cases of primary hypertension is established.[38] Other dietary components possibly involved are calcium and potassium.[39-41] Inverse relationships between dietary calcium intake and blood pressure have been documented, while calcium supplementation lowers blood pressure in experimental models and in clinical trials.[40,41] Calcium requirements are increased in normal pregnancy, and there are data suggesting an association between inadequate calcium intake and hypertension during pregnancy.[42] Supplemental calcium does not seem to have beneficial effects on blood pressure in normal pregnancy,[43] but whether it is useful in the management of pregnant women with chronic hypertension is currently under investigation.

Environment and Behavior

Obesity and excess alcohol intake contribute to hypertension. Conversely, weight loss, increased physical activity, and decreased alcohol intake have been demonstrated to be effective strategies for lowering blood pressure.[1] As noted in Chapter 2, obesity is also an independent risk factor for preeclampsia.[44]

Physiology and Pathophysiology of Essential Hypertension During Pregnancy

The cardiovascular, renal and hemodynamic alterations in pregnancy pertinent to blood pressure regulation were summarized above. Surprisingly, few detailed investigations of the physiology of essential hypertension in pregnancy have been performed. Such individuals are an intriguing group to investigate because they have a high incidence of superimposed preeclampsia. Thus, longitudinal studies of chronic hypertensives may be helpful in elucidating early pregnancy phenomena important in the pathophysiology of preeclampsia.

Blood Pressure Patterns and Hemodynamic Measurements

Women with essential hypertension normally demonstrate the expected decrease in blood pressure in early- and midpregnancy. In women who develop superimposed preeclampsia, blood pressure may start to increase in the late second trimester, whereas women who have uncomplicated pregnancies will frequently demonstrate even lower blood pressures at this time of gestation.[9] It has been suggested that absence of a midsecond trimester decrease in blood pressure is associated with more gestational complications and predictive of development of preeclampsia. Ambulatory blood pressure monitoring techniques have not been extensively studied in pregnant women with essential hypertension, although, preliminary studies suggest that they will have limited utility in predicting superimposed preeclampsia.[45]

Cardiac function has not been investigated extensively during pregnancy in women with essential hypertension. Increased left ventricular mass has been reported in third-trimester chronic hypertensives,[46] however, longitudinal studies are needed. Other hemodynamic parameters such as plasma volume and peripheral vascular resistance have been reported to be similar to normotensive pregnant women, unless superimposed preeclampsia develops (see Chap. 9).[47]

Similarly, there is a paucity of information concerning renal function and hemodynamics during pregnancies complicated by chronic hypertension (see Chap. 8). In one study there was a normal increase in creatinine clearance and urinary calcium excretion in most women with uncomplicated essential hypertension during pregnancy, but as expected, when superimposed preeclampsia developed, renal function decreased modestly while marked hypocalciuria supervened.[48] A preliminary study of Doppler analysis of the renal artery in hypertensive pregnant women noted an increase in renal blood flow with chronic hypertension, consistent with abnormal autoregulation.[49] These intriguing observations are not surprising given the alterations that have been reported in nonpregnant essential hypertensives.

Hormonal and Biochemical Alterations

Most investigations of pregnant women with chronic essential hypertension demonstrate that until superimposed preeclampsia develops, levels of hormones and other circulating substances associated with blood pressure regulation are similar to values in normotensive pregnancy. The stimulation of the renin–angiotensin systems in these two groups are also similar,[9] as is platelet angiotensin II binding.[50] Of further interest, pregnant women with essential hypertension destined to develop superimposed preeclampsia also manifest reductions in plasma renin activity in midpregnancy, again in a fashion similar to that described in nulliparas who subsequently become preeclamptic.[9] The decrease in plasma renin activity is accompanied by a decrease in urinary aldosterone excretion, and is an expected response to increased vasoconstriction. Furthermore, some women who developed superimposed preeclampsia and had low plasma renin activity also had a marked decrease in plasma estradiol.[9] Others have reported that plasma estradiol levels are decreased in women with uncomplicated chronic hypertension in pregnancy.[51] Finally, we have noted similar plasma progesterone levels in women with chronic hypertension, with and without preeclampsia, and in normotensive pregnant women.[9]

Several studies of nitric oxide production in normal and preeclamptic pregnant women have been conducted, but as of 1999 we were aware of only one that focuses on essential hypertension in pregnancy. In this study, the authors reported significantly decreased levels of nitric acid metabolites compared to normotensive gestation.[52] This finding, consistent with observations in nonpregnant essential hypertensives, is surprising in view of the frequently observed pregnancy-induced vasodilation and decrease in blood pressure in these patients.

Platelet intracellular calcium concentration has been reported to be increased in nonpregnant essential hypertensives, as well as in preeclamptics.[53] The rationale for such studies is the belief that platelets are surrogates for vascular smooth muscle, an increase in their intracellular calcium implying similar increments in the vascular cells suggesting increased tone or vasoconstriction. Kilby et al.[54] reported increased platelet cytosolic calcium levels in five pregnant chronic hypertensives, while Hojo et al.[55] noted no differences in the lymphocyte intracellular free calcium levels of pregnant women with essential hypertension.

Pathophysiology of Superimposed Preeclampsia

While there is evidence that women with essential hypertension are at greater risk to develop superimposed preeclampsia, the reason for this is not known. In view of the evidence for abnormalities in placental implantation and the uteroplacental circulation in the pathophysiology of preeclampsia, it is somewhat surprising that a maternal factor such as hypertension is a major risk factor. One possibility is that there may be a "shared risk factor" for both essential hypertension and preeclampsia that is only indirectly related to high blood pressure. However, having reviewed the heterogeneous factors involved in the pathogenesis of essential hypertension, it is worth considering whether some forms of essential hypertension, for example high or low renin, may be particularly predisposed to preeclampsia. This appears to be the case with secondary hypertension, for instance, women with renovascular hypertension have an extraordinarily high incidence of preeclampsia.[56] Currently, there is little information regarding this issue in essential hypertension.

Secondary Hypertension

Secondary forms of hypertension are quite rare compared with essential hypertension, and comprise only 2 to 5% of hypertensives diagnosed and treated at specialized centers. In routine care groups, however, their numbers are even lower. The most common etiologies are renal disease, renovascular hypertension, aldosteronism, Cushing syndrome, and pheochromocytoma. The prevalence of secondary hypertension in women of childbearing age has not been determined. Of importance, prognosis is best when a diagnosis of secondary hypertension is made prior to conception, because most forms of secondary hypertension are associated with increased maternal and fetal morbidity and mortality.

Renal Disease

A detailed discussion of renal disease and pregnancy is beyond the scope of this chapter. There are, however, several points to emphasize regarding the management of hypertension associated with intrinsic renal disease. Kidney disease is the most common cause of secondary hypertension, and may be due to anatomic or congenital abnormalities, glomerulonephritis, diabetes, systemic lupus erythematosus, or interstitial nephritis.

All young women with a newly diagnosed hypertension should be screened for intrinsic renal disease with blood tests for renal function, and urinalysis for detection of proteinuria or red blood cells. Those with a strong family history of renal disease should be screened with ultrasound for polycystic kidney disease. This autosomal-dominant disorder often presents with hypertension in the 3rd and 4th decades. When renal disease is detected, regardless of its cause, these women should be counseled about the increased maternal and fetal risks associated with impaired renal function (preconception serum creatinine level $\geq$ 1.4 mg/dL) or poorly controlled hypertension.

Women with renal disease should be managed by a multidisciplinary team of obstetricians and nephrologists. This is particularly appropriate for renal transplant recipients, in whom concerns regarding immunosuppression and risk of infection and rejection require coordinated specialty care. Therapy of hypertension is similar to that in gravidas with essential hypertension, although many nephrologists treat hypertension more aggressively during pregnancy when there is underlying renal disease.

Renovascular Hypertension

This entity refers to hypertension caused by anatomic lesions of the renal arteries. The narrowing of the lumen leads to diminished blood flow to one or both kidneys, with resulting renal ischemia, stimulation of the renin–angiotensin system, and ensuing hypertension. It is important to emphasize that not all anatomic lesions of the renal artery result in hypertension, because they may not be severe enough to compromise renal blood flow. Thus, demonstration (by angiography) of a lesion does not necessarily establish the diagnosis of renovascular hypertension, though cure of hypertension after revascularization remains the most reliable proof of renovascular hypertension.[57]

The causes of renovascular hypertension are many. *Atherosclerotic renovascular disease* is primarily observed in postmenopausal women, especially those with a history of tobacco use and diffuse vascular disease, whereas *fibromuscular dysplasia* is more likely to be present in young women, making it the form most likely to be encountered in pregnancy.[58] The latter lesion, three times more common in women than men (but infrequent in black or Asian populations), is a nonatherosclerotic, noninflammatory vascular occlusive disease, most often presenting as *medial fibroplasia*.[58] Fibromuscular dysplasia has a prevalence of approximately 1% in hypertensive populations. Although the renal arteries are most commonly involved, other vessels including carotid, coronary, abdominal aorta, and peripheral arteries may also be affected.

Clinical clues suggestive of renovascular hypertension are severe hypertension, which may be resistant to medical therapy, and which first appears in the second, third, or fourth decades. Abdominal bruit and a high peripheral venous plasma renin activity are among the findings traditionally associated with the disorder. Several noninvasive screening tests are also useful. These include captopril renography and Doppler ultrasonography of the renal arteries.[59] The definitive test, unfortunately invasive, remains angiography.[59] These tests are justified for use in pregnant women because the hypertension is potentially curable with either angioplasty or surgery, and without adequate treatment these women often do poorly in pregnancy. In addition, captopril is administered only once, and the fetal radiation dose during angiography is extremely small and in the range permissable for pregnancy. We prefer angiography to noninvasive testing, as the latter may not detect the smaller branch lesions which are more frequent when fibromuscular dysplasia is present. Angiography in the latter disorder typically reveals multiple stenotic images with intervening aneurysmal outpouchings, the "string of beads" image, or occasionally, a pattern of solitary focal stenoses. Magnetic resonance angiography with gadolinium enhancement is currently being investigated, and may have potential usefulness in pregnancy.[60]

Renal angioplasty is a highly effective method in treating nonpregnant patients with fibromuscular dysplasia. There is a high rate of technical success, cure, or improvement exceeding 80%.[61]

Knowledge of renovascular hypertension in pregnancy is based on a handful of case reports and a few limited series of patients totaling approximately 25 cases. Many of the patients manifested early and severe preeclampsia and poor pregnancy outcomes.[62-66] A recently published retrospective comparison of pregnancy outcomes in four patients with known renovascular hypertension matched to 20 women with essential hypertension[56] demonstrated that those with renovascular hypertension were younger (age 25 vs. 36) and had higher blood pressure levels during pregnancy. Of interest, the four women with renovascular hypertension all developed superimposed preeclampsia in contrast to 30% of those with essential hypertension. Plasma renin activity in one woman with renovascular hypertension was, as expected, quite elevated when measured early in pregnancy, but decreased when preeclampsia developed.

Also, of interest are sporadic cases of early pregnancy detection of renovascular hypertension, and successful revascularization during midpregnancy, with good pregnancy outcome.[65-67] We have also documented the experiences of two women with untreated renovascular hypertension whose pregnancies were complicated by severe preeclampsia. Both had successful angioplasty postpartum and their subsequent pregnancies were normal. In view of the dramatic clinical improvement which usually follows revascularization, as well as the anecdotal experience described above, it seems justified to rule out renovascular hypertension before conception in young women with suggestive clinical features. Furthermore, based on these observations, the role of renal ischemia and renin-mediated hypertension in the pathogenesis of preeclampsia warrants further investigation.

In summary, pregnant women with renovascular hypertension who have not undergone revascularization are at considerable risk, especially for superimposed preeclampsia and fetal complications. Temporizing therapy with angiotensin-converting enzyme inhibitors or angiotensin II receptor blocking agents are precluded for use in pregnancy, but treatment of hypertension with other drugs that suppress renin secretion is possible. Those most likely to be effective are methyldopa and beta-adrenergic receptor blockers.

Primary Aldosteronism

This form of hypertension results from increased secretion of aldosterone, and may be due to a solitary adrenal adenoma (Conn syndrome) or bilateral adrenal hyperplasia. There is also a variant, labeled nodular hyperplasia, characterized by enlargement of the adrenal glands which contain one or more adenomas which secrete most of the aldosterone. Another form, which is hereditary, is glucocorticoid remediable aldosteronism. This disease results from a chromosomal crossover producing a chimeric gene which causes aldosterone to be synthesized by the adrenal fasciculata, and regulated by adrenocorticotropic hormone (ACTH).

Primary aldosteronism may not be that rare, but the milder forms are frequently overlooked.[68] The classic clinical features are hypertension, hypokalemia, suppressed plasma renin activity, excessive urinary potassium excretion, hypernatremia, and metabolic alkalosis. Manifestation of each of these features is variable, and even hypokalemia, once thought as the sine qua non for diagnosing aldosterone excess, may be initially absent in as many as 25% of patients.[68] Diagnosis is made by demonstrating biochemical and hormonal abnormalities, followed by computerized tomography (CT) of the adrenal gland (helpful in differentiating an adenoma from hyperplasia). If an adenoma is detected, radiologic imaging may be followed by adrenal vein sampling to document unilateral aldosterone secretion prior to surgery.[69] Surgery is indicated for unilateral disease, with a cure rate of about 65%, and an improvement in an additional 33%. Medical therapy with spironolactone (in nonpregnant populations) is usually effective for patients with hyperplasia, although high doses may be necessary. Calcium channel blockers have also been reported to be effective.[70]

Several cases of aldosteronism have been reported in pregnancy.[71-81] Some of these have been complicated by considerable morbidity, including severe hypertension, hypokalemia, preeclampsia, and poor fetal outcome, but there are also instances where hypertension and hypokalemia have been ameliorated during gestation.[76,81] It is hypothesized that such improvement, when it occurs, is a consequence of the high levels of progesterone which antagonize the actions of aldosterone.[76]

Primary aldosteronism may be difficult to diagnose in pregnant women because of the marked alterations in the renin–angiotensin–aldosterone system that occur in normal pregnancy. Both renin and aldosterone production are markedly increased with a fivefold increase in urine aldosterone excretion compared to that observed in nonpregnant patients with primary aldosteronism.[82] Moreover, mild hypokalemia is not unusual in the course of a normal pregnancy. Greater degrees of hypokalemia (≤ 3 mEq/L), however, are unusual and should be investigated. In one case involving a pregnant women with an aldosteronoma, reported by us[82] (Fig. 19–2), plasma renin activity was not totally suppressed, but became undetectable postpartum. Her plasma renin levels, however, were approximately one-third to one-half of those routinely observed in other pregnant women with essential hypertension.[9] Her urinary aldosterone excretion was well above the increases recorded in most women with uncomplicated gestations.

Treatment of aldosteronism diagnosed during pregnancy is controversial.[78-81] If blood pressure improves spontaneously or is easily controlled with antihypertensive drugs, then it is reasonable to postpone surgical intervention until postpartum. Spironolactone, reported to cause virilization in rodent fetuses exposed in utero, should be avoided.[83] The use of antihypertensive medications in pregnancy is detailed in Chapter 18, and in this respect there are reports of the beneficial effects of calcium channel blockers in nonpregnant patients with aldosteronism.[70] Thus, we would prescribe these latter agents, especially if methyldopa proved ineffective. However, when faced with severe hypertension resistant to therapy, and marked hypokalemia requiring very large replacement doses, it may be prudent to consider surgery. During pregnancy, magnetic resonance imaging (MRI) is preferable to CT, as the former does not use ionizing radiation. Adrenal vein sampling does not seem to have been reported in pregnancy, and is unadvisable since too many X-rays are required to perform this procedure. Thus, documentation of a unilateral adenoma during pregnancy may be suboptimal, which is one reason why surgery may be indicated for treatment failure alone. In this respect, there are several reports of surgical removal of adenomas during the second trimester followed by favorable maternal and fetal outcomes.[73,78,79,81]

Pheochromocytoma

Pheochromocytoma is rare, but when unrecognized may have fatal consequences.[84] On the other hand, there are many apparently benign pheochromocytomas revealed only as an incidental finding at autopsy.[85] Pheochromocytomas arise from

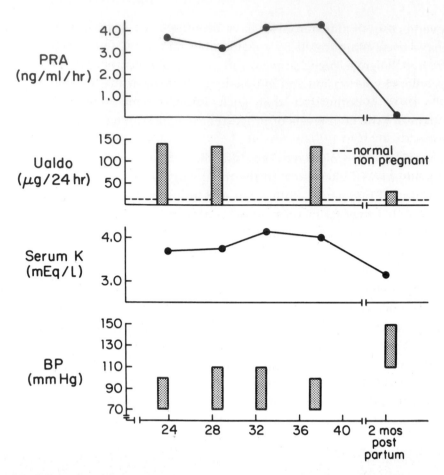

Figure 19–2. Plasma renin activity (PRA), urine aldosterone excretion, serum potassium, and blood pressure during pregnancy and 2 months postpartum in a woman with primary aldosteronism. Hypertension and hypokalemia resolved during pregnancy therapy and recurred after delivery. PRA was higher during pregnancy compared with postpartum values, although it was relatively low compared with women with essential hypertension. Urine aldosterone excretion was higher than normal for pregnancy. (*Reprinted, with permission, from August PA, Sealy JE: The renin–angiotensin system in normal and hypertensive pregnancy and in ovarian function. In: Laragh JH, Brenner BM, eds. Hypertension: Pathology, Diagnosis, and Management. New York: Raven Press; 1990:1761–1778.*)

chromaffin cells, a tissue which has differentiated from neural crest stem cells and which synthesizes and stores catecholamines. Although the majority of these tumors are in the adrenal glands, as many as 10 to 15% are extraadrenal in association with sympathetic nerves, mainly in the abdomen (Fig. 19–3) and pelvis, but very rarely in the thorax or in the neck.

The clinical manifestations of pheochromocytoma may be dramatic. They result from catecholamine excess or complications of severe hypertension, and include headache, sweating, palpitations, and anxiety in association with paroxysmal or sustained hypertension.[85] Any patient presenting with such symptoms should be screened for pheochromocytoma, preferably prior to conception, thus avoiding concerns regarding fetal x-ray exposure, and making therapeutic strategies easier. Additional features that may be suggestive of pheochromocytoma are hyperglycemia, orthostatic hypotension, and weight loss. The two most reliable screening procedures are the measurement of 24-hour urinary metanephrines and plasma catecholamines. If biochemical evidence of pheochromocytoma is present, then CT, or preferably MRI, of the abdomen (Fig. 19–3) should be performed. Specialized nuclear medicine tests utilizing iodine 131-metaiodobenzylguanidine may be helpful in identifying extraadrenal pheochromocytomas.[84] Appropriate treatment in nonpregnant individuals is preoperative alpha-blockade, followed by surgical removal of the tumor.

Over 100 cases of pheochromocytoma presenting during pregnancy or in the immediate puerperium have been reported, and both maternal and fetal morbidity and mortality are extremely high when the presence of the tumor is unknown prior to delivery.[86-90] Instances of unsuspected pheochromocytoma presenting as myocardial infarction in pregnant women are also on record.[91,92] Other serious complications include cardiac arrhythmias, shock, pulmonary edema, cerebral hemorrhage, and hemorrhaging into the tumor. In several instances the presenting signs and symptoms, late pregnancy-accelerated hypertension, proteinuria, and seizures, were indistinguishable from preeclampsia and/or eclampsia.[93-95] In fact, there is a suggestion that the clinical manifestations may be more dramatic as pregnancy progresses because the enlarged uterus is more apt to compress the tumor.

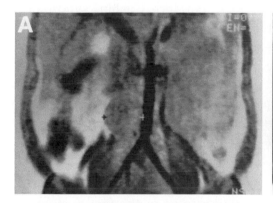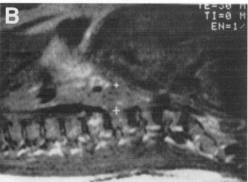

Figure 19–3. Magnetic resonance images of an extraadrenal pheochromocytoma in a 27-week pregnant patient who presented during gestational week 19 with severe hypertension alternating with hypotension even at bed rest. Plasma norepinephrine levels were ≥ 8000 pg/mL in this patient who was managed medically with phenoxybenzamine and propranolol through her 36th gestational week, at which time a 2900-g healthy boy was delivered by cesarean section followed by successful exterpation of the tumor. Coronal section, A, demonstrates that the tumor, 4–5 cm in diameter (between the +s), is located above the bifurcation of the aorta, and just behind the enlarged uterus shown in the sagittal section (again between the +s) and virtually on the vena cava. Despite its proximity to the great vessels, the pheochromocytoma presented few problems at surgery. (*Modified, with permission, from Greenberg M, Moawad AH, Wieties BM, et al: Extraadrenal pheochromocytoma: Detection during pregnancy using MR imaging.* Radiology *1986;161:475–476.*)

Surgical removal is the therapy of choice when a pheochromocytoma is diagnosed in the initial two trimesters, although successful medical management throughout the entire pregnancy has been reported.[88] Preoperative management includes alpha-blockade with either phenoxybenzamine[89,90] or combinations of alpha- and beta-blockers. Placental transfer of phenoxybenzamine has been reported, and may lead to perinatal depression and hypotension in newborns.[95] Labetalol, an alpha- and beta-blocker, has also been used successfully during gestation.[88]

The approach to treatment in the third trimester is more variable and includes combined cesarean delivery and tumor resection, tumor resection followed by delivery, and delivery followed by tumor resection at a later date. Once the predicted fetal survival is high, we prefer the combined procedure of cesarean delivery and immediate tumor resection.[89,94]

Cushing Syndrome

Cushing syndrome is also quite rare in pregnant hypertensives, possibly because patients with this disorder have a variety of menstrual irregularities.[96] Also, the syndrome may be difficult to diagnose because the hormonal alterations of normal pregnancy mimic those of the disease.[96] Most of the pregnancy-associated cases have been due to either adrenal adenomas, or pituitary-dependent adrenal hyperplasia. In several instances the disease has appeared during pregnancy, and remitted or improved postpartum, leading to suggestions that a placental ACTH-like compound may have caused the disease.[96-98] Of importance, Cushing syndrome is associated with excessive maternal morbidity, with hypertension, superimposed preeclampsia, diabetes, and congestive heart failure being the most common complications. There is also a high incidence of preterm delivery, growth restriction, and fetal demise. Management includes surgical resection during the first trimester or surgery after delivery in the third trimester. Therapeutic approaches in the second trimester are more complex, as the risks of surgery must be weighed against the risks of medication to treat hypercortisolism.[99]

Postpartum Hypertension

Hypertension associated with preeclampsia may resolve in the first postpartum week, although with more severe cases blood pressure may continue to rise after delivery and the hypertension may persist for 2 to 4 weeks postpartum.[100,101] Ferrazzani et al.[101] stress that the time required for the blood pressure to normalize postpartum correlates both with laboratory markers indicative of renal impairment and with early delivery. Of interest, blood pressure in normotensive women is higher during the first 5 postpartum days,[102] and it has been proposed that this may relate to the shifting of fluid from the interstitial space to the intravascular volume which occurs in the immediate puerperium. We are unaware of large clinical treatment trials that focus uniquely on hypertension in the immediate puerperium. This is unfortunate because severe hypertension in the setting of resolving vasospasm may potentially interfere with cerebral autoregulation resulting in seizures or cerebrovascular accidents. Thus, in the absence of more definitive data we recommend that systolic blood pressure levels $\geq$ 160 mm Hg and diastolic levels $\geq$ 100 mm Hg be treated in the puerperium (see below). Women with postpartum hypertension should not receive bromocriptine because of anecdotal reports that such therapy paradoxically exacerbates the hypertensive syndrome and may cause cerebrovascular accidents.[103]

New Onset Hypertension in the Puerperium

Hypertension may first be diagnosed in the postpartum period. When this occurs, the differential diagnosis includes postpartum preeclampsia or eclampsia, unrecognized chronic hypertension that was masked by pregnancy, and rarely, microangiopathic syndromes such as hemolytic uremic syndrome or thrombotic thrombocytopenic purpura.

Postpartum preeclampsia or eclampsia is uncommon, and in some cases, careful scrutiny of antepartum records reveals evidence of preeclampsia prior to delivery. However, there are instances of well-documented normotensive deliveries where hypertension in association with laboratory features of preeclampsia has appeared late in the first postpartum week or afterward. Late postpartum *eclampsia* has also been observed, the seizures occurring after the first postpartum week.[104-106] The pathogenesis of these phenomena is poorly understood, and certainly is at odds with the traditional concept of preeclampsia–eclampsia as disorders observed only during pregnancy or the immediate puerperium caused by abnormalities in placental development. Currently no standard protocols exist for the management of these late postpartum syndromes; some authorities use the traditional approach of parenteral magnesium sulfate, others concerned about previously subclinical epilepsy use phenytoin. In most instances the disease resolves within 48 to 72 hours. Periodic suggestions that corticosteroids and/or uterine curettage be used are also offered, especially when severe systemic disease is present.[106] We do not recommend these approaches.

Hypertension appearing de novo in the puerperium without laboratory abnormalities suggestive of preeclampsia is most likely due to undiagnosed chronic hypertension. In some cases the blood pressure had normalized during gestation as a response to the physiologic vasodilation that accompanies pregnancy. In most instances the underlying disorder is essential hypertension, however, secondary causes should be considered when there are unusual features such as severe hypertension, hypokalemia, or symptoms suggestive of pheochromocytoma (see above).

MANAGEMENT PRINCIPLES

The purpose of treating chronic hypertension in pregnancy is to ensure a successful term delivery of a healthy infant without jeopardizing maternal well being. This contrasts the treatment philosophy for nonpregnant subjects where the primary concern is prevention of long-term cardiovascular morbidity and mortality. In the latter population blood pressure control is essential, the recent report of the Joint National Committee on Prevention, Detection, Evaluation, and Treatment of High Blood Pressure[1] recommending levels be maintained between 120 to 135 mm Hg systolic and 75 to 85 mm Hg diastolic, respectively. Management also includes aggressive attention to modifying other cardiovascular risk factors such as blood lipid and glucose levels, body weight, and smoking. Some of these concerns are relevant during pregnancy (e.g., smoking, blood glucose), but others are not. For example, the level of blood pressure control tolerated during pregnancy may be higher, because the risk of exposure of the fetus to additional antihypertensive agents may outweigh the small benefits to the mother of complete normalization of her pressure during a 9-month period. Excessive weight loss is not recommended during pregnancy, nor is vigorous cardiovascular exercise which may reduce uteroplacental perfusion.

Preconception Counseling

Management ideally begins prior to conception, and includes ruling out and treating, if detected, secondary causes of hypertension. Women in whom hypertension is known to have been present for 5 years or more require careful evaluation for evidence of target organ damage, i.e., left ventricular hypertrophy, retinopathy, and azotemia. Pregnant women 35 years of age or older, particularly those with chronic illnesses, should be screened for occult coronary disease, and this is particularly important in women with type 1 diabetes with evidence of vascular complications. Ideally, adjustment of medications should also precede conception, discontinuing, of course, drugs with known deleterious fetal effects (especially angiotensin-converting enzyme inhibitors and angiotensin II receptor antagonists). Risks posed by pregnancy are best discussed, and less emotionally evaluated, prior to conception. For example, women with stage 1 and 2 hypertension should be informed of the high likelihood of a favorable outcome, but should still be apprised of the risks of superimposed preeclampsia and the fetal complications associated with this disorder. This is also the best time to emphasize the importance of compliance and that frequent visits increase the likelihood of detecting preeclampsia and other complications well before they become life-threatening to mother or fetus. Patient education, by increasing compliance, should a priori improve outcome. Women with small children, and those in the workforce, should be informed of the possibility that lifestyle adjustments will be necessary especially if complications develop. This will allow them to plan ahead for increased support both at home and at work. Finally, early planning, including the assembling of a multidisciplinary team consisting of obstetrician and internists optimize the chances of a successful outcome in hypertensive women with other medical complications (e.g., renal transplant recipients, diabetic nephropathy, systemic lupus erythematosus).

Nonpharmacologic Management

Pregnant hypertensives, in contradistinction to their nonpregnant counterparts, are not advised to exercise vigorously, although careful studies of the effects of aerobic exercise on pregnancy outcome have not been performed. However, moderate exercise, such as walking program 3 to 5 times a week, is acceptable. The major concern regarding vigorous exertion is that women with chronic hypertension are at risk for preeclampsia, a condition characterized by decreased uteroplacental blood flow, and such exercise may compromise blood flow even further.

Excessive weight gain, of course, is not advisable, but again, in contradistinction to therapy in nonpregnant populations, obese women should not be advised to lose weight during pregnancy. Dietary adjustments in pregnant women with chronic hypertension have not been extensively investigated. Salt restriction, an important component of management in nonpregnant populations, is less so in gestation, where extremely low sodium intakes (≤ 2 g NaCl) may even jeopardize the physiologic plasma volume expansion which normally occurs. However, in women with "salt-sensitive" hypertension, successfully managed with a low sodium diet prior to conception, it is reasonable to continue such diets during pregnancy, limiting restriction to between 60 to 80 mEq/d. Increased dietary calcium intake (i.e., greater than the recommended 1200 mg/d) may be beneficial in nonpregnant hypertensives, but data with respect to pregnancy, however, are inconclusive. In this respect, meta-analyses of small trials of the efficacy of supplementation to prevent preeclampsia in normotensive women were encouraging,[107] while a large, carefully conducted, randomized placebo-controlled trial failed to detect any beneficial actions of added calcium to diets of normotensive primiparous women.[43] Still needed are studies of calcium supplementation to prevent superimposed preeclampsia in women with chronic hypertension. Other dietary approaches, such as supplementation with magnesium or fish oil, have been investigated in normotensive pregnant women with negative results, but have not been studied in women with chronic hypertension.[108]

Pharmacologic Management (see Chap. 18)

Guidelines for antihypertensive therapy during gestation are less clear than those for nonpregnant hypertensives. For the latter, there are compelling data from large population studies to document the benefits of lowering blood pressure with medication, even in women with only mild hypertension.[1] During pregnancy, however, though maternal safety remains the primary concern, there is also a desire to minimize exposure of the fetus to drugs, given their unknown long-term effects on growth and development. Therefore, permissible maternal blood pressure levels are analyzed in terms of preventing complications during the relatively short duration of the pregnancy, rather than the long-term cardiovascular risk. Another debatable issue is whether lowering blood pressure will prevent superimposed preeclampsia, but at present there is little or no convincing evidence to support this contention.[109,109a] Thus, it is permissible to tolerate higher blood pressure levels during gestation, which do not harm in the short run, while limiting use of antihypertensive drugs. In this respect, most pregnant women with chronic hypertension have only mild or very moderate elevations in blood pressure and require little or no medication at all. However, "appropriate" or "tolerable" levels of blood pressure during gestation for these patients seem to have been set empirically, and multicenter clinical trials are needed to support or reject such practices.

We recommend the guidelines of the National High Blood Pressure Education Program's Working Group Report on High Blood Pressure in Pregnancy[2] in which antihypertensive drug treatment is only commenced when maternal blood pressure reaches diastolic levels of ≥ 100 mm Hg. There are exceptions, however, including parenchymal renal disease, and evidence of target organ damage (e.g., retinopathy and cardiac hypertrophy), in which case therapy is recommended once levels are ≥ 90 mm Hg.

It is in regard to fetal well being where the argument of whether to treat is more debatable. While the evidence is far from conclusive, it suggests fetal benefits when mild to moderate hypertension is treated with antihypertensive drugs during pregnancy.[110] For instance in one frequently cited trial, treatment with methyldopa was associated with a reduction in perinatal mortality, primarily midtrimester loss,[111] but a similar benefit was not evident in another large trial.[112]

In summary, the unknown but potential hazards of antihypertensive treatment during pregnancy are sufficient reasons for withholding drug treatment when mild hypertension (diastolic levels of 90–99 mm Hg) is present, particularly during the initial trimester. As noted, many of these patients experience a physiologic decrease in blood pressure which on occasion reaches normotensive levels. Patients whose levels are ≥ 100 mm Hg, however, should be treated, while evidence of renal disease or end-organ damage requires initiation of treatment at lower levels (≥ 90 mm Hg).

Specific Antihypertensives

The pharmacology, safety, and efficacy of antihypertensive drugs in pregnancy are addressed in detail in Chapter 18. For most agents the evaluations are sporadic, and there are almost no follow-up data regarding the children exposed to the drug in utero. In fact, the only antihypertensive for which credible follow-up exists is methyldopa,[113] where no adverse effects were documented, an important reason why this agent is considered one of the safest drugs for use during pregnancy. Methyldopa is usually prescribed alone, but on occasion the direct-acting vasodilator hydralazine has been added to the regimen, and this drug also has a long history of use in gestation and appears safe.[113] A brief summary regarding other groups of antihypertensive agents follows.

Beta-adrenoreceptor blockers have been used extensively to lower blood pressure in pregnancy, although there are only a few placebo-controlled clinical trials, as well as one very brief follow-up of the offspring.[114] Most reports are of women enrolled as patients relatively late in pregnancy, in the second or third trimesters, but there is one small, carefully conducted, placebo-controlled study of women treated with atenolol prior to 24 weeks' gestation in which a significant reduction in birth weight was noted.[115] In summary, the preponderance of data through 1997 attests to the overall safety of beta-blockers, but when treatment is commenced early in pregnancy, there may be lower birth weight.

Labetalol, a combined beta- and alpha-adrenergic blocker, has been used widely in pregnancy, with periodic claims to its superiority to other agents. In comparative trials with methyldopa, it appears to have similar efficacy and similar incidence of maternal side effects,[116,117] though when compared to placebo, significant fetal benefits have not been demonstrated.[118] Thus, it is used by us as a "second-line" antihypertensive agent in the treatment of gravidas with chronic hypertension.

Limited trials have been conducted regarding the efficacy of calcium channel blockers in pregnant women, many of which are uncontrolled and limited to treatment in an acute setting.[119-121] One concern about prescribing these agents relates to the high incidence of superimposed preeclampsia in chronic hypertensives, a complication that often requires initiation of parenteral magnesium therapy. Since magnesium also interferes with calcium-dependent, excitation-contraction coupling, and there is the potential for severe hypotension and neuromuscular blockade in women receiving both calcium channel blocking agents and magnesium, and indeed, anecdotal reports of these complications have appeared,[122] we prescribe calcium channel blockers to pregnant women as "third-line" agents.

Angiotensin-converting enzyme (ACE) inhibitors are contraindicated in pregnancy, their association with fetopathy and neonatal renal failure and death were documented in Chapter 18. These observations have led to similar rejection of the use of angiotensin II receptor antagonists in pregnancy, although there are no comparable human pregnancy data with these drugs.

Only limited experience with alpha-blockers has been reported in pregnancy. Because of their efficacy in controlling the signs and symptoms of pheochromocytoma, they are indicated in the medical management of this condition. Finally, use of diuretics in pregnancy has been controversial, mainly because of concern that saluretic therapy interferes with the physiologic volume expansion of normal pregnancy (proof of this, however, is limited). The National High Blood Pressure Education Program Working Group condemned using diuretics in preeclampsia, but noted they need not be discontinued if the woman was receiving these drugs prior to conception. Since most pregnant patients have but mild or moderate hypertension, we tend to discontinue diuretic therapy, especially in view of the "physiologic" declines in pressure during the initial trimesters. We do however use these drugs in women who appear refractory to our first-line medication because of salt sensitivity.

Antihypertensive Medications and Lactation

Studies of the possible effects of antihypertensive agents on breastfeeding infants are limited. In general, drugs that are bound to plasma proteins are not transferred to breast milk.[123] Lipid-soluble drugs may achieve higher concentrations compared with water-soluble drugs.[124] Methyldopa is considered safe, and preliminary data suggest that the levels in breast milk are low. Several beta-blockers are concentrated in breast milk, with atenolol and metoprolol resulting in high levels, and propranolol and labetalol resulting in very low levels.[125] Although captopril levels in breast milk have been reported as low, in view of the adverse effects of ACE inhibitors on neonatal renal function, we do not recommend these agents to lactating women. There are only limited reports of calcium channel blockers and their transfer into breast milk, however, no adverse effects have been reported.[126,127] Finally, although the concentration of diuretics in breast milk is usually low, these agents may reduce the quantity of milk production and interfere with the ability to successfully breast feed.[124]

REFERENCES

1. The Sixth Report of the Joint National Committee on Prevention, Detection, Evaluation, and Treatment of High Blood Pressure: *Arch Intern Med* 1997;157:2413–2446.
2. National High Blood Pressure Education Program Working Group Report on High Blood Pressure in Pregnancy. *Am J Obstet Gynecol* 1990;163:1689–1712.
3. Fisher KA, Luger A, Spargo BH, et al: Hypertension in pregnancy: Clinical–pathological correlations and remote prognosis. *Medicine* 1981;60:267–276.
4. Chesley LC: *Hypertensive Disorders in Pregnancy*. New York: Appleton Century Crofts; 1978.
5. Berkowitz RS, Goldstein DP: Chorionic tumors. *N Engl J Med* 1996;335:1740–1748.
6. Bader ME, Bader RA: Cardiovascular hemodynamics in pregnancy and labor. *Clin Obstet Gynecol* 1968;1:924–939.
7. Wilson M, Morganti AA, Zervoudakis I, et al: Blood pressure, the renin–aldosterone system and sex steroids throughout normal pregnancy. *Am J Med* 1980;68:97–104.
8. Poppas A, Shroff SG, Korcarz CE, et al: Serial assessment of the cardiovascular system in normal pregnancy. Role of arterial compliance and pulsatile arterial load. *Circulation* 1997;95:2407–2415.
9. August P, Lenz T, Ales KL, et al: Longitudinal study of the renin–angiotensin–aldosterone system in hypertensive pregnant women: Deviations related to development of superimposed preeclampsia. *Am J Obstet Gynecol* 1990;163:1612–1621.
10. Schobel HP, Fischer T, Heuszer K, et al: Preeclampsia—a state of sympathetic overactivity. *N Engl J Med* 1996;335:1480–1485.
11. August P, Muller FB, Sealey JE, Edersehim TG: The stimulated renin angiotensin system in pregnancy maintains blood pressure. *Lancet* 1995;345:896–898.
12. Baylis C, Beinder E, Suto T, August P: Recent insights into the roles of nitric oxide and renin–angiotensin in the pathophysiology of preeclampsia pregnancy. *Semin Nephrol* 1998; 18:208–230.
13. Gangula PR, Supowit SC, Wimalawansa SJ, et al: Calcitonin gene-related peptide is a depressor in NG-nitro-L-arginine methyl ester-induced hypertension during pregnancy. *Hypertension* 1997;29:248–253.
14. Sturgiss SN, Dunlop W, Davison JM: Renal haemodynamics and tubular function in human pregnancy. *Clin Obstet Gynaecol* (Bailliére) 1994;8:209–234.
15. Dunlop JCH: Chronic hypertension and perinatal mortality. *Proc Royal Soc Med* 1966; 59:838–841.
16. Rey E, Couturier A: The prognosis of pregnancy in women with chronic hypertension. *Am J Obstet Gynecol* 1994;171:410–416.
17. Ananth CV, Savitz DA, Williams MA: Placental abruption and its association with hyper-

tension and prolonged rupture of membranes: A methodologic review and meta-analysis. *Obstet Gynecol* 1996;88:309–318.

18. Mabie WC, Pernoll ML, Biswas MK: Chronic hypertension in pregnancy. *Obstet Gynecol* 1986;67:197–205.

19. Sibai BM, Abdella TN, Anderson GD: Pregnancy in 211 patients with mild chronic hypertension. *Obstet Gynecol* 1983;61:571–576.

20. Sibai BM, Mabie WC, Shamsa F, et al: A comparison of no medication versus methyldopa or labetalol in chronic hypertension during pregnancy. *Am J Obstet Gynecol* 1990;162:960–967.

21. Sibai BM, Anderson GD: Pregnancy outcome of intensive therapy in severe hypertension in first trimester. *Obstet Gynecol* 1986;67:517–522.

21a. Sibai B, Lindheimer MD, Hauth J, et al: Risk factors for preeclampsia, abruptio placenta, and adverse neonatal outcome in women with chronic hypertension. *N Engl J Med* 1998;339:667–671.

22. Caritis S, Sibai B, Hauth J, and The National Institute of Child Health and Human Development Network of Maternal–Fetal Medicine Units: Low-dose aspirin to prevent preeclampsia in women at high risk. *N Engl J Med* 1998;338:701–705.

23. Ness RB, Roberts JM: Heterogeneous causes constituting the single syndrome of preeclampsia: A hypothesis and its implications. *Am J Obstet Gynecol* 1996;175:1365–1370.

24. Duley L: Maternal mortality associated with hypertensive disorders of pregnancy in Africa, Asia, Latin America and the Caribbean. *Br J Obstet Gynaecol* 1992;99:547–553.

25. Williams GH, Fisher NDL: Genetic approach to diagnostic and therapeutic decisions in human hypertension. *Curr Opin Nephrol & Hypertens* 1997;6:199–204.

26. Jeunemaitre X, Soubrier F, Kotelevstsev YV, et al: Molecular basis of human hypertension: Role of angiotensinogen. *Cell* 1992;71:169–180.

27. Casari G, Barlassina C, Cusi D, et al: Association of the α-adducin locus with essential hypertension. *Hypertension* 1995;25:320–326.

28. Ward K, Hata A, Jeunemaitre X, et al: A molecular variant of angiotensinogen associated with preeclampsia. *Nature Genet* 1993;4:59–61.

29. Arngrimsson R, Purandare S, Connor M, et al: Angiotensinogen: A candidate gene involved in pre-eclampsia? *Nature Genet* 1993;4:114–115.

30. Sealey JE, Blumenfeld JD, Bell GM, et al: On the renal basis for essential hypertension: Nephron heterogeneity with discordant renin secretion and sodium excretion causing a hypertensive vasoconstriction-volume relationship. *J Hypertens* 1988;6:763–777.

31. Mackenzie HS, Garcia DL, Anderson S, Brenner BM: The renal abnormality in hypertension: A proposed defect in glomerular filtration surface area. In: Laragh JL, Brenner BM, eds. *Hypertension: Pathophysiology, Diagnosis, and Management*, ed 2. New York: Raven Press; 1995: 1539–1552.

32. Coleman TG, Bower JD, Langford HG, Guyton AC: Regulation of arterial pressure in the anephric state. *Circulation* 1970;42:509–514.

33. Mueller FB, Laragh JH: First-line and combination antihypertensive drug therapy. In: Laragh JH, Brenner BM, eds. *Hypertension: Pathophysiology, Diagnosis, and Management*. New York: Raven Press; 1990:2107–2115.

34. Goldstein DS. Kopin IJ: The autonomic nervous system and catecholamines in normal blood pressure control and in hypertension. In: Laragh JH, Brenner BM, eds. *Hypertension: Pathophysiology, Diagnosis and Management*. New York: Raven Press; 1990:711–747.

35. Roberts JM, Taylor RN, Musci TJ, et al: Preeclampsia: An endothelial cell disorder. *Am J Obstet Gynecol* 1989;161:1200–1204.

36. DeFronzo RA, Ferrannini E: Insulin resistance. A multifaceted syndrome responsible for NIDDM, obesity, hypertension, dyslipidemia, and atherosclerotic cardiovascular disease. *Diabetes Care* 1991;14:173–194.

37. Solomon CG, Graves SW, Greene MF, Seely EW: Glucose intolerance as predictor of hypertension in pregnancy. *Hypertension* 1994;23:717–721.

38. Elliott P: Observational studies of salt and blood pressure. *Hypertension* 1991;17(suppl 1): I3–I8.

39. McCarron DA, Morris CD, Henry HJ, Stanton JL: Blood pressure and nutrient intake in the United States. *Science* 1984;224:1392–1397.

40. Grobee DE, Hofman A: Effect of calcium supplementation on diastolic blood pressure in young people with mild hypertension. *Lancet* 1986;2:703–707.

41. Appel LJ, Moore TJ, Obarzanek E, et al (for the DASH Collaborative Research Group): A clinical trial of the effects of dietary patterns on blood pressure. *N Engl J Med* 1997;336: 117–124.

42. Hojo M, August P: Calcium metabolism in normal and hypertensive pregnancy. *Semin Nephrol* 1995;15:504–511.

43. Levine RJ, Hauth JC, Curet LB, et al: Trial of calcium to prevent preeclampsia. *N Engl J Med* 1997;337:69–76.

44. Sibai BM, Gordon T, Thom E, et al and the NICHD Network of Maternal–Fetal Medicine Units: Risk factors for preeclampsia in healthy nulliparous women: A prospective multicenter study. *Am J Obstet Gynecol* 1995;172:642–648.

45. Benedetto C, Zonca M, Marozio L, et al: Blood pressure patterns in normal pregnancy and in pregnancy-induced hypertension, preeclampsia and chronic hypertension. *Obstet Gynecol* 1996;88:503–510.

46. Thompson JA, Hays PM, Sagar KB, Cruikshank DP: Echocardiographic left ventricular mass to differentiate chronic hypertension from preeclampsia during pregnancy. *Am J Obstet Gynecol* 1996;155:994–999.

47. Sibai BM, Abdella TN, Anderson GD, McCubbin JH: Plasma volume determination in pregnancies complicated by chronic hypertension and intrauterine fetal demise. *Obstet Gynecol* 1982;60;174–178.

48. Taufield P, Ales KL, Resnick LM, et al: Hypocalciuria in preeclampsia. *N Engl J Med* 1987; 316:715–718.

49. Kublickas M, Lunell NO, Nisell H, Westgren M: Maternal renal artery blood flow velocimetry in normal and hypertensive pregnancies. *Acta Obstet Gynecol Scand* 1996;75:715–719.

50. Baker PN, Pipkin FB: Platelet angiotensin II binding in pregnant women with chronic hypertension. *Am J Obstet Gynecol* 1994;170:1301–1302.

51. Warren WB, Gurewitsch ED, Goland RS: Corticotropin-releasing hormone and pituitary-adrenal hormones in pregnancies complicated by chronic hypertension. *Am J Obstet Gynecol* 1995;172:661–666.

52. Nobunaga T, Tokugawa Y, Hashimoto K, et al: Plasma nitric oxide levels in pregnant patients with preeclampsia and essential hypertension. *Gynecol Obstet Invest* 1996;41:189–193.

53. Haller H, Oeney T, Hauck U, et al: Increased intracellular free calcium and sensitivity to angiotensin II in platelets of preeclamptic women. *Am J Hypertens* 1989;2:238–243.

54. Kilby MD, Pipkin FB, Symonds EM: Platelet cytosolic calcium in human pregnancy complicated by essential hypertension. *Am J Obstet Gynecol* 1993;169:141–143.

55. Hojo M, Suthanthiran M, Helseth G, August P: Increased intracellular free calcium concentration in lymphocytes from preeclamptics: A consequence of extracellular calcium deficit? *Am J Obstet Gynecol*: accepted 1999.

56. Hennessy A, Helseth G, August P: Renovascular hypertension in pregnancy: Increased incidence of severe preeclampsia. *JASN* 1997;8:316A.

57. Wilkinson R: Epidemiology and clinical manifestations. In: Novick AC, Scoble J, Hamilton G, eds. *Renal Vascular Disease*. London: WB Saunders; 1996:171–184.

58. Stanley JC: Arterial fibrodysplasia. In: Novick AC, Scoble J, Hamilton G, eds. *Renal Vascular Disease*. London: WB Saunders; 1996:21–35.

59. Mann SJ, Pickering TG: Detection of renovascular hypertension. State of the art: 1992. *Ann Intern Med* 1992;117:845–853.

60. Le TT, Haskal ZJ, Holland GA, Townsend R: Endovascular stent placement and magnetic resonance angiography for management of hypertension and renal artery occlusion during pregnancy. *Obstet Gynecol* 1995;85:822–825.

61. Tegtmeyer CJ, Selby JB, Hartwell GD, et al: Results and complications of angioplasty in fibromuscular disease. *Circulation* 1991;83:I155–I161.

62. Hotchkiss RL, Nettles JB, Wells DE: Renovascular hypertension in pregnancy. *South Med J* 1971;64:1256–1258.

63. Koskela O, Kaski P: Renal angiography in the follow-up examination of toxemia of late pregnancy. *Acta Obstet Gynecol Scand* 1971;50:41–43.

64. Roach CJ: Renovascular hypertension in pregnancy. *Obstet Gynecol* 1973;42:856–860.
65. McCarron DA, Keller FS, Lundquist G, Kirk PE: Transluminal angioplasty for renovascular hypertension complicated by pregnancy. *Arch Intern Med* 1982;142:1727–1728.
66. Easterling TR, Brateng D, Goldman ML, et al: Renovascular hypertension during pregnancy. *Obstet Gynecol* 1991;78:921–925.
67. Diego J, Guerra J, Pham C, Epstein M: Management of renovascular hypertension complicating pregnancy. *JASN* 1996;7:1549.
68. Bravo EL, Tarazi RC, Dustan HP, et al: The changing clinical spectrum of primary aldosteronism. *Am J Med* 1983;74:641–651.
69. Blumenfeld JD, Vaughan ED Jr: Adrenal hypertension. In: Brady HR, Wilcox CS, eds. *Therapy in Nephrology and Hypertension: A Companion to Brenner and Rector's The Kidney*. Phildelphia: Saunders; 1999:451–462.
70. Nadler JL, Hsueh W, Horton R: Therapeutic effect of calcium channel blockade in primary aldosteronism. *J Clin Endocrinol Metab* 1985;60:896–899.
71. Crane MG, Andes JP, Harris JJ, et al: Primary aldosteronism in pregnancy. *Obstet Gynecol* 1964;23:200–208.
72. Neerhof MG, Shlossman PA, Poll DS, et al: Idiopathic aldosteronism in pregnancy. *Obstet Gynecol* 1991;78:489–491.
73. Gordon RD, Fishman LM, Liddle GW: Plasma renin activity and aldosterone secretion in a pregnant woman with primary aldosteronism. *J Clin Endocrinol Metab* 1967;27:385–388.
74. Lotgering FK, Derkx FMH, Wallenburg HCS: Primary hyperaldosteronism in pregnancy. *Am J Obstet Gynecol* 1986;155:986–988.
75. Colton R, Perez GO, Fishman LM: Primary aldosteronism in pregnancy. *Am J Obstet Gynecol* 1984;150:892–893.
76. Biglieri EG, Slaton PE: Pregnancy and primary aldosteronism. *J Clin Endocrinol Metab* 1976;27:1628–1632.
77. Merrill RH, Dombrowski RA, MacKenna JM: Primary hyperaldosteronism during pregnancy. *Am J Obstet Gynecol* 1984;150:786–787.
78. Solomon CG, Thiet MP, Moore F, Seely EW: Primary hyperaldosteronism in pregnancy. A case report. *J Reprod Med* 1996;41:255–258.
79. Aboud E, de Swiet M, Gordon H: Primary aldosteronism in pregnancy—should it be treated surgically? *Irish J Med Sci* 1995;164:279–280.
80. Webb JC, Bayliss P: Pregnancy complicated by primary aldosteronism. *South Med J* 1997;90:243–245.
81. Baron F, Sprauve ME, Huddleston JF, Fisher AJ: Diagnosis and surgical treatment of primary aldosteronism in pregnancy: A case report. *Obstet Gynecol* 1995;86:644–645.
82. August PA, Sealey JE: The renin–angiotensin system in normal and hypertensive pregnancy and in ovarian function. In: Laragh JH, Brenner BM, eds. *Hypertension: Pathophysiology, Diagnosis and Management*. New York: Raven Press; 1990:1761–1778.
83. Hecker A, Hasan SH, Neumann F: Disturbances in sexual differentiation of rat foetuses following spironolactone treatment. *Acta Endocrinol* 1980;95:540–545.
84. Lie JT, Olney BA, Spittel JA: Perioperative hypertensive crisis and hemorrhagic diathesis: Fatal complication of clinically unsuspected pheochromocytoma. *Am Heart J* 1980;100:716–722.
85. Manger WM, Gifford RW: Pheochromocytoma: A clinical overview. In: Laragh JH, Brenner BM, eds. *Hypertension: Pathophysiology, Diagnosis, and Management*, ed 2. New York: Raven Press; 1995:2225–2244.
86. Leak D, Carroll JJ, Robinson DC, Ashworth EJ: Management of pheochromocytoma during pregnancy. *Can Med Assoc J* 1977;116:371–375.
87. Schenker JG, Chowers I: Pheochromocytoma and pregnancy. Review of 89 cases. *Obstet Gynecol Surv* 1971;26:739–747.
88. Lyons CW, Colmorgen GH: Medical management of pheochromocytoma in pregnancy. *Obstet Gynecol* 1988;72:450–451.
89. Burgiss GE: Alpha blockade and surgical intervention of pheochromocytoma in pregnancy. *Obstet Gynecol* 1979;53:266–270.
90. Stenstrom G, Swolin K: Pheochromocytoma in pregnancy. Experience of treatment with phenoxybenzamine in three patients. *Acta Obstet Gynecol Scand* 1985;64:357–361.

91. Jessurun CR, Adam K, Mosie KJ, Wilansky S: Pheochromocytoma-induced myocardial infarction in pregnancy. A case report and literature review. *Tex Heart Inst J* 1993;20:120–122.

92. Hamada S, Hinokio K, Naka O, et al: Myocardial infarction as a complication of pheochromocytoma in a pregnant woman. *Eur J Obstet Gynecol Reprod Biol* 1996;70(2):197–200.

93. Easterling TR, Carlson K, Benedetti TJ, Mancuso JJ: Hemodynamics associated with the diagnosis and treatment of pheochromocytoma in pregnancy. *Am J Perinatol* 1992;9:464–466.

94. Freier DT, Thompson NW: Pheochromocytoma and pregnancy: The epitome of high risk. *Surgery* 1993;114:1148–1152.

95. Santeiro ML, Stromquist C, Qyble L: Phenoxybenzamine placental transfer during the third trimester. *Ann Pharmacother* 1996;30:1249–1251.

96. Buescher MA, McClamrock HD, Adashi EY: Cushing syndrome in pregnancy. *Obstet Gynecol* 1992;79:130–137.

97. Kreines K, Perin E, Salzer R: Pregnancy in Cushing's syndrome. *J Clin Endocrinol Metab* 1969;24:75–79.

98. Reschini F, Giustina G, Crosignani PG, D'Alberton A: Spontaneous remission of Cushing's syndrome after termination of pregnancy. *Obstet Gynecol* 1978;51:598–602.

99. Van der Spuy ZM, Jacobs HS: Management of endocrine disorders and pregnancy. Part II. Pituitary, ovarian and adrenal disease. *Postgrad Med J* 1984;60:312–320.

100. Walters BNJ, Walters T: Hypertension in the puerperium (letter). *Lancet* 1987;2:330.

101. Ferrazzani S, Caruso A, De Carolis S, et al: The duration of hypertension in puerperium of preeclamptic women relates to fetal growth, renal impairment and week of delivery. *Am J Obstet Gynecol* 1994;171:506–512.

102. Walters BNJ, Thompson ME, de Swiet M: Blood pressure in the puerperium. *Clin Sci* 1986;71:589–594.

103. Makdassi R, De Cagny B, Lobjoie E, et al: Convulsions, hypertension crisis and acute renal failure in postpartum: Role of bromocriptine? *Nephron* 1996;72:732–733.

104. Lubarsky SL, Barton JR, Friedman SA, et al: Late postpartum eclampsia revisited. *Obstet Gynecol* 1994;83:502–505.

105. Brady WJ, De Behnke DJ, Carter CT: Postpartum toxemia: Hypertension, edema, proteinuria and unresponsiveness in an unknown female. *J Emerg Med* 1995;13:643–648.

106. Magann EF, Martin JN: Complicated postpartum preeclampsia–eclampsia. *Obstet Gynecol Clin North Am* 1995;22:337–356.

107. Bucher HC, Guyatt GH, Cook RJ, et al: Effect of calcium supplementation on pregnancy-induced hypertension and preeclampsia: A meta-analysis of randomized controlled trials. *JAMA* 1996;275:1113–1117.

108. Lindheimer MD: Pre-eclampsia–eclampsia 1996: Preventable? Have disputes on its treatment been resolved? *Curr Opin Nephrol & Hypertens* 1996;5:452–458.

109. Redman CWG: Controlled trials of antihypertensive drugs in pregnancy. *Am J Kidney Dis* 1991;17:149–153.

109a. Sanchez-Ramos L, Mora CS: Effect of antihypertensive therapy on superimposed preeclampsia in patients with chronic hypertension: A meta-analysis. *Am J Obstet Gynecol* (in press Jan 1999 [abstr.]).

110. Fletcher AE, Bulpitt CJ: A review of clinical trials in pregnancy. In: Rubin PC, ed. *Hypertension in Pregnancy*, vol 10. (*Handbook of Hypertension* series, Birkenhager WH, Reid JL, eds.). New York: Elsevier; 1988:186–201.

111. Redman CWG, Beilin LJ, Bonnar J: Treatment of hypertension in pregnancy with methyldopa: Blood pressure control and side effects. *Br J Obstet Gynecol* 1977;84:419–426.

112. Gallery EDM, Ross MR, Gyory AZ: Antihypertensive treatment in pregnancy: Analysis of different responses to oxprenolol and methyldopa. *Br Med J* 1985;29:563–566.

113. Ounsted M, Cockburn J, Moar VA, Redman CWG: Maternal hypertension with superimposed pre-eclampsia: Effects on child development at $7\frac{1}{2}$ years. *Br J Obstet Gynaecol* 1983;90:644–649.

114. Reynolds B, Butters L, Evans J, et al: First year of life after the use of atenolol in pregnancy associated hypertension. *Arch Dis Child* 1984;59:1061–1063.

115. Butters L, Kennedy S, Rubin PC: Atenolol in essential hypertension during pregnancy. *Br Med J* 1990;301:587–589.

116. Plouin PF, Breart G, Maillard F, et al: Comparison of antihypertensive efficacy and perinatal safety of labetalol and methyldopa in the treatment of hypertension in pregnancy: A randomized controlled trial. *Br J Obstet Gynecol* 1988;95:868–876.

117. Symonds EM, Lamming GD, Jadoul F, et al: Clinical and biochemical aspects of the use of labetalol in the treatment of hypertension in pregnancy: Comparison with methyldopa. In: Riley A, Symonds M, eds. *The Investigation of Labetalol in the Management of Hypertension in Pregnancy*. Amsterdam: Exerpta Medica; 1982:62–76.

118. Sibai BM, Gonzalez AR, Mabie WC, Moretti M: A comparison of labetalol plus hospitalization versus hospitalization alone in the management of preeclampsia remote from term. *Obstet Gynecol* 1987;70:323–327.

119. Lindberg B, Lindeberg S, Marsal K, Andersson KE. Calcium channel blockade (isradipine) in treatment of hypertension in pregnancy: A randomized placebo-controlled study. *Am J Obstet Gynecol* 1995;173:872–878.

120. Jannet D, Carbonne B, Sebban E, Milliez J: Nicardipine versus metoprolol in the treatment of hypertension during pregnancy: A randomized comparative trial. *Obstet Gynecol* 1994; 84:354–359.

121. Magee LA, Schick B, Donnenfeld AE, et al: The safety of calcium channel blockers in human pregnancy: A prospective multicenter cohort study. *Am J Obstet Gynecol* 1996;174: 823–828.

122. Waisman GD, Mayorga LM, Camera MI, et al: Magnesium plus nifedipine: Potentiation of hypotensive effect in preeclampsia? *Am J Obstet Gynecol* 1988;159:308–309.

123. Committee on Drugs: The transfer of drugs and other chemicals into human milk. *Pediatrics* 1994;93:137–150.

124. White WB: Management of hypertension during lactation. *Hypertension* 1984;6:297–300.

125. Atkinson H, Begg EJ: Concentrations of beta-blocking drugs in human milk (letter). *J Pediatr* 1990;116:156.

126. Ehrenkranz RA, Ackerman BA, Hulse JD: Nifedipine transfer into human milk. *J Pediatr* 1989;114:478–480.

127. Anderson P, Bondesson U, Mattiasson I, Johansonn BW: Verapamil and norverapamil in plasma and breast milk during breast feeding. *Eur J Clin Pharmacol* 1987;31:625–627.

Index

Page numbers followed by t and f indicate tables and
figures, respectively.

Page numbers followed by *t* and *f* indicate tables and
figures, respectively.

Page numbers followed by *t* and *f* indicate tables and
figures, respectively.

Chorionic villi. *See also* Anchoring villi
  in placentation, 377–379
Chromium, endothelial cell activation and, 407–408,
    408f
Chronic hypertension
  abatement in pregnancy, Chesley on, 27–28
  characteristics of, 546–547
  definition of, 544t, 606
    by NHBPEP's Working Group, 25
  diagnosis of, 606–607
  effects on mother, 609
  and fetal outcome, 58, 610–611
  and preeclampsia risk, 48–49
  preeclampsia superimposed on. *See*
      Superimposed preeclampsia
  in pregnancy
    diagnosis of, 215
    differential diagnosis of, 215–216
    management of, 605–628
  prevalence of, 605–606
  renal handling of uric acid in, 293–297, 295t
Circulatory function
  in preeclampsia–eclampsia, 327
  in pregnancy, 112–113, 136–147
    adequacy, global assessment of, 145–147
Cirrhosis, hepatic, blood volume and circulatory
    state in, 104–105, 143–144, 157–158
Classification, of hypertensive disorders in
    pregnancy
  Chesley on, 19–21
  current controversies about, 23–26
Clonidine
  mechanism of action, 586–587
  use in pregnancy, 588
cM. *See* Centimorgan
Coagulation cascade
  factors, in normal vs preeclamptic pregnancy,
      358f, 358–361, 360t
  pathways of, 358, 358f
  in preeclampsia, 191–192
Coagulation index, 366
Coagulopathy
  in normal vs preeclamptic pregnancy, 358–365,
      360t, 367
  in preeclampsia–eclampsia, 189–190, 202, 203f,
      349–350
Collagen, type IV, glomerular, in preeclamptic
    nephropathy, 250
Colloid therapy
  benefits, in preeclampsia, 333–335
  contraindications to, 177, 571, 573
Coma
  after eclamptic convulsions, 554–556
  in preeclampsia–eclampsia, 188
Combative state, after eclamptic coma, 555
Common iliac artery, volumetric flow in, in
    pregnancy, 97
Complement fraction β_1-A–C, serum levels
  in normal pregnancy, 297–298
  in preeclampsia, 301
Computed tomography (CT)
  contraindications to, 619
  cranial
    in cerebral edema, 188, 188f
    in eclampsia, 185, 186f
Congenital adrenal hypoplasia, and preeclampsia,
    440

Conn syndrome, 618
Consanguinity studies, in preeclampsia, 436–437
Contraception, and preeclampsia, 51–52
Controls, in studies of preeclampsia–eclampsia,
    difficulties with, 59
Creatinine clearance, in pregnancy, 267–269, 268f
Cryofibrinogen levels, in normal vs preeclamptic
    pregnancy, 361
Crystalloid therapy, contraindications to, 177, 333,
    573
Cushing syndrome, in pregnancy, 622
Cyclic adenosine monophosphate (cAMP), platelet,
    in normal vs preeclamptic pregnancy, 351t,
    355–357
Cyclic guanosine monophosphate (cGMP)
  and endothelial cell dysfunction, 502
  platelet, in normal vs preeclamptic pregnancy,
      357
  and renal hemodynamics, 274
Cyclin B, cytotrophoblast expression of, 383, 384f
Cyclooxygenase, and hemodynamic changes in
    pregnancy, 94
Cytokines
  and endothelial cell activation, 413–414
  and reset osmostat in pregnancy, 121–122
Cytotrophoblasts
  adhesion molecule repertoire of
    in normal pregnancy, 386–389
    in preeclampsia, 389–391
  differentiation of
    in situ, 381–382
    in vitro, 381–386
    preeclampsia and, 389–390
  in normal placentation, 377–379, 378f–379f, 380
  in preeclampsia, 380–381
  proliferation of, 381–386
  protein expression by, 383, 384f
  stage-specific antigen expression by, 381–382

Death
  fetal. *See* Fetal loss
  maternal, after eclamptic convulsions, 56, 57f, 556
Dehydroepiandrosterone sulfate, clearance rate, and
    placental perfusion, 193
Delivery
  blood loss at, 573
  convulsions during, 556
  magnesium sulfate and, 562
  postponing, hazards of, 551
  for preeclampsia, 549–551, 572–573
Dexamethasone, contraindications to, 177
Diabetes insipidus
  animal model of, 115
  syndrome, in late pregnancy, 126
  transient, in preeclampsia, 179
Diabetes insipidus gravidarum, 126
Diabetes mellitus
  animal models of, 507
  and preeclampsia, 48–49
    perinatal outcome in, 58–59
  retinopathy of, preeclampsia and, 187–188
  risk of, after preeclampsia–eclampsia, 56
  type II, and essential hypertension, 613
Diazepam, for eclamptic convulsions, 530, 534, 536t,
    563, 564f, 565t

Page numbers followed by t and f indicate tables and
figures, respectively.

Page numbers followed by *t* and *f* indicate tables and
figures, respectively.

Page numbers followed by *t* and *f* indicate tables and figures, respectively.

Page numbers followed by t and f indicate tables and figures, respectively.

Page numbers followed by *t* and *f* indicate tables and
figures, respectively.

Page numbers followed by t and f indicate tables and
figures, respectively.